FRAZIER'S A TEXTBOOK OF FOOD MICROBIOLOGY

OTHER RELATED TITLES IN LIFE SCIENCES

FRAZIER'S A TEXTBOOK OF FOOD MICROBIOLOGY

EIGHTH EDITION

Edited and Revised by

K.R. Aneja

MSc, PhD, Post Doc (UK), FBS, FPSI, FIMS, FMSI, FSBA

Honorary Professor & Research Advisor
Sardar Bhagwan Singh University
Dehradun (Uttarakhand)

Former Professor and Chairman
Department of Microbiology
Kurukshetra University, Kurukshetra
Haryana, India

MedTech Science Press
A Division of Scientific International
Engaging Sciences—Developing Minds!

FRAZIER'S
A TEXTBOOK OF
FOOD MICROBIOLOGY

MedTech Science Press
A Division of
Scientific International Pvt. Ltd.

Eighth Edition: 2026

ISBN: 978-93-6363-936-2

Published by: Rajan Jain, Scientific International (Pvt.) Ltd.

Registered Office: • **New Delhi:** 4222/1, Ansari Road, Daryaganj, New Delhi-110002

Branch Office: • **Bengaluru:** House No. 1665, Ground Floor, 18th Main, BSK 2nd Stage, Bengaluru-560070

Printed in India

Preface

Food microbiology, the applied branch of microbiology, is a crucial discipline that bridges the gap between microbiology and food science, playing a vital role in ensuring food safety, quality, and preservation. Globally, there is a rising demand for plant, animal and microbial foods, free from food spoilage microorganisms and/ or toxins, and added with a proper preservative to increase the shelf-life, that do not cause health problems in humans, such as allergy, infection, poisoning or cancer, leading into a healthier and longer life. Microbiological analysis is important to determine the safety and quality of food. Application of molecular tools and sensors has improved our understanding of the responses of pathogens (e.g., bacterial, fungal, viral and protozoan) to foods and food environment. Keeping this in mind, a new chapter" **detection of foodborne pathogens by conventional and advanced techniques** has been added in the Part-V11 Detection of Microorganisms in Food in this edition Additionally, most of the figures have been replaced with new explainatory figures for better understanding of the readership. This new edition of the book has been carefully structured to provide a comprehensive understanding of microbial interactions with food, contamination sources, and strategies for preservation, safety and dection of foodborne pathogens. It is designed to serve as a valuable tool for students, researchers, and professionals in the fields of microbiology, food science, environmental secience, public health and biotechnology.

The book is divided into 7 parts, each addressing critical aspects of food microbiology.

Part I introduces the fundamental concepts of microbial growth in food and the key microorganisms relevant to food science. It explores how food serves as a medium for microbial proliferation and examines the essential microbes involved in food production, spoilage, and fermentation. Additionally, it discusses food contamination sources and preventive measures, ensuring readers grasp the foundational knowledge required to understand food microbiology.

Part II focuses on food preservation techniques, including both traditional and modern methods. It covers heat-based preservation, high-temperature treatments, moisture removal, and the use of food additives to extend shelf life. These chapters highlight the science behind these preservation strategies and their applications in maintaining food safety and quality.

Part III delves into the specific contamination and preservation challenges associated with different food categories, including cereals, grains, sweeteners, fruits, vegetables, meat, fish, seafood, eggs, poultry, dairy, and canned foods. Each chapter provides insights into the microbial risks associated with these foods and the best preservation methods to mitigate contamination and spoilage.

Part IV explores the role of microorganisms in food fermentation and production. It discusses microbial cultures used in fermentation, microbial transformations in food processing, and the applications of microbial enzymes in food production. This section highlights the beneficial aspects of microorganisms in food biotechnology and their significance in producing fermented foods.

Part V addresses foodborne diseases, focusing on bacterial and nonbacterial foodborne illnesses, including poisoning and infections. It also covers the investigation of foodborne disease outbreaks, providing essential knowledge for public health professionals and food safety investigators.

Part VI emphasizes food sanitation and safety regulations. It discusses microbiological principles in food sanitation and the regulatory frameworks that govern food safety, ensuring compliance with industry standards.

Finally, **Part VII** deals with the detection of foodborne pathogens, such as bacteria, fungi, protozoa, helminths and viruses using **conventional techniques** (e.g., culture-based method, biochemical methods, immunological-based detection methods, nucleic-acid based methods) ;**rapid methods** based on traditional methods ; and **advanced methods** (e.g.,hybridization, DNA microarray, spectroscopy and biosensor-based methods).

With this book, I aim to provide a thorough understanding of food microbiology, equipping readers with the knowledge and tools to ensure food safety, quality, and sustainability. I hope this resource proves beneficial for both academic and professional pursuits in this essential field.

—Author

Contents

Part-I

Microbial Interactions in Food

To fully comprehend the interactions between microorganisms and food, it is essential to recognize that the composition of the food determines the microorganisms present. A solid understanding of a food's chemistry is crucial to grasping its microbiological aspects. Chapter 1 highlights the key food parameters that influence their microbiological properties. Chapter 2 focuses on the primary categories of foodborne microorganisms. The topic of food contamination by microorganisms is briefly introduced in Chapter 3, as it will be revisited in detail in later sections of the text. Likewise, Chapter 4 provides an overview of spoilage principles, with more specific discussions on individual commodities in subsequent chapters.

1 Food as a Medium for Microbial Growth

To fully comprehend the interactions between microorganisms and food, it is essential to recognize that the composition of the food determines the microorganisms present. A solid understanding of a food's chemistry is crucial to grasping its microbiological aspects. Chapter 1 highlights the key food parameters that influence their microbiological properties. Chapter 2 focuses on the primary categories of foodborne microorganisms. The topic of food contamination by microorganisms is briefly introduced in Chapter 3, as it will be revisited in detail in later sections of the text. Likewise, Chapter 4 provides an overview of spoilage principles, with more specific discussions on individual commodities in subsequent chapters.

The interactions between microorganisms, plants and animals are natural and constant. The ecological role of microorganisms and their importance in all geochemical cycles of nature are well documented. Since human food consists mainly of plants and animals or products derived from them, it is understandable that our food may contain microorganisms that interact with food.

Food provides an ideal environment for microbial growth due to its nutrient-rich composition, moisture content, and temperature. Microorganisms such as bacteria, fungi, and yeast thrive in foods that contain high levels of proteins, carbohydrates, fats, and other nutrients, which they use for growth and reproduction. The pH level of food also plays a significant role in microbial development; foods with neutral or slightly acidic pH, such as meats, dairy products, and some fruits, are particularly susceptible to microbial contamination.

In most cases, microorganisms use our food as a source of nutrients for themselves. growth. This can certainly lead to food spoilage. By increasing their numbers, using nutrients, producing enzymatic changes, and contributing to off-flavor through the breakdown of a product or the synthesis of new compounds, they can "spoil" a food. This is a normal consequence of the action of microorganisms, because one of their functions in nature is to convert the reduced forms of carbon, nitrogen, and sulfur from dead plants and animals into the oxidized forms needed by plants. which in turn are consumed by animals. So just by "doing their job" in nature, they can often make our food supply unsafe to eat. To avoid this, we minimize contact between microorganisms and our food (prevent contamination) and also eliminate microorganisms from our food, or at least adjust storage conditions to prevent their growth (storage).

When the microorganisms involved are pathogenic, their association with our food is essential from a public health perspective. Many of our foods support the growth of pathogenic microorganisms or at least serve as a vector for their development. Again, we try to prevent them from entering and growing in our foods or to eliminate them through processing.The interactions between microorganisms and our foods are sometimes beneficial, as evidenced by the many cultivated products consumed and evaluated.

What are the determining factors of these interactions? Why is this interaction beneficial at some times and not at others? Why do some foods support the growth of microorganisms more readily than others? Why are some foods very stable with respect to microbial spoilage? The food is the substrate, so its characteristics are an important element to consider. The type of microorganisms present and the environmental conditions are also important. However, the food or substrate determines what can or cannot grow. By understanding the characteristics of a food or substrate, predictions can be made about the microbial flora that may develop. Knowledge of the factors that promote or inhibit the growth of microorganisms is essential to understanding the principles of food spoilage and preservation. The main compositional factors of a food that affect microbial activity are the concentration of hydrogen ions, moisture, redox potential (O-R), nutrients, and the presence of inhibitory substances or barriers.

In addition to nutrients, the moisture content of food is another critical factor. Foods with high water activity, such as fresh meats, vegetables, and fruits, provide favorable conditions for microorganisms to grow. Conversely, dehydrated foods with low moisture content are less conducive to microbial growth but may still support certain types of microorganisms like molds. Temperature is also a key determinant—most microorganisms grow best at temperatures between 20°C and 45°C, making improperly stored food, especially perishable items, particularly vulnerable to contamination.

The presence of oxygen further influences microbial growth. Aerobic bacteria and fungi require oxygen to thrive, while anaerobic bacteria can proliferate in low-oxygen environments, such as in vacuum-sealed packages or canned foods. When microorganisms colonize food, they may cause spoilage, leading to undesirable changes in taste, smell, appearance, and texture. Some foodborne pathogens, such as Salmonella, *E. coli*, and Listeria, pose significant health risks, leading to foodborne illnesses if consumed. Therefore, understanding the conditions that promote microbial growth in food is essential for ensuring food safety and preventing contamination through proper storage, handling, and processing techniques.

HYDROGEN-ION CONCENTRATION (pH)

Every microorganism has a minimum, maximum, and optimum pH for its growth. Microbial cells are significantly affected by the pH of foods because they apparently have no mechanism to regulate their internal pH. In general, yeasts and molds are more tolerant of acidity than bacteria. The natural pH of foods varies, although most foods are neutral or acidic. Foods with a low pH are more sensitive to acidity. 5) are generally not easily spoiled by bacteria and are more susceptible to spoilage by yeast and mold. A food with an inherently low pH tends to be more microbiologically stable than a neutral food. The excellent keeping quality of the following foods is linked to their limiting pH-fruit, soda, fermented milk, sauerkraut and gherkins. Some foods have a low pH because of their acidity; others, for example , fermented products, have a low pH due to the acidity developed by the accumulation of lactic acid during fermentation.

Molds can grow over a wider range of pH values than most yeasts and bacteria, and many molds grow at acidity levels that are too high for yeast and bacteria. Most fermentation yeasts favor a pH of about 4.0 to 4.5, such as in fruit juices, and skin yeasts grow well in acidic foods, such as sauerkraut and cucumbers. In contrast, most yeasts do not grow well in alkaline substrates and must adapt to such environments. Most bacteria are favored by a pH close to neutral, although some, such as acidifiers, are favored by moderate acidity, and others, such as active proteolytic bacteria, can grow in high (alkaline) pH environments, such as that found in stored egg whites.

Buffers in food, i. Compounds that are resistant to pH changes are important not only for their buffering capacity, but also for their ability to be particularly effecti e within a certain pH range. Buffers allow acidic (or alkaline) fermentation to continue for longer with higher yields of products and organisms than would otherwise be possible. Vegetable juices have a low buffering capacity, which allows a significant decrease in pH with the production of small amounts of acid by lactic acid bacteria at the beginning of the fermentation of sauerkraut and pickles. This allows lactic acid bacteria to suppress unwanted pectin hydrolysis and competing proteolytic organisms. A low buffering capacity allows a variety of microorganisms to appear more rapidly during fermentation than a high buffering capacity. Milk, on the other hand, is quite high in protein (a good buffe) and therefore allows considerable growth and acid production by lactic acid bacteria in fermented milk production before the growth of the initial culture is finally suppressed

The pH of a product can be easily determined with a pH meter, but this value alone may not be sufficien to predict microbial responses. It is also desirable, for example, to know the acid responsible for a given pH, because some acids, especially organic acids, are more inhibitory than others. The inhibitory properties of many organic acids, including acetic, benzoic, citric, lactic, propionic, and sorbic acids, make them widely used as acidulants or preservatives in foods. Furthermore, changes in titratable acidity are not always evident from pH measurements.

Not only are the growth rates of microorganisms affected by pH, but also survival rates during storage, heating, drying, and other forms of processing. Furthermore, the initial pH may be suitable, but due to competing flora or the growth of the organism itself, the pH may be unfavorable. Conversely, the initial pH may be limiting, but the growth of a limited number of microorganisms can shift the pH to a range more favorable for the growth of many other microorganisms.

MOISTURE REQUIREMENT: THE CONCEPT OF WATER ACTIVITY

Moisture is a critical factor for microbial growth in food, and the concept of water activity (aw) is used to measure the availability of water for microorganisms. Water activity refers to the amount of free water in a food that is available for microbial use, distinct from the total moisture content of the food. While all foods contain water, not all of it is available to microbes for growth. Water activity ranges from 0 (completely dry) to 1.0 (pure water), with higher values indicating more available water for microbial growth.

Most bacteria, molds, and yeasts require a water activity of around 0.90 or higher to grow and reproduce. Foods with high water activity, such as meats, dairy products, and fresh fruits, are more prone to microbial contamination. On the other hand, foods with lower water activity, such as dried fruits, grains, and salted or sugar-preserved foods, are less susceptible to microbial growth, as the water is bound to other components like sugars and salts, making it unavailable for microorganisms.

By understanding and controlling water activity, food processors can extend the shelf life of products and reduce the risk of spoilage and foodborne illness. Techniques like dehydration, salting, or adding sugar can lower water activity in foods, thus inhibiting microbial growth and ensuring food safety.

Water activity (a_w) is the partial vapor pressure of water in a solution divided by the standard state partial vapor pressure of water. In the field of food science, the standard state is most often defined as pure water at the same temperature. Using this particular definition, pure distilled water has a water activity of exactly one. Water activity is the thermodynamic activity of water as solvent and the relative humidity of the surrounding air after equilibration. As temperature increases, aw typically increases, except in some products with crystalline salt or sugar.

Water migrates from areas of high aw to areas of low aw. For example, if honey ($a_w \approx 0.6$) is exposed to humid air ($a_w \approx 0.7$), the honey absorbs water from the air. If salami ($a_w \approx 0.87$) is exposed to dry air ($a_w \approx 0.5$), the salami dries out, which could preserve it or spoil it. Lower aw substances tend to support fewer microorganisms since these get desiccated by the water migration.

The definition of

$$a_w \equiv \frac{p}{p^*}$$

where p is the partial water vapor pressure in equilibrium with the soltion, and p* is the (partial) vapor pressure of pure water at the same teperature.

An alternate definition can b

$$a_w \equiv l_w x_w$$

where l_w is the activity coefficien of water and x_w is the mole fraction of water in the aqueous fraction.

Relationship to Relative Humidity: The relative humidity (RH) of air in equilibrium with a sample is also called the Equilibrium Relative Humidity (ERH) and is usually given as a percentage.It is equal to water activity according to ERH = a_w ×100%. The estimated mold-free shelf life (MFSL) in days at 21 °C depends on water activity according to

$$MFSL = 10^{7.91-8.1a_w}$$

Water becomes unavailable in several ways:

- **Solutes and Ions Bind Water in Solution:** Therefore, an increase in the concentration of dissolved substances, such as sugars and salts, actually constitutes drying of the material. Not only is water bound by solutes, but water tends to leave microbial cells by osmosis if there is a higher concentration of solutes outside the cells than inside.
- **Hydrophilic Colloids (gels) Make Water Unavailable:** For example, 3 to 4 percent agar in a medium can inhibit bacterial growth by leaving very little moisture available.
- **Water of Crystallization or Hydration is Generally Not Available to Microorganisms:** Water itself, when crystallized as ice, can no longer be used by microbial cells. The Aw of ice-water mixtures (the vapor pressure of ice divided by the vapor pressure of water) decreases with decreasing temperature below 0 °C. The aw values of pure water are 1.00 at 0 °C, 0.953 at -5 °C, 0.907 at -10 °C, 0, 846 at -15 ° C, 0.823 at -20 °C, and so on. In a food, such as the form of ice, the concentration of solutes in unfrozen water increases, decreasing its aw.

The reduction in aw by a solute depends mainly on the total concentration of solute molecules and ions, each of which is surrounded by water molecules more or less closely. The solution then has a lower freezing point and a lower vapor pressure than pure water.

Organisms must compete with these particles for water molecules. The drop in vapor pressure for an ideal solvent follows Raoult's law: the vapor pressure of the solution relative to that of the pure solvent is equal to the mole fraction of the solvent; thus, pp0 = n2/n1 + n2, where p and p0 are the vapor pressures of the solute and solvent and n1 and n2 are the number of moles of solute and solvent, respectively. Although, a_w varies with temperature, the changes are only small in the temperature range that allows microbial growth. However, as the solute concentration increases, a change in temperature becomes more important compared to aw because of an increasing effect on ionization

Here is a table showing the principal groups of foods and their approximate water activity (a_w):

Table. Principal Groups of Foods and Their a_w

Food Group	Approximate Water Activity (a_w)
Fresh fruits and vegetables	0.95 - 1.00
Meat (fresh)	0.97 - 0.99
Dairy products (fresh milk)	0.98 - 0.99
Canned foods (vegetables, meat, fish	0.85 - 0.95
Breads and baked goods	0.95 - 1.00
Processed cheeses	0.85 - 0.95
Fats and oils	0.00
Dry grains and cereals	0.60 - 0.80
Sugar and syrups	0.60 - 0.75
Confectionery (candies, chocolates)	0.60 - 0.75
Pickled foods	0.85 - 0.90
Fermented foods	0.90 - 0.95

This table provides an overview of the water activity levels of common food groups, which are critical for determining microbial growth potential and spoilage.

Each microorganism has specific limits for water activity (a_w) that dictate its growth, including a maximum, optimum, and minimum a_w. This range depends on various factors discussed later. As a_w decreases from the optimum level, the microorganism experiences a longer lag phase, slower growth, and reduced synthesis of cellular substances—these changes vary by organism and the solute used to lower a_w.

Factors influencing the $_w$ requirements of microorganisms include:

- **Temperature**: Most microorganisms show the highest tolerance to low aw at their optimal temperatures.
- **Oxygen Availability:** Aerobic organisms grow at a lower aw when oxygen is present, while anaerobic organisms grow at a lower aw in the absence of oxygen.
- **Type of Solute Used to Reduce a_w**: For many organisms, particularly molds, the lowest aw for growth is relatively unaffected by the type of solute. However, some organisms have lower limiting a_w values with certain solutes. For example, potassium chloride is less toxic than sodium chloride and has a lower inhibitory effect than sodium sulfate
- **Nutritive Value of the Culture Medium**: Generally, a better medium for growth allows for a lower limiting a_w.
- **pH:** Organisms are typically more tolerant of low a_w at neutral pH compared to acidic or alkaline conditions.
- **Inhibitors:** The presence of inhibitors reduces the range of aw within which microorganisms can grow.

Methods for controlling a_w include: (1) equilibration with controlling solutions, (2) determining the water-sorption isotherm for the food, and (3) adding solutes. Measuring aw can be done through freezing-point determinations, manometric techniques, or electrical devices. Freezing-point methods are only suitable for liquid foods with high aw values. Manometric techniques, which directly measure vapor pressure in the food's vapor space, are highly accurate. Electrical devices measure aw indirectly by assessing relative humidity in the vapor space surrounding the food. A collaborative study comparing aw measurement methods (Labuza et al., 1976) found manometric vapor-pressure determinations to be the most accurate.

Most bacteria thrive in environments where aw is close to 1.00 (e.g., between 0.995 and 0.998), such as in low concentrations of sugar or salt. However, some bacteria can grow in higher concentrations. For example, culture media for bacteria typically contain no more than 1% sugar and 0.85% sodium chloride. In concentrations as low as 3-4% sugar and 1-2% salt, some bacteria may be inhibited.

The optimal a_w and lower growth limits depend on factors like food, temperature, pH, oxygen levels, carbon dioxide, and inhibitors. For example, the lower limit aw for growth of certain food bacteria is 0.97 for Pseudomonas, 0.96 for Escherichia coli, 0.95 for Bacillus subtilis, 0.945 for Enterobacter aerogenes, 0.86 for Staphylococcus aureus, and 0.93 for Clostridium botulinum. Other bacteria can grow at aw values below 0.90. These figures would vary with different growth conditions. Optimal aw values for some food bacteria are 0.99 to 0.995 for Staph. aureus and Salmonella spp., 0.995 for E. coli, and 0.982 for Streptococcus faecalis.

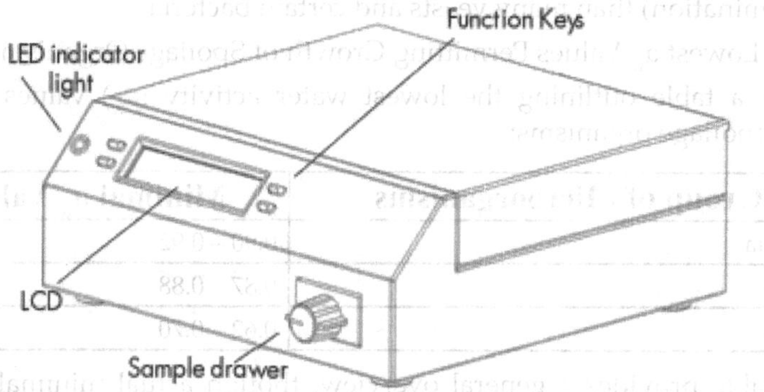

Fig 1.1. An Image of Water Activity Meter

Molds differ significantly in the range of optimum aw and aw for asexual spore germination. The range of spore germination is greatest at temperatures close to the germination optimum and in better culture conditions. The minimum Aw for spore germination has been found to be as low as 0.62 for some molds and as high as 0.93 for others (e.g., molds). For example, Mucor, Rhizopus and Botrytis. Each mold also has an optimal aw and aw range for growth. Examples of optimal aw are 0.98 for Aspergillus sp. , 0.99 to 0.98 for a Rhizopus sp. and 0.99 for a Penicillium sp. aw should be less than 0.62 to stop any possibility of mold growth, although an a_w < 0.70 inhibits most food spoilage molds and an a_w < 0.94 inhibits molds such as Rhizopus and less than 0.85 inhibits Aspergillus spp. A decrease in aw below the optimum for a mold retards spore germination and reduces the growth rate and can therefore be an important factor in food preservation. Many molds can grow on average with an aw close to 1.00 (pure water).

A consideration of the moisture requirements of microorganisms leads to several general conclusions:

- Each organism has its own optimum aw characteristic and its own aw range for growth under a given set of environmental conditions. Factors affecting the moisture requirements of organisms are- (a) the nutritional properties of the substrate, (b) its pH, (c) its content of inhibitory substances, (d) the availability of free oxygen, and (e) temperature. The range of aw that allows growth is reduced if one of these environmental factors is not optimal, and further reduced if two or more conditions are not favorable.
- Unfavorable Aw not only leads to a decrease in growth rate, but also to a decrease in maximum cell yield.
- The more unfavorable the aw of the substrate, the greater the delay (delay) in the initiation of growth or germination of spores. This is often important in food preservation by reducing the growth rate of the organism.
- In general, bacteria require more moisture than yeast, and yeast more than mold, as shown in table which shows the lower aw limits for bacteria, yeast, and mold. There are notable exceptions to this generalization, however, as some molds have a higher minimum aw for growth (and spore germination) than many yeasts and certain bacteria.

Table Lowest a_w Values Permitting Growth of Spoilage Organism

Here's a table outlining the lowest water activity (a_w) values permitting growth of spoilage organisms:

Group of Microorganisms	Minimal a_w Value
Bacteria	0.90 – 0.92
Yeasts	0.87 – 0.88
Molds	0.62 – 0.70

This table provides a general overview, though actual minimal aw values can vary depending on specific species within each group and environmental conditions.

Microorganisms capable of thriving in environments with high solute concentrations, such as sugar and salt, naturally have a low minimal aw. Halophilic bacteria need specific levels of dissolved sodium chloride to grow, while osmophilic yeasts flourish in high sugar concentrations.

OXIDATION-REDUCTION POTENTIAL

Oxidation-reduction potential (ORP) is an important factor influencing microbial growth in food, as it measures the ability of a food environment to accept or donate electrons, which affects microbial metabolism. The ORP is typically expressed in millivolts (mV), and it determines the oxygen availability and the overall redox state of the food. A high ORP indicates an aerobic (oxygen-rich) environment, while a low ORP indicates an anaerobic (oxygen-poor) environment.

Microorganisms vary in their oxygen requirements, and ORP helps to determine which types of microbes can thrive in a particular food. Aerobic microorganisms, such as certain bacteria and molds, prefer higher ORP values and require oxygen for growth. These microbes are typically found in foods exposed to air, such as fresh fruits and vegetables. In contrast, anaerobic microorganisms, including harmful pathogens like Clostridium botulinum, grow in low-ORP environments where oxygen is limited, such as in vacuum-sealed or canned foods.

By controlling ORP through factors like packaging, processing, and storage conditions, food manufacturers can influence the microbial environment and reduce the risk of spoilage or contamination. For example, vacuum packing and canning lower ORP, creating conditions that inhibit aerobic microbial growth and favor anaerobic preservation, thus extending food shelf life and enhancing safety.

The oxygen tension or partial pressure around a food and the O-R potential, or reducing and oxidizing power of the food itself, affect the type of organisms that grow and thus the changes produced in the food. The O-R potential of a food is determined by (1) the O-R potential characteristic of the original food, (2) the equilibrium capacity, i.e. resistance to change in the food potential, (3) the oxygen tension of the atmosphere surrounding the food, and (4) the access of the atmosphere to the food. Air has a high oxygen tension, but the headspace in an "evacuated" can would have a low oxygen tension.

From the standpoint of their ability to utilize free oxygen, microorganisms are classified as aerobic when they require free oxygen, anaerobic when they grow best in the absence of free oxygen, and facultative when they grow well either aerobically or anaerobically. Molds are aerobic, most yeasts grow best aerobically, and bacteria of various types can be aerobic, anaerobic, or facultative. From an O-R potential perspective, a high (oxidizing) potential favors aerobes but will allow the growth of facultative organisms, and a low (reducing) potential favors anaerobic or facultative organisms. However, some organisms considered aerobic can grow (but not well) at surprisingly low O-R potentials. The growth of an organism can change the O-R potential of a food enough to limit other organisms. Anaerobes, for example, can lower the O-R potential to a level that is inhibitory to aerobes.

Most fresh plant and animal foods have a low and balanced Q&A potential in-plants due to reducing substances such as ascorbic acid and reducing sugars and animal tissues due to -SH (sulfhydr l) and other reducing groups. While plant or animal cells are respiring and remain active, they tend to maintain the O-R system at a low level, resisting the effect of oxygen diffusion from the outside. Therefore, a piece of fresh meat or a Whole fresh fruit only presents aerobic conditions at and near the surface. The meat can support aerobic growth of mucus- or acid-forming bacteria on the surface, while anaerobic decay occurs inside. This situation can be modified by processing processes. Heating can reduce the acidifying power of food by destroying or changing reducing and oxidizing substances and also allows more rapid diffusion of oxygen to the inside, either by destroying. acidifying substances, or by changing the physical structure of the food. The treatment may also remove oxidizing or reducing substances; thus, pure fruit juices lose reducing substances that were removed during extraction and filtration and therefore become more favorable for yeast growth than sugar containing the original pulp.

In the presence of limited amounts of oxygen, the same aerobic or facultative organisms can produce incompletely oxidized products, such as organic acids, from carbohydrates, while with plenty of oxygen available, complete oxidation to carbon dioxide and water may result. Protein degradation under anaerobic conditions may result in putrefaction, while under aerobic conditions the products are likely to be less palatable.

NUTRIENT CONTENT

The types and proportions of nutrients in foods are essential in determining which organism is most likely to thrive. Attention should be paid to (1) foods that produce energy, (2) foods that promote growth, and (3) auxiliary nutrients or vitamins that may be needed for energy or growth.

Foods for Growth

Microorganisms vary in their ability to utilize different nitrogenous compounds as a nitrogen source for growth. Some organisms cannot break down proteins independently and rely on proteolytic organisms to access nitrogen. The effecti eness of a protein as a nitrogen source depends on the hydrolysis products it generates, such as peptides and amino acids. While some microorganisms can utilize simpler nitrogenous compounds like peptides, amino acids, urea, or ammonia, their ability to do so often depends on the environmental conditions. Certain lactic acid bacteria, for example, thrive on polypeptides but cannot break down casein or grow effecti ely with only a few types of amino acids available. When fermentable carbohydrates are present in a substrate, acid fermentation occurs, suppressing proteolytic bacteria and conserving nitrogen compounds while preventing the formation of unpleasant nitrogenous by-products.

Although, many molds are proteolytic, relatively few bacterial genera and even fewer yeast species exhibit active proteolytic activity. Generally, proteolytic bacteria grow best at neutral pH and are inhibited by acidity, with exceptions such as acid-proteolytic bacteria that hydrolyze proteins while producing acid.

Carbon for microbial growth is typically derived from organic compounds, although it may occasionally come from carbon dioxide. While the minerals required for microbial growth are usually available in adequate amounts, some essential minerals can become inaccessible, insufficient or lacking. For instance, milk contains inadequate iron to support the pigmentation of Penicillium roqueforti spores. Similarly, bacteria that cause septicemia often bind iron from the bloodstream, and only strains capable of competing for transferrin-bound iron thrive in human blood.

Foods for Energy

Carbohydrates, especially sugars, are mainly used as a source of energy, but other carbon compounds can be used, such as esters, alcohols, peptides, amino acids, organic acids and their salts. Complex carbohydrates, for example , cellulose, can be used by few organisms, and starch can be hydrolyzed by only a limited number of organisms. Microorganisms also vary in their ability to utilize some of the simpler sugars. Many organisms cannot utilize the disaccharide lactose (milk sugar) and therefore do not grow well in milk. Maltose is not attacked by some yeasts. Bacteria are often identified and classified based on their ability or inability to utilize various sugars and alcohols. Most organisms, if they use sugars, can use glucose.

The ability of microorganisms to hydrolyze pectin, characteristic of some types of bacteria and many molds, is certainly important for the softening or decay of fruits and vegetables or fermented products derived from them.

A limited number of species of microorganisms can obtain their energy from fat, but only if there is no more available energy source, such as sugar. First, the fat must be hydrolyzed by lipase into glycerol and fatty acids, which can serve as an energy source for the hydrolyzing organism or other organisms. In general, aerobic microorganisms are more often involved in the breakdown of fat than anaerobic ones, and lipolytic organisms are usually also proteolytic. Direct oxidation of fats containing unsaturated fatty acids is generally chemical

The products of protein hydrolysis, peptides and amino acids, for example, serve as an energy source for many proteolytic organisms when a better energy source is lacking and as an energy source for other non-proteolytic organisms. Meat, for example, may be low in carbohydrates and therefore break down into proteolytic species, e.g. Pseudomonas spp. , with a subsequent increase in weakly proteolytic or non-proteolytic species that can utilize the products of protein hydrolysis. Organisms vary in their ability to utilize individual amino acids for energy. This is because it is the number of sugar molecules (or moles) that affects aw, and a percentage is usually expressed as weight per unit volume.

It is not only the type of energy supply that is important, but also its concentration in solution and thus the osmotic effect and the amount of moisture available. For a given percentage of sugar in solution, the osmotic pressure will vary according to the weight of the sugar molecule. Thus, a 10% glucose solution has approximately twice the osmotic pressure of a 10% sucrose or maltose solution; that is, it holds twice the moisture. In general, mold can grow in higher concentrations of sugars and yeast in fairly high concentrations, but most bacteria grow best in fairly low concentrations. Of course, there are notable exceptions to this generalization-osmophilic yeasts grow in sugar concentrations similar to molds, and some bacteria can grow in fairly high sugar concentrations.

An adequate supply of nutrients for growth will promote the use of these foods as a source of energy. A good nitrogen diet will allow you to use more carbohydrates than if nitrogen is poor in nature or quantity. Organisms that require additional growth supplements may be prevented from growing if One or more of these "vitamins" are lacking, which could change the entire course of decomposition.

Essential Micronutrients and Vitamins

Essential micronutrients and vitamins play a crucial role in supporting microbial growth in food. Microorganisms require various vitamins, minerals, and trace elements to carry out their metabolic processes, grow, and reproduce. Foods rich in micronutrients provide an ideal environment for microbial growth, as these nutrients act as cofactors for enzymes involved in cellular processes such as energy production, protein synthesis, and DNA replication.

Vitamins such as B vitamins (e.g., B1, B2, B12, and folic acid) are essential for many microbes, particularly bacteria and yeast, as they help with energy metabolism and cell division. B vitamins, for instance, are involved in key enzymatic reactions that allow microbes to convert nutrients into usable energy. Similarly, vitamins like vitamin C (ascorbic acid) and vitamin K also support various microbial activities, including antioxidant defense and biosynthesis of essential molecules. These vitamins are typically abundant in fresh fruits, vegetables, and dairy products, which are also susceptible to microbial contamination and spoilage.

Minerals like iron, magnesium, and zinc are equally important. Iron, for example, is required by many bacteria and fungi for oxygen transport and energy production, and it is often a limiting factor in microbial growth. Magnesium acts as a cofactor in over 300 enzymatic reactions, helping with processes like protein synthesis and nucleic acid synthesis. Zinc is involved in regulating microbial metabolism and is essential for the growth of many pathogenic bacteria.

The availability of these essential micronutrients in food can significantly impact microbial growth. Foods that are rich in vitamins and minerals, such as meats, dairy, fruits, and vegetables, provide an excellent medium for microorganisms, supporting their growth and reproduction. In contrast, foods that are deficient in these nutrients are less conducive to microbial growth, limiting the survival and proliferation of microbes. Understanding the role of micronutrients in microbial growth helps food producers implement effecti e preservation techniques, such as reducing nutrient availability or altering environmental conditions, to minimize spoilage and foodborne illnesses.

Thus, bacteria differ in the foods they can use for energy-some can use a variety of carbohydrates, for example, coliform bacteria and Clostridium spp. , and others only one or two, while some can use other carbon compounds such as organic acids and their salts, alcohols and esters (Pseudomonas spp.). Some bacteria can hydrolyze complex carbohydrates, while others cannot. Similarly, the nitrogen needs of bacteria such as Pseudomonas spp. can be met by simple compounds such as ammonia or nitrates; or more complex compounds such as amino acids, peptides, or proteins may be used or even required, as is the case for lactic acid bacteria. Bacteria also differ in their requirements for additional vitamins or growth factors; some (staph. aureus) synthesize some and others (Pseudomonas or E. aureus) all the necessary factors, and others must have them all (lactic acid bacteria and many pathogens). It should be noted that in general, the better the living environment of an organism, the wider the range of temperature, pH and Aw in which growth can occur.

NATURAL INHIBITORS AND BIOLOGICAL BARRIERS

Inhibitory substances, either naturally present in food, added intentionally or accidentally, or developed by the growth of microorganisms or by processing methods, can inhibit the growth of all microorganisms or, more commonly, can inhibit specific types. Examples of natural inhibitors include lactenins and anticoliform factor in fresh milk, lysozyme in egg whites, and benzoic acid in cranberries.

A microorganism growing in a food may produce one or more inhibitory substances other organisms, products such as acids, alcohols, peroxides, and even antibiotics. Propionic acid produced by propionic bacteria in Swiss cheese is a mold inhibitor; alcohol formed in large quantities by wine lees inhibits competitors; and nisin produced by some strains of Streptococcus lactis may be useful in inhibiting lactate-fermenting clostridia, which form gas during cheese ripening, and undesirable in retarding some of the essential lactic acid streptococci during the production process. There is also the risk of destruction of inhibitory compounds present in foods by microorganisms. Some molds and bacteria are able to destroy some of the phenolic compounds added to meat or fish by smoking or benzoic acid added to foods; sulfur dioxide is destroyed by yeasts that are resistant to it; and lactobacilli can inactivate nisin. Heating foods can result in the formation of inhibitory substances-heating lipids can accelerate autoxidation and make them inhibitors, and frying concentrated sugar syrups can result in the production of furfural and hydroxymethyl furfural, which are inhibitors of fermenting organisms. Prolonged storage at high temperatures can produce similar results.

The effect of the biological structure of foods on the protection of food from spoilage has been observed. The internal parts of healthy tissues of living plants and animals are sterile or poor in microbes. Therefore, if they are not given the opportunity to penetrate, spoilage organisms may be few or absent. Often foods are covered with a protective covering, for example eggshells, poultry skins, nut shells and fruit and vegetable peels or skins, or we may have surrounded the food with an artificial covering, for example. , plastic, or wax. This physical protection of food can not only help preserve it, but also determine the type, rate, and course of spoilage. Layers of fat in meat can protect this part of the meat, or scales can protect the exterior of fis . On the other hand, an increase in exposed surface area caused by peeling, skinning, flaking, or chopping can serve not only to disperse decaying organisms but also to release fluids containing food material for invaders. Frozen tissue can achieve a similar result.

In meat, the growth of spoilage bacteria occurs primarily in the liquid between the small fibers of the meat and only after rigor mortis that most of this food matter is released from the fibers to become a ailable to spoilage organisms.

Synergistic Influences on Microbial Growt

The compositional factors of food—such as water activity (aw), pH, oxidation-reduction (O-R) potential, and nutrient content—play a crucial role in shaping the microbial flora. These factors often interact, making it essential to consider the overall ecological environment of the food. For instance, a microorganism growing at its optimal pH is more resilient to changes in aw compared to one growing near its minimum or maximum pH. Consequently, the combined inhibitory effect of unfavorable pH and aw can be observed. To inhibit or slow microbial growth, multiple factors can be adjusted simultaneously rather than relying on a single inhibitory condition.

Studies on factors affecting the germination of Clostridium botulinum spores have revealed interactions between aw, pH, temperature, O-R potential, and concentrations of sodium chloride and sodium nitrate. Due to the challenge of collecting extensive data across a wide range of variables, mathematical models are often used to design effecti e preservation strategies. For example, predictive techniques considering the combined effects of pH, aw, and temperature have been utilized to assess the risk of microbial hazards, such as the growth of Staphylococcus aureus and Salmonella typhimurium (Broughall and Brown, 1984).

2 Key Microorganisms in Food Science

Key microorganisms in food science include bacteria, yeasts, molds, and viruses, each playing distinct roles in food production, preservation, and spoilage. Bacteria such as *Lactobacillus* and *Bifidobacterium* are essential in the fermentation of dairy products like yogurt and cheese. *Escherichia coli* and Salmonella are harmful bacteria that can cause foodborne illnesses. Yeasts, such as Saccharomyces cerevisiae, are vital in baking and brewing, helping to ferment sugars into alcohol and carbon dioxide. Molds like *Aspergillus* and *Penicillium* are used in food processing, especially in cheese production, but can also cause spoilage in stored food. Viruses, though less common in food science, can cause contamination, with Norovirus being a prominent example of a foodborne virus. Understanding these microorganisms helps in improving food safety, quality, and the development of functional foods.

Food microbiologists need to be familiar with the important microorganisms in foods, at least to the extent that they can identify the major types using what is known about their characteristics and comparing their results with those of sequencing researchers. The first section of this chapter briefly describes the identification and classification of food molds, since these organisms are not studied extensively in the usual introductory microbiology course. We discuss some aspects of the classification of yeasts, but we do not attempt to cover determinant bacteriology, a subject to which the student usually receives an adequate introduction in the first icrobiology course.

UNDERSTANDING MOLDS

Mold on food, with its cloudy or cottony appearance, sometimes colored, is familiar to everyone, and foods with a moldy or "mold" coating are generally considered unsafe to eat. While it is true that mold is involved in the spoilage of many types of food, specific molds are useful in the production of certain foods or food ingredients. Thus, some types of cheese are made with mold, for example blue, Roquefort, Camembert, Brie, Gammelost, etc. , and molds are used in the preparation of oriental dishes, such as soy sauce, miso, soy sauce and others that we will discuss later. Molds are cultivated as animal feed and are used to produce products used in food, such as amylase for bread production or citric acid used in beverages. Some molds produce various toxic metabolites (mycotoxins), which are discussed in Chapter 25.

Common Characteristics of Molds

The term "mold" is commonly used to refer to certain multicellular filamentous fungi whose growth on food is usually easily recognized by its fluff or cottony appearance. Most of the growth usually appears white, but it may be colored, dark, or smoky. Colored spores are typical of some mature molds and provide color to part or all of the growth. The thallus, or vegetative body, is characteristic of thallophytes, which lack true roots, stems, and leaves.

Morphological Characteristics

In identifying and classifying molds, their morphology, which includes shape and structure, is assessed through both macroscopic and microscopic examination. The mold thallus comprises a network of branched and intertwined filaments called hyphae (singular-hypha), collectively referred to as the mycelium. Hyphae may grow underground or within food (subterranean) or above the surface (aerial). They can be categorized as vegetative, primarily responsible for nutrient absorption, or fertile, involved in reproductive structures. Fertile hyphae are usually aerial but can also be subterranean in some molds. Hyphae may vary in appearance, being either smooth and full or thin and ragged. Some molds produce sclerotia, dense clusters of modified, thick-walled hyphae, which are highly resistant to heat and adverse conditions, making them significant in processed food contexts.

Microscopic examination of hyphae reveals distinctive characteristics useful for mold identification. Molds are classified into septate molds, with transverse walls dividing the hyphae into cells, and non-septate (coenocytic) molds, where hyphae appear as cylindrical structures without cross-walls. Non-septate hyphae contain nuclei dispersed along their length and are considered multicellular. Hyphae may range in color from colorless and transparent under the microscope to dark or smoky in larger masses.

Septate hyphae grow either at the tip (apical growth) or along the hypha (intercalary growth), with the type of growth being characteristic of the mold. In non-septate hyphae, nuclear division is accompanied by filament elongation. Specific mycelial structures, such as the rhizoids of *Rhizopus* and *Absidia*, the stem cells of *Aspergillus*, and the Y-shaped branching of *Geotrichum*, are key to mold identification

Molds primarily reproduce asexually through spores but may also form sexual spores. Sexual reproduction is characteristic of "perfect" fungi, classified as *Oomycetes, Zygomycetes* (non-septate), *Ascomycetes, Basidiomycetes* (septate). In contrast, "imperfect" fungi (Fungi Imperfecti), typically septate, reproduce only via asexual spores. Molds can also propagate from fragments of transplanted mycelium.

Sexual Spores

Molds that produce sexual spores are classified based on their spore formation process and the type of spores they generate. Nonseptate molds, known as

Phycomycetes, produce oospores and are categorized as *Oomycetes.* These molds are mainly aquatic, but the group also includes significant plant pathogens, such as the "downy mildews" responsible for potato late blight and tomato buckeye rot. Oospores are formed by the union of a small male gamete with a larger female gamete. In contrast, Zygomycetes form *zygospores* through the fusion of two hyphal tips, which can arise from the same or different mycelia. Both oospores and zygospores are encased in a thick wall, making them resistant to prolonged drying.

Ascomycetes, characterized by septate hyphae, produce sexual spores called ascospores. These spores form after the fusion of two cells from either the same or separate mycelia, followed by cell division. Ascospores are enclosed within a sac-like structure called an ascus, which typically holds eight spores. These asci may occur individually or be clustered within a protective structure called an ascocarp, formed by intertwining hyphae. *Basidiomycetes,* which include mushrooms, plant rusts, and smuts, produce a unique type of sexual spore known as the basidiospore.

Asexual Spores

their small size, lightweight nature, and resistance to desiccation. These spores are easily dispersed through the air and can germinate to form new molds when conditions are favorable. The three primary types of asexual spores are (1) conidia (singular-conidium), (2) arthrospores or oidia, and (3) sporangiospores. Conidia are formed on specialized fertile hyphae called conidiophores and are typically exposed rather than enclosed.

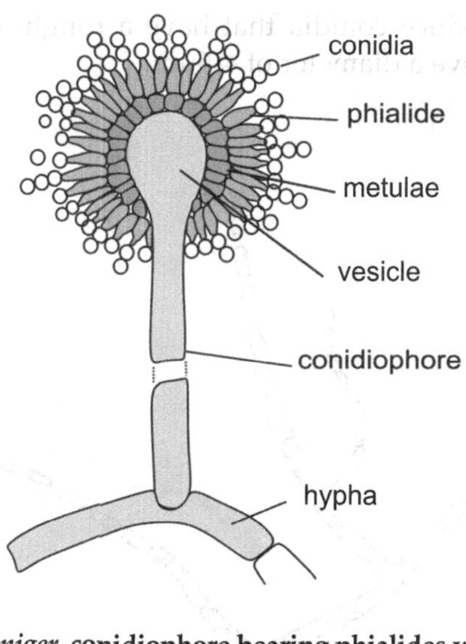

Fig 2.1. ***Aspergillus niger*, conidiophore bearing phialides with catenate conidia.**

In contrast, sporangiospores are contained within a sac-like structure called a sporangium (plural-sporangia) located at the tip of a fertile hypha called a sporangiophore. Arthrospores develop through the fragmentation of hyphae, where the individual hyphal cells transform into arthrospores. Examples of these spore types are discussed in the context of significant mold genera

Additionally, a fourth type of asexual spore, known as chlamydospores, is produced by many molds. These are formed when certain cells within the mycelium accumulate food reserves, swell, and develop a thicker wall compared to surrounding cells. Chlamydospores, or resting cells, are better equipped to endure unfavorable conditions and can germinate into new molds when the environment becomes favorable.

Aspergillus niger is a filamentous fungus, forming filamented hyphae that make them appear like small plants.

Macroscopic observation of *A.niger* reveals that their growth is initially white but they change to black after a few days producing conidial spore. The edges of the colonies appear pale yellow producing radial fissures.

A microscopic view of *A.niger* reveals that *A.niger* has smooth colored conidiophores and conidia. The conidiophores are protrusions from a septate and hyaline hyphae. The conidial heads appear radial and they split into columns (biseriate). the conidiophore vesicle produces sterile cells known as metulae which support the phialides on the conidiophores,

- The Conidiophores are 400-3000μm long, they are smooth and hyaline.
- The conidiophore becomes dark at the apex and terminating in a globose vesicle which is 30-75μm in diameter.
- The metulae and phialides cover the vesicle.

The phialides produce conidia that have a rough texture, are dark brown colored, and have a diameter of 4-5μm.

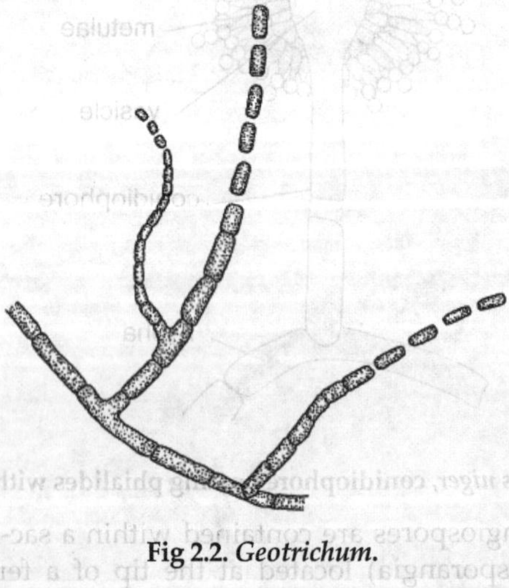

Fig 2.2. *Geotrichum.*

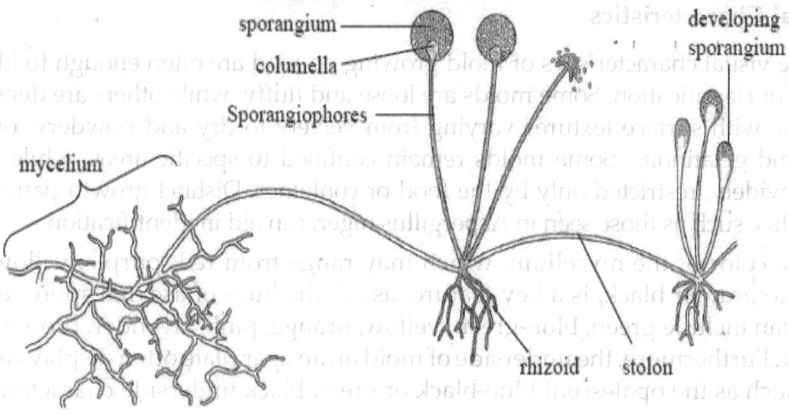

Fig 2.3. Detailed view of sporulating structure of *Rhizopus*.

Physiological Characteristics

The physiological characteristics of molds are briefly summarized here and will be explored in detail later.

- **Food Requirements:** Molds can utilize diverse nutrients, from simple to complex compounds. Many produce hydrolytic enzymes such as amylases, pectinases, proteinases, and lipases and are often cultivated for these enzymes.
- **Moisture Requirements:** Molds generally need less available moisture than yeasts or bacteria. For instance, maintaining a moisture content below 14–15% in foods like flour or dried fruits can effecti ely inhibit or delay mold growth.
- **Temperature Requirements:** Most molds are mesophilic, thriving at moderate temperatures, with an optimal range of 25–30°C. However, some, such as Aspergillus species, can grow well at 35–37°C or higher. Certain molds are psychrotrophic, capable of growing at refrigeration temperatures and even slowly below freezing, with reports of growth as low as −5 to −10°C. A few are thermophilic, preferring higher temperatures for optimal growth.
- **Oxygen and pH Requirements**: Molds are aerobic organisms, requiring oxygen to grow. They can adapt to a wide pH range (2 to 8.5), with acidic conditions being particularly favorable.
- **Inhibitors:** Some molds secrete inhibitory substances, like penicillin from Penicillium chrysogenum and clavacin from Aspergillus clavatus. Additionally, chemical agents like sorbic acid, propionates, and acetates can suppress mold growth (mycostatic) or eliminate it entirely (fungicidal).

Although mold growth typically starts slower than that of bacteria or yeasts, it accelerates rapidly once conditions become favorable.

Cultural Characteristics

The visual characteristics of mold growing on food are often enough to identify its type or classification. Some molds are loose and fluffy while others are dense and compact, with surface textures varying from velvety to dry and powdery, or even moist and gelatinous. Some molds remain confined to specific areas, while others spread widely, restricted only by the food or container. Distinct growth patterns on the thallus, such as those seen in Aspergillus niger, can aid in identification

The color of the mycelium, which may range from red, purple, yellow, and brown to gray or black, is a key feature, as are the hues of asexual spore masses, which can include green, blue-green, yellow, orange, pink, lavender, brown, gray, or black. Furthermore, the underside of mold on an agar plate often displays unique traits, such as the opalescent blue-black or green-black underside characteristic of Cladosporium.

CLASSIFICATION AND IDENTIFICATION OF MOLDS

Molds are classified as organisms within the kingdom Myceteae, lacking roots, stems, leaves, and chlorophyll. They belong to the Eumycetes, or true fungi, and are further categorized into subdivisions, classes, orders, families, and genera.

The primary criteria for distinguishing and identifying molds include:

- **Sexual Spore Production:** Presence and type of sexual spores, such as oospores, zygospores, or ascospores.
- **Asexual Spore Types**: Classification into sporangiospores, conidia, or arthrospores (oidia).
- **Hyphae Structure:** Whether hyphae are septate or nonseptate.
- **Mycelium Characteristics**: Clarity (clear or dark) and color (colored or colorless).

Spore Head Features

For sporangia- size, shape, color, and location.

For conidia-bearing spore heads: structure (single conidia, chains, budding, or masses), arrangement of sterigmata or phialides, and adhesion of conidia.

- **Microscopic Spore Features:** Characteristics of asexual spores, especially conidia, including shape, size, color, texture (smooth or rough), and whether they are one-, two-, or multi-celled.
- **Special Structures:** Presence of unique features like stolons, rhizoids, foot cells, apophysis, chlamydospores, or sclerotia.
- **Sporangiophore or Conidiophore Structure:** Whether simple or branched, types of branching, size and shape of the columella, and arrangement (single or in bundles).

An in-depth guide to food-borne fungi, including illustrations, photomicrographs, photographs of molds on agar, and an identification key, has been created by Samson et al. (1984).

Molds of Industrial Importance

Several molds of industrial importance are outlined by genus, with typical morphological structures presented in the accompanying Figures.

Mucor

Mucor are involved in the spoilage of some foods and the manufacture of others. A widely distributed species is *M. racemosus. M. rouxii* is used in the "Amylo" process for the saccharification of starch, and mucors help ripen some chesses (e.g., Gammelost) and are used in making certain Oriental foods.

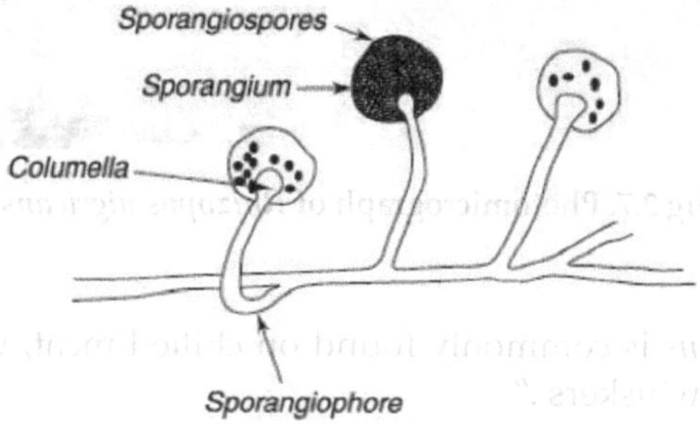

Fig 2.4. Sporangiophores bearing columellate sporangia in *Mucor*.

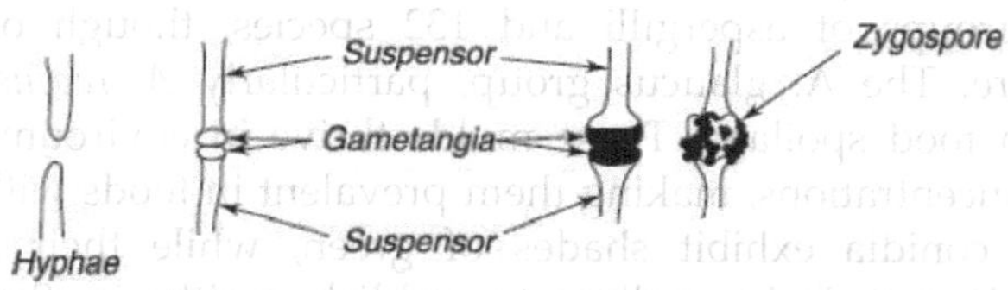

Fig 2.5. Zygospore formation in *Mucor*.

Zygorrhynchus

These soil molds are similar to *Mucor* except that the zygospore suspensors are markedly unequal in size.

Rhizopus

Rhizopus stolonifer, the so-called bread mold, is very common and is involved in the spoilage of many foods: berries, fruits, vegetables, bread, etc.

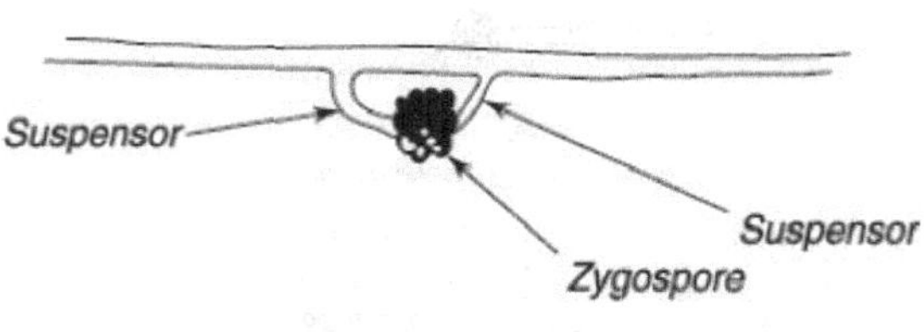

Fig 2.6. Zygospore formation in *Zygorrhynchus*.

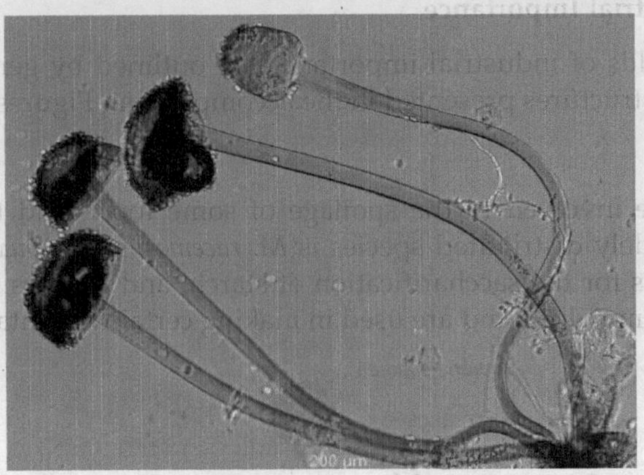

Fig 2.7. Photomicrograph of *Rhizopus nigricans*.

Thamnidium

Thamnidium elegans is commonly found on chilled meat, where it causes a condition known as "whiskers ."

Aspergillus

Aspergillus species are widely distributed, with many contributing to food spoilage, while others play a role in food production. Raper and Fennell (1965) identified 18 groups of aspergilli and 132 species, though only a few are noteworthy here. The A. glaucus group, particularly *A. repens*, is frequently associated with food spoilage. These molds thrive in environments with high sugar or salt concentrations, making them prevalent in foods with low moisture content. Their conidia exhibit shades of green, while their ascospores are contained within asci inside yellow to reddish perithecia. Some researchers classify these molds as Ascomycetes within the genus *Eurotium*, a designation used for species with a perfect (sexual) reproductive stage.

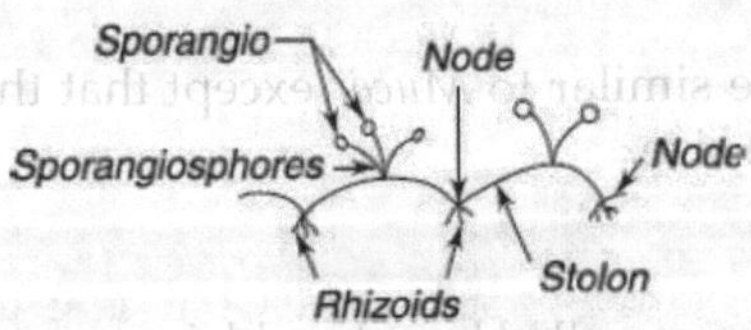

Fig 2.8. Diagram of *Absidia*, showing locations of sporangiophores and rhizoids.

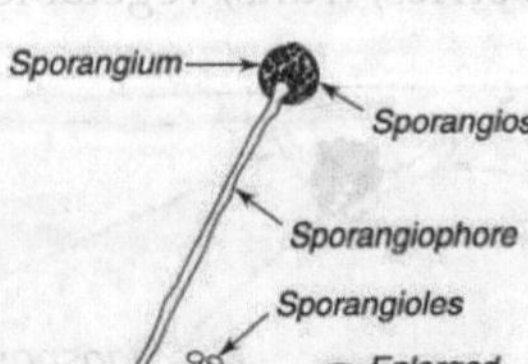

Fig 2.9. Sporulating structure in *Thamnidium*.

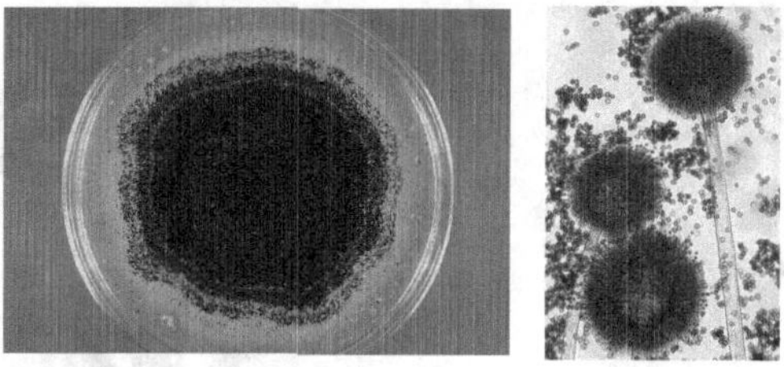

A B

Fig 2.10. *Aspergillus niger.* (A) Fungal colony growing on Czapek agar (B) Photomicrograph of conidiphore with vesicle having catenate conidia on phialdes .

The *A. niger* group, with *A. niger* as a leading species, is widespread and may be important in foods. The spore-bearing heads are large, tightly packed, and globular and may be black, brownish-black, or purple-brown. The conidia are rough, with bands of pigment.

Many strains have sclerotia, colored from buff to gray to blackish. Selected strains are used for the commercial production of citric and gluconic acids and in a variety of enzyme preparations. The *A. flavus-oryzae* group includes molds important in the marking of some Oriental foods and the production of enzymes, but molds in this group often are involved in the spoilage of foods. Conidia give various yellow to green shades to the spore heads, and dark sclerotia may be formed.

Penicillium

This genus is widely distributed and holds significant relevance in food contexts. It is categorized into groups and subgroups, with numerous species identified. Classification is based on the branching patterns of the spore-bearing structures, known as penicilli, which resemble small brushes. These structures, or verticillata, consist of clusters of three or more components: sterigmata, metulae (subbranches), and branches. Notable species include *P. expansum*, a blue-green-spored mold that causes soft rot in fruits, and *P. digitatum*, characterized by olive- or yellowish-green conidia, which leads to soft rot in citrus fruits. *P. italicum*, known as the "blue contact mold" with blue-green conidia, also affects citrus fruits, while P. camemberti, with grayish conidia, is instrumental in ripening Camembert cheese. Similarly,

P. roqueforti, with bluish-green conidia, plays a role in the ripening of blue cheeses like Roquefort. Some species produce asci containing ascospores within cleistothecia, and a few exhibit sclerotia, which have occasionally caused issues in canned acidic foods.

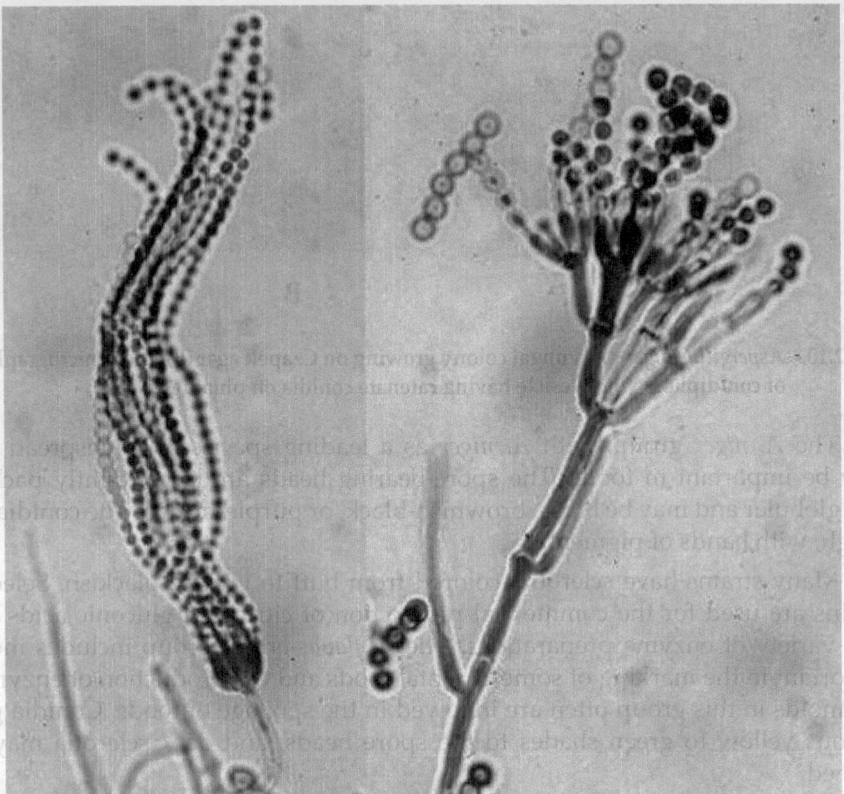

Fig 2.11. Photomicrograph showing penicillus in *Penicillium* sp.

Trichothecium

The common species, *T. roseum,* is a pink mold which grows on wood, paper, fruits such as apples and peaches, and vegetables such as cucumbers and cantaloupes. This mold is easily recognized by the clusters of two-celled conidia at the ends of short, erect conidiophores. Conidia have a nipplelike projection at the point of attachment, and the smaller of the two cells of each conidium is at this end.

Geotrichum (Oospora* or *Oidium)

Some authors classify this genus among yeastlike fungi, while others place it with molds. Species can appear white, yellowish, orange, or red, initially forming a firm, felt-like mass that eventually becomes soft and creamy. *Geotrichum candidum* (also known as *Oospora lactis*), commonly referred to as "dairy mold," produces white to cream-colored growth. The hyphae are septate and typically dichotomously branched in common species. The asexual spores are arthrospores (oidia), which can appear rectangular when formed from submerged hyphae and oval when produced from aerial hyphae.

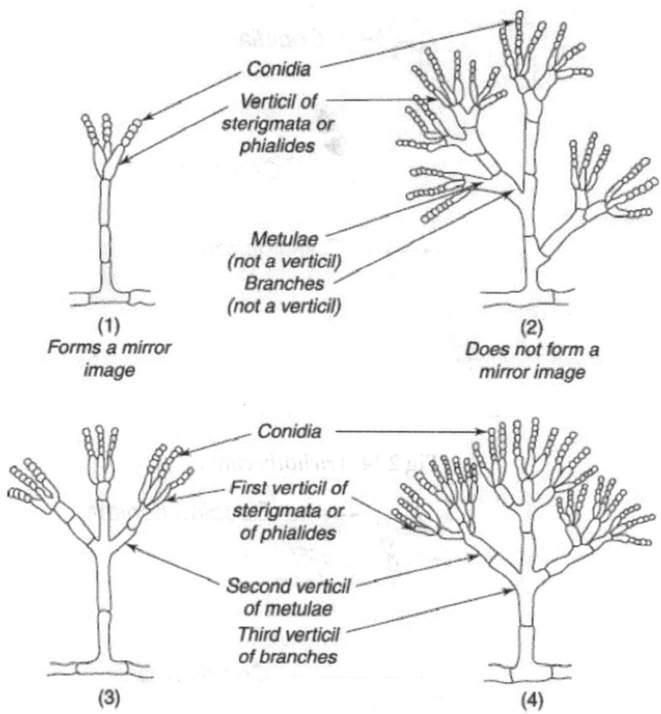

Fig 2.12. Diagram showing different types of penicillus heads in different *Penicillium* spp.: (1) monoverticillata symmetrica, (2) monoverticillata asymmetrica, (3) biverticillata symmetrica, and (4) polyverticillata symmertrica.

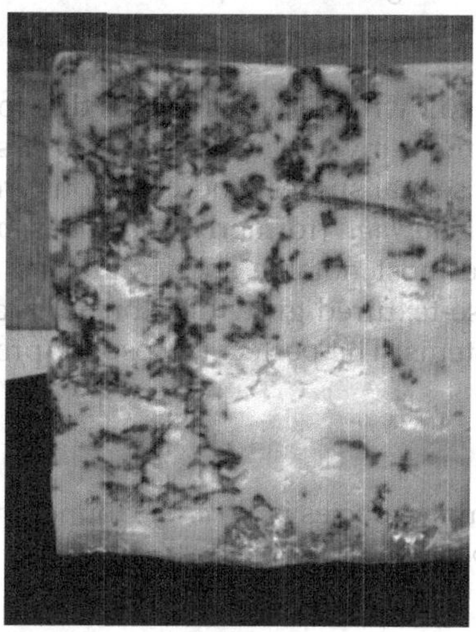

Fig 2.13. Photograph of Penicillium roqueforti on moldy cheese.

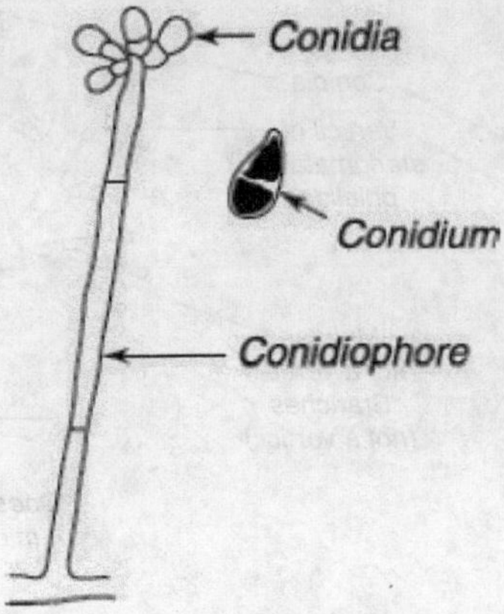

Fig 2.14. *Trichothecium.*

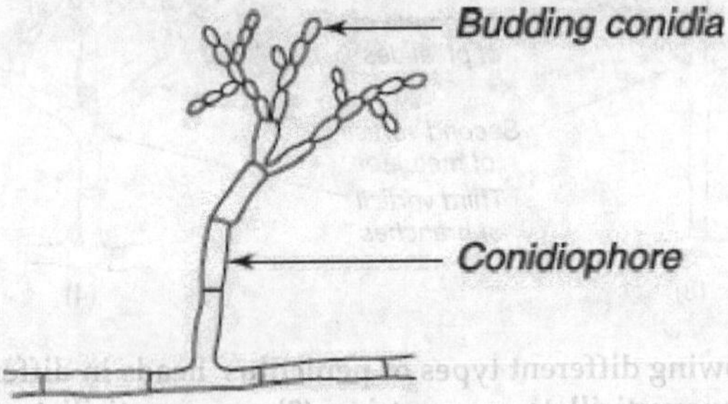

Fig 2.15. *Neurospora (Monilia).*

Neurospora (Monilia)

This genus has been known by several names due to confusion regarding its classification. However, most mycologists agree that it should be classified as a perfect mold (producing sexual spores) and commonly refer to it as Neurospora. The species *Neurospora sitophila* (formerly *Monilia sitophila*), often called the "red bread mold," is the most notable species in food applications, frequently appearing as a pink, loose-textured growth on bread. It also grows on sugarcane bagasse and other food items. The perfect (ascospore-producing) stage is seldom observed.

Sporotrichum

Among the saprophytic species is *S. carnis*, found growing on chilled meats, when it causes "white spot."

Botrytis

One species important in foods is *B. cinerea*. It causes a disease of grapes but may grow saprophytically on many foods.

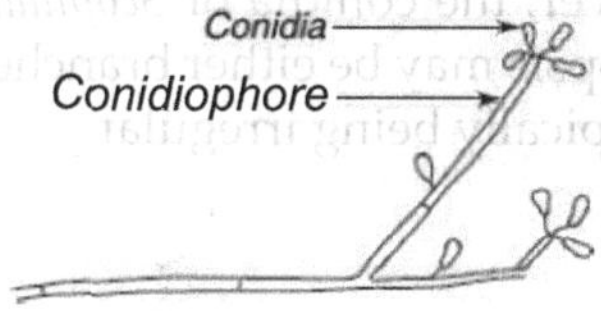

Fig 2.16. *Sporotrichum.*

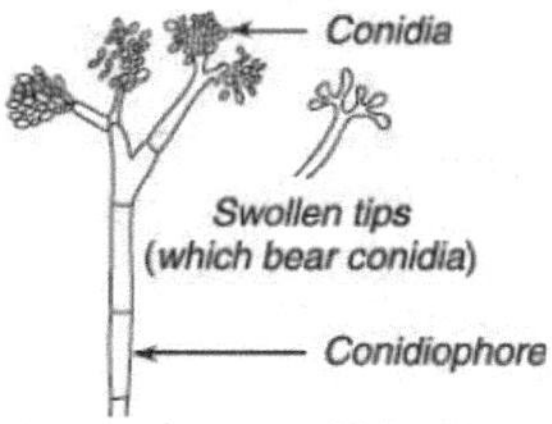

Fig 2.17. *Botrytis cinerea.*

Cephalosporium

C. acremonium is a common species, as is *Trichoderma viride*. The fully developed mold appears bright green due to the clusters of green conidia being bound together, with tufts of sterile hyphae protruding above the conidiophores.

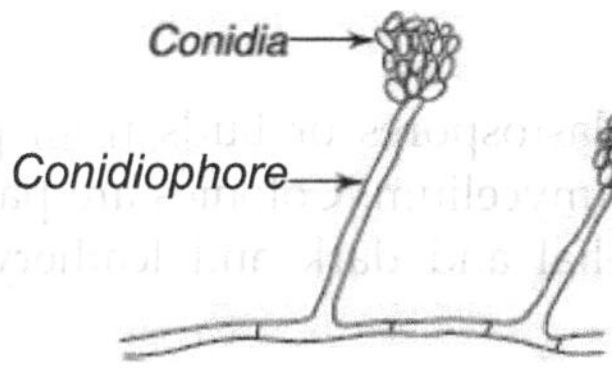

Fig 2.18. *Cephalosporium.*

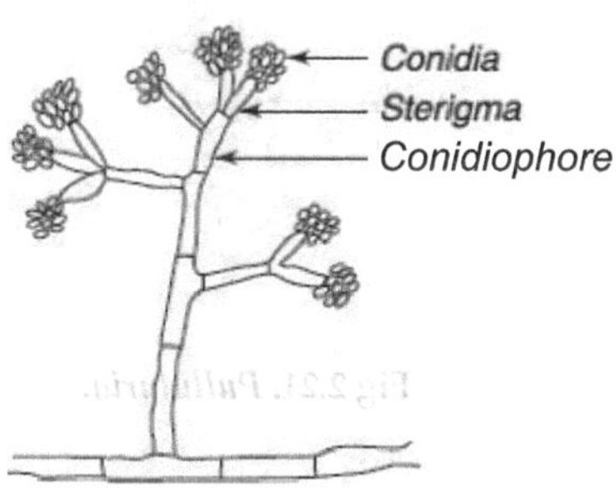

Fig 2.19. *Trichoderma.*

Scopulariopsis

S. brevicaulis is a commonly found species. This genus can be confused with *Penicillium,* as both feature brush-like penicilli and chains of spores detached from the sterigmata. However, the conidia of *Scopulariopsis* are never green. The conidiophores in Scopulariopsis may be either branched or unbranched, simple or complex, with branching typically being irregular.

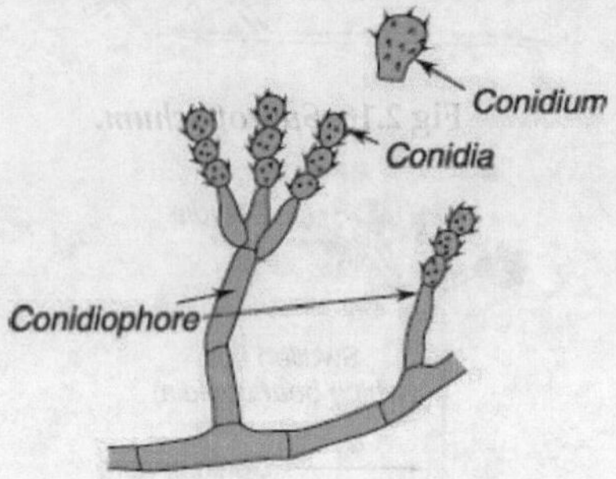

Fig 2.20. ***Scopulariopsis.***

The spore-bearing structures can range from complex, branching systems with penicilli to single sterigmata emerging from short aerial hyphae branches. The spores have a distinct microscopic appearance; they are not green but typically yellowish-brown, lemon-shaped, thick-walled, spiny, and pointed at one end, with a thick ring at the opposite end. The colonies are brownish and cotton-like in texture.

Pullularia

Ovate, hyaline conidia (blastospores or buds from preexisting cells) borne as lateral buds on all parts of the mycelium. Colonies are pale and slimy and yeastlike when young, becoming mycelial and dark and leathery in age. *P. pullulans* is a common species.

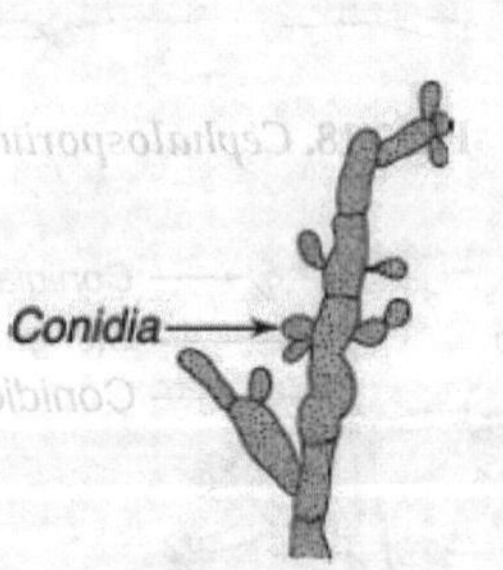

Fig 2.21. ***Pullularia.***

Cladosporium

C. herbarum is a prominent species. These dark molds are responsible for causing "black spot" on various foods, cellar walls, and other surfaces. Colonies of *C. herbarum* exhibit restricted growth and have a thick, velvety texture, with colors ranging from olive to gray-green. The reverse side of the colony displays a striking opalescent blue-black to greenish-black hue.

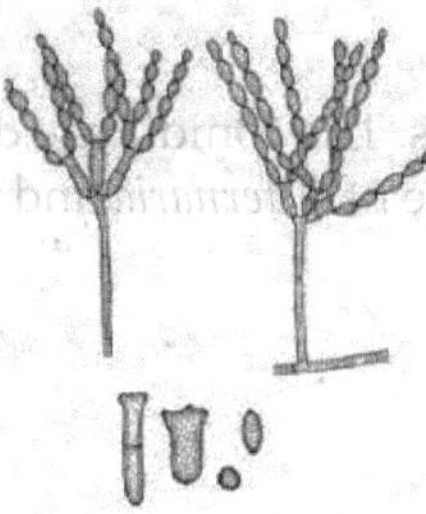

Fig 2.22. *Cladosporium.*

Helminthosporium

Species of this genus are for the most part plant pathogens but may grow saprophytically on vegetable materials.

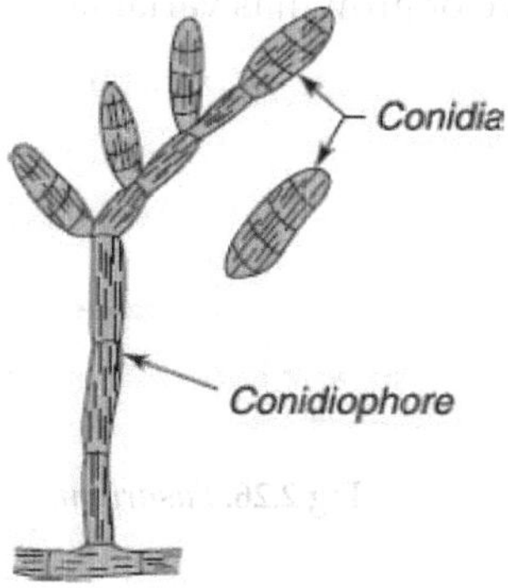

Fig 2.23. *Helminthosporium.*

Alternaria

Molds from this genus are frequent culprits in food spoilage. Common species include A. citri (which causes rot in citrus fruits), *A. tenuis* (*A. alternata*) *and A. brassicae.*

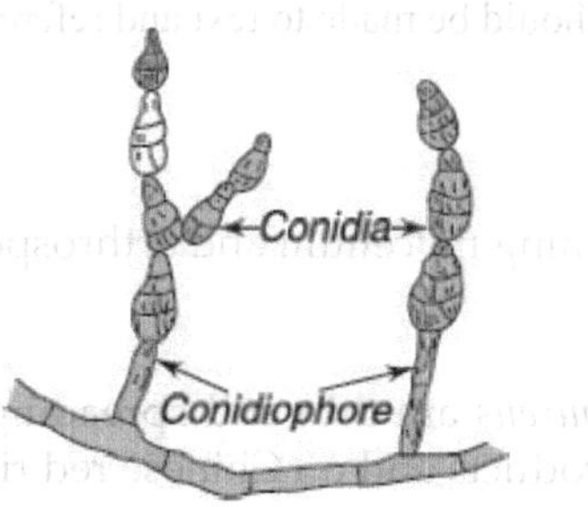

Fig 2.24. *Alternaria.*

The mycelial mass typically appears as a dirty gray-green, although the hyphae often appear nearly colorless under a microscope. The brown, multicellular conidia are arranged in chains on the conidiophore.

Stemphylium

This, too, is a common genus. The conidia are dark and multicellular but have fewer cross walls than those of *Alternaria* and are rounded at both ends.

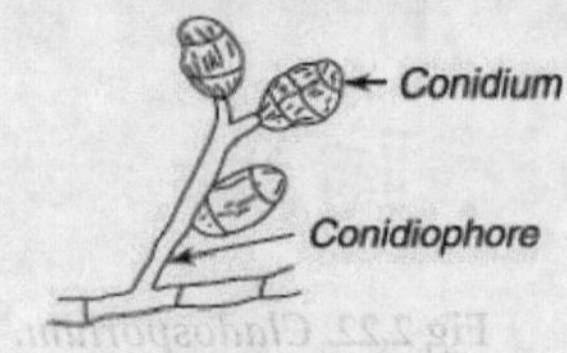

Fig 2.25. *Stemphylium.*

Fusarium

Molds of this genus often grow on foods. The species are very difficul to identify, and the appearance of growth is variable.

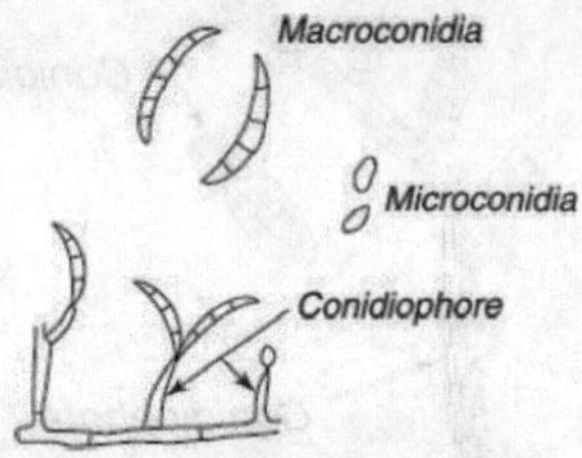

Fig 2.26. *Fusarium.*

Sclerotinia

Some species are responsible for rotting vegetables and fruits, typically appearing in the conidial stage. The lemon-shaped conidia are arranged in chains, with a "plug" separating each conidium. In the previous discussion of molds important in food spoilage, genera that grow only occasionally on specific foods have been excluded but will be addressed alongside those foods.For the descriptions of these genera, reference should be made to text and reference books on fungi listed at the end of this chapter.

Endomyces

Yeastlike fungi, forming mycelium and arthrospores. Some species rot fruits.

Monascus

Colonies of *M. purpureus* are thin and spreading and reddish or purple in color. Found on dairy products and on Chinese red rice (ang-khak).

YEASTS AND YEAST LIKE FUNGI

The term "yeast" is often used but is difficul to define. In this context, it refers to fungi that are typically unicellular, ovoid or spherical in shape, and do not form filaments. These fungi reproduce by budding or fissio

Yeasts are unicellular fungi widely used in food science for fermentation, producing bread, beer, wine, and other fermented products. Saccharomyces cerevisiae is the most significant yeast, valued for its role in alcohol production and dough leavening. Yeastlike fungi, such as *Candida* and *Rhodotorula,* can spoil food by growing on dairy, fruits, and processed products, causing discoloration and off-flavor

Beneficial yeasts contribute to probiotics and enzyme production, while spoilage yeasts pose challenges in food preservation. Proper storage, hygiene, and microbial control are vital to managing their impact in food systems.

Key Features of Yeasts

Yeasts are primarily classified based on their morphological traits, though their physiological characteristics are more significant to food microbiologists

Cultural Characteristics

In general, the appearance of yeast growth in large masses is not particularly helpful for identifying yeast species. However, growth as a film on the surface of liquid media can suggest an oxidative or film-forming yeast, while the production of a carotenoid pigment can indicate the genus *Rhodotorula.* The appearance of yeast growth becomes more important when it leads to colored spots on food. Differentiating yeast colonies from bacterial ones on agar plates can be challenging; microscopic examination is the only reliable method. Most young yeast colonies are moist and slightly slimy, though some may appear mealy. Typically, colonies are white, but they can also be cream-colored or pink. Some colonies remain relatively unchanged as they age, while others become dry and wrinkled.

Yeasts can be classified as oxidative, fermentative, or both. Oxidative yeasts may form a film, pellicle, or scum on the surface of a liquid, and are referred to as film yeasts. Fermentative yeasts usually grow throughout the liquid and produce carbon dioxide.

Morphological Characteristics

Yeast morphology is identified through microscopic examination. Yeasts exhibit a range of shapes, such as spherical, ovoid, lemon-shaped, pear-shaped, cylindrical, triangular, or even extended into a false or true mycelium. They also differ in size. Key structural components include the cell wall, which may be metachromatic, albuminous, or starchy. Special staining methods are needed to visualize the nucleus.

Reproduction

Most yeasts reproduce asexually through multilateral or polar budding, in which a portion of the protoplasm protrudes through the cell wall, grows, and ultimately forms a new yeast cell. In certain yeasts, such as some fil yeasts, the bud arises from a tubelike extension of the mother cell. The nuclear material is replicated and divided between the mother and daughter cells. A few yeast species reproduce by fission, while one species uses a combination of fission and budding

Sexual reproduction in "true" yeasts (*Ascomycotina*) involves the creation of ascospores, where the yeast cell functions as the ascus. This process usually follows the conjugation of two cells, although some yeasts can form ascospores without conjugation, followed by conjugation of the ascospores or smaller daughter cells. The number of spores per ascus and the features of the ascospores—such as color, wall texture (smooth or rough), and shape (round, oval, reniform, bean-shaped, sickle-shaped, Saturn-shaped, hemispherical, angular, fusiform, or needle-shaped)—differ for each type of east.

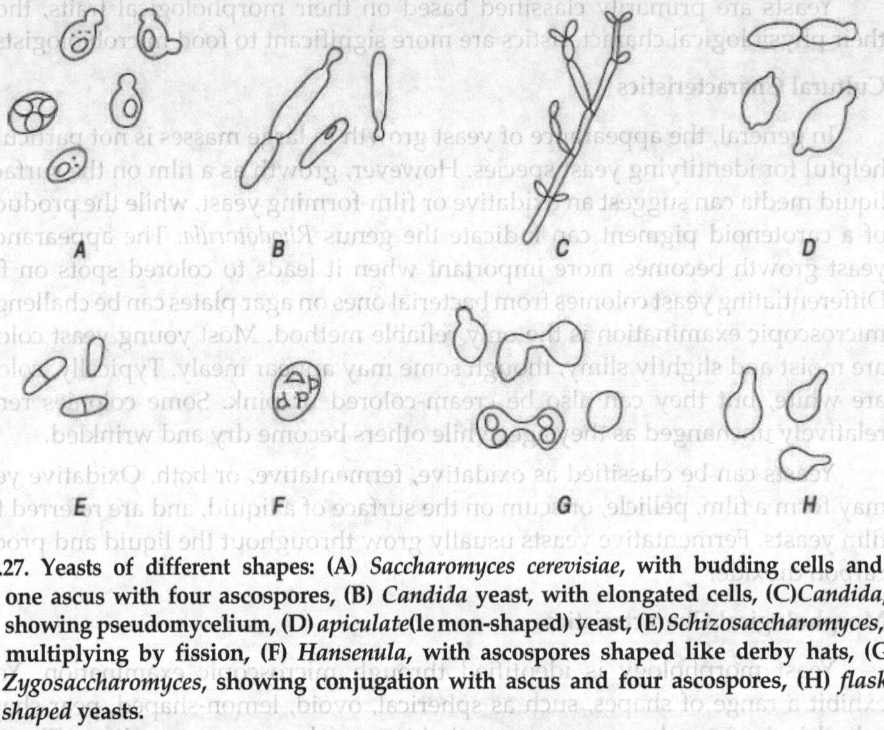

Fig. 2.27. Yeasts of different shapes: (A) *Saccharomyces cerevisiae*, with budding cells and one ascus with four ascospores, (B) *Candida* yeast, with elongated cells, (C)*Candida*, showing pseudomycelium, (D) *apiculate*(le mon-shaped) yeast, (E) *Schizosaccharomyces*, multiplying by fission, (F) *Hansenula*, with ascospores shaped like derby hats, (G) *Zygosaccharomyces*, showing conjugation with ascus and four ascospores, (H) *flask-shaped* yeasts.

"False" yeasts, which produce no ascospores or other sexual spores, belong to the Fungi Imperfecti. Cells of some yeasts become chlamydospores by formation of a thick wall about the cell, for example, *Candida*, *Rhodotorula*, and *Cryptococcus*.

Physiological Characteristics

While yeast species can vary significantly in their physiology, industrially important yeasts share enough common characteristics to allow for generalizations, though exceptions should always be considered. Most common yeasts thrive when moisture is abundant, but many can grow in environments with higher concentrations of solutes like sugar or salt, requiring less moisture than most bacteria, though still more than molds. Based on water activity (aw), yeasts are classified as either ordinary or osmophilic. Ordinary yeasts typically grow in environments with an aw between 0.88 and 0.94, such as beer, condensed milk, and baker's yeast. In contrast, osmophilic yeasts can grow in low aw environments (0.62-0.65), such as syrups, although some are inhibited around 0.78 in salt brine or sugar syrup. The optimal aw for yeast growth depends on environmental factors, including substrate nutrition, pH, temperature, oxygen availability, and potential inhibitors.

Yeasts generally thrive at temperatures between 25 to 30°C, with a maximum growth range of 35 to 47°C. Some yeasts can even grow at or below 0°C. They typically prefer an acidic pH of around 4 to 4.5 and are less effecti e in alkaline environments unless adapted. While most yeasts require oxygen for optimal growth, fermentative types can grow anaerobically, though more slowly. Sugars serve as the primary energy source for yeasts, although some, like film yeasts, can oxidize organic acids and alcohols. The carbon dioxide produced by bread yeasts aids in leavening, while alcohol produced by fermentative yeasts is key in making products like wine, beer, and industrial alcohol. Yeasts also contribute to flavor development in wines.

Yeasts can utilize a range of nitrogenous compounds, from simple forms like ammonia and urea to more complex amino acids and polypeptides. Additionally, they need various growth factors to thrive. Yeasts, especially true yeasts with sexual reproduction, can undergo physiological changes, including breeding for specific traits or mutations leading to new forms. Many yeast strains, such as Saccharomyces cerevisiae, are tailored for different applications, including baking, brewing, winemaking, and high-alcohol production.

CLASSIFICATION AND IDENTIFICATION OF YEASTS

True yeasts belong to the subdivision *Ascomycotina,* while false or asporogenous yeasts are classified under the subdivision *Fungi Imperfecti* or *Deuteromycotina.* For further details on the classification and identification of yeasts, refer to Barnett et al. (1983). The equivalent names of some yeasts are given in the table below.

Table. Equivalent Names of Some CommonYeasts

Genus	Species (Old Name)	Species (New Name)
Saccharomyces	*S. uvarum*	*S. pasgorialus*
Saccharomyces	*S. fragilis*	*Kluyveromyces marxianus*
Saccharomyces	*S. lactis*	*Kluyveromyces marxianus var. lactis*
Saccharomyces	*S. rouxii*	*Zygosaccharomyces rouxii*
Saccharomyces	*S. mellis*	*Zygosaccharomyces rouxii*
Saccharomyces	*S. nussbaumeri*	*Zygosaccharomyces rouxii*
Debaryomyces	*D. kloeckeri*	*D. hansenii*

This table reflects the reclassification of several *Saccharomyces* species, as noted in the reference by Lodder (1984).

Certain yeasts are classified under two different genera depending on whether they reproduce sexually. Some examples of these yeasts, with equivalent names, are listed in Table. The primary criteria for identifying and classifying yeast genera include the following:

Formation of Ascospores

- Method of Ascospore Production:
  - o Parthenogenetically (without conjugation of yeast cells), followed by conjugation of ascospores or small daughter cells.
  - o After isogamic conjugation (conjugating cells are similar).
  - o After heterogamic conjugation (conjugating cells diffe).
- **Appearance of Ascospores:** Shape, size, and color. Most are spheroidal or ovoid, but some species (e.g., *Hansenula*) have distinct shapes.
- **Number of Ascospores per Ascus:** Typically one, two, four, or eight.
- **Appearance of Vegetative Cells:** Shape, size, color, and inclusions.

Method of Asexual Reproduction

- Budding
- Fission
- Combined budding and fissio
- Arthrospores (oidia)
  - o **Presence of Mycelium:** Whether a mycelium, pseudomycelium, or no mycelium is formed.

Growth Characteristics

Growth as a film over the surface of liquids (film yeasts) or throughout the medium.

Color of Macroscopic Growth

Physiological Characteristics (used for differentiating species or strains within a species):

- Nitrogen and carbon sources
- Vitamin requirements
- Oxidative or fermentative properties

Lipolysis, urease activity, acid production, or formation of starchlike compounds

Yeasts of Industrial Importance

Most industrial yeasts belong to the genus *Saccharomyces*. The term "wild yeast" refers to any yeast other than the one being actively used or encouraged.

Thus, a yeast employed in one process could be considered wild in another. Most troublesome wild yeasts are asporogenous or false yeasts.

Genus *Schizosaccharomyces*

Schizosaccharomyces is a genus of fission yeasts known for their unique division by binary fission rather than budding. *S. pombe* is the most studied species, used in traditional African brewing and scientific research. These yeasts tolerate acidic and high-sugar environments, making them valuable in alcoholic fermentation and food preservation.

Genus *Saccharomyces*

Yeast cells in this genus can be round, ovate, or elongated and may form pseudomycelium. They reproduce by multipolar budding or ascospore formation, which can occur after conjugation or from diploid cells in the vegetative stage. S. cerevisiae is the most well-known species, used in food industries for bread leavening, ale, wine, and alcohol production.

- **Top Yeasts:** These are active fermenters that grow rapidly at 20°C, forming clumps and producing CO_2, which causes them to float to the surface
- **Bottom Yeasts:** These grow more slowly and ferment best at 10-15°C. They do not clump and settle at the bottom of the fermentation essel.

Saccharomyces cerevisiae var. *ellipsoideus* is a high-alcohol variety used for industrial alcohol and wine production. Other species like *S. uvarum* (used in beer making) and *S. fragilis* and *S. lactis* (important for lactose fermentation in dairy products) are also significant. Some *Saccharomyces* species, such as *S. rouxii* and *S. mellis*, are osmophilic.

Lodder (1984) reclassified many *Saccharomyces* species, including *S. uvarum* (now considered a variant of *S. cerevisiae*), *S. fragilis* (now *Kluyveromyces marxianus*), and *S. lactis* (now K. *marxianus* var. *lactis*). Other reclassifications include *S. rouxii, S. mellis*, and *S. nussbaumeri* (now *Zygosaccharomyces rouxii*) and *Debaryomyces kloeckeri* (now *D. hansenii*).

Genus Kluyveromyces

These yeasts reproduce by multilateral budding and release ascospores upon maturity. Species like *S. fragilis* and *S. lactis* are now classified under this genus.

Genus Zygosaccharomyces

Some researchers consider *Zygosaccharomyces* a subgenus of *Saccharomyces*. These yeasts are osmophilic and grow in high sugar concentrations, causing spoilage in honey, syrups, molasses, and in the fermentation of soy sauce and certain wines. *Z. nussbaumeri* is known for growing in honey.

Genus Debaryomyces

These round or oval yeasts form pellicles on meat brines, with ascospores having a warty surface. *D. kloeckeri* is commonly found on cheese and sausage.

Genus *Pichia*

These yeasts are oval to cylindrical and may form pseudomycelia. Ascospores are typically round or hat-shaped, with one to four per ascus. *P. membranaefaciens* forms a pellicle on liquids like beer or wine.

Genus *Hansenula*

Similar in appearance to *Pichia,* these yeasts are more fermentative, although some species form pellicles. Ascospores are typically hat- or Saturn-shaped.

Genus *Hanseniaspora*

These lemon-shaped (apiculate) yeasts are commonly found in fruit juices. *Nadsonia* yeasts are large and lemon-shaped as well.

FALSE YEASTS (FUNGI IMPERFECTI)

Genus *Torulopsis*

Torulopsis yeasts are round to oval and characterized by multilateral budding. These fermentative yeasts can cause issues in breweries and spoil various foods. T. sphaerica ferments lactose and may spoil dairy products, while other species can spoil sweetened condensed milk, fruit juice concentrates, and acidic foods.

Genus *Candida*

Candida yeasts form pseudohyphae or true hyphae with abundant budding cells or blastospores, and some may produce chlamydospores. Many species form films and can spoil foods that are high in acid and salt. *C. utilis* is cultivated for use in food and feed, while *C. krusei* is used with dairy starter cultures to maintain activity and prolong the lifespan of lactic acid bacteria. *C. lipolytica,* a lipolytic species, can spoil butter and oleomargarine.

Genus *Kloeckera*

Kloeckera yeasts are imperfect, apiculate, or lemon-shaped. *K. apiculata* is commonly found on fruits, flowers, and in soil.

Genus *Trichosporon*

Trichosporon yeasts bud and form arthrospores, growing best at low temperatures. They are typically found in breweries and on chilled beef, with *T. pullulans* being a common species.

Genus *Brettanomyces*

Brettanomyces yeasts are typically ogive- or arch-shaped and produce high amounts of acid. They play a role in the late fermentation of Belgian lambic beer and English beers and are also found in French wines. Common species include *B. bruxellensis* and *B. lambicus.*

Genus *Rhodotorula*

Rhodotorula yeasts are red, pink, or yellow and may cause discoloration on foods, such as colored spots on meats or pink areas in sauerkraut.

Groups of Yeasts

Film yeasts, including those in the genera *Pichia, Hansenula, Debaryomyces, Candida,* and *Trichosporon,* thrive on the surfaces of acidic foods like sauerkraut and pickles. They oxidize organic acids, facilitating the growth of less acid-tolerant organisms that contribute to spoilage. *Hansenula* and *Pichia* can withstand high alcohol levels, potentially oxidizing alcohol in beverages. *Pichia* species are often encouraged to grow on Jerez and Arbois wines, where they are believed to contribute unique flavors and esters.

Debaryomyces is highly tolerant to salt and can grow on cheese brines containing up to 24 percent salt. These film yeasts generally produce little or no alcohol from sugars.Yeasts with apiculate or lemon-shaped cells, such as *Saccharomyces, Hanseniaspora, Nadsonia,* and *Kloeckera,* are considered undesirable in wine fermentation due to their tendency to produce off-flavors, low alcohol yields, and highly volatile acids.

Osmophilic yeasts, including *Saccharomyces rouxii* and *S. mellis,* thrive in environments with high osmotic pressure, such as those containing high concentrations of sugars, salts, or other solutes. These yeasts are responsible for spoilage in products like dried fruits, concentrated fruit juices, honey, maple syrup, and other sugary solutions.

Salt-tolerant yeasts can be found in curing brines, salted meats and fish, soy sauce, miso paste, and tamari sauce. Among the most salt-tolerant film yeasts are species of *Debaryomyces,* which grow in curing brines and on salted meats and cucumbers, as well as *Saccharomyces rouxii,* which can form films on brine. Other genera, such as *Torulopsis, Brettanomyces,* and others, also grow in brines. *Saccharomyces rouxii* plays a significant role in alcohol and flavor production in soy sauce, though species of *Torulopsis, Pichia, Candida,* and *Trichosporon* may also be present. Both *S. rouxii* and *Pichia* are sometimes involved in soy sauce spoilage. Similarly, yeasts are involved in miso production, with the specific types varying based on salt concentrations ranging from 7 to 20 percent.

BACTERIA

Although deterministic bacteriology (the classification and identification of bacteria) is beyond the scope of this book and should be discussed in other textbooks, some of the morphological, cultural, and physiological characteristics of bacteria will be briefly mentioned because of their relevance to the preservation or potency of food.

Morphological Characteristics in Food Bacteriology

One of the first steps in the identification of bacteria in a food is microscopic examination to ascertain the shape, size, aggregation, structure, and staining reactions of the bacteria present. The following characteristics may be of special significance.

Encapsulation

The presence of capsules or slime may account for sliminess or ropiness of a food. In addition, capsules serve to increase the resistance of bacteria to adverse conditions, such as heat or chemicals. To the organism they may serve as a source of reserved nutrients. Most capsules are polysaccharides of dextrin, dextran, or levan.

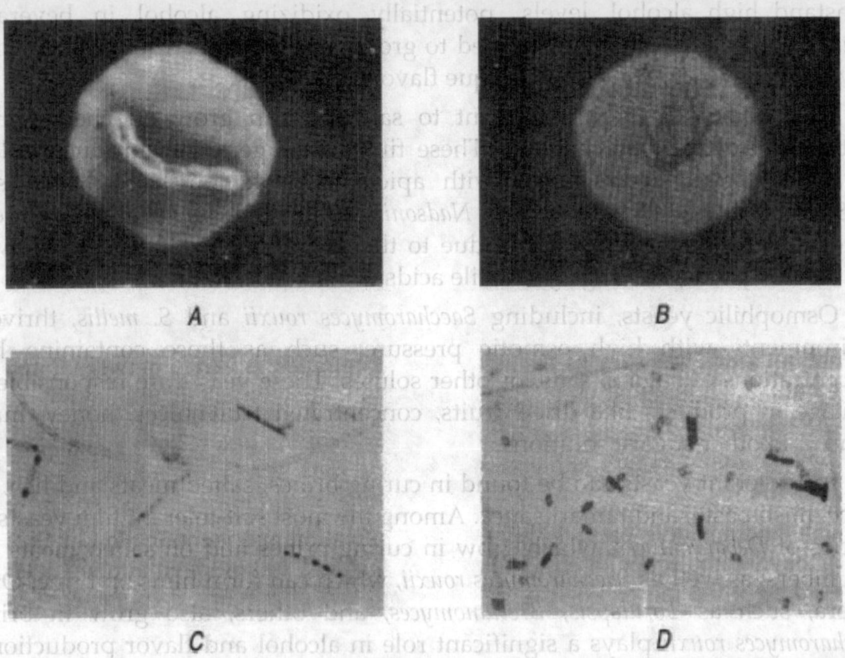

Fig. 2.28. Bacterial structures: (A) capsules, (B)flagella, (C) granules in *Lactobacillus bulgaricus, (D) spores of *Bacillus subtilis*. (Courtesy of P. R. Elliker).**

Formation of Endospores

Bacteria of the genera *Bacillus, Clostridium, Desulfotomaculum, Sporolactobacillus* (rods), and *Sporosarcina* (cocci) share the ability to form endospores . Spore-forming species of the genera *Bacillus* (aerobes and some facultative anaerobes) and *Clostridium* (anaerobes) are of particular interest to the food microbiologist. Endospores form in an intracellular zone, are highly refractive, and are resistant to heat, ultraviolet light, and desiccation. Lysis of vegetative cells releases free endospores, which can lie dormant without detectable metabolism for years. The complete cycle of the vegetative cell, from sporulation to free spore, through eventual prolonged dormancy, to germination and growth of the spore within the vegetative cell, is extremely complex.

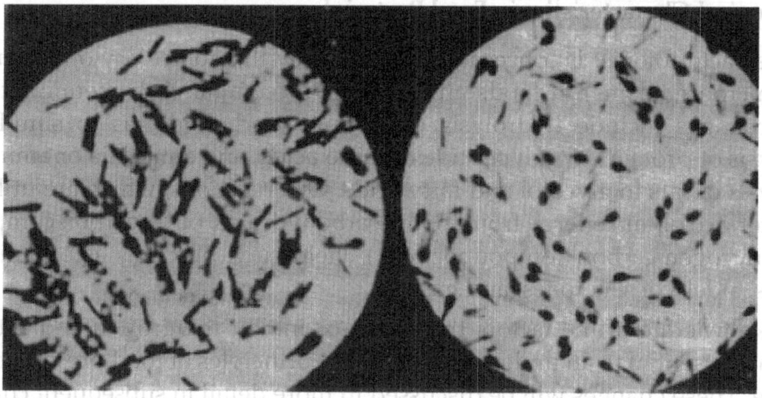

Fig. 2.29. Photomicrograph showing terminal endospores in a rod. The spores are clear in the left-hand field and stained in the right-hand field (X1300).

Sporulation usually occurs at the end of the log phase of growth, possibly due to nutrient depletion or product accumulation. During this transition from vegetative cell to spore, the spore becomes refractory, there is a massive uptake of Ca^{2+} ions, and the synthesis of dipicolinic acid (DPA), a compound absent in vegetative cells, occurs. The acquisition of heat resistance by the forming spore is closely linked to the formation of DPA and the uptake of Ca^{2+}.

Germination is generally favored under conditions favorable to the growth of vegetative cells, but it can occur under conditions that do not allow such growth, e.g. , at low temperatures. It is caused by mixtures of amino acids, Mg^{2+} and Mn^{2+} ions, glucose, dipicolinic acid plus Ca^{2+} ions, and heat shock or thermal activation, which activates dormant enzymes. The optimum temperature and duration of heat shock depend on the type of spore, with heat treatment being more important for thermophilic spores, for example, than for mesophiles. Germination is inhibited by sorbic acid at acidic pH, by certain divalent cations, by starch, and by oleic and linoleic acids.

Spore "dormancy" is defined as delayed germination (and growth) under apparently favorable conditions. The spores do not germinate, possibly due to unfavorable conditions such as inhibitors in the environment or a lack of essential nutrients, such as amino acids. Some spores may germinate but not grow, and some may have been damaged by heat, radiation, or other agents, so they require a more complex or specialized growth environment than their ancestors. For example, delayed spore germination of days to months has been reported. eg., dormancy from a few days to 3 or 4 months with *Bacillus megaterium* spores and from 15 days to 72 months with *Clostridium botulinum* spores.

Formation of Cell Aggregates

It is characteristic of some bacteria to form long chains and of others to clump under certain conditions. It is more difficul to kill all bacteria in intertwined chains or sizable clumps than to destroy separate cells.

Physiological Characteristics in Food Bacteriology

The bacteriologist is concerned with the growth and activity of bacteria (and other microorganisms) in foods and with the accompanying chemical changes. These changes include hydrolysis of complex carbohydrates to simple ones; hydrolysis of proteins to polypeptides, amino acids, and ammonia or amines; and hydrolysis of fats to glycerol and fatty acids. O-R reactions, which are utilized by the bacteria to obtain energy from foods (carbohydrates, other carbon compounds, simple nitrogen-carbon compounds, etc.), yield such products as organic acids, alcohols, aldehydes, ketones, and gases.

A knowledge of the factors that favor or inhibit the growth and activity of bacteria is essential to an understanding of the principles of food preservation and spoilage. These changes will be discussed in more detail in subsequent chapters.

Cultural Characteristics in Food Bacteriology

Bacterial growth in and on foods often is extensive enough to make the food unattracti e in appearance or otherwise objectionable. Pigmented bacteria cause discolorations on the surfaces of foods films may cover the surfaces of liquids; growth may make surfaces slimy; or growth throughout the liquids may result in undesirable cloudiness or sediment.

Genera of Bacteria Important in Food Bacteriology

This discussion focuses on bacterial genera important in food, highlighting their characteristics without delving deeply into classification and identification. Classification follows the system presented in Bergey's Manual of Systematic Bacteriology (vols. I and II, 1984 and 1986). Obsolete names are marked with an asterisk and discussed in the appendix.

Genus *Acetobacter*

Acetobacter species oxidize ethyl alcohol into acetic acid. They are rod-shaped, motile, and commonly found on fruits, vegetables, souring fruits, and alcoholic beverages. These bacteria are a significant spoilage concern in alcoholic drinks.

Genus *Aeromonas*

Aeromonas consists of gram-negative rods that thrive at an optimum temperature of 22 to 28°C. They are facultative anaerobes and can tolerate cold temperatures. Frequently isolated from aquatic environments, *A. hydrophila* is pathogenic to humans as well as to fish, frogs, and other mammals.

Genus *Alcaligenes*

Alcaligenes bacteria typically produce an alkaline reaction in their growth medium. *A. viscolactis* causes ropiness in milk, while *A. metalcaligenes* leads to slimy growth on cottage cheese. These bacteria are commonly found in manure, feeds, soil, water, and dust. Some species were formerly classified under the genus *Achromobacter*.

Genus *Bacillus*

Bacillus species are aerobic to facultative anaerobic, forming endospores that do not swell the rods in which they are formed. The genus includes both mesophilic and thermophilic species, with some being proteolytic or nonproteolytic. *B. subtilis* spores are less heat-resistant compared to those of thermophilic species like B. *stearothermophilus*. *Bacillus* species can cause spoilage and are significant in food testing for sterilization methods.

Genus *Brevibacterium*

Brevibacterium linens is important in the surface smear of certain cheeses, such as Limburger or brick cheese, where it contributes to the characteristic orange-red pigmentation and aids in the ripening process.

Genus *Brochotrix*

Brochotrix species are gram-positive rods that form long, filamentous chains, often knotted. They thrive at 20 to 25°C and can grow at a range of pH values and in the presence of NaCl. They are responsible for spoilage in refrigerated meats and meat products stored aerobically or vacuum-packed.

Genus *Alteromonas*

This genus includes several species previously classified under *Pseudomonas*. *Alteromonas* species are marine organisms, potentially important in seafood spoilage.

Genus *Arthrobacter*

Predominantly a soil organism, *Arthrobacter* is generally inert in foods. However, some species can grow at 5°C, classifying them as psychrotrophs.

Genus *Campylobacter*

Originally classified under *Vibrio, Campylobacter* species are oxidase-positive, catalase-positive, gram-negative, and exhibit a curved, spiral shape. These bacteria prefer reduced oxygen conditions. *C. fetus* subsp. *jejuni* is a major cause of gastroenteritis in humans.

Genus *Clostridium*

Clostridium species are anaerobic or microaerophilic bacteria that often cause food spoilage due to their fermentation of carbohydrates, producing acids and gases. *C. perfringens* and other species can disrupt curds in milk, while species like *C. butyricum* cause late gas in cured cheese. Soil is a primary source of these bacteria.

Genus *Corynebacterium*

Corynebacterium includes C. *diphtheriae*, which can be transported by foods. C. bovis is a commensal organism found on the cow's udder and may contribute to bovine mastitis.

Genus *Desulfotomaculum*

Desulfotomaculum species are gram-negative rods that swell when they form endospores. These bacteria are found in soil, fresh water, and the rumen. They reduce sulfur compounds to hydrogen sulfide, contributing to spoilage in canned foods (e.g., *C. nigrificans* now classified as *D. nigrificans*).

Genus *Erwinia*

Erwinia species are plant pathogens causing necrosis, galls, and soft rots in vegetables and fruits. *E. carotovora* is associated with bacterial soft rot in various plants.

Genus *Escherichia*

Escherichia species, primarily found in the intestinal tracts of warm-blooded animals, are part of the coliform group. Some strains, like *E. coli*, can be pathogenic to humans.

Genus *Enterobacter*

Previously classified as *Aerobacter, Enterobacter* species are part of the coliform group and are widely distributed in nature.

Genus *Flavobacterium*

Species of *Flavobacterium* are yellow- to orange-pigmented and can cause spoilage in meats, shellfish, poultry, eggs, butter, and milk. Some species are psychrotrophic and can grow on thawing vegetables.

Genus *Gluconobacter* (formerly *Acetomonas*)

Gluconobacter species oxidize ethanol to acetic acid. *G. oxydans* can cause ropiness in beer through viscous growth.

Genus *Halobacterium*

Halobacterium species are obligate halophiles, commonly found in high-salt environments such as salted fish. They can cause discolorations in foods high in salt. Several bacteria previously classified under Flavobacterium are now included in this genus.

Genus *Klebsiella*

Many *Klebsiella* species are capsulated and typically found in the respiratory and intestinal tracts of humans. *K. pneumoniae* is a causative organism for bacterial pneumonia in humans.

Family *Lactobacillaceae* - Genus *Lactobacillus*

Lactobacillus species are rods that form chains and are microaerophilic or anaerobic. They ferment sugars primarily into lactic acid, and can be either homofermentative or heterofermentative. Species like *L. bulgaricus* and *L.*

helveticus are important in the dairy industry, as they help ferment lactose into lactic acid. *Lactobacillus* is primarily found on plant surfaces, in manure, and in dairy products.

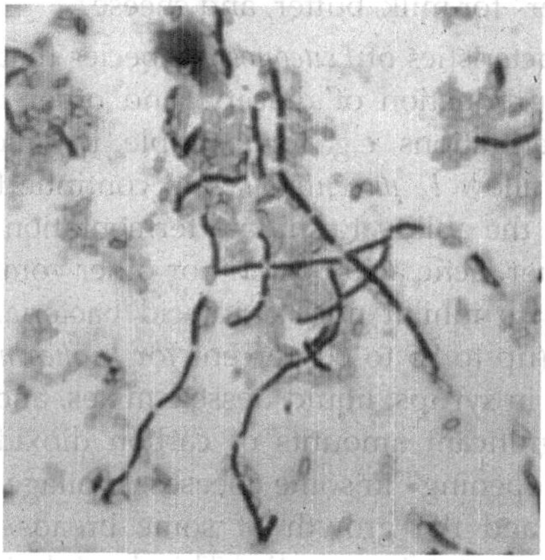

Fig. 2.30. Photomicrograph of Gram- stained *Lactobacillus bulgaricus*.

Characteristics that make the lactobacilli important in foods are as follows:

- Their ability to ferment sugars with the production of considerable amounts of lactic acid, making it possible to use them in the production of fermented plant and dairy products or the manufacture of industrial lactic acid but resulting in the deterioration of some products, e.g., wine or beer,
- Production of gas and other volatile products by heteroferenative species, sometimes with damage to the quality of food, as with L. fermentum growing in Swiss cheese or *L. hilgardii* or *L. trichodes** in wines,
- Their inability to synthesize most of the vitamins they require, making them unable to grow well in foods poor in vitamins but useful in assays for the vitamin content of foods, and
- The heat resistance, or thermoduric properties, of most of the high-temperature lactobacilli, enabling them to survive pasteurization or other heating processes, such as that given the curd in the manufacture of Swiss and similar cheeses.

Species of *Lactobacillus* different from the ones already mentioned have been found growing in refrigerated meats, but only a few names for these lactobacilli have been suggested, e.g., *L. viridescens* for one causing greening of sausage and *L. salinmandus** for one growing in sausage. These lactobacilli are exceptional because of their ability to grow at low temperatures.

Genus *Leuconostoc*

This genus, named *Betacoccus* by Orla-Jensen, contains heterofermentative lactic streptococci, which ferment sugar to lactic acid, as well as considerable amounts of acetic acid, ethyl alcohol, and carbon dioxide. The ability of *L.*

*dextranicum** and *L. cremoris** to ferment citric acid from milk and produce the desired flavoring substance diacetyl (the lesser acetoin and 2,3-butanediol are also produced) and to stimulate lactic streptococci has led to their involvement as the so-called "Lactic starter" for milk, butter, and cheese.

Some of the characteristics of *Leuconostoc* species that make them important in foods are (1) the production of diacetyl and other flavoring products, (2) tolerance to salt concentrations, e.g. for example, in sauerkraut and dill pickle fermentations, which allow *L. mesenteroides* to continue the early part of lactic acid fermentation, (3) the ability to initiate fermentation in vegetable products more rapidly than other lactic acid bacteria or other competing bacteria. and to produce enough acid to inhibit non-lactic acid bacteria, (4) tolerance to high sugar concentrations (up to 55 to 60 percent for *L. mesenteroides)*, which allows the organism to grow in syrups, liquid dessert mixes, and ice creams, etc. . ., (5) the production of significant amounts of carbon dioxide from sugars, which leads to undesirable "opening" in some cheeses, spoilage of foods rich in sugars (syrups, mixes, etc.) and the growth of some breads, (6) significant sludge production in sucrose-containing media. This is a desirable characteristic for dextran production, but a hazard in sucrose-rich materials such as in the production of sucrose from sugar cane or beet.

The habitat of this genus is the surface of plants.

Genus *Listeria*

These bacteria are gram-positive, non-spore-forming rods with tumbling motility. L. monocytogenes can cause food-borne disease outbreaks (Chapter 24)

Genus *Microbacterium*

Bacteria of this genus are important because of their resistance to adverse conditions and their use in production of vitamins. They are small, nonmotile, gram-positive, asporogenous, catalase-positive, aerobic, homofermentative, lactic acid-producing rods, which sometimes produce palisade arrangements. *M. lacticum* is the species usually encountered. Microbacteria are very resistant to heat for non-spore-forming bacteria, surviving pasteurization of milk readily and even temperatures of 80 to 85°C for 10 min. They therefore are among the thermodurics that give high counts in pasteurized dairy products, such as market milk and dry milk. Their range of temperature for growth is 15 to 35°C, and their optimum is about 30°C. Therefore, in plating for these organisms, incubation of plates should be at below 35 °C, preferably at about 30°C.

Genus *Micrococcus*

Micrococci are spherical bacteria that form irregular clusters, tetrads, or packets. They are typically gram-positive, aerobic, and catalase-positive. These bacteria thrive at temperatures around 25 to 30°C and grow well on standard laboratory media. However, their characteristics can vary significantly between species. Some key traits that make micrococci relevant in food production include:

- Salt tolerance, enabling growth in meat-curing brines and brine tanks.
- Thermoduric nature, allowing survival of pasteurization processes, as seen with *M. varians*.
- Pigmentation, with species like *M. luteus* producing yellow and *M. roseus* producing pink colors.
- Utilization of ammonium salts or other simple nitrogenous compounds for nitrogen.
- Fermentation of sugars to produce moderate amounts of acid.
- Some species are acid-proteolytic, such as *M. freudenreichii*.
- Ability to grow in cooler temperatures, such as around 10 °C or lower.
- Micrococci are widespread in nature and commonly found in dust, water, and on poorly sanitized food utensils and equipment.

Genus *Mycobacterium*

Mycobacterium tuberculosis, the causative agent of tuberculosis, can be spread through contaminated foods, particularly raw milk from infected cows.

Genus *Pediococcus*

Pediococcus are gram-positive, catalase-negative, and microaerophilic cocci that occur singly, in pairs, or in short chains. These bacteria are homofermentative, primarily producing lactic acid from sugars, and are capable of growing in salt brines up to 5.5%. Their optimal temperature range is 25 to 32°C, although they can grow between 7 and 45°C.

Key traits include:

- Salt tolerance, acid production, and the ability to thrive in cool temperatures.
- Involvement in the fermentation of brined vegetables and spoilage of alcoholic beverages such as beer, where *P. damnosus* can cause off-flavo like diacetyl.
- *P. cerevisiae* has been used as a starter culture in fermented sausages.

Genus *Photobacterium*

This genus consists of coccobacilli and occasional rods, some of which are luminescent. *Photobacterium phosphoreum* is known to cause phosphorescence in meats and fish.

Genus *Propionibacterium*

Propionibacteria are small, nonmotile, gram-positive rods, often coccoid, that are catalase-positive and anaerobic to aerotolerant. These bacteria ferment lactic acid, carbohydrates, and polyalcohols to produce propionic and acetic acids and carbon dioxide.

In Swiss cheese, *Propionibacterium freudenreichii* ferments lactates, contributing to gas formation that creates holes in the cheese and adds to its flavor. Pigmented propionibacteria can also cause color defects in cheese.

Genus *Pseudomonas*

Pseudomonas species are gram-negative, motile, asporogenous rods that can cause food spoilage. They are characterized by their ability to utilize a wide variety of noncarbohydrate carbon compounds and produce a range of products that negatively affect food flavo

Genus *Proteus*

Species of *Proteus* are involved in the spoilage of meats, seafood, and eggs. Their presence in large numbers in unrefrigerated foods raises concerns about their role in food poisoning.

Notable traits include:

- Ability to grow in low temperatures (refrigeration).
- Production of various pigments, including greenish fluorescence from *P. fluorescens* and Various colors from other species.
- Resistance to many disinfectants and sanitizers.
- Some species can grow in low moisture environments, but they are limited by a high aw (0.97 to 0.98).

Genus *Salmonella*

Salmonella species are enteric pathogens that can grow in foods and cause food infections. They are typically transmitted via contaminated food.

Genus *Serratia*

Serratia species, such as *S. marcescens*, produce a pink or magenta pigment and are responsible for red discoloration on food surfaces.

Genus Shigella

Shigella species cause bacillary dysentery and can be transported by foods, posing a risk for foodborne illness.

Genus *Sporolactobacillus*

Lactobacillus inulinus has been reclassified as *Sporolactobacillus inulinus* due to its ability to form endospores, though it shares many characteristics with *Lactobacillus* species.

Genus *Sporosarcina*

Sporsarcina are gram-positive cocci that form endospores. Notable species include *S. ureae* and *S. halophila*.

Genus *Staphylococcus*

Staphylococcus species, such as *S. aureus*, grow in irregular, grapelike clusters and can produce enterotoxins that lead to food poisoning.

Key traits of *S. aureus* include:

- Facultative anaerobic growth.
- Production of yellow to orange colonies, though some may be white.
- Beta-hemolytic and coagulase-positive strains are pathogenic.

Genus *Streptococcus*

Streptococci are characterized by their growth in pairs or chains. They are classified into four groups based on serology-pyogenic, viridans, lactic, and enterococcus.

The **pyogenic group** includes *S. agalactiae,* causing mastitis in cows, and *S. pyogenes,* responsible for infections like septic sore throat and scarlet fever.

The **viridans group** includes *S. thermophilus,* which is important in cheese making and fermented milks like yogurt, and *S. bovis,* found in cow manure and saliva. These species are thermoduric, capable of surviving pasteurization, and grow at 45°C but not at 10°C.

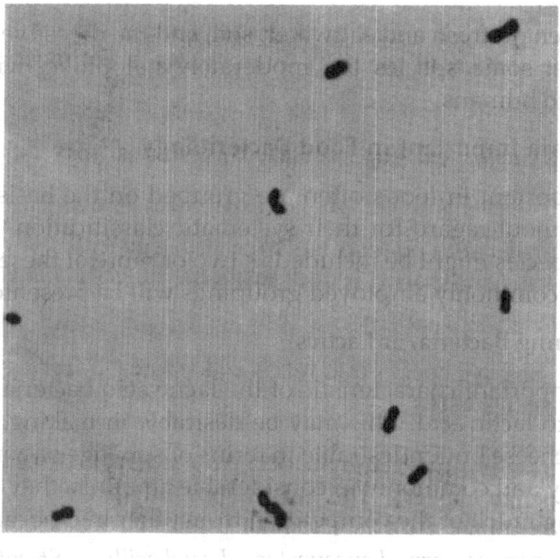

Fig. 2.31. Photomicrograph of *Streptococcus lactis (*1000).**

The **lactic group** includes significant dairy bacteria like *Streptococcus lactis* and *S. cremoris,* which thrive at 10°C but not at 45°C. These bacteria are utilized as starters in cheese, cultured buttermilk, and certain butter varieties, often alongside *Leuconostoc* species. *S. lactis* also plays a role in raw milk souring. These bacteria tolerate only 2–4% salt, making them unsuitable for the lactic fermentation of brined vegetables. Common sources include green plants, feeds, silage, and utensils.

The **enterococcus group** comprises *S. faecalis, S. faecium,* and related subspecies. While *S. faecalis* is more heat-resistant and typically human-derived, *S. faecium* is associated more with plants. Subspecies include *S. faecalis* subsp.

liquefaciens, which is acid-proteolytic, and *S. faecalis* subsp. *zymogenes*, which is beta-hemolytic. These bacteria, commonly found in raw foods, grow at both 10°C and 45° and exhibit unique features: they are thermoduric, tolerate up to 6.5% salt, grow at an alkaline pH of 9.6, and thrive across a wide temperature range (5–50°C). *S. faecalis* has been isolated from foods like bacon and often serves as an indicator of fecal contamination or plant sanitation due to its intestinal origin in humans and animals. Frequently isolated enterococci include *S. faecalis* and *S. faecium*, along with other Lancefield group D streptococci such as *S. bovis* and *S. avium*.

Genus *Yersinia*

Yersinia is found in soil, this genus includes *Y. pestis*, responsible for the plague, and *Y. enterocolitica*, which can cause foodborne illnesses. Formerly classified under *Pasteurella*, they now belong to the Enterobacteriaceae family due to their similarity to *Salmonella*.

Genus *Streptomyces*

These organisms can impart undesirable musty or earthy flavors to foods. They are aerobic bacteria that form branching filaments and chains of spores.

Genus *Vibrio*

Widely present in fresh and saltwater, soil, and the digestive tracts of humans and animals, some species are moderately halophilic, with certain types pathogenic to humans.

Groups of Bacteria Important in Food Bacteriology

Bacteria important in foods often are grouped on the basis of one common characteristic without regard for their systematic classification. It is obvious that some bacterial species might be included in two or more of these artificial groups. Examples of the commonly employed groupings will be presented.

Lactic Acid-Forming Bacteria, or Lactics

The most important characteristic of the lactic acid bacteria is their ability to ferment sugars to lactic acid. This may be desirable in making products such as sauerkraut and cheese but undesirable in terms of spoilage of wines. Because they form acid rapidly and commonly in considerable amounts, they usually eliminate for the time being much of the competition from other microorganisms.

The major genera are *Leuconostoc, Lactobacillus, Streptococcus,* and *Pediococcus*.

Acetic Acid-Forming Bacteria, orAcetics

Most acetic acid bacteria today belong to one of two genera, *Acetobacter* and *Gluconobacter*. Both oxidize ethyl alcohol to acetic acid, but *Acetobacter* is capable of oxidizing acetic acid to carbon dioxide. The characteristics that make acetic acid bacteria important are: (1) their ability to oxidize ethanol to acetic acid, which makes them useful in the production of vinegar and harmful in alcoholic beverages, (2) their strong oxidizing power, which can cause the oxidation of the desired product, acetic acid, by unwanted species or by desired species under unfavorable conditions; this oxidizing power can be useful, as in the oxidation of

D-sorbitol to L-sorbose in the preparation of ascorbic acid by synthetic methods, and (3) the excessive viscosity of some species, for example vinegar generators.

Butyric Acid-Forming Bacteria, orButyrics

Most bacteria of this group are spore-forming anaerobes of the genus *Clostridium.*

Propionic Acid-Forming Bacteria, or Propionics

Most bacteria of this group are in the genus *Propionibacterium,* although propionic cocci have been reported.

Proteolytic Bacteria

Proteolytic bacteria are a diverse group known for producing extracellular proteinases, enzymes that break down proteins outside the cell. While all bacteria have intracellular proteinases, only a few species release them extracellularly. These bacteria can be classified based on their oxygen requirements and spore-forming abilities-aerobic or facultative spore-formers, non-spore-formers, and anaerobic spore-formers. For example, *Bacillus cereus* is an aerobic, spore-forming proteolytic bacterium, while *Pseudomonas fluorescens* is non-spore-forming and facultative. *Clostridium sporogenes,* on the other hand, is an anaerobic spore-former.

Many species of *Clostridium, Bacillus, Pseudomonas,* and *Proteus* exhibit proteolytic activity. Some bacteria, known as "acid-proteolytic," can simultaneously ferment acids and hydrolyze proteins, such as *Streptococcus faecalis* var. *liquefaciens* and *Micrococcus caseolyticus.* Certain proteolytic bacteria are putrefactive, decomposing proteins anaerobically to produce unpleasant compounds like hydrogen sulfide, amines, and fatty acids. This characteristic is common in most proteolytic *Clostridium* species, as well as in some *Proteus* and *Pseudomonas* species. Additionally, some *Pseudomonas* strains produce heat-resistant proteinases that can survive ultrahigh temperature treatments.

Lipolytic Bacteria

Lipolytic bacteria produce lipase enzymes, which catalyze the breakdown of fats into fatty acids and glycerol. Many actively proteolytic bacteria are also lipolytic; for instance, *Pseudomonas fluorescens* is both strongly proteolytic and lipolytic. Lipolytic species are found in genera such as *Pseudomonas, Alcaligenes, Staphylococcus, Serratia,* and *Micrococcus.* Many microbial lipases are resistant to processing, so the absence of viable lipolytic bacteria in spoiled food does not guarantee the absence of microbial lipase activity.

Saccharolytic Bacteria

Saccharolytic bacteria hydrolyze complex carbohydrates like disaccharides and polysaccharides into simpler sugars. A subset of these bacteria, known as amylolytic, possess amylase enzymes that hydrolyze starch outside the cell, such as *Bacillus subtilis* and *Clostridium butyricum.* Only a few bacteria can break down cellulose.

Some *Clostridium* species are categorized as either proteolytic (breaking down proteins but not sugars) or saccharolytic (fermenting sugars but not proteins). For instance, *Clostridium lentoputrescens* is proteolytic and typically does not ferment carbohydrates, while *C. butyricum* is nonproteolytic but ferments sugars.

Pectinolytic Bacteria

Pectinolytic bacteria produce enzymes called pectinases that break down pectin, a carbohydrate responsible for the structural rigidity of plant cell walls. These enzymes contribute to the softening of plant tissues and the loss of gelling properties in foods. Pectinolytic species are found in genera such as *Erwinia, Bacillus, Clostridium, Achromobacter, Aeromonas, Arthrobacter,* and *Flavobacterium*. Certain molds also exhibit pectinolytic activity.

Thermophilic Bacteria

Thermophilic bacteria, or thermophiles, thrive at temperatures above 45°C, with optimal growth typically occurring at 55°C or higher. These bacteria are significant in foods stored at elevated temperatures. For instance, *Bacillus stearothermophilus* causes thermophilic flat sour spoilage in low-acid canned foods, while gaseous spoilage in canned goods can result from the growth of *Clostridium thermosaccharolyticum*.

Thermoduric Bacteria

Thermoduric bacteria are generally defined as those that can survive heat treatment such as pasteurization. Species of *Bacillus, Micrococcus**, and Enterococci can survive pasteurization of liquid eggs. Bacteria of the genera *Clostridium, Bacillus, Micrococcus, Streptococcus, Lactobacillus,* and *Microbacterium* are commonly found in foods. Occasionally, molds such as *Byssochlamys fulva* and also *Aspergillus* and *Penicillium* are thermosets. Some thermoregulatory bacteria, such as *Bacillus* and Enterococci, may also be psychrotrophic . In milk, where higher pasteurization and longer cooling times are important, these heat-resistant or thermoduric psychrotrophs can often be found.

Psychrotrophic Bacteria, or Psychrotrophs

These bacteria are able to grow at commercial refrigeration temperatures. Unlike psychrophiles, psychrotrophs do not have their optimal temperature for growth at refrigeration temperatures; rather, their optimum is usually between 25°C and 30°C. Most of the bacteria responsible for the loss of quality in nonsterile refrigerated foods, excluding seafoods, are psychrotrops. Psychrotrophic bacteria are found chiefly in the genera *Pseudomonas, Flavobacterium, Achromobacter,* and *Alcaligenes,* although *Micrococcus, Lactobacillus, Enterobacter, Arthrobacter,* and other genera may contain psychrotrophic species. Additionally, various yeasts and molds are able to grow at refrigeration temperatures.

Halophilic Bacteria, or Halophiles

Truly halophilic bacteria require certain minimum concentrations of dissolved sodium chloride to grow. These bacteria, including *Pseudomonas,*

Moraxella, Flavobacterium, Acinetobacter, and *Vibrio* species, which grow best in media containing 0.5 to 3.0% salt, are considered mildly halophilic. These microorganisms have been isolated from many species of fish and crustaceans. Bacteria isolated from foods such as salted fish, salted meat, and some salted vegetables and that grow best in environments containing 3.0 to 15% salt are called moderate halophiles. These bacteria are found in the genera *Bacillus, Micrococcus, Vibrio, Acinetobacter,* and *Moraxella.*

Sometimes in very salty foods, containing 15-30% salt, extreme halophiles such as *Halobacterium* and *Halococcus* species can be isolated. They are often also pigmented pink or red. Other bacteria are salt-tolerant, meaning that halotolerant bacteria can grow with or without salt. They are usually able to grow in foods containing 5.0% salt or more; these include several types of *Bacillus, Micrococcus, Corynebacterium, Streptococcus,* and *Clostridium.* Other important halophilic or halotolerant bacteria in foods are found in the genera *Sarcina, Pseudomonas, Pediococcus* and *Alcaligenes.*

Osmophilic or Saccharophilic Bacteria

The most frequently encountered osmophilic microorganisms in foods are various species of yeasts. Osmophilic bacteria are those which grow in high concentrations of sugar; however, most bacteria called osmophiles are merely sugar-tolerant, e.g., species of *Leuconostoc.*

Slime- or Rope-Forming Bacteria

Examples of these bacteria have already been given: *Alcaligenes viscolactis**, *Enterobacter aerogenes* and *Klebsiella oxytoca,* responsible for the viscosity of milk, and Leuconostoc spp., responsible for the formation of mucus in sucrose solutions and the viscous growth of various bacteria present in food. . Some species of *Streptococcus* and *Lactobacillus* have varieties that make milk foamy or thick. A micrococci makes meat curing solutions sticky.

Lactobacillus plantarum and other strains of lactobacilli can cause the viscosity of fruits, vegetables and various grain products, for example. for example in cider, sauerkraut and beer. Various species of *Bacillus* are responsible for the firm consistency of bread.

Gas-Forming Bacteria

Certain bacteria produce gas in such small quantities and at such a slow rate that it often goes undetected. This is sometimes the case with heterofermentative lactic acid bacteria, though gas production may be noticeable under different conditions. Genera that include gas-producing bacteria include *Leuconostoc, Lactobacillus* (heterofermentative), *Propionibacterium, Escherichia, Enterobacter, Proteus, Bacillus* (aerobic species), and *Clostridium.* Bacteria from the first three genera produce only carbon dioxide, while those from the latter genera produce both carbon dioxide and hydrogen.

Pigmented Bacteria

The colors produced by pigmented bacteria growing in or on foods span the entire visible spectrum and include both black and white. There will be many examples in a later discussion of food spoilage. All species in some genera are pigmented, such as *Flavobacterium* (yellow to orange) and *Serratia* (red). Pigmented species are found in many genera; many species of *Micrococcus* are pigmented, for example. In addition, pigmented varieties exist within some species, for example. for example, *Lactobacillus plantarum* is a rust-colored bacteria that discolors cheese. *Halobacterium* species are pigmented pink, red, or red-orange. *Halococcus* species are pigmented red or red-orange.

Coliform and Fecal Coliform Group

Coliforms are small rods defined as aerobic and facultative anaerobic, gram-negative, non-sporulating bacteria that ferment lactose with gas formation. The main types of coliform bacteria are *Escherichia coli* and *Enterobacter aerogenes*; however, up to twenty species can meet these criteria, including species of other *Enterobacteriaceae* and even species of *Aeromonas*. The group of fecal coliforms includes coliforms capable of growing at high temperatures (44.5 or 45°C). The original purpose of the high-temperature incubation tests was to differentiate coliforms of fecal origin from those of non-fecal origin. The designation "fecal coliform" or "coliform" is not taxonomically valid; rather, these terms refer to groups of bacteria that can grow under specific test conditions.

Procedures for coliform enumeration, fecal coliform enumeration, and even the enumeration of *E. coli* in foods are widely used and accepted as indicators. The use of "indicator" microorganisms began with the use of *E. coli* in water to replace the *Salmonella typhi* test. The concept is based on Shardingen's suggestion in 1892 that members of the species we now call *E. coli* should be used as an index or indicator of fecal contamination because they can be recovered with less difficulty than *Salmonella* species. Other groups of indicators or tests suggested or used include fecal streptococci or enterococci, enterobacteria, staphylococci (suggesting the possible presence of *S. aureus* enterotoxin or misuse) and the presence of *Geotrichum candidum*, the machine mold, as an indicator of the hygiene of contaminated plant and equipment.

Some of the characteristics that make coliform bacteria important in food spoilage are (1) their ability to grow well on a variety of substrates and to utilize a number of carbohydrates and other organic compounds as fuel for energy and a number of relatively simple nitrogen compounds. as a source of nitrogen, (2) its ability to synthesize most of the necessary vitamins, (3) the ability of the group to grow well over a fairly wide range of temperatures, from <10°C to about 46°C, (4) its ability to produce significant amounts of acid and gas from sugars,(5) its ability to cause off-flavors often described as "dirty" or "barnyard", and (6) the ability et E. aerogens to make foods viscous or stringy.

3 Food Contamination and Prevention

Food contamination occurs when harmful microorganisms, chemicals, or foreign substances are introduced into food, posing risks to health. Contamination can happen at any stage of food production, from harvesting and processing to storage, transportation, and preparation. The primary sources of contamination include bacteria, viruses, fungi, parasites, and toxic chemicals, all of which can cause foodborne illnesses.

Bacterial contamination is the most common form, with pathogens like *Salmonella, Escherichia coli,* and *Listeria* being major culprits. These microorganisms multiply quickly under favorable conditions, particularly in moist, warm environments. Viruses like norovirus and hepatitis A can also contaminate food, typically through contaminated water or improper handling. Fungal contamination, such as molds, can occur in food products like grains and fruits, leading to the production of mycotoxins, which are toxic compounds harmful to human health.

Prevention of food contamination begins with good hygiene practices throughout the food production chain. Proper handwashing, sanitization of equipment, and use of safe water are essential steps. In agriculture, maintaining cleanliness in fields and ensuring proper storage and transport conditions help reduce contamination risks. Additionally, controlling temperatures during food storage and cooking is critical, as many harmful microorganisms thrive in the danger zone (40°F to 140°F or 4°C to 60°C).

Food safety regulations, including Hazard Analysis and Critical Control Points (HACCP), are widely used in food industries to identify and control potential contamination points. Education and awareness campaigns also play a significant role in reducing foodborne illnesses, empowering consumers and food handlers to practice safe food handling techniques. Overall, a multi-faceted approach involving proper sanitation, temperature control, and regulatory oversight is essential to preventing food contamination and ensuring food safety.

Chemical contamination may occur through exposure to pesticides or industrial chemicals, while physical contamination typically results from accidents during packaging or food handling. Growing plants host a characteristic microbiota on their surfaces and can become contaminated by external sources. Similarly, animals possess a typical surface microbiota as well as an intestinal one, release microorganisms through excretions and secretions, and can also be contaminated from outside sources. Plants and animals suffering from parasitic diseases carry the pathogens responsible for those diseases. However, studies indicate that the inner, healthy tissues of plants and animals typically contain few or no living microorganisms.

Preventing food contamination is essential for ensuring food safety. This involves proper sanitation practices, such as washing hands and utensils, and cooking food to the right temperature to kill harmful pathogens. Food should also be stored at the correct temperature to prevent bacterial growth. Additionally, sourcing food from reputable suppliers and adhering to food safety regulations help reduce the risk of contamination.Education on food safety practices is crucial, especially in food industries and households, to mitigate contamination risks. Awareness campaigns, strict adherence to safety standards, and the use of modern technology like food sensors can further enhance food safety. Ensuring food is free from contamination is vital to protect public health and maintain food quality.

FROM GREEN PLANTS AND FRUITS

Green plants and fruits are susceptible to contamination by microorganisms, which can occur during growth, harvesting, processing, storage, or handling. Microbial contamination in plants and fruits typically involves bacteria, fungi, and viruses. Bacteria like *Salmonella* and *E. coli* can be introduced through contaminated soil, water, or handling practices. Fungi, such as molds and yeasts, thrive on fruits, leading to spoilage and the production of mycotoxins, which are harmful to human health.

To prevent contamination, it is essential to implement proper agricultural practices, including the use of clean water, avoiding the use of untreated manure, and practicing crop rotation to reduce the buildup of harmful microorganisms in the soil. During harvesting, care should be taken to minimize physical damage to fruits, as damaged areas are more susceptible to microbial invasion.

Post-harvest handling is critical in reducing contamination. Proper washing and sanitizing of fruits, along with maintaining the right temperature during storage and transportation, help inhibit microbial growth.

Additionally, consumers should wash fruits thoroughly before consumption, and ensure they are stored at appropriate temperatures to prevent contamination and spoilage. Effecti e food safety practices throughout the entire food supply chain are crucial for minimizing contamination risks from green plants and fruits..

FROM ANIMALS

Sources of microorganisms from animals include the surface flora, the flora of the respiratory tract, and the flora of the gastrointestinal tract. The natural surface flora of meat animals usually is not as important as the contaminating microorganisms from their intestinal or respiratory tracts. However, hides, hooves, and hair contain not only large numbers of microorganisms from soil, manure, feed, and water but also important kinds of spoilage organisms. Feathers and feet of poultry carry heavy contamination from similar sources. The skin of many meat animals may contain micrococci, staphylococci and beta-hemolytic streptococci. Staphylococci on the skin or from the respiratory tract may find their way onto the carcass and then to the final raw product. The feces and fecal-contaminated products of animals can contain many enteric organisms, including *Salmonella*. Salmonellosis in animals can result in contamination animal products or by-products and thus contaminate foods derived from them with *Salmonella*.

Table. Sources of Bacterial Contamination for a Selection of Bacteria:

Bacteria	Skin	Intestine	Feces	Other	Salt	Fresh	Soil	Foods
Acinetobacter	+	+	+	+		+	+	+
Aeromonas		+	+	+		+	+	+
Alcaligenes	+		+	+	+	+	+	+
Bacillus		+	+	+	+	+	+	+
Campylobacter	+	+	+	+	+	+	+	+
Clostridium	+	+	+	+	+	+		+
Enterobacter		+	+	+	+	+	+	+
Escherichia	+	+	+					
Lactobacillus	+	+	+	+	+	+		+
Listeria	+	+	+	+	+	+	+	+
Pseudomonas		+	+	+	+	+		+
Salmonella	+	+	+	+	+			+
Staphylococcus	+	+	+	+		+	+	+
Streptococcus	+	+	+	+	+			+
Vibrio	+	+	+	+		+		+

This table highlights where each bacteria might be found (Skin, Intestine, Feces, Other, Saltwater, Freshwater, Soil, and Foods). A "+" indicates presence in that particular source.

Pig or beef carcasses may harbor *Salmonella* bacteria, but due to subsequent processing and handling, only a small number of these bacteria cause human salmonellosis. In fact, meat from slaughtered animals is not often linked to human salmonellosis. In recent years, eggs and egg products have been identified as more common sources. The incidence of salmonellosis from eggs has decreased due to the pasteurization of egg products.

Various infectious disease agents from animals can be transmitted to humans through food, though this is just one of several possible transmission routes. Improvements in animal husbandry have significantly reduced or eliminated many of these diseases. A list of animal-derived infectious agents causing foodborne illnesses includes *Brucella, Mycobacterium tuberculosis, Coxiella, Listeria, Campylobacter*, beta-hemolytic streptococci, *Salmonella*, enteropathogenic *Escherichia coli*, parasites, and viruses.

Animals, ranging from the simplest to the most complex organisms, contribute their waste and, eventually, their bodies to the soil, water, and plants. While direct contamination of food plants from these sources has received little attention, it can occur, particularly in the case of coliform bacteria or enterococci. Insects and birds also play a role in contaminating fruits and vegetables by causing physical damage, introducing microorganisms, and creating conditions favorable for microbial spoilage.

FROM SOIL

The soil contains the greatest variety of microorganisms of any source of contamination. Whenever microbiologists search for new kinds of microorganisms or new strains for special purposes, they usually turn first to the soil. Not only numerous kinds of microorganisms but also large total numbers are present in fertile soils, ready to contaminate the surfaces of plants growing on or in them and the surfaces of animals roaming over the land.

Soil dust is whipped up by air currents, and soil particles are carried by running water to get into or onto foods. The soil is an important source of heat-resistant spore-forming bacteria. No attempt will be made to list the microorganisms important in food microbiology that could come from the soil, but it can be stated with certainty that nearly every important microorganism can come from soil. Especially important are various molds and yeasts and species of the bacterial genera *Bacillus, Clostridium, Enterobacter, Escherichia, Micrococcus, Alcaligenes, Flavobacterium, Chromobacterium, Pseudomonas, Proteus, Streptococcus, Leuconostoc*, and *Acetobacter* as well as some of the higher bacteria such as the actinomycetes and the iron bacteria.

Modern methods of food handling usually involve washing the surfaces of foods and hence the removal of much of the soil from those surfaces, and care is taken to avoid contamination by soil dust.

FROM WATER

Natural waters contain not only their native flora but also microorganisms from soil and potentially from animals or sewage. Surface waters in streams, pools, and lakes, as well as stored waters in ponds, vary greatly in microbial content, ranging from thousands of microorganisms per milliliter after a rainstorm to much lower counts resulting from self-purification in calm lakes and running water. Groundwater from springs or wells, having passed through rock and soil layers, has been filtered to a certain extent, removing most bacteria and other suspended particles. As a result, bacterial counts in these waters can range from just a few to several hundred per milliliter.

Water bacteriology is of interest to food microbiologists in two primary ways: (1) public health concerns and (2) economic considerations. From a public health perspective, water used in food production must be free from pathogens and safe to drink. Indicator bacteria tests, as outlined by the American Public Health Association (1985), can confirm the safety of water. For example, *Escherichia coli*, often of intestinal origin, can be distinguished from *Enterobacter aerogenes*, which is more commonly found in plant surfaces and soil than in intestinal contents. Some laboratories monitor water quality by performing regular total plate counts and coliform tests, increasing chlorination when abnormalities are detected. Non-fermenting bacteria, like Pseudomonas species, can thrive in waterlines and evade traditional coliform testing; therefore, total plate counts are crucial. Chlorination is practiced when there is any doubt about the water's sanitary quality, with chlorine levels typically ranging from 0.025 to 2 parts per million, depending on water composition and contamination levels.

From an economic standpoint, water for food handling or processing should have favorable chemical and bacteriological qualities. It should be free of undesirable taste, odor, color, and contaminants, and be available in sufficien quantities at the required temperature. The chemical composition, including hardness, alkalinity, and levels of organic matter, iron, manganese, and fluorine, should meet the standards for use in food processing.

In total, water used in food processing should meet both sanitary and economic standards. It should be free of harmful microorganisms, as contamination from water used in food ingredients, washing, cooling, or ice production can introduce undesirable bacteria. Coliform bacteria from cooling tank water, anaerobic gas formers from soil, and spoilage bacteria from cannery cooling water can all pose risks to food safety. For example, *Alcaligenes viscolactis* and *Enterobacter aerogenes,* which cause milk ropiness, typically come from contaminated water. Water treatment methods such as sedimentation, filtration, chlorination, ultraviolet irradiation, or boiling can help purify water, although care must be taken to prevent contamination during filtration. Proper water treatment is vital to ensure the microbial safety of water used in food production.

FROM SEWAGE

When untreated domestic sewage is used to fertilize plant crops, there is likelihood that raw plant foods will be contaminated with human pathogens, especially those causing gastrointestinal diseases. The use of "night soil" as a fertilizer still persists in some parts of the world but is rare in the United States. In addition to the pathogens, coliform bacteria, anaerobes, enterococci, other intestinal bacteria, and viruses can contaminate the foods from this source. Natural waters contaminated with sewage contribute their microorganisms to shellfish, fish, and other seafood.

Treated sewage going onto soil or into water also contributes microorganisms, although it should contain smaller numbers and fewer pathogens than does raw sewage.

FROM AIR

Airborne contamination can contribute to foodborne illnesses and spoilage, as microorganisms such as bacteria, molds, and yeasts can settle on food surfaces through dust, droplets, or airborne particles. These microbes often enter food during processing, storage, or handling, especially in environments where air quality is not controlled.

To prevent contamination from the air, maintaining proper hygiene and cleanliness in food production and storage areas is essential. Using air filtration systems, such as HEPA filters, helps reduce airborne microorganisms. Additionally, proper ventilation, temperature control, and humidity regulation limit the growth of microbes in food storage and processing environments.

In food handling, covering food during storage, minimizing exposure to open air, and practicing good personal hygiene—such as using hairnets and face masks—can further reduce airborne contamination risks. By controlling air quality and following sanitary practices, the chances of food contamination from the air are minimized, ensuring safer food handling and storage.

SOURCES OF MICROORGANISMS IN AIR

Air does not contain a natural flora of microorganisms, for all that are present have come there by accident and usually are on suspended solid materials or in moisture droplets. Microorganisms get into air on dust or lint; dry soil; spray from streams, lakes, or oceans; droplets of moisture from coughing, sneezing, or talking; and growths of sporulating molds on walls, ceilings, floors foods, and ingredients. Thus the air around a plant manufacturing yeast usually is high in yeasts, and the air of a dairy plant may contain bacteriophages or at least the starter bacteria being used there.

Kinds of Microorganisms in Air

Microorganisms in the air do not grow but merely survive, with those most resistant to desiccation tending to persist the longest. Mold spores are typically present in the air due to their small size, resistance to drying, and large numbers produced by each mold plant. Many mold spores do not absorb water easily, making them less likely to settle from humid air compared to particles that readily absorb moisture. While any type of bacterium can be suspended in the air, particularly on dust particles or within moisture droplets, certain types are more common in undisturbed air. Cocci are generally more abundant than rod-shaped bacteria, and bacterial spores are relatively rare in air that is free from dust. Yeasts, particularly chromogenic ones that do not produce spores, are commonly found in air samples. Additionally, when dust or sprays of various materials are released into the air, microorganisms typical of those materials are present-soil organisms in soil and dust, water organisms in water sprays, and plant organisms in feed or fodder dust.

Numbers of Microorganisms in Air

The numbers of microorganisms in air at any given time depend on such factors as the amount of movement, sunshine, humidity, location, and the amount of suspended dust or spray. Numbers vary from less than one per cubic foot at a mountaintop to thousands in very dusty air. Individual microorganisms and those on suspended dust or in droplets settle out in quiet air; conversely, moving air brings organisms up into it. Therefore, numbers of microorganisms in air are increased by air currents caused by movements of people, by ventilation, and by breezes. Direct rays from the sun kill microorganisms suspended in air and hence reduce numbers. Dry air usually contains more organisms than does similar air in a moist condition. Rain or snow removes organisms from the air, so that a hard, steady rainfall may practically free the air of organisms.

According to a review of airborne contamination of foods by Heldman (1974), various surveys have indicated that (1) the microbial populations of different processing plants are similar, (2) populations vary tremendously in numbers from one part of a given plant to another, (3) population in a plant are related to air quality outside the plant, and (4) population levels are related to the level of activity of workers.

Treatment of Air

It has been noted that the number of microorganisms in the air can be naturally reduced through sedimentation, exposure to sunlight, and rain or snow washing. Artificial removal of microorganisms from the air may involve these natural processes or methods like filtration, chemical treatments, heat, or electrostatic precipitation. Filtration through various fibers, such as cotton or fiberglass, or activated carbon, is the most commonly used method. These fibers are either replaced periodically or sterilized with heat or gas. Water spraying or bubbling air through water is generally ineffecti e and rarely used alone. Chemical treatments are becoming more prevalent, with techniques such as passing air through tunnels lined with ultraviolet lamps or installing these lamps in specific areas to reduce contamination. Electrostatic precipitation of dust and microorganisms has also proven successful. Heat treatment at extremely high temperatures has been effecti e but is costly. Once microorganisms are removed, precautions are necessary to prevent their return. Positive pressure in rooms helps keep outside air out, filters in ventilation or air-conditioning systems prevent the spread of organisms between areas, and ultraviolet-irradiated air locks at doors reduce the number of microorganisms brought in by workers.

DURING HANDLING AND PROCESSING

Contamination of food from the natural sources mentioned earlier can occur either before the food is harvested or gathered, or during its handling and processing. Additional contamination may result from equipment that comes into contact with the food, packaging materials, and personnel. The processor makes efforts to clean and "sanitize" the equipment to minimize contamination and selects packaging materials that help reduce it. The term "sanitize" is used instead of "sterilize" because, although the goal is to sterilize the equipment—removing all living organisms—sterility is rarely fully achieved. Contamination during the handling and processing of specific types of food will be addressed in later chapters focused on those foods.

Personnel in food processing plants can contaminate foods during handling and processing. Various workers suggest that human beings shed from 10^3 to 10^4 viable organisms per minute. The numbers and types of organisms shed are closely related to the subjects' working environment.

Table. Number of Workers Engaged in Different Occupations and Positive Cultures of Coagulase-negative and Coagulase-positive Staphylococci, Fecal Coliforms, and Enterococci Obtained from their Hands

Occupation	Number of workers examined	Workers with positive cultures	
		No.	%
Nonfood employment	200	87	43.5
Mechanized food industry	127	68	53.5
Catering service	207	151	72.9
Bakeries	27	26	96.3
Ripened cheese industry	124	114	91.9
Mean industry	129	125	96.9

Since the role of the food handler in food-borne disease outbreaks has been clearly demonstrated, from a public health aspect this source of contamination has received considerable attention. demonstrates the potential contamination of foods from the hands of various workers.

4 Key Microorganisms in Food Microbiology

Key microorganisms in food microbiology include bacteria, yeasts, molds, and viruses, each playing distinct roles in food production, preservation, and spoilage. Bacteria such as *Salmonella, Escherichia coli,* and *Listeria* are significant foodborne pathogens, capable of causing serious illnesses when food is contaminated. These bacteria thrive in warm, moist environments and multiply rapidly if food is improperly stored or handled. Lactic acid bacteria, like *Lactobacillus,* are beneficial microorganisms used in the fermentation of dairy, vegetables, and meat products, contributing to flavor development and preservation.

Yeasts, such as *Saccharomyces cerevisiae,* are crucial in baking and alcohol production due to their fermentation capabilities. However, spoilage yeasts like *Candida* can cause discoloration and off-flavors in food. Molds, including *Aspergillus* and *Penicillium,* can grow on a variety of foods, leading to spoilage and the production of mycotoxins, which are harmful to human health.

Viruses, such as norovirus and hepatitis A, can contaminate food through contact with infected food handlers or contaminated water. These microorganisms require proper hygiene, temperature control, and food safety practices to prevent contamination and ensure food safety.

FITNESS OR UNFITNESS OF FOOD FOR CONSUMPTION

When is a food safe to eat? According to Thom and Hunter (1924), "a product is safe to eat if an informed consumer, knowing the history of its production and seeing the material itself, eats it, and vice versa, the same product is spoiled when such an examiner rejects it. It is like food, by definition, the quality of food depends on the person who judges it, for what one person will eat, another, for example. like their "high" game meat, with a strong flavor developed by hanging or aging the meat, while most Americans call this spoiled meat. The buried fish, the breast rat, eaten by the Eskimos is a foul-smelling semi-liquid product that most of us would consider inedible. Hungry people may eat foods they would not normally eat.

Despite the differences between individuals in their judgments of the quality of foods, they agree on certain criteria to guarantee their quality:

- The desired stage of development or maturity. Fruits should be at a certain stage of maturity, but different; sweet corn should be young enough to be sweet and milky; Poultry should preferably come from relatively young birds.

- Absence of contamination at any stage of production or processing. Vegetables should not be eaten raw if they have been fertilized with water; oysters from water contaminated with water should be rejected; food handled by dirty or sick workers should be rejected; food contaminated by flies or rodents should be suspected
- Absence of undesirable change resulting from microbial attack or enzyme action in the food. Sometimes it is difficul to draw a line between spoilage by microorganisms and harmless growth, or the same type of change may be considered undesirable in one food and desirable in another. So the housewife says that sour milk is spoiled, but buttermilk fermented by lactic fermentation is good. The rotting of meat signifies some spoilage, but the rotting changes in Limburger cheese are normal during the ripening process. Some changes that qualify as spoilage may be merely changes in appearance or physical characteristics, as in the case of wilted lettuce or limp carrots, even though the product may not have undergone microbial spoilage and there has been little loss of nutritional value. However, each of us has our own idea of whether a food is spoiled and can usually make up our own mind without much difficult

CAUSES OF SPOILAGE

The term "spoiled" typically refers to decay or decomposition of an undesirable nature in food, while food unfit for consumption due to sanitary concerns is generally not considered spoiled. Spoilage can result from several factors:

- Growth and activity of microorganisms (occasionally involving higher organisms). Often, a sequence of organisms is involved.
- Insects
- The action of enzymes from plant or animal food sources.
- Purely chemical reactions, not influenced by enzymes from tissues or microorganisms.
- Physical changes such as those caused by freezing, burning, drying, or pressure. This discussion will primarily focus on spoilage caused by microorganisms.

CLASSIFICATION OF FOODS BY EASE OF SPOILAGE

On the basis of ease of spoilage, foods can be placed in three groups:

- **Stable or Nonperishable Foods-**These foods, which do not spoil unless handled carelessly, include such products as sugar, flour, and dry beans.
- **Perishable Foods-**This group includes most important daily foods that spoil readily unless special preservative methods are used. Meats, fish, poultry, most fruits and vegetables, eggs, and milk belong in this classification
- **Semiperishable Foods-**If these foods are properly handled and stored, they will remain unspoiled for a fairly long period, e.g., potatoes, some varieties of apples, waxed rutabagas, and nutmeats.

Most foods fall into one of these three groups, but some are near enough to the borderline to be difficult to place

FACTORS AFFECTING KINDS AND NUMBERS OF MICROORGANISMS IN FOOD

The type of spoilage caused by microorganisms and enzymes in food depends on the types and quantities of these agents present and the surrounding environmental conditions. Most raw foods naturally contain a variety of bacteria, yeasts, molds, and possibly plant or animal enzymes. Due to specific environmental factors, only a small proportion of these microorganisms will grow rapidly and cause spoilage—usually a single type, but occasionally two or three. These microorganisms may not have been the predominant ones in the original food. If spoilage by the first organisms continues unchecked, secondary spoilage by other microorganisms may occur, or a succession of organisms and changes may take place.

The presence and quantity of microorganisms on or in food will be influenced by the extent and type of contamination, prior opportunities for growth, and any pretreatments the food has undergone. Contamination can increase the microbial load in food and introduce new types of microorganisms. For instance, wash water can transfer surface-taint bacteria into butter; plant equipment can introduce spoilage organisms during processing; washing machines can contaminate eggs; and dirty boats can add bacteria to fish. This increased microbial load, especially spoilage-causing organisms, makes preservation more challenging, making spoilage more likely and rapid, and possibly causing a different type of spoilage than would have occurred without contamination.

The growth of microorganisms in or on food will naturally increase the bioburden, primarily involving the organisms most likely responsible for spoilage. A higher microbial load complicates the prevention of spoilage and can influence the form of spoilage.

Pretreatments can either remove or destroy certain microorganisms, introduce new ones, alter the proportions of existing microorganisms, or inactivate enzymes, thus limiting spoilage agents and potential types of spoilage. For instance, washing can remove organisms from the surface or introduce new ones from the wash water. If an antiseptic or germicidal solution is used for washing, the number of organisms can be greatly reduced, and some types may be eliminated. Treatments using rays, ozone, sulfur dioxide, or germicidal vapors can reduce the number of microorganisms, often selectively. High temperatures will kill more organisms, leaving fewer types alive as the temperature increases. Various storage conditions can either increase or decrease microbial presence. Any of these treatments, along with others not mentioned, will impact the quantity, type, proportion, and health of microorganisms present.

FACTORS AFFECTING THE GROWTH OF MICROORGANISMS IN FOOD

Associative Growth

Microorganisms typically interact with each other in various ways that influence spoilage or fermentation in foods. The competition between different types of bacteria, yeasts, and molds generally dictates which microorganism will dominate and cause its specific type of spoilage. In favorable conditions, bacteria usually grow faster than yeasts, and yeasts outpace molds. Yeasts only surpass bacteria when they are already the dominant organisms or when environmental conditions slow bacterial growth. Molds thrive only when the environment favors them over yeasts or bacteria. Among bacteria, different species compete, with one usually outgrowing the others. Similarly, among yeasts and molds, one species often dominates based on the prevailing conditions.

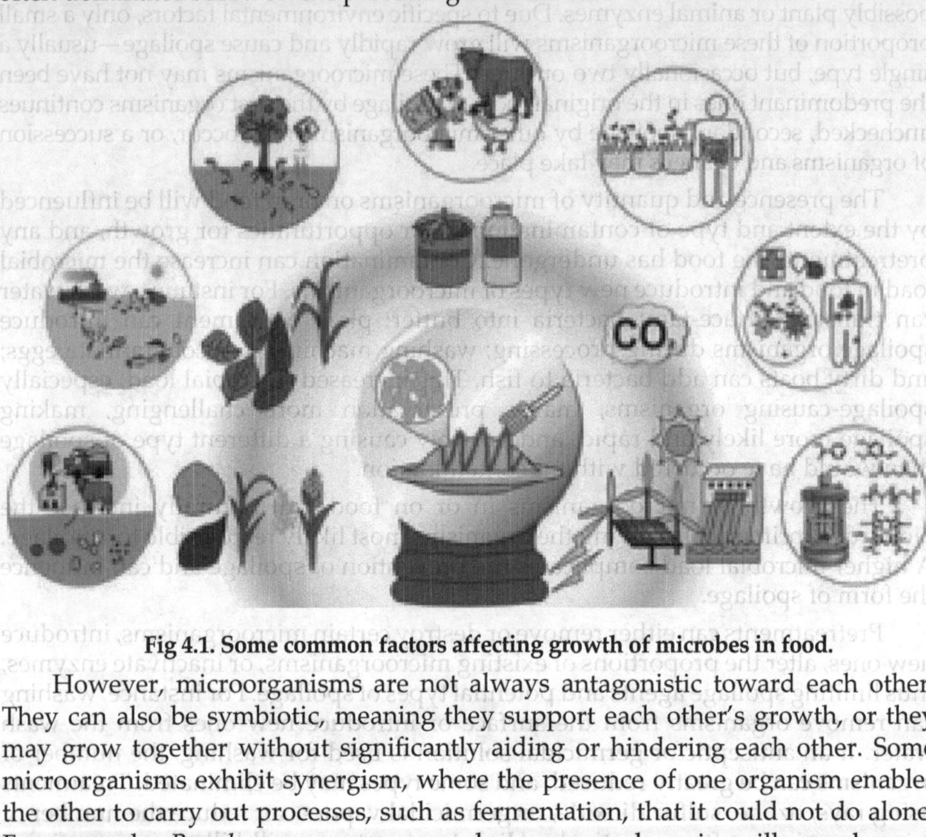

Fig 4.1. Some common factors affecting growth of microbes in food.

However, microorganisms are not always antagonistic toward each other. They can also be symbiotic, meaning they support each other's growth, or they may grow together without significantly aiding or hindering each other. Some microorganisms exhibit synergism, where the presence of one organism enables the other to carry out processes, such as fermentation, that it could not do alone. For example, *Pseudomonas syncyanea,* when grown alone in milk, produces a light-brownish tinge, while Streptococcus lactis does not alter the milk's color. However, when both organisms grow together, they produce a bright blue color due to the pH effect on the brown pigment produced by *P. syncyanea*.

An important form of microorganism interaction is metabiotic, where one organism creates conditions favorable for the growth of another. Both organisms may grow at the same time, but more commonly, one succeeds the other. This is evident in the natural fermentations or decompositions of raw foods. For instance, raw milk left at room temperature initially supports an acid fermentation by *Streptococcus lactis* and coliform bacteria, which are eventually inhibited by the acid they produce. The more acid-tolerant lactobacilli then thrive, increasing acidity until they are stopped. Yeasts and molds then grow on the surface, eventually reducing the acidity enough for proteolytic bacteria to become active. Metabiosis in sauerkraut fermentation follows a similar pattern, with a succession of microorganisms: first, miscellaneous bacteria (mainly coliforms), followed by *Leuconostoc mesenteroides*, then *Lactobacillus plantarum*, and finally *Lactobacillus brevis*.

Impact of Environmental Factors

The environment determines which of the different types of microorganisms present in a food will grow faster than others and cause their characteristic type of change or spoilage. The factors that make up this environment are interdependent and, in combination, determine which organisms will grow and what effects will occur. Among these factors, the most important are the physical and chemical properties of the food, the availability of oxygen, and temperature. The physical state and structure of the food The physical state of the food, its colloidal nature and whether it has been frozen, heated, moist, or dry, as well as its biological structure, can have a significant impact on whether a food will spoil and the type of spoilage.

Water in food, its location, and availability is one of the most important factors affecting microbial growth. Water can be considered as a chemical component necessary for growth and a part of the physical structure of food.

The moisture requirements of molds, yeasts and bacteria were discussed in Chapter 1. It was pointed out that all microorganisms need moisture to grow and that they all grow best in the presence of an abundant supply. This moisture must be available to organisms, i.e. , not related in any way, such as from solutes or from a hydrophilic colloid such as agar. Solutes such as salt and sugar dissolved in water cause osmotic pressure that tends to pull water out of cells if the concentration of solutes is greater outside the cells than inside. It is remembered that when the relative humidity of the air around the food corresponds to the humidity or water activity available to the food, the food and the surrounding air will be in equilibrium with respect to the humidity.

A dry food like bread is more likely to be spoiled by mold; syrups and honey, with their high sugar content and therefore reduced aw, promote the growth of osmophilic yeast; And Wet and neutral foods, such as milk, meat, fish and eggs are usually spoiled by bacteria. In any case, environmental factors other than humidity must be considered to predict the type of microorganism that can cause spoilage. Grape juice, for example, can support yeast because of its relatively high sugar content and low pH, but it will favor bacterial growth if the incubation temperature is too high or too low for yeast fermentation. Refrigerated foods can mold in the presence of air, but suffer from bacterial spoilage in its absence. Honey, although its sugar content is too high for most yeasts but not for some molds, is rarely spoiled by mold because of the fungistatic substances present.

An aw of up to 0.70 makes it impossible for microorganisms to spoil a food stored at room temperature. This is approximately the available moisture level in powdered milk at 8 percent total moisture, whole egg powder at 10 to 11 percent, flour at 13 to 15 percent, powdered milk at 15 percent. percent, dehydrated lean meats at 15 percent, legumes at 15 percent, dehydrated vegetables at 14 to 20 percent, dehydrated fruits at 18 to 25 percent, and starches at 18 percent (Mossel and Ingram, 1955).

It is possible that microorganisms growing on foods can change the available moisture level by releasing metabolic water or by altering the substrate in a way that releases water. For example, in the production of hardness in bread, *Bacillus subtilis* is thought to cause moisture to be released after starch decomposition and thus create more favorable conditions for its growth. Destruction of moisture-retaining tissues, such as in fruit by mold, can make water available to yeast or bacteria.

Freezing not only inhibits microbial growth if the temperature is low enough, but is also likely to damage the tissue, so the fluids released during thawing promote microbial growth. Freezing also increases the concentration of dissolved substances in the part unfrozen when the temperature drops, which slows down and eventually stops the growth of organisms capable of growing at temperatures below 0°C. Freezing also results in the removal of water from the hydrophilic colloids, which is not completely recaptured after thawing.

Heat treatment can change not only the chemical composition of the food, but also its structure, softening the tissues, releasing or maintaining moisture, destroying or forming colloidal suspensions, gels or emulsions, and modifying them. permeability of food to moisture and oxygen. Proteins can be denatured and are therefore more available to some organisms than they were in their native state. Starch or protein can gel, releasing moisture and breaking down more easily. For the reasons given, cooked foods generally break more easily than the original fresh foods.

Changes in the colloidal constituents of foods can be caused by agents other than freezing or heating processes, such as sound waves, but the results are similar. Fat-water emulsions are more likely to break down, and the breakup spreads more rapidly, when the water is the continuous phase and the fat is the discontinuous phase, as in French vinaigrette, compared to butter, when the opposite is tru

The effect of the biological structure of foods on the protection of foods from spoilage was discussed in Chapter 1.

Chemical Properties of the Food

The chemical composition of a food determines its ability to serve as a culture medium for microorganisms. Each organism has its own ability to use certain substances as an energy source, carbon source, and/or nitrogen source.

Properties of a food dictating the numbers and type of organisms that will grow in and possibly spoil a food have been discussed in Chapter 1 and include (1) pH, or hydrogen-ion concentration, (2) nutrient content, (3) moisture availability, (4) O-R potential, and (5) possible presence of inhibitory substances.

Temperature

Any non-sterile food is prone to spoilage over time if it remains moist and is not frozen. It becomes vulnerable to spoilage within a temperature range of -5 to 70°C. Given the wide variation in microorganisms' optimal, minimum, and maximum temperatures for growth, the storage temperature of food signific ntly influence the type, rate, and extent of microbial changes. A small fluct ation in temperature can favor a completely different organism, leading to a distinct form of decay. Molds and yeasts typically do not thrive above 35-37°C, so they are less relevant in foods stored at higher temperatures. However, these organisms grow well at normal room temperatures, and some even survive at freezing or slightly sub-zero temperatures. While most bacteria favor average temperatures, certain species (thermophiles) grow best at high temperatures, and others (psychrophiles and psychrotrophs) thrive in cooler environments. As a result, molds can develop in refrigerated foods, and thermophilic bacteria flou ish in warm environments. In raw milk, storage temperature determines the bacteria that initially grow-cold-resistant bacteria like *Pseudomonas* and *Alcaligenes* thrive near freezing, while at room temperature, *Streptococcus lactis* and coliform bacteria dominate; at 40-45°C, thermophilic species such as *S. thermophilus* and *S. faecalis* grow first, and at 55-60°C, *Lactobacillus thermophilus* flourishes. It's important to note that the temperature of raw food storage can influence its degr dation rate and microbial spoilage susceptibility.

In different regions, the temperatures used for food handling and storage vary significantly. In some countries, refrigeration is the norm for perishable foods, whereas, in others, it is rare to store foods this way for extended periods. This difference leads to distinct spoilage patterns in various countries. In the United in refrigeration, with psychrotrophic strains of *Pseudomonas, Flavobacterium, Alcaligenes,* and other genera, along with yeasts and molds, playing a significant role. In contrast, in areas where refrigeration is not the norm, ambient temperature becomes a key factor, with seasonal variations impacting spoilage. During milder climates, mesophilic bacteria, yeasts, and molds become more prominent, while in hot weather (26.7-43°C or higher), organisms suited for these conditions, such as coliform bacteria, *Bacillus, Clostridium, Streptococcus, Lactobacillus,* and others, thrive. Tropical climates tend to be less favorable for most yeasts and molds. In rare cases, such as during World War II, foods (especially canned varieties) were stored in conditions that favored thermophiles, as seen when canned foods were kept under tarpaulins in tropical areas.

Combinations of all the factors just mentioned and the types, numbers and sizes of microorganisms present and their environment controlled by the physical and chemical properties of the food, the oxygen tension and redox potential, and the temperature, will determine the types of microorganisms most likely to grow in a food and therefore the changes that need to be made. All of these factors must be considered when making predictions about the sustainability of longevity. maintaining the quality and microbial flora of staple foods

Table. Classification of the Major Foods in Order of Increasing Microbiological load

Stability characteristics					
Class	**"Processing including heat treatment, compositional modification, and packaging**	**Temp. °C**	**Time of spoilage-free storage**	**Examples**	**Predominant microbial flora at retail**
1	None of functional nature	<10	10-40 hr	Fresh meat, milk, fish, poultry, eggs, vegetables	Psychrotrophic, nonfermentative gram-negative rods
2	Pasteurization, followed by hermetic packaging	<10	3 days to 2 weeks	Dairy products, sliced cured meat products	Sporing rods and Lancefield group D streptoeocci
3	Reduction of water activity to c0. 0.95. pH reduction and addition of preservation with hermetic packaging	<10	A few weeks	"Gafflebitter' and similar semi-preserved fish products	Lactobacilli, streptococci, yeasts and molds
4	Reduction of water activity to c0. 0.85 pH lactic acid combinations of equivalent microbistatic effect pasteurization	25	Many weeks	Condensed milk, mayonnaise, margarine, smoked sausage	Yeast, molds
5	Reduction of water activity to ca. 0.80, sometimes in combination with pH reduction	25	Unlimited, i.e., until chemical reactions interfere	Shelf-stable products such as salami, stockfish, sauces.	Molds
6	Reduction of water activity, to <0.60	35	Unlimited	Dehydrated foods	Bacilli, group D streptococci, mold spores
7	Appertization	35	Unlimited	Canned cured meat producers and fruits	An occasional spore, i.e, counts of $<10^2$/g
8	Sterilization	Any	Unlimited	Canned milk, soups, meat, vegetables, and fis	None

Examples will be cited throughout the chapters to follow on the spoilage of specific foods. Sometimes a change in only one of the factors mentioned will be enough to limit the change to be expected, but more often several factors exert a combined effect. Thus a combination of low moisture, refrigerator temperature, high acidity, and high sugar would make mold growth more likely than growth of yeasts or bacteria. But increasing the moisture content and the temperature would change conditions to favor yeasts, and decreasing the acidity and sugar content would encourage bacteria.

CHEMICAL CHANGES CAUSED BY MICROORGANISMS

Microorganisms cause various chemical changes in food, leading to spoilage or fermentation. Bacteria, yeasts, and molds can break down carbohydrates, proteins, and lipids, producing acids, gases, and enzymes. For example, lactic acid bacteria convert sugars into lactic acid, souring dairy and vegetables. Yeasts ferment sugars into alcohol and carbon dioxide, essential in bread and alcohol production. Molds degrade proteins and lipids, often leading to the production of unpleasant flavors and mycotoxins. These biochemical changes are critical in both food preservation (e.g., fermentation) and spoilage, influencing food safety and quality.

The following discussion is concerned only with the important types of decomposition of main constituents of foods and the chief products produced.

Changes in Nitrogenous Organic Compounds

Most nitrogen in foods is in the form of proteins that must be hydrolyzed by microbial or food enzymes into polypeptides, simple peptides, or amino acids before they can serve as a nitrogen source for most organisms. Proteinases catalyze the hydrolysis of proteins into peptides, which can make the food taste bitter. Peptidases catalyze the hydrolysis of polypeptides into simpler peptides and ultimately into amino acids. The latter impart desirable or undesirable flavors to certain foods, e.g. , amino acids contribute to the aroma of ripened cheeses.

In most cases, these hydrolyses will not produce particularly objectionable products. However, anaerobic decomposition of proteins, peptides, or amino acids can result in the production of unpleasant odors and is called putrefaction. It produces malodorous sulfur-containing products, such as hydrogen, methyl and ethyl sulfides, and mercaptans, as well as ammonia, amines (e.g. , histamine, tyramine, piperidine, putrescine and cadaverine), indole, skatole and fatty acids.

When microorganisms act on amino acids, they can deaminate, decarboxylate, or both, resulting in the products listed in Table 4. 2. *Escherichia coli,* for example, produces glyoxylic acid, acetic acid and ammonia from glycine; *Pseudomonas* also produces methylamine and carbon dioxide; and clostridia yield acetic acid, ammonia and methane. From alanine, these three organisms produce (1) α-keto acids, ammonia and carbon dioxide, (2) acetic acid, ammonia and carbon dioxide, and (3) propionic acid, acetic acid, ammonia and carbon dioxide, respectively. From serine, *E. coli* produces pyruvic acid and ammonia, and *Clostridium* species yield propionic acid, formic acid, and ammonia. As mentioned, sulfur from sulfur-containing amino acids can be reduced to sulfides or mercaptans. *Desulfotomaculum nigrificans* (formerly *C. nigrificans*), an obligate anaerobe, can reduce sulfate to sulfur. and produces hydrogen sulfide from cystine.

Table. Products from the Microbial Decomposition of Amino Acids

Chemical process	Products
Oxidative deamination	Keto acid + NH_3
Hydrolytic deamination	Hydroxy acid + NH_3
Reductive deamination	Saturated fatty acid + N_3
Desaturation deamination (at a and b positions)	Unsaturated fatty acid + N_3
Mutual O-R between pairs of amino acids	Keto acid + fatty acid + N_3
Decarboxylation	Amine + GO_2
Hydrolytic deamination + decarboxylation	Primary alcohol + NH_3 + CO_2
Reductive deamination + decarboxylation	Hydrocarbon + NH_3 + CO_2
Oxidative deamination + decarboxylation	Fatty acid + NH_3 + CO

Other nitrogenous compounds decomposed include: (1) amides, imides, and urea, from which ammonia is the principal product, (2) guanidine and creatine, which yield urea and ammonia, and (3) amines, purines, and pyrimidines, which may yield ammonia, carbon dioxide, and organic acids (chiefly lactic or acetic).

Changes in Nonnitrogenous Organic Compounds

The main nonnitrogenous foods for microorganisms, mostly used to obtain energy but possibly serving as sources of carbon, include carbohydrates, organic acids, aldehydes and ketones, alcohols, glycosides, cyclic compounds, and lipids.

Carbohydrates

Carbohydrates, when available, are generally preferred by microorganisms over other energy sources. Complex di-, tri-, or polysaccharides are usually hydrolyzed to simple sugars before use. A monosaccharide, such as glucose, will be aerobically oxidized to carbon dioxide and water and undergo anaerobic decomposition involving one of six main types of fermentation: (1) alcoholic fermentation, such as that of yeast, with ethanol and carbon dioxide as the main products. (2) simple lactic fermentation, such as that of homofermentative lactic acid bacteria, with lactic acid as the main product, (3) mixed lactic acid fermentation, such as that of heterofermentative lactic acid bacteria, with lactic and acetic acid, ethanol, glycerol, and carbon dioxide. as the main products, (4) coliform type fermentation, such as that of coliform bacteria, with lactic, acetic and formic acids, ethanol, carbon dioxide, hydrogen and possibly acetoin and butanediol as possible products, (5) propionic fermentation, by propionic bacteria, which produces propionic, acetic and succinic acids and carbon dioxide, or (6) butyric-butyl-isopropyl fermentation, by anaerobic bacteria, which produces butyric and acetic acids, carbon dioxide, hydrogen and, in some cases, acetone, butylene glycol, butanol and 2-propanol. A variety of other products are possible from sugars when several microorganisms are active, including higher fatty acids, other organic acids, aldehydes and ketones.

Organic Acids

Many organic acids are commonly found in foods as salts are oxidized by organisms to carbonates, making the environment more alkaline. Aerobically, organic acids can be completely oxidized to carbon dioxide and water, as in the case of yeasts. The acids can be oxidized to other simple acids or other similar sugar products. Saturated fatty acids or lower ketone derivatives are split into acetic acid, two carbons at a time, assisted by coenzyme A. Unsaturated or hydroxy fatty acids can be partially split in a similar manner, but must be converted to a saturated acid (or ketone derivative) for complete beta oxidation.

Other Compounds

Alcohols usually are oxidized to the corresponding organic acid, e.g., ethanol to acetic acid. Glycerol may be dissimilated to products similar to those from glucose. Glycosides, after hydrolysis to release the sugar, will have the sugar dissimilated characteristically. Acetaldehyde may be oxidized to acetic acid or reduced to ethanol. Cyclic compounds are not readily attacked.

Lipids

In food microbiology, lipids are essential components of both microbial cell structures and the food itself. While lipids themselves are not microorganisms, they play a crucial role in the growth, survival, and metabolic processes of microorganisms involved in food production, spoilage, and fermentation.

Microorganisms, particularly certain bacteria and molds, can metabolize lipids for energy. Lipolytic bacteria, such as *Pseudomonas* and *Bacillus*, break down fats in food, leading to spoilage and the development of rancid flavors. Similarly, molds like *Aspergillus* and *Penicillium* can produce lipases that degrade lipids in dairy products, meats, and oils, causing deterioration.

On the positive side, lipids are vital in the production of fermented foods, such as cheese, where microbial activity affects the texture and flavor profile. Yeasts also contribute to lipid metabolism during fermentation, especially in products like beer and wine. Controlling lipid breakdown is essential for food preservation. Proper storage, temperature control, and sanitation practices are critical in minimizing the action of spoilage microorganisms on lipids, preserving the sensory quality and safety of food products.

Pectic Substances

Protopectin, the water-insoluble pectin substance of plants, is converted to pectin, a water-soluble polymer of galacturonic acid containing methyl ester bonds and varying degrees of neutralization by various cations. Mix with sugar and acid. Pectinesterase hydrolyzes the methyl ester bond of pectin to produce pectic acid and methanol. Polygalacturonases break the bonds between the galacturonic acid units of pectin or petic acid to produce smaller chains and eventually release D-galacturonic acid, which can be broken down into simple sugars.

Part-II

Fundamentals of Food Preservation

This section discusses the principles, particularly the microbiological ones, involved in various food preservation methods. Thanks to advancements in preservation and transportation techniques, our diets have become more diverse and nutritionally balanced. Perishable foods are now available year-round rather than seasonally, meal preparation has become more convenient, and overall food production is cleaner and more sanitary. Furthermore, these enhanced preservation and transportation methods have enabled countries with surplus food to assist nations in need by providing high-quality food supplements.

5 Fundamentals of Food Preservation

Food preservation is the process of handling and treating food in a way that prolongs its shelf life by preventing or delaying deterioration, loss of quality, edibility, or nutritional value. Generally speaking, preservation entails stopping the growth of bacteria, fungi (like yeasts), and other microorganisms in addition to delaying the oxidation of fats that results in rancidity.

Aseptic techniques focus on preventing contamination during food handling, packaging, and storage. By maintaining a sterile environment These techniques prevent or reduce the entry of microorganisms that can cause foodborne damage or illness. This is especially important in industries such as canned food, where careful sterilization and hygiene are key to ensuring product safety. The use of aseptic packaging, in which food is placed in sterilized containers without exposure to air. It also preserves product quality and extends shelf life.

Disposal methods include drying, refrigeration and filtration techniques, physical or chemical operations to remove elements that allow microbial growth. For example, drying will It removes moisture, which is an important factor in the survival and spread of bacteria, yeast, and mold. Refrigeration, on the other hand, slows down the metabolic activity of microorganisms. By maintaining the freshness of perishable foods Prevent contamination early on. Filtration removes contaminants from liquids, such as in water purification or juicing. This ensures that the final product is free of harmful microorganisms

Foods for human consumption can be divided into eight main groups, four of plant and four of animal origin, and several lesser groups. The eight main classes of foods are as follows:

Plant-Origin Foods	Animal-Origin Foods
1. Cereals and Grains Examples: Wheat, rice, oats	1. Meat and Poultry Examples: Beef, chicken, lamb, turkey
2. Vegetables Examples: Spinach, carrots, potatoes	2. Fish and Seafood Examples: Salmon, shrimp, tuna, cod
3. Fruits Examples: Apples, bananas, oranges	3. Dairy Products Examples: Milk, cheese, yogurt, butte
4. Legumes and Pulses Examples: Beans, lentils, chickpeas	4. Eggs Examples: Chicken eggs, duck eggs

In addition to the foods of plant origin, spices, flavoring agents, nuts, and edible fungi (such as yeasts, molds, and mushrooms) can also be included. Sodium chloride serves as a mineral food, a flavor enhancer, an essential nutrient, and a chemical preservative. Certain foods may be fortified with minerals, such as the addition of iron and calcium compounds to flour. Some coloring and flavoring substances in foods are artificially synthesized. Vitamins are generally found in foods, but they can also be added or taken separately after being chemically synthesized or produced by microorganisms.

Most kinds of food are readily decomposed by microorganisms unless special methods are used for their preservation.

METHODS OF FOOD PRESERVATION

There are several preventative techniques that can be applied to completely stop, postpone, or otherwise lessen food spoiling. With the help of preservatives, food can have a longer shelf life and be harvested, processed, sold, and stored in the home of the consumer for a longer period of time.

The main methods of food preservation are:

- Asepsis, or keeping microorganisms.
- Elimination of microorganisms.
- Maintain anaerobic conditions, for example in a sealed container and under vacuum.
- The use of high temperatures.
- The use of low temperatures.
- Drying; this includes the fixation of water by dissolved substances, hydrophilic colloids, etc.
- The use of chemical preservatives, developed by microorganisms or added.
- Radiation.
- Mechanical destruction of microorganisms, e.g. , with grinding, high pressure, etc. (not used industrially).
- Combination of two or more of the above methods. It is rare that a single method is effecti e and generally several are combined. For example, canned food is preserved by heat treatment in a vacuum-sealed can. When preservation methods are combined, the intensity required for each is generally reduced to a lower level than that required for preservation by a single agent. When benzoate or sorbate is added to fruit juices, less heat is required to sterilize these products. If salt, sugar, and vinegar are added to ketchup, pickles, or condiments, each can be used in a lower concentration than if it were added alone. Foods previously irradiated with gamma rays or treated with the antibiotic tylosin require less heat for sterilization than foods not treated in this way.

PRINCIPLES OF FOOD PRESERVATION

The preservation of foods through various methods involves the following principles:

- Prevention or slowing down of microbial spoilage
  - o By preventing the entry of microorganisms (asepsis)
  - o By removing microorganisms, such as through filtratio
  - o By inhibiting microbial growth and activity, for instance, using low temperatures, drying, anaerobic environments, or chemicals
  - o By eliminating microorganisms, such as through heat or radiation
- Prevention or delay of food's natural decay:
  - o By destroying or deactivating food enzymes, such as through blanching
  - o By preventing or delaying chemical reactions, for instance, using antioxidants to prevent oxidation
- Prevention of damage from insects, animals, mechanical factors, etc., which is not covered in this text. Methods to control microorganisms are generally effecti e in inhibiting enzymatic activities or chemical reactions within the food. However, techniques like drying or using low temperatures may still allow self-decomposition unless additional precautions are taken. For instance, most vegetables are blanched (heated) to deactivate their enzymes before freezing.

Delay of Microbial Decomposition

Many common methods of food preservation depend not on the destruction or removal of microorganisms but on delay in the initiation of growth and hindrance to growth once it has begun.

A summary of the major preservation factors and their mode of action and achievement is presented in Table.

Growth Curve of Microbial Cultures

When microorganisms are introduced into a food and conditions are suitable, they begin to multiply and progress through several growth phases. By periodically counting the organisms and plotting the logarithms of their numbers per milliliter against time, a growth curve can be obtained. This curve is typically divided into distinct phases: (1) the lag phase (A to B), where growth is absent or numbers may even decrease, (2) the positive acceleration phase (B to C), where the growth rate increases continuously, (3) the logarithmic or exponential growth phase (C to D), where the multiplication rate is at its fastest and remains constant, (4) the negative acceleration phase (D to E), where the rate of growth begins to slow, (5) the stationary phase (E to F), where the population stabilizes, (6) the accelerated death phase (F to G), (7) the death phase (G to H), where the number of organisms decreases faster than new cells are produced, and (8) the survival phase (H to I), where no new cells are formed, but the remaining cells persist on internal nutrients. For many microorganisms, the population does not decline at a consistent rate until zero, as the solid line in the figure suggests. Instead, it tapers off slowly, with a few viable cells remaining for a prolonged period, as shown by the broken line.

Table. Classification of Preservation Factors

Mode of action	Preservation factor	Mode of achievement
Prevention of Microbial Growth	Asepsis	Keeping microorganisms out of the food (e.g., sterile packaging)
	Removal of Microorganisms	Filtration, washing, or other methods to physically remove microorganisms
	Low Temperature	Refrigeration or freezing to inhibit microbial growth
	Drying	Dehydration to reduce water content and inhibit microbial activity
	Anaerobic Conditions	Creating oxygen-free environments to hinder microbial growth
	Chemical Inhibitors	Adding preservatives to prevent or slow down microbial growth
Destruction of Microorganisms	Heat (Thermal Processing)	Pasteurization, sterilization, or cooking to kill microorganisms
	Radiation	Use of ionizing radiation to destroy microorganisms
Inactivation of Enzymes	Blanching	Heat treatment to deactivate enzymes that cause spoilage
	Chemical Inhibitors	Addition of chemicals to prevent enzymatic activity (e.g., antioxidants)
Prevention of Chemical Reactions	Antioxidants	Use of substances to prevent oxidation and chemical deterioration
Physical Protection from Damage	Packaging	Using physical barriers to protect from mechanical, insect, or animal damage
	Atmospheric Control	Modifying atmospheric conditions (e.g., vacuum sealing) to reduce spoilage

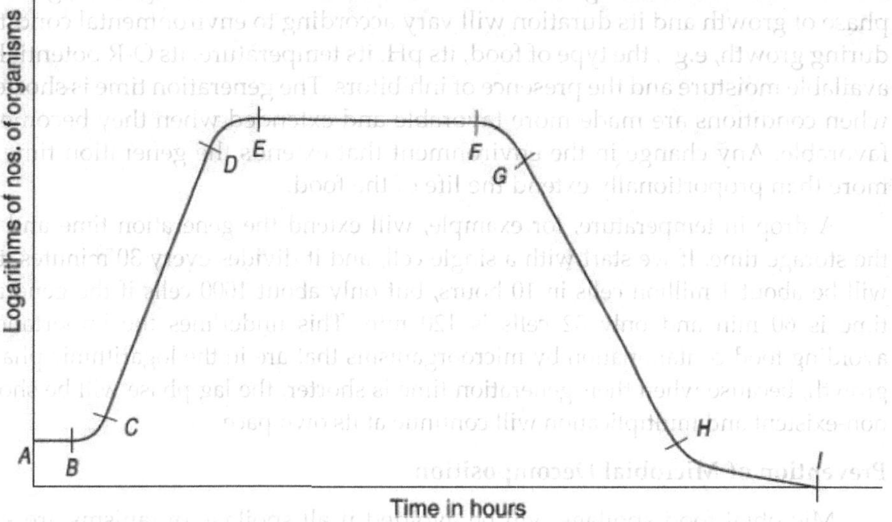

Fig 5.1. **Growth curve. A to B, lag phase; B to C, phase of positive acceleration; C to D, logarithmic or exponential phase; D to E, phase of negative acceleration; E to F, maximal stationary; F fo G, accelerated death phase; G to H, death phase; and H to I, survival phase.**

Applications to Food Preservation

Especially important in food preservation (i.e., prevention of spoilage) is the lengthening, as much as possible, of the lag phase and the phase of positive acceleration. This can be accomplished in different ays:

- By introducing as few spoilage organisms as possible, i.e., by reducing the amount of contamination; the fewer organisms present, the longer the lag phase.
- By avoiding the addition of actively growing organisms (from the logarithmic phase of growth). Such organisms might be growing on unclean containers, equipment, or utensils that come in contact with foods.
- By one or more unfavorable environmental conditions: unfavorable foods, moisture, temperature, pH, or O-R potential, or presence of inhibitors. The more unfavorable the conditions, the longer the delay of the initiation of growth.
- By actual damage to organisms by processing methods such as heating or irradiation.

Thus, for example, bacteria or their spores subjected to sublethal heat treatments have been found to require a better culture medium for growth than do the unheated organisms. Often a combination of methods for delaying the initiation of growth is enough to give a food the desired storage life.

From the growth curve, we can calculate the generation time of organisms, that is, the time that passes between the formation of a daughter cell and its division into two new cells. The generation time will be shorter during the logarithmic phase of growth and its duration will vary according to environmental conditions during growth, e.g. , the type of food, its pH, its temperature, its O-R potential, the available moisture and the presence of inhibitors. The generation time is shortened when conditions are made more favorable and extended when they become less favorable. Any change in the environment that extends the generation time will more than proportionally extend the life of the food.

A drop in temperature, for example, will extend the generation time and thus the storage time. If we start with a single cell, and it divides every 30 minutes, there will be about 1 million cells in 10 hours, but only about 1000 cells if the generation time is 60 min and only 32 cells is 120 min. This underlines the importance of avoiding food contamination by microorganisms that are in the logarithmic phase of growth, because when their generation time is shorter, the lag phase will be short or non-existent and multiplication will continue at its own pace.

Prevention of Microbial Decomposition

Microbial food spoilage will be avoided if all spoilage organisms are killed (or eliminated) and recontamination is avoided. However, simply stopping the growth of microorganisms does not necessarily prevent decomposition, since viable organisms or their enzymes may still be active.

As we will note in the following chapters, most agents kill microorganisms more easily when they are present in small numbers than in large amounts; this also highlights the importance of pollution. Particularly important is the introduction or accumulation of microorganisms resistant to the lethal agent used, for example heat-resistant bacterial spores when foods have to be treated with heat. Vegetative cells of organisms in their logarithmic phase of growth are less resistant to lethal agents and are more resistant in the late lag phase or the maximum stationary phase of growth.

ASEPSIS

In nature, there are many examples of asepsis, or protection against microorganisms, used as a factor of preservation. The internal tissues of healthy plants and animals are usually free of microorganisms, and if microorganisms are present, they are unlikely to cause spoilage. If the food is covered with a protective covering, microbial decomposition is delayed or prevented. Examples of such coverings are the shells of nuts, the skins of fruits and vegetables, the husks of corn, the shells of eggs, and the skin, membranes, or fat of meat or fish. Only when the protective covering is damaged or the decomposition spreads from the outer surface do the internal tissues undergo decomposition by microorganisms.

In the food industry, increasing attention is being paid to preventing food contamination from raw materials to finished products. The food technologist is interested in the "bioburden" of microorganisms present in or on a food and considers the types and numbers of organisms present. Species are important as they can include spoilage organisms, those desired in food fermentation, or even pathogenic microorganisms. The number of microorganisms is important because the more spoilage organisms there are, the more likely the food will spoil, the more difficul it is to preserve the food, and the more likely it is to harbor pathogens. Bioburden can be the result of contamination, the growth of organisms, or both. The quality of many types of food is judged in part by the number of microorganisms present. Here are some examples of the importance of aseptic methods in the food industry.

Food packaging is a widely used application of asepsis. Packaging can range from a carton or grain package, which primarily prevents contamination during handling, to a tightly sealed canned food container, which, if undamaged, protects the processed contents from contamination by microorganisms.

In the dairy industry, contamination by microorganisms is avoided as much as possible in the production and handling of drinking milk and milk intended for other purposes, and the quality of the milk is judged by its bacterial content.

In the canning industry, the bioburden or microbial load determines the thermal process necessary to preserve a food, especially if the contamination introduces heat-resistant spoilage organisms, such as sporulated thermophiles that can come from the crew; and the sealed box prevents recontamination after heat treatment.

In the meat packing industry, sanitary methods of slaughtering, handling and processing reduce the burden and thus improve the quality of keeping the meat or meat products.

In industries that involve the controlled fermentation of food, for example in the manufacture of cheese, the fewer competing organisms in the fermentation material, the more likely that the fermentation will be successful.

REMOVAL OF MICROORGANISMS

In most cases, the removal of microorganisms is not very effecti e for food preservation, but under special conditions it can be useful. Removal can be accomplished by filtration, centrifugation (sedimentation or clarification), washing, or cutting

Filtration is the only effecti e method for complete removal of organisms and its use is limited to clear liquids. The liquid is filtered through a previously sterilized "antibacterial" filter made of sintered glass, diatomaceous earth, unglazed porcelain, membrane covers, or similar materials, and the liquid is penetrated by positive or negative pressure. This method has been used successfully for fruit juices, beer, soft drinks, wine, and water.

Centrifugation, or sedimentation, is generally not very effecti e, as some, but not all, microorganisms are removed. Sedimentation is used in drinking water treatment, but by itself is not sufficient When centrifugation (clarification) is applied to milk, the primary objective is not to remove bacteria, but to remove other suspended matter, although high-speed centrifugation removes most spores.

Washing raw foods can be beneficial for their preservation, but can be harmful under certain conditions. Washing heads of cabbage or cucumbers before fermentation into sauerkraut and pickles, respectively, removes most of the microorganisms from the surface of the soil and thus increases the percentage of desirable lactic acid bacteria in the total flora. Washing fresh fruits and vegetables helps to remove soil organisms that may be resistant to the heat preservation process. It is clear that the removal of organisms and food intended for these organisms from food contact equipment, followed by microbial treatment of the equipment, is an essential and effecti e procedure when handling all types of foods. Washing food can be hazardous if the water adds spoilage organisms or increases humidity to encourage the growth of spoilage organisms.

Cutting off spoiled parts of a food or discarding spoiled samples is important from a food law perspective and can be beneficial for food preservation. Even if a large number of spoilage organisms are eliminated in this way, serious contamination of the remaining food may occur. It is recommended to cut off the outer leaves of the cabbage heads to make sauerkraut.

MAINTENANCE OF ANAEROBIC CONDITIONS

Anaerobic conditions in containers can be a factor in the preservation of packaged and sealed foods. Completely filling, evacuating the headspace (the free space in a box), or replacing the air with carbon dioxide or an inert gas such as nitrogen will cause anaerobic conditions. The spores of some aerobic spores are particularly resistant to heat and can survive in canned foods, but they are unable to germinate or grow in the absence of oxygen. Production of carbon dioxide during fermentation and accumulation on the surface serve to create anaerobic conditions and prevent the growth of aerobes.

Heat-Based Food Preservation Methods

6

Heat-based food preservation methods involve using high temperatures to kill or deactivate microorganisms, enzymes, and spoilage agents. Common techniques include pasteurization, sterilization, and blanching. Pasteurization involves heating food to a specific temperature (typically 60-85°C) for a set time to kill harmful microorganisms without affecting the food's nutritional quality. This method is commonly used in dairy products, juices, and canned vegetables.

Sterilization uses higher temperatures (above 100°C) to destroy all microorganisms, ensuring long-term shelf life, as seen in canned foods and some sauces. This process often involves pressure cooking or autoclaving. Blanching involves briefly immersing food in boiling water or steam, followed by rapid cooling. This technique is commonly used for vegetables before freezing to inactivate enzymes and reduce microbial load without significantly affecting texture or color.

These heat treatments are crucial in reducing the risk of foodborne illness, preserving flavor, and extending the shelf life of food products

Depending on the method of heat application, it may kill only some of the vegetative cells, most or all of the cells, part of the bacterial spores, or all of them. The chosen heat treatment will depend on the types of microorganisms to be eradicated, other preservation methods used, and the impact of heat on the food.

FACTORS INFLUENCING HEAT RESISTANCE (THERMAL DEATH TIME)

The thermal death time (TDT) of microorganisms refers to the time required to kill a specific number of microbes at a given temperature. Several factors influence the heat resistance of microorganisms, affecting the effecti eness of heat-based food preservation methods.

Cells and spores of microorganisms differ widely in their resistance to high temperatures. Some of these differences are the result of factors that can be controlled, but others are characteristic of the organisms and cannot always be explained. There are differences in heat resistance within a population of cells or spores, as illustrated by the frequency distribution curve. A small number of cells have low resistance (points A to B); most of the cells have a medium resistance (points B to C); and a small number have high resistance (points C to D). Conditions of growth may favor one or the other of these groups, and, by selection, cultures that are more or less heat-resistant than usual can be produced.

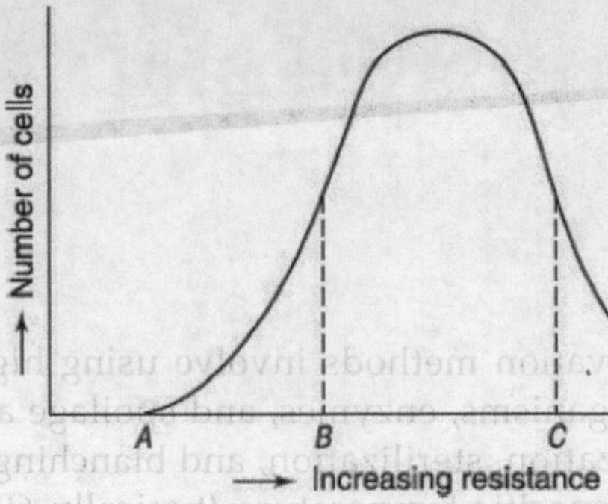

Fig 6.1. Frequency distribution curve depicting heat resistance in a culture.

Several factors are known to impact the heat resistance of cells or spores, and these should be considered when comparing microorganisms or planning heat treatments for their destruction. The main factors include:

Temperature-time Relationship: The time required to kill cells or spores decreases as the temperature increases. This is demonstrated in Table 6.1, which presents the findings of Bigelow and Esty (1920) for 115,000 spores of flat sour bacteria per milliliter in corn juice at pH 6.1.

Previous History of the Cells or Spores: The growth conditions of the cells and the method of spore production, along with any treatments received afterward, will affect their heat resistance

Initial Concentration of Spores (or Cells): A higher concentration of spores or cells necessitates a more intense heat treatment to ensure complete destruction. Bigelow and Esty's study on thermophilic spores from spoiled canned food in corn juice at pH 6.0 at 120°C, shown in Table, illustrates this.

Table . Effect of Temperature of Heating on Time Needed to Kill Spores of Flat Sour Bacteria

Temperature, °C	Thermal death time, or time to destroy all spores, minutes
100	1,200
105	600
110	190
115	70
120	19
125	7
130	3
135	1

Table. Effect of Initial Numbers of Spores on Time Required to Kill them

Initial concentration of spores, number/ml	Thermal death time, or time required to kill all spores, min at 120°C
50,000	14
5,000	10
500	9
50	8

- **Culture Medium***:* The environment in which growth occurs plays a critical role. The type and quantity of nutrients in the medium affect the organism's heat resistance, with the general trend being that the better the growth medium, the more resistant the cells or spores tend to be. The presence of essential growth factors typically promotes the formation of heat-resistant cells or spores. This may explain why substances like vegetable infusions and liver extract enhance heat resistance. According to Curran (1935), spores grown and aged in soil or oats are more resistant compared to those cultivated in broth or agar. The influence of carbohydrates, amino acids, and organic acid radicals is variable and difficul to predict. For instance, a small amount of glucose in the medium might increase heat resistance, but excess sugar can lead to acid accumulation, which reduces resistance. Certain salts, such as phosphate and magnesium ions, are believed to lower the heat resistance of bacterial spores grown in mediums containing them. Additionally, prolonged exposure to metabolic byproducts tends to decrease the heat resistance of cells and spores.
- **Temperature of Incubation:** The temperature of growth of cells and the temperature of sporulation influences their heat resistance. In general, resistance increases as the incubation temperature is raised toward the optimum for the organism and for many organisms increases further as the temperature approaches the maximum for growth. Escherichia coli, for example, is considerably more heat-resistant when grown at 38.5°C, which is near its optimal temperature, than at 28°C. Spores of Bacillus subtilis, grown at different temperatures in 1 percent peptone water, were heated with the results shown in Table.

Table. Effect of Temperature of Formation of Spores of *Bacillus subtilis* on their Heat Resistance

Temperature of spore formation	Heat resistance	Comments
20°C	Low	Spores formed at this temperature have reduced heat resistance.
30°C	Moderate	Heat resistance begins to increase with a higher formation temperature.

Temperature of spore formation	Heat resistance	Comments
40°C	High	Spores formed at 40°C exhibit significantly higher heat resistance
50°C	Very High	Spores formed at this higher temperature show maximum heat resistance.
60°C	Extremely High	Heat resistance is at its peak, spores are highly resistant to heat damage.
70°C	Variable	Some spores may begin to lose heat resistance at this extreme temperature.

This table outlines how the heat resistance of *Bacillus subtilis* spores increases with the temperature at which they are formed, showing the correlation between formation temperature and resistance to heat.

- **Phase of Growth or Age**: The heat resistance of vegetative cells changes depending on their growth stage, while the heat resistance of spores is influenced by their age. Bacterial cells exhibit their highest resistance during the late lag phase and similarly high resistance during the maximum stationary phase, with resistance declining afterward (refer to Chapter 5). Cells are most susceptible to heat during the logarithmic growth phase. Immature spores are less heat-resistant compared to mature ones. Some spores gain heat resistance during the first few weeks of storage, but this resistance begins to decline over time.
- **Desiccation**: Dried spores of some bacteria are harder to kill by heat than are those kept moist, but this apparently does not hold for all bacterial spores.

Composition of the substrate in which cells or spores are heated. The material in which the spores or cells are heated is so important that it must be stated if a thermal death times is to have meaning.

- **Moisture:** Moist heat is far more effecti e at killing microorganisms than dry heat, meaning that dry materials require higher temperatures for sterilization compared to moist ones. In a bacteriological lab, sterilization of common materials is achieved in about 15 to 30 minutes at 121°C using the moist heat of an autoclave. However, when dry heat from an oven is used, the process takes 3 to 4 hours at temperatures between 160 to 180°C. For example, spores of *Bacillus subtilis* are destroyed in under 10 minutes at 120°C in steam, but sterilization in anhydrous glycerol requires 30 minutes at 170°C.
- **Hydrogen-ion Concentration (pH):** In general, cells or spores are most heat resistant in a substrate that is at or near neutrality. An increase in acidity or alkalinity hastens killing by heat, but a change toward the acid side is more effecti e than a corresponding increase in alkalinity. Spores

of *B. subtilis* heated at 100°C in 1-15 m phosphate solutions, adjusted to various pH values, gave the results shown in Table. Other examples will be given in the discussion of the heat processing of canned foods.

Table. Effect of pH on Heat Resistance of Spores of *Bacillius subtilis*

pH Level	Heat resistance of spores
4.0	Low resistance to heat
5.0	Moderate resistance to heat
6.0	Increased heat resistance
7.0	Optimal heat resistance
8.0	High heat resistance
9.0	Very high heat resistance
10.0	Heat resistance begins to decrease

This table highlights the relationship between pH and the heat resistance of *Bacillus subtilis* spores. As the pH shifts from acidic to slightly alkaline, the heat resistance generally increases, peaking around neutral pH and then beginning to decline in highly alkaline environments.

Cameron (1940) categorized canned foods into two main groups based on their pH values-acid foods with a pH below 4.5 and low-acid foods with a pH above 4.5. Acid foods typically include common fruits and certain vegetables, while low-acid foods include meat, seafood, milk, and most vegetables. Cameron further subdivided low-acid foods into four categories:

- **Low-acid foods** with a pH above 5.3, such as peas, corn, lima beans, meats, fish, poultry, and milk (though Cameron originally included only vegetables and fruits in his grouping).
- **Medium-acid foods** with a pH between 5.3 and 4.5, such as spinach, asparagus, beets, and pumpkin.
- **Acid foods** with a pH between 4.5 and 3.7, including tomatoes, pears, and pineapple.
- **High-acid foods** with a pH of 3.7 or below, such as berries and sauerkraut.

The effect of pH on food is influenced by the fact that heating at high temperatures lowers the pH of low- or medium-acid foods. The higher the initial pH, the more significant the decrease in pH during heating. Foods with an initial pH of less than 5.5 to 5.8 show little change in acidity after heating

- **Other Constituents of the Substrate:** The only salt present in appreciable amounts in most foods is sodium chloride, which in low concentrations has a protective effect on some spores.

Sugar seems to protect some organisms or spores but not others. The optimal concentration for protection varies with the organism- it is high for some osmophilic

Table. Effect of Protective Substances on Heat Resistance of Bacteria

	Temperature		
Substance	***S. lactis***	***E. coli***	***L. bulgaricus***
Cream	69-71	73	95
Whole milk	63-65	69	91
Skim milk	59-63	65	89
Whey	57-61	63	83
Broth	55-57	61	

It can be observed that as the levels of protective substances (such as proteins and fats) in the media decrease, the temperature required to kill the organism within 10 minutes also decreases (Brown and Peiser, 1916). The temperature needed for killing varies depending on the organism, being high for spores and low for non-osmophilic cells. The protective effect of sugar may be linked to a decrease in water activity (aw), as reduced aw typically increases heat resistance.

Different solutes impact bacteria in distinct ways. For instance, glucose offers more protection against heat to *Escherichia coli* and *Pseudomonas fluorescens* compared to sodium chloride at aw levels close to the minimum for growth. Conversely, glucose provides little to no protection and may even be harmful to *Staphylococcus aureus*, while sodium chloride is highly protective.

Given that solute concentration can influence the heat treatment required for sterilization, food processors sometimes categorize foods into high-soluble-solids foods, such as syrups and concentrates, and low-soluble-solids foods, such as fruits, vegetables, and meats.

Colloidal substances, particularly proteins and fats, act as heat protectants. This is clearly demonstrated in the work of Brown and Peiser (1916), who observed thermal death points. Additionally, antiseptic or germicidal substances in the medium can assist heat in eliminating organisms. For example, the combination of hydrogen peroxide and heat is used to reduce bacterial content in sugar, a process also applied in milk processing.

THERMAL RESISTANCE OF MICROORGANISMS AND THEIR SPORES

Microorganisms' heat resistance is typically measured in terms of their thermal death time, which refers to the time required at a specific temperature to kill a certain number of organisms (or spores) under defined conditions. This is sometimes called the absolute thermal death time to differentiate it from the majority thermal death time, which refers to the time needed to kill most of the cells or spores, and the thermal death rate, which indicates the rate at which killing occurs.

Although, the term thermal death point is rarely used today, it originally referred to the temperature required to kill all organisms within 10 minutes.

Studies comparing the heat resistance of various yeasts, molds, bacteria, and their spores vary, mainly due to differences in the cultures used and the conditions during heating. As a result, only broad conclusions will be drawn, with specific examples from various researchers included.

HEAT RESISTANCE OF MOLDS AND MOLD SPORES

Most molds and their spores are destroyed by moist heat at 60°C within 5 to 10 minutes, though some species exhibit significantly higher heat resistance. Asexual spores are generally more heat-resistant than the mycelium, requiring temperatures 5 to 10°C higher to be destroyed within the same time frame. Species such as *Aspergillus* and certain *Penicillium* and *Mucor* molds are more heat-resistant than others. A particularly heat-resistant mold found on fruits is *Byssochlamys fulva* (*Paecilomyces*), which has resilient ascospores. The pasteurization processes used for milk typically kill all molds and their spores, although some aspergilli spores, not typically present in milk, might survive such treatments.

Sclerotia are particularly challenging to kill with heat, as some can endure temperatures of 90 to 100°C for short periods and cause spoilage in canned fruits. For example, destroying sclerotia from a *Penicillium* species required 1,000 minutes at 82.2°C or 300 minutes at 85°C. Mold spores also show considerable resistance to dry heat, with research indicating that dry heat at 120°C for up to 30 minutes may not be sufficient to eliminate some of the more resistant spore

Heat Resistance of Yeasts and Yeast Spores

The resistance of yeasts and their spores to moist heat varies depending on the species, strain, and the substrate in which they are heated. Generally, the ascospores of yeasts require only 5 to 10°C more heat to be destroyed compared to the vegetative cells from which they originate. Most ascospores are killed by heating at 60°C for 10 to 15 minutes, although a few may exhibit greater resistance. None, however, can survive even brief exposure to 100°C. Vegetative yeasts are typically destroyed at temperatures between 50°C and 58°C for 10 to 15 minutes. Both yeasts and their spores are killed during pasteurization processes, such as heating milk at 62.8°C for 30 minutes or 71.7°C for 15 seconds, and yeasts are easily killed during bread baking, where the interior temperature reaches about 97°C.

Heat Resistance of Bacteria and Bacterial Spores

The heat resistance of bacterial vegetative cells varies significantly depending on the species, ranging from easily killed delicate pathogens to thermophiles that may need several minutes at temperatures between 80 to 90°C. A few general observations about the heat resistance of bacterial vegetative cells include- (1) cocci are generally more heat-resistant than rods, although there are exceptions, (2) bacteria with higher optimal and maximal growth temperatures are more likely to be heat-resistant, (3) bacteria that tend to clump or form capsules are more difficul to kill than those that do not, and (4) cells with high lipid content are more resistant to heat than other types of cells.

A few examples of thermal death times of bacterial cells are shown in Table.

It should be kept in mind that these thermal death times (and those to be given later for spores) are for various concentrations of cells (or spores), heated in different substrates, and might be higher or lo er under other conditions.

Table. Thermal Death Times of Bacterial Cells

Bacterial species	Temperature (°C)	Time to kill	Note
Escherichia coli	55°C	10-15 minutes	Easily killed at lower temperatures.
Staphylococcus aureus	60°C	5-10 minutes	Resistant compared to E. coli.
Salmonella enterica	60°C	10-15 minutes	Similar resistance to E. coli.
Clostridium botulinum	80°C	2-3 minutes	Highly resistant spores.
Bacillus subtilis	85°C	5-7 minutes	Resistance varies with spore maturity.
Listeria monocytogenes	70°C	10-12 minutes	Can survive pasteurization.
Campylobacter jejuni	55°C	15-20 minutes	Relatively heat-sensitive.
Pseudomonas aeruginosa	60°C	10-15 minutes	Moderately resistant to heat.
Mycobacterium tuberculosis	75°C	15-30 minutes	Highly heat-resistant due to cell wall.

This table summarizes the thermal death times for various bacterial species under specific heat conditions. The time required to kill the bacteria depends on factors like the species, strain, and environmental conditions during heating.

The heat resistance of bacterial spores varies greatly with the species of bacterium and the conditions during sporulation. Resistance at 100°C may vary from less that 1 min to over 20 hr. In general, spores from bacteria with high optimal and maximal temperatures for growth are more heat-resistant than those from bacteria growing best at lower temperatures. Or a sporeformer growing with another of higher heat resistance may have increased resistance, e.g., *Clostridium perfringens* growing with *C sporogenes*. Examples of thermal death times of bacterial spores are given in Table.

Table. Thermal Death Times of Bacterial Spores

Spores of Bacterial	Time (minutes) to kill at 100°C
Bacillus anthracis	1.7
Bacillus subtilis	15–20
Clostridium botulinum	100–330
*Clostridium calidotolerans**	520
Flat sour bacteria	Over 1,030

Heat Resistance of Enzymes

While most food and microbial enzymes are deactivated at 79.4°C, certain enzymes can survive higher temperatures, particularly when high-temperature-short-time treatments are used. A key objective of thermal processing (Witter, 1983) is to deactivate enzymes that could cause product spoilage during storage. Generally, processes aimed at killing microorganisms also deactivate problematic enzymes.

However, there are significant exceptions. For instance, some hydrolases (proteinases and lipases) can maintain considerable activity after ultrahigh-temperature treatment. The remaining activity of these enzymes could spoil the product over extended storage periods. Additionally, bovine phosphatase is used as a "marker" in milk pasteurization. The presence of this enzyme in processed milk typically indicates improper pasteurization. False positives may occur if high microbial phosphatase levels are present.

Determination of Heat Resistance (Thermal Death Time)

A detailed description of all the procedures and equipment used for determining the heat resistance of bacterial spores is beyond the scope of this text. For a comprehensive discussion on the methods for suspending and heating spores, as well as the equipment involved, refer to Nickerson and Sinskey (1972). Additionally, the National Canners Association Manual (1968) offers an extensive review of all aspects of thermal resistance determinations.

This text will provide an overview of Esty and Meyer's (1922) simple glass-tube method for determining thermal death time, while only briefly touching upon the more complex techniques used in canning laboratories. In this method, a standardized suspension of spores (or cells) in a buffer solution or food liquor is sealed in small glass tubes, which are then heated in a thermostatically controlled bath set to the desired temperature. The tubes are periodically removed, cooled immediately, and either incubated directly or subcultured into an appropriate medium for incubation to check for survivor growth. A basic outline of the method is provided.

Preparation of the Spore (or Cell) Suspension

Various bacteria are utilized as "test organisms," depending on the specific process used (Table 6.8). These organisms are cultured in a medium under conditions (temperature and time) that promote the formation of resistant spores (or cells). They are then harvested from solid media or centrifuged from liquid media, washed, and prepared into a suspension. To ensure consistency, it is important to break up or eliminate any clumps, as this can lead to irregular results. This is typically achieved by shaking the suspension with glass beads or sand, or by filtering through materials like cotton, gauze, or filter pape

In some cases, the spore suspension is reincubated for 24 hours to complete the sporulation process. The suspension is then pasteurized to kill any vegetative cells, which could offer protection. Following this, the concentration of spores (or cells) per unit volume is determined using a cultural or direct counting method. This stock suspension is diluted in the heating medium to achieve the desired concentration for the test, and the suspension is dispensed in 1- milliliter portions into glass vials, which are sealed and refrigerated. The heating medium can be a buffered phosphate solution, food, or food liquor. The volume of the suspension added should be minimal (1 to 2 percent) to avoid altering the composition of the heating substrate. A concentration of about 1 million (1 × 10^6) cells or spores per milliliter or gram is recommended.

Table. Bacteria Used as Test Organisms

Bacteria used	Processing of test purpose
Clostridium sporogenes (P.A. 3679)	Inoculated pack studies
*Bacillus subtilis var niger** (syn. *B. globigii*, ATCC 9372)	Hot air and ethylene oxide studies
Bacillus pumilus (ATCC 27142)	Cobalt or gamma radiation sterilization
Bacillus stearothemophilus (ATCC 7953)	Steam sterilization
Bacillus subtilis (ATCC 6633)	Steam sterilization

Heating to Determine the Thermal Death Time

- The heating of the vials is done in an agitated and thermostatically controlled bath of oil for higher temperatures or water for temperatures below 100°C. Tubes are heated at one temperature for varying intervals of time. The following precautions are taken:
- The vials are brought to a definite temperature before introduction into the bath, usually at 0°C, obtained in a bath of ice water. An arbitrary preheating time, for example, 30 sec, is allowed before timing begins. Vials of resistant spores sometimes are preheated to 100°C in boiling water before being introduced into the bath.
- When using an oil bath, it is important to wipe the vials dry before placing them in the bath and to seal them carefully, as water can cause the oil to foam. If a large number of iced vials are added simultaneously, the cooling effect on the bath must be taken into account
- For accurate results, the multiple- tube method is recommended. A minimum of fi e replicate vials should be used in exploratory trials, and

twenty- fi e to thirty vials when tubes are removed at short intervals. Fewer replicates increase the likelihood of "skips," where killing occurs after a certain period, followed by survival after a longer heating period.

Test for Viability (Survival)

If the substrate used for heating provides a good culture medium for the organism and the organism can grow anaerobically, the vials can be incubated to check for the growth of survivors.

Otherwise, the vial contents are subcultured into a suitable culture medium and incubated under optimal conditions for the organism. To determine the number of survivors, a quantitative count is performed using methods like the agar plate or other cultural techniques. The composition of the survival testing medium is critical, as spores or cells exposed to extreme heat may have stricter nutritional requirements than before heating. Instead of vials, the American Can Company uses special flat cans that can be evacuated, sealed, and then heated and cooled in small steam sterilizers. The National Food Processors Association laboratories employ a unit with valves that allows periodic sample withdrawals under aseptic conditions. This method is useful for determining thermal death rates. Several of these procedures are described by Lopez (1981).

Thermal Death Time (TDT) Curves

One method for obtaining data and plotting TDT curves is referred to as the growth- no- growth method. An example of data that might be obtained by this procedure using a series of six tubes or vials at each time interval is presented in Table 6.9. At a heating temperature of 110°C for 110 min none of six tubes contained survivors, but there were survivors following 80 min of heating. Thus for these specific conditions (number of spores, heating menstruum, etc.) the thermal death time at 110°C is greater than 80 min but less than or equal to 110 min.

Table. Thermal Death Time Data

Temperature	Corrected heating time, min	Number of samples	
		Heated	Positive
110 °C (230 °F)	25	6	6
	40	6	6
	60	6	6
	80	6	5
	110	6	0
	140	6	0
115.6 °C (240 °F)	10	6	6
	14	6	6
	18	6	6
	22	6	2

	28	6	0
	36	6	0
121 °C (250 °F)	3	6	6
	4	6	6
	5.5	6	2
	7.5	6	0
	10	6	0
	13	6	0

Source- Condensed from National Canners Association (1968). Data on PA 3679 in strained peas.

If the TDT values from Table are plotted on semilogarithmic paper, the curve in Figure results. Temperature is plotted using arithmetic values, while time in minutes is plotted logarithmically. In this method, a single line (line A) is drawn above all survivor points and below all destruction points. Alternatively, survivor points are connected with one line, and destruction points with another. Then, the average slope of these two lines is used to create a single line.

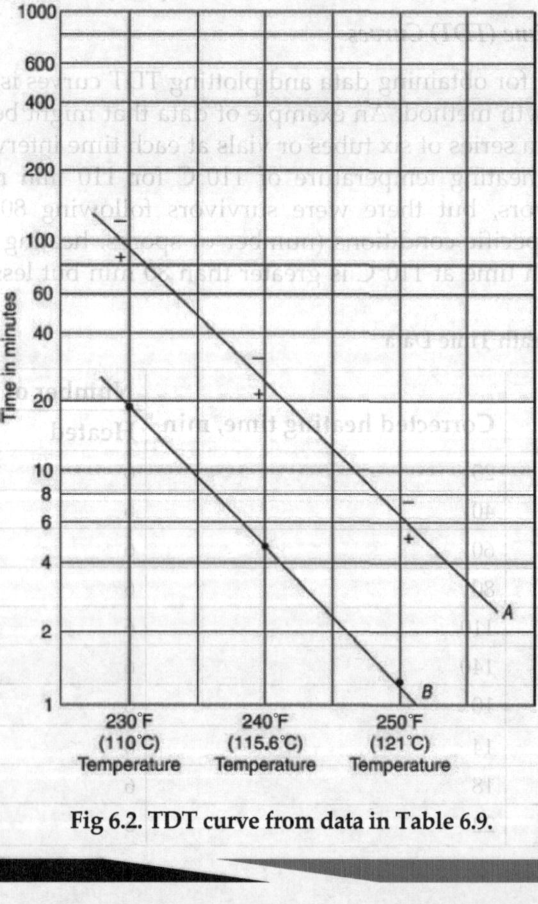

Fig 6.2. TDT curve from data in Table 6.9.

The classical endpoint method of Bigelow and Esty (1920) is similar, except that survival is observed in only one of several tubes at each temperature. For instance, their original study used a spore population of 6×10^9 per tube and heating continued until only one tube out of ten had one or more survivors. This approach reflects a population of 6×10^{10} being reduced to about 1. The time required can be used as the thermal death time (TDT), and TDTs can be plotted to generate a TDT curve.

Another approach involves first determining death rate or survivor curves at various temperatures. For instance, by counting survivors at different time intervals during the heating of a spore population, a survivor curve is plotted with the number of survivors on a logarithmic scale and time on an arithmetic scale.

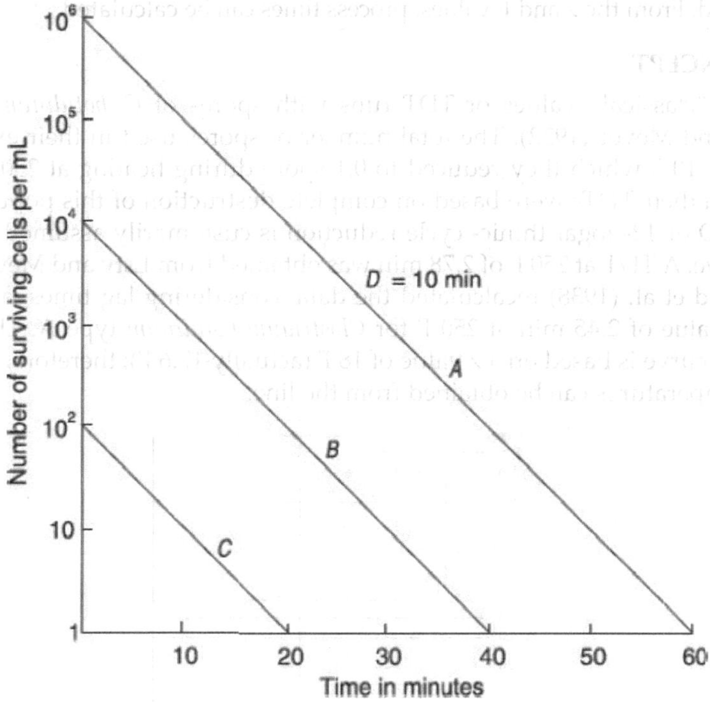

Fig 6.3. Hypothetical survivor curves

The death rate curve is represented by the line, and the symbol D denotes the decimal reduction time— the time needed to reduce the viable spore count by 90%. A TDT curve for a given spore suspension can be constructed if D values at several temperatures are known. By plotting D values (in minutes) on a logarithmic scale and temperature in degrees Fahrenheit on an arithmetic scale, a line can be drawn to represent the TDT curve. This line, however, is referred to as a "phantom" TDT curve because it shows the correct slope but not the exact position when compared to points derived from complete destruction times for a specific spore concentration.

Whether an endpoint method or a growth- no- growth method is used or D values, TDTs are plotted to give a TDT curve. The straight line indicates that the order of death by heat is logarithmic, in other words, that the death rate is constant. From the straight line obtained or an extension of it, TDTs for temperatures and times not listed can be estimated. The slope of the line is termed the z value and is the interval in temperature, in degrees Fahrenheit, required for the line to pass through one logarithmic cycle on the semilogarithmic paper. In other words, z represents the degrees Fahrenheit required to reduce the TDT tenfold. The z value can also be expressed in degrees Celsius but should be stated as z C. F is the time in minutes required to destroy the organism in a specified medium at 250 F (121.1°C). The uncorrected z value. and the F value1 is 16.4 min. These vales will vary with the heat resistance and concentration of the test organism and with the medium in which it is heated. From the z and F values, process times can be calculated.

12D CONCEPT

The "classical" values or TDT runs with spores of *C. botulinum* are those of Esty and Meyer (1922). The total number of spores used in their experiments was 6.0×10^{10}, which they reduced to 0.1 spore during heating at 250 F (121°C). Although their TDTs were based on complete destruction of this population, the value 12D or 12- logarithmic- cycle reduction is customarily assumed from their TDT curve. A TDT at 250 F of 2.78 min was obtained from Esty and Meyer's curve. Townsend et al. (1938) recalculated the data, considering lag times, and arrived at an F value of 2.45 min at 250 F for *Clostridum botulinum* type A. The slope of this TDT curve is based on a z value of 18 F (actually 17.6 F); therefore, F values at other temperatures can be obtained from the line.

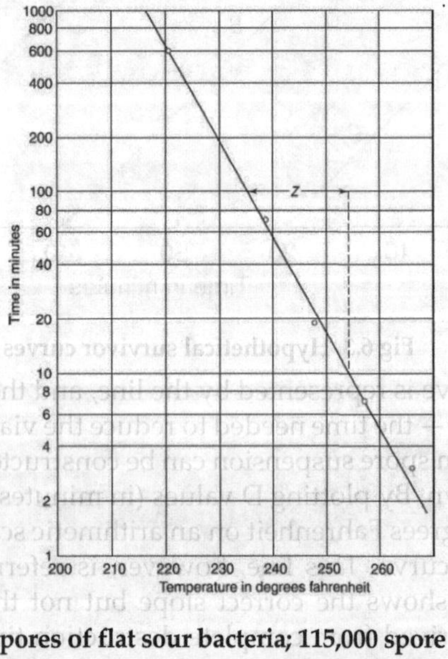

Fig 6.4. TDT curve for spores of flat sour bacteria; 115,000 spore per milliliter in corn at pH 6. (z = 19).

As a safety measure, the canning industry has recommended a 12D heat treatment for *C. botulinum* spores in low- acid foods, i.e., enough heat or process lethality to reduce 10^{12} spores to one spore per milliliter. In reality, starting populations would never approach 1×10^{12} spores per milliliter or gram; therefore, 12D reflects processing to extreme fractions of a spore or one spore surviving in one can among an extremely large number of cans processed. Stumbo (1964) presented an illustration of the 12D concept as follows- assuming that D has a value of 0.21 min for *C. botulinum* at 250 F and that each can of food contains one spore, a process at 250 F for 2.52 min would reduce *C. botulinum* spores to one spore in 10^{12} cans. This can be shown mathematically as follows:

$$F0 = D250(\log a - \log b)$$
$$= 0.21\ (\log 1 - \log 10{-}12)$$
$$= 0.21 \times 12 = 2.52$$

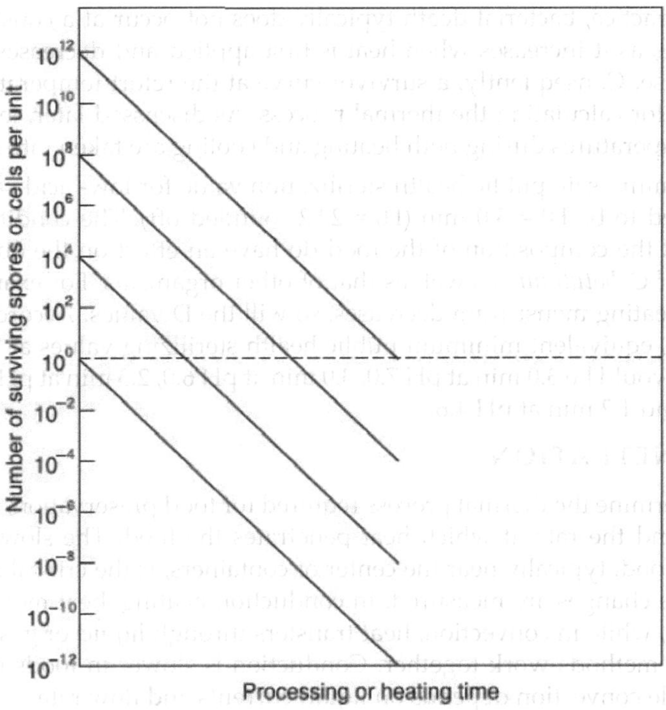

Fig 6.5. Extrapolation of hypothetical survivor curves illustrating a 12D or 12- log-cycle reduction.

When it is considered that processes employed commercially usually exceed this F0 value (treatments of F0 = 6.0 to 8.0 are not unusual) to eliminate the more heat- resistant thermophilic sporeformers, an additional safety margin is realized. The 12D concept is therefore somewhat arbitrary but universally used. The understanding of D values and length of time to reduce a given population when a given D value is known or assumed can be further clarified by consulting Figure.

As illustrated, the higher the initial count of cells or spores, the longer it takes to reduce the number to one per milliliter. For instance, with a D value of 10 minutes as shown in the figure, it would take 60 minutes to reduce the spore count from 1 million to 1 spore per milliliter, whereas only 20 minutes would be needed if there were 100 spores initially. After 80 minutes, theoretically, there would be 0.01 spores per milliliter, or 1 spore per 100 milliliters of the heating medium. This concept of processing to achieve fractions of a spore per unit or one spore per multiple units. Survivor curves, however, do not always follow the straight- line pattern shown. Convex curves may occur due to the clumping of cells or spores, or because injured cells can repair some of the damage.

Concave curves are believed to result from varying resistance among individual cells or spores. A shoulder at the beginning of the curve might suggest a slower inactivation rate of cells or spores, while a tailing effect after significant reductions in numbers indicates that some cells or spores are more resistant than others. In practice, bacterial death typically does not occur at a constant heating temperature, as it increases when heat is first applied and decreases during the cooling phase. Consequently, a survivor curve at the retort temperature alone is insufficien for calculating the thermal process. As discussed later, lethal rates at varying temperatures during both heating and cooling are taken into account.

A minimum safe public health sterilization value for low- acid canned foods is considered to be F0 = 3.0 min (F0 = 2.52 rounded off). The conditions during heating and the composition of the food do have an effect on the observed heat resistance of *C. botulinum* as well as that of other organisms. For example, as the pH of the heating menstruum decreases, so will the D values. According to Pflug et al. (1985), equivalent minimum public health sterilizing values at 250 °F for C. botulinum would be 3.0 min at pH 7.0, 3.0 min at pH 6.0, 2.3 min at pH 5.5, 1.6 min at pH 5.0, and 1.2 min at pH 4.6.

HEAT PENETRATION

To determine the thermal process required for food preservation, it's essential to understand the rate at which heat penetrates the food. The slowest- heating part of the food, typically near the center of containers, is the critical area, and its temperature changes are measured. In conduction heating, heat moves molecule to molecule, while in convection, heat transfers through liquid or gas movement. Often, both methods work together. Conduction is slower in foods but faster in metals, while convection depends on liquid currents and flow rate

When both conduction and convection are present, they may act simultaneously or in succession. In suspensions of solid food particles in liquid, conduction heats the particles, and convection heats the liquid. Some foods, like sugar syrups or tomato juices, change consistency during heating, causing irregular heating curves.

Several factors affect the time needed to heat food in a container to sterilizing temperature:

- **Initial Food Temperature**: The initial temperature of the food in the can has minimal effect on the time to reach the retort temperature, but food at a higher initial temperature spends more time in the lethal range for microorganisms and heats more uniformly.

- **Retort Temperature**: Food reaches the retort temperature at similar times, but the fastest heating occurs in the hottest retort, reaching lethal temperatures quickly.
- **Container Material**: Glass heats slower than metal cans.
- **Size and Shape of the Container**: Larger cans take longer to heat due to greater distance to the center and lower surface- to- volume ratio. Slim, cylindrical cans heat faster than compact ones.
- **Consistency of Food**: The consistency and size of food pieces influenc heat penetration, requiring classification based on how pieces behave during cooking.
    - o Pieces that retain their identity, i.e., do not cook apart. Examples are peas, plums, beets, asparagus, and whole- grain corn. If the pieces are small and in brine, as with peas, heating is almost as in water. If the pieces are large, heating is delayed, because the heat must penetrate to the center of the pieces before the liquor can reach the retort temperature. Large beets or large stalks of asparagus heat more slowly than small ones.
    - o Pieces that cook apart and become mushy or viscous. These heat slowly, because heat penetration becomes mostly by conduction rather than convection. This takes place in cream- style corn, squash, pumpkin, and sweet potatoes.
    - o Pieces that layer. Asparagus layers vertically; hence, convection currents travel mostly up and down. Spinach layers horizontally, producing a "baffle board effect", which interferes with convection currents. Layering is greatly affected by the degree of fill of the can

The consistency of the contents in the can is influenced by the addition of certain sauces. For example, tomato sauce on baked beans slows heat penetration more than plain sauce. Starch, when its concentration rises toward 6%, increasingly interferes with heat transfer, but beyond this concentration, additional starch has little further impact. Sodium chloride, when added, does not reach concentrations high enough to significantly affect the heating rate. The rate of heat penetration also decreases with higher sugar concentrations; however, this effect is somewhat offset by the substantial reduction in the viscosity of sugar solutions— even thick ones— as the temperature increases.

Rotation and agitation. Rotating or agitating the container during heat processing can speed up heat penetration if the food is fluid, but it may also lead to undesirable physical changes in some foods. It has minimal impact on foods with free convection currents and small particles, such as peas. However, agitation is beneficial for foods that tend to layer, like spinach, tomatoes, and peach halves. Older equipment typically limits can rotation from 10 to 12 rpm, but newer methods of end- over- end rotation allow higher speeds.

Rotation is effecti e for canned evaporated milk, and shaking is used for pastes or purees. A process for brined, whole- kernel corn uses a continuous cooker with high- boiling liquid, where the can contents are mixed by rotating on a reel or rollers. Cooling follows similar heat transfer principles, with rapid, controlled cooling being preferred. Slow cooling can lead to overcooking and allow thermophiles to grow.

DETERMINATION OF THERMAL PROCESSES

The following data are needed for the calculation of thermal processes for a canned food- (1) the TDT curve for the most heat- resistant organism likely to be present in the food; in low- acid foods this usually would be for the spores of a thermophile, e.g., the flat sour organism, and (2) the heat penetration and cooling curves for the food in the size and type of container to be used. One of three methods is used to determine the heat process: (1) the graphical method, (2) the formula method, or (3) the nomogram method.

By each of these methods equivalent processes can be calculated, i.e., heat processes that effect the same killing of microorganisms in the food.

The principle is similar for all three of the methods for the calculation of thermal processes, but since the graphical method is the simplest to explain, it will be outlined and the others will be only briefly mentioned.

General Method for Calculation of Process Time

To calculate the time in minutes t necessary to destroy a certain number of test organisms (or spores) in a given container of a food by heating at the temperature T, knowing the values for z and F, the following equations are employed (t/F = time to destroy organism at temperature T if F = 1; F/t = lethal rate at T):

then

$$\frac{\log t - \log F}{\log 10\ (=1)} = \frac{250 - T}{z}$$

or

$$\log \frac{t}{F} = \frac{250 - T}{z} \quad \text{and} \quad \frac{t}{f} = \text{antilog}\ \frac{250 - T}{z}$$

$$t = F\ \text{antilog}\ \frac{250 - T}{z}$$

The Graphical Method

Briefly, the graphical method, as described by Bigelow et al. (1920), is as follows:

- The TDT curve for the most heat- resistant spoilage organism in the food being canned is established. TDT values from this curve are then converted into lethal rates for various heating temperatures. The lethal rate for a specific temperature is the inverse of the TDT. For example, if it takes 400 minutes at 210°F to eliminate all the spores, the lethal rate is 1/400 = 0.0025.

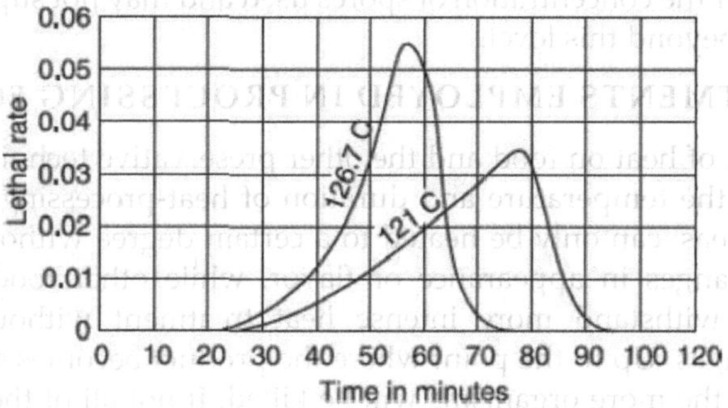

Fig 6.6. Equivalent lethality curves with retort at 126.7°C and 121°C. Corn in no. 2 cans; 50,000 spores per milliliter.

- The heat-penetration (and cooling) curve for the specific food and can size is determined.
- Lethal rates for different temperatures at the can's center during both heating and cooling are plotted on the heat- penetration (and cooling) curve. Lethal rates are 0.01 unit per side of a square, with times set to 10 minutes per side. An area equal to ten squares beneath the lethality curve signifies complete destruction of all spores (or cells). If this area is less than ten squares, the process is insufficient if it exceeds ten squares, the process is excessive. The area under the curve is measured using a planimeter.

The Formula Method

The thermal process is mathematically calculated using the formula method, which applies data from the TDT and heat penetration curves to an equation. See Ball and Olson (1957) for specifics on this approach

The Nomogram Method

The nomogram method is the quickest way to estimate heat treatment time. It involves applying TDT and heat penetration data to a graphical representation of these numerical relationships and has an advantage over the methods described previously in that the "growth time" of steam pressure sterilizers is taken into account. The original paper by Olson and Stevens (1939) should be consulted for a description of this method.

Regardless of the method used for this calculation of heat treatment times, they are verified by actual tests on canned foods. An experimental package is inoculated with a known concentration of spores of the spoilage- resistant organism. These plates and uninoculated controls are treated for several time intervals close to that calculated for the selected temperature, incubated to test for spoilage, and subcultured to test for sterility.

A safety margin is usually allowed beyond the minimum treatment to kill the tested spores when recommendations are made regarding the time of heat treatment. It should be borne in mind that the recommended procedures will be effecti e only for the concentration of spores used and may not support significant contamination beyond this level.

HEAT TREATMENTS EMPLOYED IN PROCESSING FOODS

The impact of heat on food and the other preservative techniques to be used will determine the temperature and duration of heat-processing. Certain foods, like milk and peas, can only be heated to a certain degree without experiencing unfavorable changes in appearance or flavor, while other foods, like corn or pumpkin, can withstand more intense heat treatment without experiencing significant changes. Up to the point where the product becomes sterile, the more heat treatment, the more organisms will be killed. If not all of the organisms are eliminated, either the food must be handled to stop the growth of any remaining spoilage organisms or the heating must eliminate all possible spoilage organisms.

While most of the spoilage organisms are killed during pasteurization, some survive and must be inhibited by low temperatures or another preservative method in order to prevent spoiling. In canning, every effort is made to eliminate any organisms that could cause the food to spoil during subsequent handling. One could categorize the different levels of heating applied to food into three groups: (1) pasteurization, (2) heating at approximately 100 degrees Celsius, and (3) heating above 100 degrees Celsius.

Pasteurization

Pasteurization is a heat treatment process that kills a portion of the microorganisms present but not all, typically using temperatures below 100°C. The heating may be done with steam, hot water, dry heat, or electric currents, and the product is cooled quickly afterward. Pasteurization is used in several situations: (1) when more intense heat treatments could damage the product, such as market milk, (2) when the goal is to kill pathogens, as with market milk, (3) when the primary spoilage organisms are not very heat-resistant, like yeasts in fruit juices, (4) when surviving spoilage organisms will be controlled by additional preservation methods, as in the chilling of market milk, and (5) when unwanted organisms are eliminated to allow for desired fermentation, as in cheese- making, often with the introduction of starter cultures.

To complement pasteurization, various preservation methods are employed, such as (1) refrigeration (e.g., for milk), (2) preventing microorganisms from entering by packaging in sealed containers, (3) maintaining anaerobic conditions in evacuated, sealed containers, (4) adding high concentrations of sugar, as in sweetened condensed milk, and (5) using chemical preservatives, like organic acids in pickles.

The pasteurization times and temperatures vary depending on the method used and the food being processed. The high- temperature- short- time (HTST) method uses high temperatures for short periods, while the low- temperature: long- time (LTH) or holding method uses lower temperatures for longer periods. For example, market milk is minimally treated at 62.8°C for 30 minutes in the LTH method, 71.7°C for at least 15 seconds in the HTST method, and 137.8°C for at least 2 seconds in the ultrapasteurized method. The treatment is selected based on the thermal resistance of the rickettsia responsible for Q fever, *Coxiella burnetti*, which may be transmitted via milk. The heat treatment may be more intense for milk used for other purposes but may be less so in cheese making, where aging of the cheese is required if raw milk is used.

Ice cream mix is pasteurized at higher temperatures than market milk, for instance, at 71.1°C for 30 minutes or 82.2°C for 16 to 20 seconds. Grape wines may be pasteurized for 1 minute at 82 to 85°C in bulk, while fruit wines are sometimes heated to over 62.8°C and bottled while hot. Beer is pasteurized at 60°C or higher, with the time depending on the temperature. Dried fruits are pasteurized in the package at 65.6 to 85°C for 30 to 90 minutes, with the duration varying depending on the type of fruit and package size. For fruit juices, pasteurization depends on acidity and whether they are in bulk or bottled. Bottled grape juice is recommended to be pasteurized at 76.7°C for 30 minutes or flash- treated in bulk at 80 to 85°C, while apple juice may be treated at 60°C for bottling or at 85 to 87.8°C for 30 to 60 seconds in bulk. Carbonated juices typically undergo an average heat treatment of 65.6°C for 30 minutes. Vinegar is pasteurized in the bottle in a water bath to at least 65.6°C, while flash- pasteurization ensures the vinegar reaches 65.6 to 71.1°C when the bottle is sealed. In bulk, vinegar is held at 60 to 65.6°C for 30 minutes

Heating at About 100°C

In the past, home canners processed foods at temperatures below 100°C for varying periods, which was enough to kill most microorganisms except for bacterial spores. This method was often sufficien for preserving low- and medium- acid foods. However, nowadays, home canners typically use pressure cookers for less acidic foods. Many acidic foods, such as sauerkraut and highly acidic fruits, can still be processed successfully at temperatures below 100°C. This is achieved by boiling the food, immersing the container in boiling water, or exposing it to flowing steam. Some very acidic foods, like sauerkraut, may be preheated to just under 100°C, packaged hot, and not further heat- processed. Blanching vegetables before freezing or drying involves brief heating at approximately 100°C.

During baking, the internal temperature of bread, cakes, and other baked goods approaches but does not exceed 100°C, as long as moisture is present, despite the oven being much hotter. The temperature of unsealed canned goods in the oven cannot surpass the boiling point of the liquid inside. Bacterial spores that survive the baking process (with a maximum temperature of about 97°C) can lead to spoilage, such as ropiness. Simmering refers to gentle boiling, with a temperature around 100°C.

In roasting meat, the internal temperature typically reaches about 60°C for rare beef, up to 80°C for well- done beef, and 85°C for pork roast. Frying heats the outer surface of the food very hot, but the center usually does not reach 100°C. In general, "cooking" is a vague term, but in the food industry, it refers to a specific time and temperature for thermal processing. Warming food can mean anything from a slight increase in temperature to heating it to 100°C.

Heating Above 100°C

Steam under pressure is typically used in steam-pressure sterilizers or retorts to reach temperatures above 100°C. As steam pressure rises, the retorts' temperature rises as well. At sea level, the temperature is therefore 100°C without pressure, 109°C with 5 lb of pressure, 115.5°C with 10 lb, and 121.5°C with 15 lb. High steam pressures are used to apply a high temperature for a few seconds when sterilizing liquid foods before putting them into sterile cans.

Using steam injection or infusion, followed by "flash evaporation" of the condensed steam and quick cooling, milk can be heated to temperatures of up to 150°C. This type of milk processing has been called ultrahigh-temperature, or UHT, processing. The procedure would "sterilize" the milk if the holding times were long enough, on the order of a few seconds. The next section will go into more detail about the heat treatments used in the production of canned goods.

Canning

Canning is the preservation of food in sealed containers, often involving heat treatment to prevent spoilage. Traditionally, most canning was done in tin- coated steel cans or glass containers, but newer materials such as aluminum, plastics, and composite materials are now also used. The term "canning" is often replaced with "hermetically sealed containers" to describe this preservation method.

The practice of preserving food by heating it in sealed containers dates back to 1765, when Spallanzani first experimented with this technique. However, it was Nicolas Appert, often regarded as the "father of canning," who developed and refined the method in the late 18th and early 19th centuries. In 1809, Appert won a French government prize for his book The Book for All Households, which detailed how to preserve a wide range of foods in cork- stoppered, wide- mouthed glass bottles by heating them in boiling water. Appert's methods, although not based on knowledge of microorganisms, laid the foundation for canning as we know it, and his process was later called "Appertization."

Over time, improvements in canning focused on better heat processing methods, the construction of more durable containers, and more precise calculations of heat treatment. By 1850, canners began using oil, salt brine, and calcium chloride baths to achieve temperatures above 100°C, which significantly reduced processing times. The closed and controlled retort, developed by Schriver in 1874, allowed for safer and more efficien steam processing. In the last century, innovations like equipment for rotating containers during processing and high-temperature- short- time heating methods have advanced the process further.

Initially, Appert's glass jar was the main container, but the tin can, patented by Peter Durand in 1810, became more widely used. The modern tin can, now made of steel coated with tin, has evolved with features such as double- crimped tops and improved gaskets to ensure better sealing. Enamels are often applied to the interior of cans to prevent discoloration or corrosion, especially for products like fruits, vegetables, and meats.

Glass containers, which Appert originally used, continue to be popular in canning, while aluminum containers, though not as durable under mechanical stress, are now used for products like beer and frozen foods. Flexible pouches made of plastic or laminated with foil are also becoming more common for packaging frozen, dried, and hot- packaged foods, and steam- pressure sterilization has been successfully applied to these pouches.

Canning has continuously evolved, with improvements in both packaging materials and heat- processing technologies ensuring longer shelf lives and better preservation of food quality.

The Canning Procedure

The general procedures in the canning of food will be mentioned only briefly here. A reference on food technology or canning such as Lopez (1981) should be consulted for technical details. Raw food for canning should be freshly harvested, properly prepared, inspected, graded if desired, and thoroughly washed before introduction into the can. Many vegetable foods are blanched or scalded briefly by hot water or steam before packaging. The blanching washes the food further, "sets" the color, softens the tissues to aid- packing, helps form the vacuum, and kills some microorganisms. A brine, consisting of salt solution or salt plus sugar, is added to some canned vegetables; and sugar syrups may be added to fruits. The container is evacuated before sealing, usually by heating the head space, or unfilled part of the container, but often by mechanical means.

The Heat Process

The calculation of heat processes for canned foods aims to achieve sterilization, but it is not always complete. The goal is not necessarily to kill all microorganisms, but to eliminate those that could cause spoilage under normal storage conditions. The result is that the food may not be fully sterile but is often termed "commercially sterile," "practically sterile," or "bacterially inactive," meaning that harmful microorganisms are eliminated, but some may still survive without the ability to grow.

The required heat processes depend on factors such as the heat resistance of the most resilient spoilage organisms and the factors influencing heat penetration. The National Food Processors Association (NFPA) publishes guidelines for the minimal heat treatment required for various foods, considering their size and packaging. For example, low- acid foods are addressed in Bulletin 26- L. With higher retort temperatures, the required processing times are shorter, but they vary based on the food's variety, sauce used, can size and shape, the initial temperature of the food, and other variables.

One advanced method, the "Strata- Cook" process, shortens the heat process for foods containing a mix of discrete particles and finely divided components, such as creamed corn. In this method, the components are stratified and kept separate during heating. The reason this is effecti e is that foods with a smaller thickness or thinner layers heat faster due to more efficien heat penetration, as small differences in water content don't significantly affect conduction- based heating.

Foods with a more liquid consistency generally require less heat treatment than those that are more densely packed. Acidic foods, like sauerkraut, require less heat than those with a neutral pH, and some foods, such as globe artichokes, are acidified before processing to allow for a lower- temperature treatment, preventing heat damage.

Table. Process Times Recommended for Some Vegetables in can Size 307 x 409

Food	Temperature °C		Minutes at retort temperature
	minimum initial	Retort	
Asparagus spears (tips down, in brine)	48.9	115.6	26
Beans, lima (in brine)	48.9	115.6	36
Beans in heavy sauce	60.0	115.6	115
Corn, cream style	60.0	115.6	105
Corn, whole kernel (in brine)	60.0	115.6	46
Potatoes sweet, solid pack	65.6	115.6	100
Pumpkin	60.0	115.6	86

Heating is usually carried out in autoclaves, with or without steam pressure depending on the requirements of the food. HTST thermal processes, now used for some liquid foods, require special equipment to sterilize bulk foods, to sterilize containers and lids, and to fill and seal sterile containers under aseptic conditions.

The Dole process is an example of the HCF (heat- cool- fill) method. In Martin's HTST sterile preservation system, mixed liquid and solid portions are heated directly by contact with high- temperature steam before aseptic preservation. When there is concern about a particularly heat-resistant spoilage organism, HTST treatment may be given to a liquid food before canning, followed by a milder heat treatment of the food in the can. French For example, tomato juice can be presterilized at 121 to 132°C to kill Bacillus coagulans spores before canning, and then sealed cans of juice are subjected to gentler heating.

In the SC process, or sterilize and seal, food sterilization is performed before the can is sealed. In the PFC method, or full pressure cooker, the food is sterilized with high- pressure steam and poured into cans; then the can is closed and the heat treatment continues for the required time before cooling. In dehydrocanning, for example. , from apple slices, the food is dried to half its original weight before canning.

Other methods of heating milk are by direct gas flame, by steam injection, by heating in a fluidized bed of solid particles, and by the hydrostatic sterilizer, which consists of a vertical tank with conveyors that carry cans through a foot of water. , up into live steam, then up and out through a second foot of water. In the "Flash 18" method, canning is done in a high- pressure chamber (18 psi). The product is subjected to HTST treatment to bring it to processing temperature, and the cans are filled, sealed, and partially cooled to room temperature.

Heat is also combined with other preservatives, e.g., For example, antibiotics, radiation, or chemicals such as hydrogen peroxide. So far, most of this work has been experimental.

PRESSURIZED PACKAGED FOODS

Pressurized packaged liquids or pastes, called aerosols, are packed under pressure of a propellant gas, usually carbon dioxide, nitrogen, or nitrous oxide, so as to dispense the food as a foam, spray, or liquid. Many foods are now being so packaged, e.g., whipped cream and other toppings, beverage concentrates, salad dressings, condiments, oils, jellies, and flavoring substances. The pressurized foods are subject to microbial spoilage unless adequate preservative methods are employed. Acid foods may be heated, canned, and then gassed, but the gassing process may contaminate the food.

Aseptic canning is a possibility for low- and medium- acid foods. Process requirements for pasteurized foods, e.g., whipped cream and other toppings, are similar with or without gas pressure. The gas used as a propellant may have an influence on the kinds of organisms likely to grow. Nitrogen, for example, would not inhibit aerobes if a little oxygen were present, but carbon dioxide would be inhibitory under the same condition. Carbon dioxide under pressure inhibits many microorganisms, including aerobic bacteria and molds, but does not inhibit lactic acid bacteria, Bacillus coagulans, Streptococcus faecalis, or yeasts. Nitrous oxide represses some fungi.

The Cooling Process

Following the application of heat, the containers of food are cooled as rapidly as is practicable. The cans may be cooled in the retort or in tanks by immersion in cold water or by a spray of water. Glass containers and large cans are cooled more gradually to avoid undue strain or even breakage. This tempering process involves the use of warm water (or spray), the temperature of which is lowered as cooling progresses. Final cooling of containers usually is by means of air currents.

The leakage of cooling water through imperfections in the container or its seal and the resultant spoilage will be discussed later (Chapter 19).

Canning in the Home

For many years, home canners have used processes similar to Appert's, with a heating temperature of no more than 100°C. This is done by one of three methods: (1) a boiling water bath in which the jars are immersed, (2) a steamer in which the jars are exposed to steam, or (3) heat from an oven. When jars are heated in the oven, the temperature cannot exceed the boiling point of the food unless the containers are sealed and pressure builds up, causing the jars to burst.

These processes are adequate for acidic foods such as fruit, but are not considered adequate for low-acid foods such as peas, corn, and meat. Modern home canning methods use pressure cookers for heat treatment of low-acid foods, according to guidelines available in state and federal home canning bulletins.

In the cold preservation method, the food is not heated before being placed in a jar or other container, unlike the hot preservation method, where the food is pre-cooked, hot when transferred to the container and immediately treated with heat. It is clear that cold packaged foods require more heat treatment in the container than hot packaged foods. The cold preservation method is not recommended for vegetables and meat.

7 High-Temperature Food Preservation

Low temperatures are employed to slow down chemical reactions, enzyme activity, and microbial growth in food. The colder the temperature, the slower the chemical processes, enzyme functions, and the growth of microorganisms. A sufficientl low temperature can prevent microorganisms from growing altogether.

Raw plant and animal foods generally contain a range of bacteria, yeasts, and molds that, under the right conditions, can cause undesirable changes. Each microorganism has an ideal temperature for growth and a minimum temperature below which it cannot multiply. As the temperature decreases from the optimal point towards this minimum, the growth rate of the organism slows, and it becomes slowest at the minimum temperature. While cooler temperatures prevent growth, some metabolic activity may still occur.

Therefore, cooling food from room temperature impacts different organisms in varying ways. A 10° drop may halt the growth of some organisms while merely slowing others, and a further 10° decrease would stop more organisms from growing and slow the others even more. Thus, low- temperature storage can significantly affect the type of spoilage organisms that dominate. The below table shows common types of bacteria that cause spoilage in chicken meat.

Table: Types of Bacteria Causing Spoilage of Chicken Meat

Bacteria	Description	Effects on Chicken Mea
Salmonella	A common bacterium found in raw poultry.	Causes foodborne illness, leading to symptoms like diarrhea, fever, and abdominal cramps.
Campylobacter	One of the most common causes of foodborne illness linked to chicken.	Results in gastroenteritis with symptoms including diarrhea, cramps, and fever.
Escherichia coli (E. coli)	Some strains, like *E. coli* O157-H7, can cause illness in undercooked chicken.	Can cause severe food poisoning with symptoms such as bloody diarrhea and kidney failure in severe cases.
Clostridium perfringens	Common in improperly cooked or stored chicken.	Leads to food poisoning with symptoms including abdominal cramps and diarrhea.

Bacteria	Description	Effects on chicken meat
Listeria monocytogenes	Often found in improperly stored or contaminated chicken.	Can cause listeriosis, which leads to fever, muscle aches, and gastrointestinal symptoms. It can be severe, especially for pregnant women, newborns, and immunocompromised individuals.
Staphylococcus aureus	Found in improperly handled or stored chicken.	Produces toxins that cause rapid onset of food poisoning, including nausea, vomiting, and abdominal cramps.
Pseudomonas spp.	Often present in refrigerated chicken that is improperly stored.	Leads to spoilage with off odors, slimy texture, and discoloration.
Bacillus cereus	Found in improperly cooked or stored chicken, especially if reheated.	Can cause foodborne illness with symptoms including vomiting (due to the emetic toxin) and diarrhea (due to the diarrheal toxin).
Enterococcus spp.	Found in chicken meat, especially in undercooked or contaminated products.	May cause spoilage with sour odors and slime formation, though it is less likely to cause illness compared to other bacteria.

The growth and metabolic reactions of microbes depend on enzymes, and the rate of enzyme reactions is directly affected by temperature. The most important aspect of this temperature effect is reflected in a decrease in the rate of growth of a microbes when the temperature is lowered, as can be seen in Table 7.2.

Table: Growth Rate of *Pseudomonas fragi* at Various Temperatures

Temperature (°C)	Growth rate	Notes
0°C	Very slow growth or no growth	Growth is severely limited at refrigeration temperatures.
5°C	Slow growth	Can grow, but at a slow rate in chilled environments.
10°C	Moderate growth	Growth increases slightly at cooler storage temperatures.
15°C	Moderate to good growth	Growth rate is significantly faster at this temperature.
20°C	Good growth	Thrives at this moderate temperature.
25°C	Very good growth	Optimal growth temperature, producing rapid bacterial replication.
30°C	Good growth	Still within the optimal range, though growth rate may decrease slightly.

Temperature (°C)	Growth rate	Notes
35°C	Moderate growth	Growth slows as temperatures rise beyond the optimal range for *P. fragi*.
40°C	Slow growth	At higher temperatures, the growth rate significantly decreases
45°C	No growth or very minimal growth	*P. fragi* is typically unable to grow above this temperature.

This table provides an overview of how the growth of *Pseudomonas fragi* varies with temperature, helping to understand its behavior in different storage conditions.

MICROBIAL GROWTH BEHAVIOR AT REDUCED TEMPERATURES

Most foodborne microorganisms cannot grow when frozen, and growth rates are slowed by refrigeration temperatures. Many foodborne pathogens can be effectively inhibited from growing at commercial refrigeration temperatures, which are below 5 to 7.2°C. *Clostridium botulinum* type E is a notable exception, requiring a minimum temperature of approximately 3.3°C to grow (Table 7.3).

Yersinia enterocolítica can survive and grow at temperatures as low as 0 to 3°C (Stern and Pierson, 1979). An earlier reference suggested a minimum temperature of 1 to 7°C (Table). Although, concern has been expressed about the low temperature growth limits of *Salmonella* (Table), Mossel et al. (1981) examined the growth potential of numerous strains and found that only one strain, *S. panama* R IV 1917, could grow at 4°C. Other bacterial foodborne pathogens have a minimum temperature for growth below 7.2°C, and refrigeration therefore may not be depended on to prevent significant growth indefinitely.

Table: Low Temperature Growth of Some Foodborne Bacterial Pathogens

Bacterial pathogen	Temperature range for growth (°C)	Optimal growth temperature (°C)	Notes
Salmonella spp.	5°C - 47°C	37°C	Can grow in refrigeration but slower.
Escherichia coli	7°C - 50°C	37°C	Growth is significantly slo er at low temperatures.
Listeria monocytogenes	-0.4°C - 45°C	30°C - 37°C	Can grow at refrigeration temperatures, making it a concern for cold- storage foods.

Bacterial pathogen	Temperature range for growth (°C)	Optimal growth temperature (°C)	Notes
Campylobacter jejuni	30°C - 47°C	42°C	Slow growth at low temperatures.
Vibrio vulnificus	5°C - 43°C	37°C	Slower growth at refrigerated temperatures.
Clostridium botulinum	3°C - 45°C	37°C	Growth slowed at low temperatures, but can still be a risk in improperly stored foods.
Bacillus cereus	4°C - 50°C	30°C - 37°C	Slower growth in cold storage but spores can survive.
Staphylococcus aureus	7°C - 48°C	37°C	Can grow at refrigeration temperatures but at a slower rate.

A few examples, reported by various workers, of low- temperature growth of microorganisms are of interest. Of the molds, *Cladosporium* and *Sporotrichum* have been found growing on foods at −6.7°C and *Penicillium* and *Monilia* at −4°C. Growth by one yeast has taken place at −34°C, and two others grew at −18°C (Michener and Elliott, 1964). Bacteria have been reported growing at temperatures as low as −5°C on meats, −10°C on cured meats, −11°C on fish, −12.2°C on vegetables (peas), and −10°C in ice cream; yeast at −5°C on meats and −17.8°C on oysters; and molds at −7.8°C on meats and vegetables and −6.7°C on berries.

Optimal Temperature Conditions for Low-Temperature Storage

Many of the terms used in connection with low- temperature storage are applied rather loosely; e.g., the term "cold storage" may refer to the use of temperatures above or below freezing, although the application of mechanical refrigeration is implied. More often it is considered to be storage above 0°C. The term "frozen storage" is more obvious; the product is stored in a frozen state, but the exact temperature would depend on the product. Most commercial storage freezers are at or below −18°C.

Common, or Cellar, Storage

Common, or cellar, storage temperatures are rarely lower than 15°C and are typically not much lower than the ambient temperature. Apples, celery, potatoes, cabbage, root crops, and the like can be stored for a short time.

Although, it happens more slowly than it would at room temperature, the deterioration of such fruits and vegetables by microbes and their own enzymes is not avoided. An excessively high humidity encourages microbial spoiling, while an excessively low humidity causes moisture loss from the food being stored in the storage cellar. It is common practice to store all foods in areas without refrigeration.

Chilling, or "Cold Storage"

Chilling storage involves keeping temperatures just above freezing, typically achieved through ice or mechanical refrigeration. It can serve as the primary preservation method for foods or as a temporary solution until another preservative process is applied. Many perishable items such as eggs, dairy, meats, seafood, vegetables, and fruits can be stored in chilling conditions for a short period with minimal alteration to their original state. While enzymatic and microbial changes are not completely halted, they are significantly slowed. Key factors to consider when using chilling storage include the storage temperature, relative humidity, air velocity, atmosphere composition in the storage area, and the potential use of ultraviolet or other types of radiation.

Temperature

The cost of storage increases as the temperature decreases. Although most foods maintain their quality best just above their freezing point, they are not typically stored at this low temperature. Instead, the chilling temperature is chosen based on the type of food and the duration and conditions of storage. Some foods have an optimal storage temperature or range that is higher than freezing, and they may be damaged by lower temperatures. For example, bananas should not be stored in the refrigerator and are best kept at around 13.3 to 16.7°C. Certain apple varieties may experience "low- temperature breakdown" near freezing, while sweet potatoes store best at 10 to 12.8°C. Refrigerator temperatures are controlled mechanically but can vary across different areas, typically ranging from 0 to 10°C

Relative Humidity

The food being stored and environmental variables like temperature, atmosphere composition, and ray treatments all affect the ideal relative humidity of the atmosphere in chilling storage. A low relative humidity causes fruits to shrink, vegetables to wilt and soften, and weight loss due to moisture loss. Microorganisms that cause spoiling thrive in environments with excessive relative humidity. Most bacterial growth on food surfaces requires the highest humidity, close to saturation; yeasts require less moisture, roughly 90 to 92 percent, and molds require even less, as they can grow in a relative humidity of 85 to 90 percent. Changes in humidity, as well as in temperature, during storage may cause "sweating," or precipitation of moisture, on the food. A moist surface favors microbial spoilage, e.g., slime on the moist surface of sausage.

Examples of how the optimal relative humidity and the temperature for chilling storage vary with the food stored are given in Table 7.4.

Ventilation

Ventilation or control of air velocities of the storage room is important in maintaining a uniform relative humidity throughout the room, removing odors, and preventing the development of stale odors and flavors. The rate of air circulation affects the rate of drying of foods. If adequate ventilation is not provided, food in local areas of high humidity may undergo microbial decomposition.

COMPOSITION OF STORAGE ATMOSPHERE

The levels and proportions of gases in the storage environment play a crucial role in preserving food through chilling. Typically, the composition of the atmosphere is not actively controlled, although plant foods continue to respire, consuming oxygen and releasing carbon dioxide. Recently, however, there has been growing interest in "gas storage," where the atmosphere is regulated by adding carbon dioxide, ozone (on an experimental basis), or other gases, or by removing carbon dioxide. Gas storage is generally used in conjunction with chilled storage. Research has shown that with the right concentrations of carbon dioxide or ozone, foods can (1) stay fresh for longer periods, (2) maintain a higher relative humidity without negatively impacting their quality, or (3) be stored at slightly higher temperatures without reducing their shelf life compared to conventional chilling methods. This approach is particularly beneficial as it allows for higher humidity levels without increasing the risk of microbial spoilage, helping many foods retain their quality by minimizing moisture loss.

Table: Optimal Relative Humidities and Storage Temperatures for Raw Foods

Food type	Optimal storage temperature (°C)	Optimal relative humidity (%)
Meat (Beef, Pork, Lamb)	0 to 2	85 to 90
Poultry (Chicken, Turkey)	0 to 2	85 to 90
Fish (Fresh)	- 1 to 0	85 to 90
Shellfis	0 to 2	85 to 90
Fruits (Apples, Pears)	0 to 4	85 to 95
Vegetables (Leafy Greens, Carrots, Broccoli)	0 to 4	95 to 100
Root Vegetables (Potatoes, Sweet Potatoes)	4 to 10	90 to 95
Eggs	0 to 5	75 to 85
Dairy Products (Milk, Cheese)	0 to 4	85 to 90

This table provides the optimal storage conditions to maintain the quality and freshness of raw foods. Temperature and humidity levels are critical in preserving their texture, flavor, and nutritional alue.

The optimal concentration of carbon dioxide in the atmosphere varies with the food stored, from the approximately 2.5 percent reported to be best for eggs and 10 percent for chilled beef up to the 100 percent for bacon. For some foods, e.g., apples, the concentration of oxygen as well as that of carbon dioxide is significant, and a definite ratio of these gases is sought. Respiring plant cells may evolve too much carbon dioxide into the storage room for some foods, and then part of it must be removed.

Irradiation

The combination of ultraviolet irradiation with chilling storage helps preserve some foods and may permit the use of a higher humidity or storage temperature than is practicable with chilling alone. Ultraviolet lamps have been installed in rooms for the storage of meat and cheese.

Freezing or "Frozen Storage"

Freezing has been a vital method of food preservation for centuries, especially in regions with naturally low temperatures. With the advent of mechanical refrigeration and rapid freezing techniques, the frozen food industry has grown significantly. Freezing has also become widespread in households, thanks to the availability of home deep freezers. When foods are stored frozen, microbial growth is completely halted, and the activity of food enzymes is significantly slowed. The colder the storage temperature, the slower the chemical and enzymatic reactions, though these processes can still occur at any temperature used for freezing. As a result, it is common practice to inactivate enzymes in vegetables by scalding or blanching them before freezing, when feasible.

Selection and Preparation of Foods for Freezing

The quality of the food to be frozen is of great importance because frozen food cannot be better than it was before it was frozen. Fruits and vegetables are selected based on their suitability and ripeness for freezing, then washed, cut, diced or otherwise handled as necessary. Most vegetables are charred or blanched, and fruit may be packed in syrup. Meats and seafood are selected for quality and treated to minimize enzymatic and microbial changes. MOST certain foods are packed before freezing, but some foods in small pieces, e.g. Strawberries, for example, can be frozen before packaging.

Blanching or blanching of vegetables is usually done with hot water or steam, with the extent of treatment varying with the food. This brief heat treatment is intended to accomplish the following tasks- (1) inactivating most plant enzymes that would otherwise cause hardness, discoloration, mold, loss of flavor, softening, and loss of nutritional value, (2) reducing (up to 99%) the number of microorganisms present in the food, (3) improving the green color of vegetables such as peas, broccoli, and spinach, (4) decolorizing leafy greens such as spinach, making them easier to wrap, and (5) displacing air trapped in the fabric.

Freezing of Foods

The speed of freezing food depends on several factors, such as the method used, the temperature, the air circulation or refrigerant, the size and shape of the packaging, and the type of food. Forced freezing generally refers to air freezing with only natural air circulation or, at best, with electric fans. The temperature is usually -23.3°C or lower, but can range from -15 to : 29°C, and freezing can last from 3 to 72 hours. It is sometimes called slow freezing to contrast with quick freezing, in which the food freezes in a relatively short time. Flash freezing is defined in various ways, but generally involves a freezing time of 30 minutes or less and usually involves the freezing of small packages or food units. Flash freezing is accomplished by one of three general methods: (1) direct immersion of the food or packaged food in a refrigerant, as in the freezing of fish in brine or berries in special syrups, (2) indirect contact with the refrigerant, where the food or packaging is in contact with a passage through which the refrigerant circulates at a temperature of - 17.8 to - 45.6°C, or (3) blast freezing, where freezing air circulates at a temperature of - 17.8 to - 34°C. 4°C is above the temperature for the food to be frozen.

One method of shipping frozen and packaged food products overseas is to freeze the packaged food with nitrogen in a special aluminum case and store it normally on the ship. The low initial temperature and insulation ensure that the food remains frozen for the desired period of time. Some fruits and vegetables, fish, shrimp and mushrooms are now frozen with liquid nitrogen. For dehydration, about half of the moisture is removed from the fruits and vegetables before freezing.

The advantages of quick freezing over slow freezing are- (1) smaller ice crystals are formed, resulting in less mechanical destruction of intact cells in the food, (2) the solidification period is shorter and therefore the diffusion of soluble materials. and the separation of ice takes less time, (3) microbial growth is inhibited more quickly, and (4) enzyme action is slowed down more quickly. Therefore, quick-frozen foods are supposed to thaw to a state closer to that of the original food than frozen foods. This seems to be true for some foods, for example vegetables, but not necessarily for all foods. Research on fish, for example, has shown that quick freezing has a slight advantage over slow freezing.

CHANGES DURING PREPARATION FOR FREEZING

The rate and kind of deterioration of foods before freezing will depend on the condition of the food at harvesting or slaughter and the methods of handling thereafter. The temperatures at which the food is held and other environmental conditions will determine the kinds of microorganisms to grow and the changes to be produced. The condition of the food at the time of freezing will determine the potential quality of the frozen food.

Changes During Freezing

The flash freezing process rapidly slows down chemical and enzymatic reactions in food and stops microbial growth. A similar effect is produced by quick or slow freezing, but less rapidly. The physical effects of freezing are of great importance. The volume of frozen food increases and ice crystals form and grow. These crystals are generally larger with slow freezing and more ice accumulates between tissue cells than with quick freezing and can crush the cells. Water is taken up by the cells to form this ice, resulting in an increase in the concentration of solutes in the unfrozen liquid, whose freezing point continuously drops to a steady state. Ice crystals are claimed to destroy tissue cells or even microorganisms, but some researchers minimize the importance of such an effect. The increased concentration of soluble substances in the cells accelerates the release, dehydration and denaturation of proteins and causes irreversible changes in colloidal systems, such as syneresis of hydrophilic colloids. It is also believed to be responsible for the destruction of microorganisms.

Changes During Thawing

Most of the changes that appear to occur during thawing are the result of freezing and storage, but are not apparent at first. As the ice crystals melt, the liquid is either reabsorbed into the tissue cells or released from the food. Slow, well-controlled thawing generally results in a better return of moisture to the cells than rapid thawing and results in a food that is more similar to the original food that was frozen. The pink or red liquid that comes out of meat during thawing is called dripping, or Bleeding and the liquid that runs out of fruits or vegetables during thawing is called oozing. The wilting or weakness of vegetables and the softness of fruits during thawing are primarily the result of physical damage during freezing. During thawing, the rate of enzyme action in the food will increase, but the time of action will be relatively short if the food is used quickly.

If thawing is rapid enough and the food is used quickly, there should be little problem with the growth of microorganisms, as the temperatures will be too low for noticeable growth. Only when thawing is very slow or when thawed foods are left at room temperature is there a possibility of significant growth and activity of microorganisms. The types of organisms that grow depend on the thawing temperature and how long the food was allowed to sit after thawing.

Changes During Storage

During storage of food in a frozen state, chemical and enzymatic reactions occur slowly. Proteins from meat, poultry, and fish can be irreversibly dehydrated, red myoglobin in meat can be oxidized (especially on the surface) to brown metmyoglobin, and fats in meat and fish can be oxidized and hydrolyzed. Concentrated, thawed solutions of sugars, salts, etc. can leak from concentrated fruit or packaging during storage as a viscous material called metacryotic fluid. Fluctuations in storage temperature lead to an increase in ice crystal size and physical damage to the food. Surface cracking of foods is likely to occur during storage. When ice crystals evaporate from a surface, a defect called freeze burn occurs on fruits, vegetables, meat, poultry, and fish. The area usually appears dry, grainy, and brown; in this area, the chemical changes mentioned above occur and the tissues become dry and hard.

At freezing temperatures, vegetative cells of microorganisms that are unable to reproduce eventually die. There is a slow but steady decline in the number of viable microorganisms as storage continues, with some species dying more quickly than others, but representatives of most species survive for months or even years.

Disposal of Thawed Foods

Sometimes power failures lead to partial or complete thawing of foods in freezers. Thawed fruits may be refrozen. Flesh foods and vegetables may be refrozen if the packages still contain some ice. Refrozen foods will contain large ice crystals and may show leakage of liquid (syneresis) and mushiness. If thawed, flesh foods can be used if their temperature is below 3.3°C. In case of doubt, the food should be discarded.

Precooked Frozen Foods

Pre-cooked frozen meals include such a variety of food types and food products that can be presented together. Most of these foods are meat, fish or poultry products, for example soups, cream products, stews, pies, fish or poultry fritters, chow mein, barbecued meat, meat and chicken a la king. However, some bread products, fruits and vegetables can be cooked and then frozen. The pre: cooking process is usually sufficien to kill any pathogens present in the raw material and to significantly reduce the total number of microorganisms present. Most samples of frozen pre- cooked foods examined by several researchers suggest that these foods can be commercially prepared with a total count of less than 50,000 per gram. The cooking process does not destroy the personnel toxins present in the food. Enterococci survive freezing and persist longer during storage than coliform bacteria and are therefore recommended as "indicator bacteria" for possible fecal contamination.

It is particularly important to prevent contamination of foods after pre-cooking, as any subsequently introduced pathogens or pests will have significantly reduced competition from other organisms and cooked foods may be a better culture medium than the original raw food if given the opportunity to grow. It is therefore important to cool and refreeze quickly after cooking to avoid any chance of spread.

If these precooked frozen foods are kept at warm temperatures for too long after thawing, food poisoning organisms can grow and produce toxins, although no such cases have been reported. Final cooking or "reheating" of these products at home or in a restaurant does not always constitute sufficien heat treatment to significantly reduce the number of organisms present or to ensure that all pathogens present are killed or toxins destroyed.

IMPACT OF SUBFREEZING AND FREEZING CONDITIONS ON MICROBIAL GROWTH

Discussing the effects of freezing on microorganisms is challenging due to the many variables and observed outcomes. A key issue is that it's impossible to study the effects of freezing on cells without also considering the effects of cooling (decreasing to 0°C) and thawing. Marth (1973) summarized the freezing process for microorganisms as involving (1) cooling of cells to 0°C, (2) additional cooling leading to extra- and possibly intracellular ice- crystal formation, (3) concentration of solutes both inside and outside the cells, (4) storing cells in a frozen state, and (5) thawing the cells and substrate.

Freezing typically leads to a significant reduction in viable microorganisms within food. This decrease in recoverable organisms can be due to either lethal or sublethal effects

Lethal Effect

Freezing kills many cells, though it does not sterilize. Freezing and storing cultures, typically in liquid nitrogen, is a common preservation method. Lethal effects are believed to result from the denaturation or aggregation of essential cell proteins or enzymes, likely caused by the increased concentration of solutes in unfrozen water, or potentially due to physical damage from ice crystals. Rapid cooling from an optimal temperature to 0°C can also cause cell death, referred to as cold shock. This is thought to occur due to changes in lipid structure in the cell membrane, disrupting permeability, or the release of inhibitors for repair enzymes, such as ribonuclease inhibitors.

Sublethal Effect

In typical microbiological counting of frozen foods, a reduction in microbial numbers doesn't always indicate the actual death of cells. Some cells might be injured or damaged, preventing them from being counted. These cells are referred to as freeze- injured, frost- injured, or metabolically injured. Freezing microorganisms in food can thus lead to cryoinjury. These injured cells can recover if given time or additional nutrients, meaning they are not truly dead.

The focus on cryoinjury in frozen foods stems from concerns about bacteriological standards for such items, the accuracy of enumeration techniques, the pathogenicity of injured pathogens, and how to interpret the viable microorganism count in frozen foods.

Response of Microorganisms to Freezing

The following variables or factors occur during freezing and perhaps dictate why some microorganisms die, some are injured, and some are not damaged.

- **The kind of microorganism and its state:** The resistance of microorganisms to freezing depends on their type, growth phase, and whether they are vegetative cells or spores. Christophersen (1973) classified microorganisms based on their freezing sensitivity into three categories:
  - susceptible,
  - moderately resistant,
  - insensitive.

Vegetative cells of yeast, molds, and many gram- negative bacteria fall into the first category. Gram- positive organisms, such as staphylococci and enterococci, belong to the second group. The third group mainly consists of spore- forming bacteria, as spores of bacilli and clostridia are highly resistant to freezing. Bacteria in the logarithmic growth phase are more likely to be killed than those in other phases.

- **The Freezing Rate:** There appears to be a critical range of temperatures which result in lethal effects; therefore, faster freezing rates would tend to be less destructive since the critical range would be passed through faster.
- **The Freezing Temperature:** High freezing temperatures are more lethal. More organisms are inactivated at −4 to −10°C than at −15 to −30°C.
- **The Time of Frozen Storage:** The initial killing rate during freezing is rapid, but it is followed by a gradual reduction of microorganisms and is referred to as storage death. The number of viable organisms decreases with lengthened time of storage. Storage of frozen foods in the critical range of temperatures would result in a more rapid reduction than at higher or lower freezing temperatures.
- **The kind of Food:** The composition of the food influences the rate of death of organisms during freezing and storage. Sugar, salt, proteins, colloids, fat, and other substances may be protective, whereas high moisture and low pH may hasten killing.
- **Influence of Defrosting:** The response of microorganisms to the rate of defrosting varies. Rapid warming has been found to be harmful to some bacteria.
- **Alternate Freezing and Thawing**: Alternate freezing and thawing is reported to hasten the killing of microorganisms but apparently does not always do so.
- **Possible Events During Freezing of the Cell:** As the temperature decreases, a larger portion of the water freezes. Consequently, the unfrozen water at each temperature becomes increasingly concentrated with solutes such as salts, proteins, and nucleic acids. This concentration can affec the pH of cellular matter, concentrate electrolytes, alter colloidal states, denature proteins, and increase viscosity. Ice crystals can form outside the cell (extracellular ice), drawing water out and causing dehydration or a concentration effect. Intracellular ice crystals may also form, growing or crystallizing within the cell, leading to changes in permeability or the formation of "holes" in the cell membrane and wall. Intracellular ice is generally considered more damaging to cells than extracellular ice.

8 Moisture Removal for Preservation

Moisture removal is one of the oldest and most effecti e methods of preserving food, preventing spoilage and extending shelf life by reducing the water content that microorganisms and enzymes require for growth. The process of drying or dehydration removes moisture from food, thereby inhibiting the growth of bacteria, molds, and yeasts, which are the primary agents of decay. By reducing the water activity (a_w) in food, drying significantly slows down the chemical reactions and microbial activities that lead to spoilage.

Food preservation through drying has been used for centuries. Certain foods, like grains, are naturally dry enough when harvested, or with minimal drying, can be stored for extended periods without spoiling, provided proper storage conditions are maintained. However, most foods retain enough moisture to support enzymatic activity and microbial growth.

To preserve these foods through drying, it is essential to remove or bind the moisture, often through the addition of solutes. Table presents a comparison of the moisture content of various foods before and after drying, showing the level of moisture that ensures the product's stability.

The history of moisture removal for preservation can be traced back to ancient civilizations, where methods such as sun drying, smoking, and salting were used to preserve fruits, vegetables, meats, and fish. With advancements in technology, modern techniques like freeze- drying, spray- drying, and vacuum drying have become widely used in the food industry, allowing for more efficient uniform, and controlled drying processes that better preserve the nutritional value, flavor, and texture of the food.

Drying also plays a crucial role in convenience foods, as it significantly reduces the volume and weight of food, making it easier to store, transport, and use. This method is commonly applied to products such as dried fruits, herbs, powdered dairy, and instant meals.

Despite its many benefits, drying must be carefully controlled to avoid nutrient loss, product discoloration, or undesirable changes in texture. In this chapter, we will explore the different drying methods, their applications, and the factors that influence the effect eness of moisture removal for food preservation.

Table: Moisture Content of Various Foods before and after Drying

Food item	Moisture content before drying (%)	Moisture content after drying (%)
Fresh Apples	85-90%	15-25%
Fresh Carrots	85-88%	6-10%
Fresh Tomatoes	95-96%	5-8%
Fresh Fish (e.g., Salmon)	75-80%	12-20%
Fresh Beef	70-75%	15-25%
Fresh Grains (e.g., Wheat)	12-20%	10-12%
Fresh Milk	85-88%	3-5%
Fresh Herbs (e.g., Basil)	70-80%	5-8%
Fresh Potatoes	80-85%	10-15%
Fresh Mushrooms	90-92%	7-10%

Drying is typically achieved by removing water, but any process that reduces the available moisture or lowers the water activity (a_w) in food can be considered a form of drying. For instance, dried fish may be heavily salted, which draws moisture out of the flesh and binds it with the salt, making it unavailable to microorganisms. Similarly, sugar is often added to foods like sweetened condensed milk to reduce the available moisture.

Various methods can be used to remove moisture from foods, ranging from the ancient technique of sun drying to modern artificial drying methods. Many terms related to food drying are somewhat vague. For example, sun- dried foods are those dried by exposure to the sun without artificial heat or control over temperature, humidity, or air movement. On the other hand, dehydrated or desiccated foods are dried using artificial heat under controlled conditions, including temperature, humidity, and airflow. The term "condensed" typically refers to moisture being removed from liquid foods, while "evaporated" may be used interchangeably with "dehydrated" or may have a similar meaning.

METHODS OF DRYING

Methods of drying will be mentioned only briefly- references on food technology should be consulted for details. The drying of individual foods will be discussed in the chapters on the preservation of these foods. Table summarizes various forms of drying applied to several foods.

Table: Types of Dryer used for Various Foods, Food by- products, and Wastes

Product	Type of dryer
Vegetables, confectionery, fruits, pectin	Compartment and tunnel tray
Grass, grain, vegetables, fruit, nuts, breakfast cereals	Conveyor band

Product	Type of dryer
Grass, grain, apple pomace, lactose, poultry manure, peat, starch (vacuum)	Rotary
Coffee, milk, tea, fruit purees	
Milk, starch, predigested infant foods, soups, brewery and distillery by- products	Film drum
Starch, fruit pulp, distillery waste products, crops	Pneumatic
Coffee, essences, meat extracts, malted and other confectioneries	Freeze dryers and vacuum dryers

Solar Drying

Solar drying is suitable only in regions with a hot, dry climate and is typically used for specific fruits like raisins, prunes, figs, apricots, nectarines, pears, and peaches. These fruits are placed on trays and may need to be turned during the drying process. Additionally, fish, rice, and various grains can also be dried using the sun. Other specialized drying methods will be covered later.

Drying by Mechanical Dryers

Most artificial drying techniques involve passing heated air with controlled humidity over the food or moving the food through such air. Various devices are used to regulate air circulation and allow for the reuse of air in certain processes. The simplest form of drying is the evaporator or kiln, often used on farms, where natural drafts created by rising heated air facilitate the drying of food. Forced-draft drying systems use heated air currents that flow across the food, typically in tunnels. Alternatively, the food may be transported on conveyor belts or trays in carts through the heated air.

For liquid foods like milk, juices, and soups, evaporation can occur at relatively low temperatures under a vacuum using a vacuum pan or similar apparatus. Another option is drum- drying, where the liquid passes over a heated drum, with or without vacuum, or spray- drying, where the liquid is sprayed into a stream of dry, heated air.

Freeze Drying

Freeze drying, or the sublimation of water from a frozen food by means of a vacuum plus heat applied at the drying shelf, is being used for a number of foods, including meats, poultry, seafood, fruits, and vegetables. Frozen thin layers of foods of low sugar content may be dried without vacuum by sublimation of moisture during passage of dry carrier gas.

Drying During Smoking

As indicated in Chapter 9, most of the preservative effect of the smoking of foods is due to the drying of the food during the process. Indeed, some workers maintain that drying is the main preservative factor, especially drying at the surface of the food.

Other Methods

Electronic heating has been suggested for the removal of still more moisture from a food already fairly well dried. Foam- mat drying, in which liquid food is whipped to a foam, dried with warm air, and crushed to a powder, is receiving attention, as is pressure- gun puffing of partially dried foods to give a porous structure that facilitates further drying. Tower drying in dehumidified air at 30°C or lower has been successful with tomato concentrate, milk, and potatoes.

FACTORS IN THE CONTROL OF DRYING

Factors that influence the control of drying include several key considerations:

- **Air Velocity:** The speed at which air moves over or through the food is an important factor in the drying process.
- **Temperature:** The temperature used in drying depends on both the type of food and the drying method.
- **Relative Humidity of Air:** This factor varies according to the food being dried, the drying method, and the stage of the drying process. Humidity tends to be higher at the beginning of the drying process and decreases as drying progresses.
- **Drying Time:** The length of time the food is subjected to drying also plays a crucial role in achieving the desired results.

If these factors are not properly controlled, it can lead to case: hardening, which occurs when moisture evaporates too quickly from the surface, while the interior remains moist. This results in the formation of a hard, impermeable surface layer that prevents further moisture removal from the food.

TREATMENTS OF FOODS BEFORE DRYING

Several pretreatments of foods to be dried are important in their effect on the microbial population, as will be discussed. These preliminary treatments may include: (1) sorting and grading based on size, maturity, and strength, (2) washing, especially of fruits and vegetables, (3) peeling of fruits and vegetables by hand, machine, in a dye bath, or by abrasion, (4) halving, slicing, slicing, or dicing, (5) alkaline soaking, which is used primarily for fruits such as raisins, grapes, and plums (for sun drying) and using 0.1 to 1.5 percent hot wort or sodium carbonate, (6) blanching or scalding of vegetables and some fruits (apricots, peaches), and (7) sulfurization of light- colored fruits and some vegetables. The fruits are sulfurized by exposure to sulfur dioxide gas produced by burning sulfur so that a level of 1000 to 3000 ppm is absorbed, depending on the fruit. Vegetables can be sulfurized after blanching in the same way or by dipping or spraying with a sulfite solution. Sulfur helps maintain a nice light color, preserves vitamin C and possibly vitamin A, and repels insects; it also kills many microorganisms present.

Procedures After Drying

The procedures after drying vary with the kind of dried food.

Sweating

"Sweating" is storage, usually in bins or boxes, for equalization of moisture or read- dition of moisture to a desired level. It is used primarily with some dried fruits and some nuts (almonds, English walnuts).

Packaging

Most foods are packaged soon after drying for protection against moisture, contamination with microorganisms, and infestation with insects, although some dried foods (e.g., fruits and nuts) may be held as long as a year before packaging.

Pasteurization

Pasteurization is primarily applied to dried fruits, where it eliminates any pathogens and prevents spoilage by killing microorganisms. Typically, the fruit undergoes pasteurization while still in its packaging. The process, which can last anywhere from 30 to 70 minutes, involves exposing the fruit to temperatures between 65.6°C and 85°C, with a relative humidity of 70 to 100 percent, depending on the type of fruit.

MICROBIOLOGY OF DRIED FOODS

Before Reception at the Processing Plant

The microbiology of foods before they arrive at the processing plant is generally similar, regardless of whether they are to be dried, chilled, frozen, canned, or processed in another way. Fruits and vegetables often carry soil and waterborne microorganisms, along with their own natural surface flora. Spoiled sections may contain the bacteria responsible for decay. If environmental conditions allow, some microorganisms may grow before the food reaches the processing facility. For instance, piled vegetables may warm up, promoting the growth of slime-producing, flavor- damaging, or rotting organisms

Meats and poultry are typically contaminated by soil, intestinal contents, handlers, and equipment, while fish carry contamination from water, their own slime, intestinal contents, and handlers. Growth can occur before they reach processing plants. Eggs can be contaminated by the hen, nests, and handlers, and without proper handling, microbial growth may occur. Milk, from the time it is secreted by the cow to its arrival at the plant, can also support the growth of psychrotrophic bacteria.

In the Plant before Drying

Microbial growth that begins on foods before they reach the drying plant can continue within the plant until the drying process begins. Additionally, equipment and workers may introduce further contamination. Various pretreatments may either reduce or increase the microbial load, but contamination can still occur after these treatments. The grading, selection, and sorting processes of foods, particularly fruits, vegetables, eggs, and milk, play a significant role in determining the types and amounts of microorganisms present. Removing spoiled fruits, vegetables, or parts helps decrease the microbial load in the food intended for drying, as does discarding cracked, dirty, or spoiled eggs, and rejecting milk that fails to meet bacteriological quality standards. Washing fruits and vegetables helps remove soil and other contaminants, which in turn reduces microorganisms, though it may also introduce new ones if the water quality is poor.

Additionally, moisture left on the surface can promote microbial growth if not properly handled. Washing eggs may be counterproductive unless done promptly, as the added moisture can allow bacteria to penetrate the shell. Peeling fruits or vegetables, particularly using steam or lye, typically reduces microbial numbers, as most organisms are concentrated on the outer surfaces. Slicing or cutting food does not inherently increase microbial counts but can do so if the equipment used is not properly cleaned and sanitized. Pre- sun drying treatments such as dipping in alkali can lower microbial levels.

Blanching or scalding vegetables results in a significant reduction in bacterial populations, sometimes as much as 99%, though bacterial growth may resume afterward due to contamination from equipment and available growth conditions. Finally, sulfuring fruits and vegetables reduces microbial numbers and helps prevent microbial growth in the final dried product

During the Drying Process

The application of heat during a drying process results in a reduction in the total number of microorganisms, but the effecti eness varies depending on the types and numbers of organisms initially present and the drying process used. In general, all yeasts and most bacteria are destroyed, but bacterial and mold spores usually survive, as do the vegetative cells of some heat- resistant types of bacteria. As we will see later, inappropriate drying conditions can also allow microorganisms to grow.

More microorganisms are killed by freezing than by dehydration during the lyophilization process. Any method that involves sudden and dramatic changes in temperature, either an increase during heat drying or a decrease during freeze drying, is likely to cause metabolic damage to some organisms, making them more demanding for food.

After Drying

If the drying process and storage conditions are suitable, there will be no growth of microorganisms in dried foods. During storage, the number of organisms decreases slowly, faster at first and slower later. Microorganisms that are resistant to drying will survive better; therefore, the percentage of these organisms will increase. Bacteria and mold spores, some micrococci and microbacteria are particularly resistant to storage under dry conditions. There may be some possibility of contamination of dried foods during packaging and other handling after drying.

Special treatments given to certain dry foods affect the number of microbes. Sweating dried fruit to equalize moisture can allow microbial growth. Pasteurization of dried fruit reduces the number of microorganisms. Some products are repackaged for retail, for example. , figs in the Middle East and are then subject to contamination.

Microbial content and the temperature of the water used to rehydrate dry foods will affect the shelf life of the rehydrated product. Bacteria in freeze-dried chicken are further reduced in number by rehydration with water at 50°C and almost eliminated when the water is at 85 to 100°C. Bacterial growth in rehydrated meat occurs at a temperature favorable, but the shelf life is better at 4°C. *Staphylococcus aureus* has been found to survive freeze-drying and rehydration at 60°C; therefore, rehydration at 100°C is recommended.

MICROBIOLOGY OF SPECIFIC DRIED FOODS

Dried Vegetables

On dried vegetables, the number of microorganisms can range from very small to millions per gram. The percentage killed by the dehydrating process is typically lower than with the more acidic fruits, and the numbers on the vegetable right before drying may be high due to contamination and growth after blanching. Inappropriate loading of drying trays may cause lactic acid bacteria to sour vegetables like potatoes and onions, leading to a noticeable rise in bacterial populations throughout the drying process. Onions are more dangerous because they aren't blanched.

Chiefly bacteria are found on dried vegetables. A number of investigators have listed the genera of bacteria found (summarized by Vaughn, 1951) to include *Escherichia, Enterobacter, Bacillus, Clostridium, Micrococcus, Pseudomonas,* and *Streptococcus.* Vaughn found *Lactobacillus* and *Leuconostoc* species predominant in many samples of dehydrated vegetables.

Dried Eggs

Dried eggs can contain from a few hundred microorganisms, mostly bacteria, per gram to over 100 million, depending on the broken eggs and the methods used. Since the contents of good quality fresh eggs are normally free of microorganisms or contain only a few, dried eggs should have a low microbial content. However, the inclusion of poorly washed eggs, eggs that have sweated, dirty and cracked eggs, and eggs already overgrown with microorganisms can add a large number of organisms; in addition, contamination and growth can occur during crushing and other handling prior to drying.

The drying process can reduce the number by ten to a hundredfold, but still allows a large number to survive. A variety of types of organisms have been found in dried eggs, including micrococci, streptococci, coliforms, spores, and molds. When egg whites have been pretreated through a fermentation process, the microbial count in the dried product can be high. Egg yolk is a better growth medium than egg white and is likely to have higher microbial counts at rest and better growth support prior to drying

Dried Fruits

The numbers of microorganisms on most fresh fruits range from comparatively few to many, depending on pretreatments, and on most dried fruits they vary from a few hundred per gram of fruit to thousands; in whole fruits they are mostly on the outer surfaces. Spores of bacteria and molds are likely to be the most numerous. When part of the fruit has supported growth and sporulation of mold before or after drying, mold spores may be present in large numbers.

Dried Milk

The number of microorganisms in dry milk may vary from a few hundred per gram to millions, depending on the milk being dried and the drying process. Roller or drum drying kills more organisms than does the spray process. The predominant kinds of organisms in dry milk are thermoduric streptococci, micrococci, and sporeformers.

INTERMEDIATE-MOISTURE FOODS

A variety of commercially prepared foods, which typically contain 20 to 40 percent moisture and are stable without refrigeration, are classified as intermediate- moisture products. These include items such as soft candies, jams, jellies, honey, many dried fruits, certain bakery goods, and even meat products like pepperoni, country ham, jerky, and some dried fish. These products are low in moisture, can be consumed directly without requiring preparation or rehydration, and do not have the typical taste of dehydrated foods. The pet food industry has been particularly successful in developing these products, sparking widespread interest across the food sector.

The stability of intermediate- moisture foods is partly due to their low water activity (aw), with such products often being referred to as reduced- water activity foods. As mentioned in Chapter 1, all microorganisms have optimal and minimal water activity levels for growth. By adjusting the aw of a product—either by adding solutes or removing water—below the minimal aw required by normal spoilage microorganisms, these products become microbiologically stable. It is important to note that many of these products may still contain viable microorganisms and spores, but these cannot reproduce or germinate due to the restrictive aw. When creating a product with reduced aw, other factors that influence microbial growth must be considered, such as pH, oxygen levels, temperature, nutrient content, and the presence of preservatives, whether natural or added.

On a commercial scale, stability is not solely reliant on reducing the aw. For instance, if only water activity reduction were used, the foods would need to have an aw of 0.65 to 0.70, resembling dehydrated products. However, most intermediate- moisture products have an aw between 0.75 and 0.85. This aw is typically adjusted through drying, the addition of solutes (like sugar, salt, and glycerol), or a combination of both methods. A prime example of intermediate-moisture food technology is moist pet food, packaged in flexible pouches, which has an aw between 0.83 and 0.85, is pasteurized, contains an antimycotic like potassium sorbate, and has a moisture content of 25 to 27 percent. Brockmann (in Van Arsdel et al., 1973) outlined the benefits of reduced water activity in food preservation, which include- (1) an aw of 0.85 inhibiting the most common food pathogens, (2) bacterial spore germination being prevented at relatively high aw values, (3) nonsporeforming organisms, which can grow at aw levels below 0.95, being susceptible to pasteurization, (4) suboptimal growth conditions causing inhibition at higher aw levels, (5) organisms that thrive in low water activities multiplying slowly, and (6) yeasts and molds being suppressed by antimycotics.

9 Enhancing Shelf Life With Food Additives

Food additives are chemicals that are added to food products during processing in order to improve their safety, extend their shelf life, and improve their organoleptic properties. Among other things, they serve as flavor enhancers, color stabilizers, antioxidants, and preservatives. Food additives keep our food safe and fresh for longer by preventing oxidation, limiting microbial growth, and preventing spoiling. It is important to remember, though, that the use of additives must always adhere to stringent guidelines and be kept within safe concentration ranges.

A food additive is defined as a substance or combination of substances, distinct from the basic food, that is present in food due to any stage of its production, processing, storage, or packaging. This definition specifically refers to intentional additives, excluding any accidental contamination (WHO, 1965). Food additives, particularly those aimed at preventing the spoilage or breakdown of food, are often termed chemical preservatives. Such spoilage may be triggered by microorganisms, food enzymes, or chemical reactions. One of the primary roles of chemical preservatives is to inhibit microbial growth and activity. These preservatives may work by disrupting microbial cell membranes, enzyme functions, or genetic processes.

Additionally, preservatives can function as antioxidants to prevent the oxidation of unsaturated fats, neutralizers of acidity, stabilizers to maintain physical characteristics, firming agents, or coatings to protect the food from microorganisms, moisture loss, and adverse microbial, enzymatic, or chemical actions. Beyond the chemicals deliberately added to food, various substances can unintentionally contaminate food during its production, processing, or packaging. For instance, pesticide, herbicide, and fungicide residues from agricultural practices, along with detergents used for cleaning food, utensils, and equipment, may remain in the food.

The effecti eness of chemical preservatives in killing or inhibiting microbial growth is influenced by several factors, including- (1) the concentration of the chemical, (2) the type, quantity, age, and prior exposure of the microorganism, (3) temperature, (4) duration of exposure, and (5) the chemical and physical properties of the substrate (such as moisture content, pH, solutes, surface tension, colloids, and protective substances). A chemical agent may be bactericidal at a certain concentration, merely inhibitory at a lower level, or ineffecti e at even more diluted concentrations.

CHARACTERISTICS OF AN EFFECTIVE ANTIMICROBIAL PRESERVATIVE

The increasing pressure on food supplies requires that food loss through product spoilage be minimized. Unfortunately, the countries experiencing food shortages and poor food quality are those that lack adequate preservation technology. Using a chemical preservative in this situation would have dire consequences.

Although, many countries have advanced preservation technologies, the methods are not used to their full potential or are not fully effecti e. Chemical preservatives are used, alone or in combination with other forms of preservation, to maintain a food in its original or manufactured state and to prevent excessive losses through spoilage.

Ideally, a chemical preservative should have a broad spectrum of antimicrobial activity; be nontoxic to humans or animals; be inexpensive; have no effect on the taste, flavor, or aroma of the original food; not be inactivated by the food or any substance it contains; not encourage the development of resistant strains; and kill rather than inhibit microorganisms. Most of the preservatives discussed in this chapter are inhibitors at acceptable concentrations, but only ethylene and propylene oxides and diethyl pyrocarbonate are lethal to microorganisms at concentrations normally used. In addition, the ideal chemical preservative has not been found. In fact, many of the most commonly used compounds are also old preservatives. The simple and "ideal" new preservatives that have been proposed are few in number and many of them, for one reason or another, have not been developed into commercially acceptable additives.

FOOD ADDITIVES

For decades, the food industry has constantly created new chemicals to treat, preserve and process our food. Using these chemicals, scientists are able to mimic natural flavors, color foods to make them appear «natural» or «fresh,» and keep them fresh for longer periods. Food additives are used to reduce the risk of microbial contamination. There are also food products made entirely of chemicals. Coffee creamers, sugar substitutes and sweets they are made almost entirely of artificial ingredients. Such manipulation of our diet can have a profound effect on our body's unique biochemical balance.

Additives described as generally recognized as safe (GRAS), have been in use for several years. The substances used as additives in food, should be of food grade and must meet the PFA or BIS specifications.

The different groups of food additi es are described in Table.

Table. Different Groups of FoodAdditives

Group of food additives	Purpose	Examples
Preservatives	Prevent food spoilage, extend shelf life	Sodium benzoate, Sorbic acid, Nitrites, Sulfite

Group of food additives	Purpose	Examples
Antioxidants	Prevent oxidation of fats and oils, preserve color and flavo	BHA (Butylated hydroxyanisole), BHT (Butylated hydroxytoluene), Ascorbic acid (Vitamin C)
Color Additives	Enhance or restore color of food products	Tartrazine, Carmine, Beta-carotene
Flavor Enhancers	Enhance or modify the flavor of food	Monosodium glutamate (MSG), Disodium inosinate, Sodium guanylate
Emulsifier	Help mix ingredients that would otherwise separate (e.g., oil and water)	Lecithin, Mono- and diglycerides, Polysorbates
Stabilizers and Thickeners	Improve texture, consistency, and appearance of food	Guar gum, Xanthan gum, Pectin
Acidity Regulators	Maintain or adjust the pH of food products	Citric acid, Lactic acid, Acetic acid
Sweeteners	Add sweetness without adding sugar or calories	Aspartame, Stevia, Sucralose, Saccharin
Leavening Agents	Cause dough to rise by producing gas	Baking soda, Sodium bicarbonate, Ammonium bicarbonate
Anti- caking Agents	Prevent clumping of powdered or granular substances	Silicon dioxide, Calcium silicate, Magnesium carbonate
Firming Agents	Maintain or improve the firmness of food	Calcium chloride, Calcium lactate
Humectants	Retain moisture and prevent drying out of food	Glycerol, Sorbitol, Propylene glycol
Packaging Additives	Enhance packaging materials or the food's interaction with packaging	Polyvinyl acetate, Beeswax

Table.Principal Preservative used in Various Foods

Name	Significance
Sodium chloride	Antimicrobial, dehydrating agent, used as brine
Sugar	Preservation of foods due to the high osmotic pressure
Sulfur dioxide	Prevents the growth of undesirable microbes during wine making, prevents browning of dried and cut fruits
Nitrate and Nitrite	Color stabilizer in the curing of meat and antimicrobial in action

Sorbic acid	Sodium and potassium salts inhibit the growth of moulds and yeast in cheese and bakery products, fruit juices, wines and pickles
Acetic acid	Vinegar (4% acetic acid) is used to preserve pickled vegetables, acetates of sodium, potassium and calcium are used to prevent ropiness and growth of moulds
Propionic acid	Sodium and calcium salts are effecti e against moulds and some bacteria; Controls Bacillus mesentericus causing ropy bread
Benzoic acid	Active agent against yeast and bacteria, well suited for the preservation of acid foods such as fruit juices, carbonated beverages, pickles and sauerkraut
Parabens	Effecti e inhibitors of molds and yeast, they are alkyl esters of p- hydroxybenzoic acid; Methyl, ethyl, propyl and heptyl esters are used
Epoxides	Antimicrobial cyclic esters, used as preservatives—ethylene oxide and propylene oxide; to reduce load of microbes in spices
Antibiotics	Antimicrobial agents used in the control of bacteria in fish and poultry products; Chlorotetracycline and oxytetracycline
Diethyl pyrocabonate	Used as an antimicrobial agent in fruit juices, wines and carbonated beverages

ADDED PRESERVATIVES

The Federal Food, Drug, and Cosmetic Act, amended by the Food Additives Amendment of 1958, defines a chemical preservative as any substance that, when added to food, prevents or slows its deterioration. However, this definition excludes common ingredients such as salt, sugars, vinegars, spices, oils extracted from spices, and substances like woodsmoke. The 1985 Code of Federal Regulations (Title 21) defines a food additive as any substance that, when added to food, either directly or indirectly becomes a component of the food or influences its characteristics, unless exempted by section 201(s) of the act. This also applies to materials used in packaging if they are likely to become part of the food or affect its properties. However, physical effects such as maintaining the food's shape, protecting contents, or preventing moisture loss do not qualify as affecting food characteristics. If a packaging component does not migrate into the food, it is not considered a food additive. Additionally, substances used to alter the flavor, texture, or other characteristics of the food may be classified as food additives, even if they don't become part of the food itself. Antimicrobial preservatives in food can be categorized as follows:

- **Preservatives not Legally Defined as Such:** This includes natural organic acids (like lactic, malic, citric), their salts, vinegar (acetic acid), sodium chloride, sugars, spices and their oils, woodsmoke, carbon dioxide, and nitrogen.

- **Chemicals Classified as Food Additives:** These include any substances not in the previous two categories, which can only be used when proven safe for humans or animals. Once proven safe, they fall into group 4.
- **Chemicals Approved by the Food and Drug Administration:** These are preservatives that have undergone safety testing and are authorized by the FDA.
- **Substances Generally Recognized as Safe (GRAS):** These include propionic acid and its salts, caprylic acid, sorbic acid and its salts, benzoic acid and its derivatives (such as methylparaben and propylparaben), sodium diacetate, sulfur dioxide and sulfites, and sodium nitrite, among others (limitations on some of these substances will be noted).

Preservatives intended to inhibit or kill microorganisms can be further classified based on various factors such as chemical composition, mode of action, specificity, effecti eness, and legal status. Some preservatives, like sugar, are effecti e due to their physical properties, while others, like sodium benzoate, work through chemical actions.

Some, such as sodium chloride, exert a combination of these effects. Some preservatives are used directly in food, acting as antiseptics, while others are applied to the outer surfaces of food, killing or inhibiting microorganisms. Certain preservatives are used in packaging materials, and others are used as gases or vapors around food. Some preservatives are added to ice, particularly for chilling fish and other foods. Preservatives may be highly specific, targeting certain types of microorganisms, such as molds or yeasts, with little effect on bacteria, or they may target specific groups or species of bacteria or other organisms

Most of the more common antimicrobial additives used in foods are presented in Table. Current allowable levels for some of the preservatives are given in Table .

Table: Use of Antimicrobial Additives in Various Foods

Food product	Benzoic acid	Methyl/Propyl paraben	Sorbates	Propionates	Sulfite	Acetates/Diacetates
Carbonated beverages	+	+	+		+	
Beverage syrup	+	+	+			
Fruit drink	+	+	+			
Fruit juice	+	+	+		+	
Wine and Beer		+	+		+	
Cheese and Cheese products			+	+		
Margarine	+		+			
Pie crust and Pastries		+	+	+		+

Pie fillings	+	+	+	+		
Sausage		+	+			
Preserved fish			+			
Salads, Salad Dressings	+	+	+			+
Dried fruits and Vegetables		+	+			
Fresh fruits and Vegetables						
Pickles, Relishes, Olives, Sauerkraut	+	+	+			+
Spices						
Starch						

ALLOWABLE PRESERVATIVE CONCENTRATIONS IN FOODS

Maximum allowable concentrations of antimicrobials preservative in diffrent foods as given in table.

Table: Maximum Levels of Antimicrobial Preservatives in Foods

Antimicrobial preservative	Maximum permitted level	Food types
Benzoic Acid	0.1% to 0.15% (1000- 1500 ppm)	Soft drinks, sauces, pickles, jams, jellies
Sodium Benzoate	0.1% to 0.2% (1000- 2000 ppm)	Beverages, fruit products, sauces, pickles
Sorbic Acid	0.1% to 0.3% (1000- 3000 ppm)	Cheese, bakery products, dried fruits
Potassium Sorbate	0.1% to 0.3% (1000- 3000 ppm)	Cheese, baked goods, beverages, dried fruits
Sulfur Dioxide (SO_2)	0.05% to 0.1% (500- 1000 ppm)	Dried fruits, wine, fruit juices
Sodium Nitrite	0.02% to 0.1% (200- 1000 ppm)	Meat products (sausages, bacon, ham)
Propionic Acid	0.1% to 0.2% (1000- 2000 ppm)	Baked goods, bread, cakes
Caprylic Acid	0.05% to 0.1% (500- 1000 ppm)	Dairy products, cheese
Calcium Propionate	0.1% to 0.2% (1000- 2000 ppm)	Baked goods, bread

Antimicrobial preservative	Maximum permitted level	Food types
Citric Acid	0.05% to 0.1% (500- 1000 ppm)	Beverages, sauces, pickles
Formic Acid	0.05% to 0.1% (500- 1000 ppm)	Animal feeds, bakery products
Potassium Metabisulfit	0.1% to 0.2% (1000- 2000 ppm)	Dried fruits, vegetables, wine
Dimethyl Dicarbonate (DMDC)	0.03% to 0.1% (300- 1000 ppm)	Fruit juices, wines, soft drinks

Note- The actual permitted levels of these antimicrobial preservatives can vary according to different regional and international regulations (such as the FDA, EU, or Codex Alimentarius standards). Always refer to the specific food safety regulations applicable in the region where the product is sold or consumed.

Organic Acids and Their Salts

Lactic, acetic, propionic, and citric acids or their salts may be added to or developed in foods. Their development in foods during fermentation will be discussed in a following section. Citric acid is used in sirups, drinks, jams, and jellies as a substitute for fruit flavors and for preservation. Lactic and acetic acids are added to brines of various kinds, green olives, etc.

Propionates

Sodium and calcium propionate are widely used to prevent mold growth and rope development in baked goods, as well as to inhibit mold in cheese foods and spreads. They are also used experimentally in products such as butter, jams, jellies, figs, apple slices, and malt extract. These propionates are effecti e against molds but have minimal impact on most yeasts and bacteria. Their effecti eness is pH- dependent, with optimal activity occurring in the pH range of 5 to 6. These preservatives are particularly useful in bread and baked goods, as while the baking process kills most molds, contamination can occur during slicing or wrapping, making the propionates essential.

They can be added to yeast- leavened dough without hindering the fermentation process. Propionic acid, a short- chain fatty acid (CH_3CH_2COOH), likely affects cell membrane permeability to exert its fungistatic action, although its exact mechanism remains unclear. Naturally, propionic acid is found in Swiss cheese as a developed preservative, with concentrations up to 1 percent.

Benzoates

Sodium benzoate, the sodium salt of benzoic acid, is widely used as an antimicrobial agent in foods such as jams, jellies, margarine, carbonated beverages, fruit salads, pickles, relishes, and fruit juices. Its effecti eness is greatly influenced by pH, being less effecti e at near- neutral pH levels and more potent in acidic conditions (pH 2.5 to 4.0). At these acidic pH levels, sodium benzoate can inhibit the growth of many bacteria, yeasts, and molds, as the undissociated benzoic acid is the active antimicrobial agent. Additionally, two esters of p- hydroxybenzoic acid, methylparaben and propylparaben, along with butyl and ethyl esters to a lesser extent, are also utilized in food preservation. These esters share similar antimicrobial properties to benzoic acid, with the key advantage of being effecti e at higher pH values. This increased efficac is due to the esterification of the carboxyl group, which allows the undissociated molecule to persist over a broader pH range. The precise mechanism of action for benzoates is not fully understood, but it is known that their effecti eness increases as the chain length of the ester group grows.

Sorbates

As a calcium, sodium, or potassium salt, sorbic acid is used as a coating, dip, or spray on packaging materials as well as a direct antimicrobial additive in foods. Cheeses, cheese products, baked goods, drinks, syrups, fruit juices, jams, pickles, margarine, dried fruits, and fruit cocktails all make extensive use of it.

Although, they are less effecti e against bacteria, sorbic acid and its salts are known to inhibit molds and yeast. With a maximum level of use at roughly pH 6.5, they work best at low pH values. At pH levels above 4.0, these substances work better than sodium benzoate.

Acetates

Although, some acetic acid derivatives, such as sodium diacetate, monochloroacetic acid, peracetic acid, and dehydroacetic acid, have been suggested as preservatives, not all of them have received FDA approval. Dehydroacetic acid has been used as a temporary preservative for squash and to impregnate cheese wrappers to prevent the growth of mold. Pigs' feet, mayonnaise, pickles, catsup, and pickled sausages all contain acetic acid in the form of vinegar. Acetic acid works better against bacteria and yeasts than molds, and its potency rises as pH falls, which would encourage the undissociated acid to be present.

Sodium diacetate has been used to treat butter wrappers and in cheese spreads and malt syrups.

Nitrites and Nitrates

Combinations of these various salts have been used in curing solutions and curing mixtures for meats. Nitrites decompose to nitric acid, which forms nitrosomyoglobin when it reacts with the heme pigments in meats and thereby forms a stable red color. Nitrates probably only act as a reservoir for nitrite, and their use is being restricted. Nitrites can react with secondary and tertiary amines to form nitrosamines, which are known to be carcinogenic. The assessment of the safety of nitrites in foods has been reviewed (Anonymous, 1981, 1982). The problem of possible carcinogenic nitrosamines may be greatest in bacon, and the extended future of nitrite use in foods will probably remain controversial. They are currently added in the form of sodium nitrite, potassium nitrite, sodium nitrate, and potassium nitrate.

Recent work has emphasized the inhibitory property of nitrites toward *Clostridium botulinum* in meat products, particularly in bacon and canned or processed hams. Nitrates have a limited effect on a limited number of organisms and would not be considered a good chemical preservative.

Sulfur Dioxide and Sulfites

The use of sulfur dioxide and sulfites in food preservation dates back to ancient civilizations, with the Egyptians and Romans burning sulfur to create sulfur dioxide for sanitizing wine- making equipment and storage vessels. In modern times, sulfur dioxide and various sulfites, such as sodium sulfite, potassium sulfite, sodium bisulfite, potassium bisulfite, sodium metabisulfite, and potassium metabisulfite, are used in the wine industry to sanitize equipment and reduce the microbial load in grape must.

These compounds, when dissolved in aqueous solutions, form sulfurous acid, which is the active antimicrobial agent, with its effecti eness enhanced at low pH values. Sulfurous acid is believed to affect microbial cells by reducing disulfide linkages, forming carbonyl compounds, reacting with ketone groups, and inhibiting respiratory mechanisms. The fumes from burning sulfur are commonly used to treat light- colored dehydrated fruits, while dehydrated vegetables are treated with a spray of neutral bisulfites and sulfites before drying. Sulfur dioxide is also employed in the preservation of syrups, fruit juices, and wine. In some countries, sulfites are permitted for use on meats and fish. Besides its antimicrobial properties, sulfites are also used to prevent enzymatic and nonenzymatic discoloration in certain foods.

Ethylene and Propylene Oxide

Unlike other chemical preservatives, ethylene oxide and propylene oxide are sterilants. Ethylene oxide is capable of killing all microorganisms, while propylene oxide, though effecti e against many microorganisms, is not as potent. These gases are believed to act as strong alkylating agents, attacking labile hydrogens. Their primary applications include sterilizing packaging materials, fumigating warehouses, and "cold sterilization" of various plastics, chemicals, pharmaceuticals, syringes, and hospital supplies. They have also been successfully used in the preservation of dried fruits, dried eggs, gelatin, cereals, dried yeast, and spices. The FDA limits the use of ethylene oxide to spices and processed natural seasonings, excluding mixtures that contain added salt. Propylene oxide is permitted only for fumigating dried prunes, glacé fruits, cocoa, gums, spices, starch, and processed nutmeats, but not peanuts.

Sugar and Salt

These compounds lower the aw and thus have an adverse effect on microorganisms. Sodium chloride is used in brines and curing solutions or is applied directly to the food. Enough may be added to slow or prevent the growth of microorganisms or only enough to permit an acid fermentation to take place. Salt has been reported to have the following effects- (1) It causes high osmotic pressure and hence plasmolysis of cells, the percentage of salt necessary to inhibit growth or harm the cell varying with the microorganism, (2) it dehydrates foods by drawing out and tying up moisture as it dehydrates microbial cells, (3) it ionizes to yield the chlorine ion, which is harmful to organisms, (4) it reduces the solubility of oxygen in the moisture, (5) it sensitizes the cell against carbon dioxide, and (6) it interferes with the action of proteolytic enzymes. The effectiveness of NaCl varies directly with its concentration and the temperature.

Because of their osmotic effect and capacity to render water unavailable to living things, sugars like glucose and sucrose are effecti e preservatives. Sweetened condensed milk, fruits in syrups, jellies, and candies are a few examples of foods that are preserved by high sugar concentrations.

Alcohols

Ethanol, which acts as a coagulant and denaturizer of cell proteins, is most effecti e as a germicide when used in concentrations between 70 and 95 percent. Flavoring extracts, such as vanilla and lemon extracts, are preserved due to their alcohol content. While the alcohol content in beer, ale, and unfortified wine is not high enough to prevent microbial spoilage, it does limit the types of microorganisms that can grow. In contrast, liqueurs and distilled liquors generally contain sufficien alcohol to protect them from microbial contamination. Methanol is toxic and should not be added to foods; however, the small amounts introduced through smoking are not harmful. Glycerol has antiseptic properties at high concentrations due to its dehydrating effect, though it plays a minimal role in food preservation. Propylene glycol has been utilized as a mold inhibitor and to eliminate airborne microorganisms through spraying.

Formaldehyde

The addition of formaldehyde to foods is not permitted, except as a minor constituent of woodsmoke, but this compound is effecti e against molds, bacteria, and viruses and can be used where its poisonous nature and irritating properties are not objectionable. Thus it is useful in the treatment of walls, shelves, floors, etc., to eliminate molds and their spores. Paraformaldehyde can be used to control bacterial and fungal growth in tapholes of maple trees. Formaldehyde probably combines with free amino groups of the proteins of cell protoplasm, injures nuclei, and coagulates proteins.

Woodsmoke

Smoking food typically serves two primary purposes- enhancing flavor and preserving the food. Additionally, it can result in other beneficial effects, such as improving the color of meat's interior and the exterior's glossy finish, as well as tenderizing the meat. The preservation aspect of smoking occurs through the infusion of chemical preservatives from the smoke into the food's surface, the combined effect of heat and preservatives during the process, and the drying effect, particularly at the surface. Typically, smoke is produced by burning wood, with hardwoods like hickory being preferred, though corncobs and other materials may also be used. Other woods used include apple, oak, maple, beech, birch, walnut, and mahogany. Sawdust is added to the fire to create a dense smudge. Temperature and humidity are adjusted to suit the type of food being smoked, with the smoking period varying depending on the food. For meat, smoking temperatures range from 43 to 71°C, and the process may last from several hours to days.

Woodsmoke contains numerous volatile compounds that can have bacteriostatic and bactericidal effects. Formaldehyde is considered the most potent of these compounds, followed by phenols and cresols. Other smoke compounds include aliphatic acids (from formic to caproic), primary and secondary alcohols, ketones, acetaldehyde, aldehydes, waxes, resins, and compounds such as guaiacol, catechol, methlcatechol, and pyrogallol, including its methyl ester. These substances are sometimes grouped as pyroligneous acid. Woodsmoke is generally more effecti e against vegetative cells than bacterial spores, with its germicidal action increasing with concentration and temperature, and varying depending on the type of wood used. The lingering effect of smoke on food is typically more pronounced against bacteria than molds. The concentration of compounds from woodsmoke needed to inhibit mold growth increases as the humidity in storage rises.

The use of "liquid smoke," a chemical solution similar to woodsmoke, applied to the surface of foods, offers little to no preservative effect, though it does contribute to flavor

Spices and Other Condiments

Spices and other condiments typically do not exhibit strong bacteriostatic effects at the concentrations commonly used in food preparation, but they can support other preservatives in inhibiting microbial growth. The effecti eness of spices varies depending on their origin, freshness, and whether they are stored whole or ground. The inhibitory properties of spices differ based on the type of spice and the microorganism being tested. For example, mustard flour and mustard's volatile oil are highly effecti e against *Saccharomyces cerevisiae,* yet cinnamon and cloves tend to be more potent against most bacteria. The essential oils of spices generally have a stronger inhibitory effect than the ground form of the spice.

Cinnamon and cloves, containing cinnamic aldehyde and eugenol respectively, are typically more bacteriostatic than many other spices. Ground peppercorn and allspice are less effecti e, while mustard, mace, nutmeg, and ginger show even weaker effects. Spices such as thyme, bay leaves, marjoram, savory, rosemary, and black pepper have only a mild inhibitory effect on most organisms and may even promote the growth of some, like yeasts and molds. Even in higher concentrations, more potent spices may allow the growth of some mold species while inhibiting the production of their asexual spores. Among the tested oils, mustard's volatile oil is the most effective against yeasts, followed by oils from cinnamon and cloves, while thyme and bay leaves are the least effective.

Unless spices are treated to reduce their microbial content, they can introduce high levels of undesirable microorganisms into foods. Other plant- based ingredients used in seasoning, such as horseradish, garlic, and onion, may have bacteriostatic or germicidal properties. Extracts from these plants, as well as from cabbage and turnip, have shown inhibitory effects on *Bacillus subtilis* and *Escherichia coli*. The active compounds, acrolein in onions and garlic, and butyl thiocyanate in horseradish, are volatile and can dissipate when exposed to air, resulting in a loss of bacteriostatic activity.

Others

Halogens are commonly added to water for various purposes, such as washing foods or equipment, cooling, and in some products like butter washing. Chlorine can be directly added to drinking water for chlorination, or hypochlorites or chloramines may be used. Iodine- impregnated wrappers are sometimes used to extend the shelf life of fruits, and iodophors—combinations of iodine with nonionic wetting agents and acids—are employed in sanitizing dairy utensils. Halogens kill microorganisms through oxidation, damaging cell membranes, or by directly reacting with cell proteins.

Hypochlorites, typically in the form of calcium or sodium, produce hypochlorous acid, a potent oxidizing agent, which is an effecti e germicide; however, their effecti eness diminishes when there is a significant amount of organic matte present. Hypochlorites are used to treat water in food plants for drinking, processing, and cooling, as well as for cleaning plant equipment. They have also been added to ice used for shipping fish and to ater for washing fruits and vegetables. Microorganisms are damaged either through oxidation or by direct chlorination of their proteins.

Phosphoric acid is used in certain soft drinks, such as colas. The oxidizing agent hydrogen peroxide is used as a preservative, typically in combination with heat. One process for pasteurizing milk for cheese involves adding hydrogen peroxide and applying a relatively low temperature, with any excess peroxide being decomposed by catalase. In the sugar industry, thermophiles are killed through a combination of heat and hydrogen peroxide. Other types of peroxides are used in food, though not for antimicrobial preservation.

Gas storage, discussed in Chapter 7 regarding preservation through chilling, involves gases like carbon dioxide, often combined with cooling, to preserve food. Oxygen or air under pressure, used in processes such as the Hofius process for milk, is combined with chilling. Nitrogen, an inert gas, is applied over foods that should not be exposed to air.

Boric acid and borates are still used in some countries as food preservatives, although their use is prohibited in the United States. Powdered boric acid has been dusted on foods like meats, but it is a weak antiseptic and not regarded as safe for health. Borax (sodium tetraborate) has been used to wash vegetables and fruits like oranges.

Colors

Any natural or synthetic dye, pigment or substance that can impart color when applied or added to a food, which includes stabilizers, color fixati es or color- retention agents are widely used in food industries.

Natural Colorants

- Anthocyanins comprise a diverse group of glycosidic derivatives of the 2-phenylbenzophyrylium structure, imparting blue, violet and red color to many edible fruits and vegetables.
- Carotenoids are oil: soluble pigments found in both plants and animals, composed of aliphatic and alicyclic unsaturated terpenes made up of eight isoprene units. Xanthophylls, a subgroup of carotenoids, are yellow pigments that are structurally similar to carotenes but contain keto or hydroxyl groups. Examples of carotenoids and xanthophylls found in natural extracts include Bixaorellana, which contains bixin; betalains from the red beetroot Beta vulgaris; curcumin, derived from the rhizome of Curcuma longa; annatto, obtained from the seeds of Bixa orellana; and saffron, a dicarboxylic carotenoid sourced from the stigma of the Crocus sativus flo ers.
- Cochineal and related pigments are extracted from the dried crushed bodies of the female D. coccus, just prior to egg- laying time. Carmine is used in the powder form in a variety of foods. Alkannet, extracted in alcohol from the roots of Alkanna tinctoria Tansch, is used in ice creams.
- Microbial colorants like Monascus are obtained from the *Monoascus* species, imparting a red color, used in wine making. It is soluble in oil and heat stable.
- Biliproteins from algae are soluble in water or alcohol and are used in chewing gum, identified as red phycoerythrins and the blue phycocyanins.

Synthetic Colorants

Synthetic colors are allowed only in specific food items such as ice creams, biscuits, cakes, sugar- based confectionery, sweets and savories, fruit syrups, fruit squash, soft drinks, soft- drink concentrates, jams, and ready- to- serve beverages, among others. When used, synthetic colors must be labeled, and the permissible quantity is limited to 200 mg/kg. These colors are preferred over natural alternatives due to their superior coloring strength, uniformity, stability, and cost- effecti eness. Coal- tar dyes are commonly used in gelatin desserts, candies, and baked goods. Red colors are derived from Poncean 4R, carmoisine, and erythrosine; yellow from tartrazine and sunset yellow; blue from indigo carmine; and brilliant blue and green from fast green. These colors must be pure, free from harmful substances, and sold under BIS certification. Certain dyes, such as Rhodamine B (pink), orange

RN II, and Blue VRS, are carcinogenic and harmful to organs like the kidney, liver, and spleen, while Melanin yellow causes reproductive damage and sterility. As a result, these dyes are banned in the food industry.

Flavors

The flavors of most fruits and vegetables are mixtures of aldehydes and esters of organic alcohols and acids, with a range of essential oils with complex terpenoid structures. Flavoring additives are ingredients occurring naturally and they can be added to give a characteristic flavor to almost all foods. Flavor enhancers are not flavors themselves but they amplify the flavors of other substances. Natural flavoring substances, such as spices, herbs, roots, essences, and essential oils are plant derivatives.

One of the most widely used flavor enhancer is MSG—monosodium glutamate — generally recognized as safe and manufactured all over the world but not used in infant foods. Chinese and Japanese cooking for centuries have been using MSG extracted from seaweeds and soya beans.

Sweeteners

Sucrose is often considered the perfect sweetener as it is colorless, water-soluble, has a "pure" taste, but is high in calories. The first synthetic sweetener was saccharin, though it often leaves a bitter aftertaste. As a result, cyclamates are commonly used in soft drinks and other low- calorie liquid foods. However, cyclamates were banned after high doses in rats led to bladder cancer. Glycyrrhizic acid, derived from the root of *Glycyrrhiza glabra,* is used in tobacco products, confectionery, and beverages. Acesulfame K, found in bakery products, chewing gum, gelatin desserts, and soft drinks, has been linked to possible cancer-promoting effects. Aspartame, used in soft drinks, gelatin desserts, and low- calorie frozen foods, is made from aspartic acid and phenylalanine and is 180 times sweeter than sucrose. It is not recommended for pregnant or lactating women and can be harmful to individuals with phenylketonuria. Sucralose, derived from sucrose, resembles table sugar in taste, is highly soluble in water, and remains stable at high temperatures. It is not absorbed by the digestive tract, so it does not contribute to the calorie count of foods and does not affect blood sugar levels. Neotame, a non-nutritive sweetener approved for use, is 8,000 to 13,000 times sweeter than sucrose and chemically similar to aspartame. Other commonly used sweeteners include dulcin, neohesperidin dihydrochalcone, 5- nitro- 2- propoxyaniline, ultrasweet, alitame, and fruit extracts from the African kutemfe and serendipity berry.

Emulsifiers and Stabilizers

The additives used as emulsifiers and stabilizers are surfactants, amphipathetic molecules which act at the interfaces of the two phases in the food. Mono- and diglycerides and phospholipids like lecithin are the commonly used emulsifiers. Stabilizers are macromolecules which form a dispersed matrix or gel into which other smaller molecules can be incorporated. Stabilizers and thickeners commonly used are exudates like guargum, a plant polysaccharide, gum Arabic, and gum karaya. Extracts like agar, alginate, pectin, carrageenan derived from plant sources are excellent stabilizers. Synthetic xanthan gum and chemicals like carboxymethyl cellulose, hydroxyl propyl methyl cellulose and methyl cellulose are also used.

Stabilizers and thickeners are hydrophilic and are dispersed as colloids in solution and help thicken gravies, pie fillings, cake toppings, chocolate milk drinks, jellies, puddings, etc.

Antioxidants

In addition to causing food to deteriorate, oxidation of fats in food also produces disagreeable smells. Antioxidants are added to fat and fat-containing substances to slow down oxidation and prevent spoiling of such foods. Butylated hydroxyanisole (BHA), butylated hydroxytoluene (BHT), propyl gallate (PG), and tertiary butyl hydroquinone (TBHQ) are phenolic compounds that are added to food as antioxidants.

Tocopherols are naturally occurring compounds found in plant and animal tissues that function as antioxidants. The way that antioxidants work is by blocking the chain of free radicals that is involved in lipid metabolism.

Flour Improvers

Chemical agents used are oxidizing agents, which help in bleaching the food product. Benzoyl peroxide is used as a flour- bleaching agent, which does not affect the quality of the flour. Chlorine dioxide, nitrosyl chloride, and nitrogen di and tertoxides are used as bleaching agents. Oxidizing agents used for dough improvement are potassium bromate, potassium iodate, calcium iodate, and calcium peroxide.

HUMECANTS AND ANTI-CAKING AGENTS

Humectants are substances that help retain moisture, influencing the viscosity and texture of foods, reducing water activity, preventing crystallization, and maintaining softness. These agents also enhance the rehydration of dehydrated foods, aiding in the solubilization of flavor compounds. Polyhydroxy alcohols, which are water- soluble and hygroscopic, include examples such as propylene glycol, glycerol, sorbitol, and mannitol. Most of these are naturally occurring as polyhydric alcohols and sugar derivatives, with the exception of glycol.

Anti- caking agents prevent particles from clumping together and forming solid masses, especially during humid conditions. Calcium silicate, for example, is used to prevent caking in baking powder, table salt, and various other foods. Calcium and magnesium salts of long- chain fatty acids also serve as conditioning agents for dehydrated vegetables and other powdered food products. Other common anti- caking agents include sodium silicoaluminate, tricalcium phosphate, magnesium silicate, and magnesium carbonate.

Leavening Agents

Leavening agents are responsible for making baked goods light and fluffy Yeast has traditionally been the primary natural leavening agent used. Ammonium salts are incorporated to supply nitrogen for yeast growth, while phosphate salts (like sodium and calcium phosphates) are included to help regulate pH levels.

Chemical leavening agents, such as baking soda and ammonium carbonate, are also commonly used. Baking powder, a combination of sodium bicarbonate and an acid component, decomposes when heated, releasing carbon dioxide and water. Ammonium carbonate is specifically used in baking biscuits and crackers, where ammonia escapes at high baking temperatures.

Chelating Agents

Chelating agents, also known as sequestrants, are compounds that form complexes with metal ions. When metal ions are released due to hydrolytic or other degrading reactions, they can participate in processes that lead to discoloration, oxidative rancidity, turbidity, and flavor changes in food. By adding chelating agents, these metal ions are bound, which stabilizes the food. In the food industry, common chelators include sorbic acid, polycarboxylic acids (like citric, malic, tartaric, oxalic, and succinic acids), polyphosphates (ATP and pyrophosphates), macromolecules (such as porphyrins and proteins), and EDTA. Chelating agents that inhibit polyphenol oxidase include substances like cyanide, diethyldithiocarbonate, sodium azide, 2- mercaptobenzothiazole, carbon monoxide, dimercaptopropanol, and potassium methyl xanthate.

Although chelating agents are not antioxidants, they act as metal scavengers that prevent oxidation. Citric acid inhibits polyphenol oxidase by lowering the pH and chelating the copper at the enzyme's active site. Citric and phosphoric acids are used as acidulants in soft drinks. Polyphosphates and EDTA are utilized as chelating agents in canned seafood. Additionally, sulfated polysaccharides, such as carrageenans, amylose sulfate, and xylan sulfate, are effecti e in preventing browning in apple juice and diced apples.

Curing Agents

Curing agents are additives that help preserve meats, enhance their color and flavor, inhibit microorganism growth, and prevent toxin formation. Sodium nitrite has long been used as a preservative and color stabilizer in meat and fish products. When added to meat, nitrite converts into nitric oxide, which then binds with myoglobin to form nitrosylmyoglobin, a heat- stable pigment. Nitrite curing helps prevent the growth of Clostridium and Streptococcus. However, nitrosation can occur during storage and processing, and there is evidence suggesting the formation of nitrosamines, leading to controversy over the use of nitrites in meat curing. Polyphosphates like sodium tripolyphosphate and sodium hexametaphosphate are also used in meat curing. These compounds enhance the tenderness, juiciness, and flavor of the meat and contribute to its antimicrobial properties.

Nutrient Supplements

Nutrient supplements are added to restore nutrients lost during processing or storage, or to enhance the nutritional value that nature may have provided.

For instance, when wheat is milled to produce refined flour, the brown part of the grain, which contains vitamins and minerals, is removed. To compensate for this loss, nutrients like thiamine, nicotinic acid, iron, and calcium are added back into the flour. Certain foods are also fortified with specific nutrients; for example, milk is often supplemented with Vitamin D to reduce the incidence of rickets. Baby foods are fortified to improve their nutritional content as well. Adding amino acids such as lysine and methionine, or using iodine in the form of potassium iodide in table salt, are other common examples of nutrient supplementation.

Processing Aids

Various foods are processed using humectants, gelling agents, and antifoaming agents. Humectants are used to keep foods moist and stop them from drying out unintentionally. Foods can be prevented from drying out by using glycerin, sorbitol, mannitol, dextrose, and corn syrup.

Fruit juice haziness, sediments, and oxidative deterioration products are eliminated by using clarifying agents such as bentonite, gelatin, and synthetic resins.

Other Groupings of Chemical Agents

Most of the oxidizing agents used in food preservation have been mentioned under other categories. These include peroxides, bromine, chlorine, iodine, hypochlorites, chloramines, and ozone. Some oxidizing agents used in bleaching flour, such as oxides of nitrogen, chlorine, nitrosyl chloride, nitrogen trichloride, and benzoyl peroxide, may have bacteriostatic or even bactericidal properties, but their purpose is not primarily for their antimicrobial effects

The role of chemical agents used for cleaning and sanitizing equipment will be discussed in Chapter 27. Most of these chemicals act as antiseptics, and some are germicidal at the concentrations used, but their main function in food preservation is to reduce contamination from microorganisms present on equipment that comes in contact with food. Therc should be minimal residual chemical carryover into the food, ensuring it does not significantly affect its preservation. Some of these chemicals are used to remove dirt and kill microorganisms on the surfaces of certain foods, such as fruits, vegetables, and eggs, but none of these detergents or sanitizers are incorporated into foods as preservatives.

Chemical preservatives can be categorized based on their specificity for particular microorganisms. Considerable focus has been given to compounds that are effecti e against molds and related fungi. Mycostatic agents previously mentioned include propionic acid and its salts, caprylic acid, acetic acid, dehydroacetic acid, monochloroacetic acid, sorbic acid and its salts, and propylene glycol. Among these, propionates and sorbates are the most widely used in foods. Chemical preservatives against molds are typically applied in liquid form to the outer surfaces of foods or used as vapors around them. Examples of mycostatic chemicals that have been tested in vapor or gaseous form around foods include propylene glycol, carbon dioxide, methyl bromide, and various phenolic derivatives. Antifungal antibiotics such as griseofulvin, pimaricin, fulcine, actidione, rimocidin, and nystatin are also employed.

Antimycotics allowed in food packaging materials under specific conditions include sodium and calcium propionates, sodium benzoate, sorbic acid and sorbates, and methyl: and propylparabens. Caprylic acid is sometimes used in cheese wraps. Iodine, sulfites, o- phenylphenol or sodium o- phenylphenate, biphenyl, dimethylolurea, and several other substances have been recommended for impregnating wrappers for foods. A large number of compounds have been suggested for treating the surfaces of fruits, vegetables, eggs, cheese, meats, and fish. These range from simple inorganic compounds like nitrites and sulfur dioxide (sulfurous acid), organic acids (such as crotonic, sorbic, and levulinic acids), and esters of organic acids (e.g., esters of vanillic or benzoic acid) to complex phenolic compounds. Biphenyl and sodium o- phenylphenate with ammonia, for instance, have been applied to citrus fruits to reduce fungal spoilage. Most of these compounds require approval from the Food and Drug Administration before use.

Boiler- Water Additives

Boiler- water additives that have been approved by the Food and Drug Administration must be used for steam that comes in contact with foods (Anonymous, 1960).

Antibiotics

Most of the well- known antibiotics have been tested on raw foods, particularly protein- rich ones like meats, fish, and poultry, to extend their shelf life at refrigeration temperatures. Aureomycin (chlortetracycline) has been found to be the most effective among the antibiotics tested, due to its broad spectrum of activity. Terramycin (oxytetracycline) is almost equally effective in prolonging the preservation of foods. Some success has also been observed with Chloromycetin (chloramphenicol).

These three antibiotics inhibit protein synthesis in cells. Other antibiotics such as streptomycin, neomycin, polymyxin, nisin, subtilin, bacitracin, and penicillin are less effective, with penicillin being of little use. Nisin is commonly used in Europe to inhibit anaerobic bacteria in cheese and dairy products. Natamycin, effecti e against yeasts and molds, is used in or tested on products like orange juice, fresh fruits, sausage, and cheese.

In experiments, antibiotics have been combined with heat treatments in an effort to reduce the thermal processing required for low- and medium- acid canned foods. Most experiments have involved peptides like subtilin, nisin, and tylosin. The idea is to apply a botulinum cook—sufficien heat to kill *Clostridium botulinum* spores—along with the addition of antibiotics to prevent the germination and growth of any surviving spores of heat- resistant thermophilic spoilage bacteria and anaerobes. Subtilin doesn't affect the heat resistance of bacterial spores but inhibits the outgrowth of heat- damaged cells, while nisin interferes with spore germination and the breakdown of the spore coat. Tylosin may inhibit cell growth.

Although, food bacteriologists recognize the potential benefits of using non-toxic antibiotics to preserve raw foods or combining them with lower heat in canned food processing, they raise concerns about using antibiotics as preservatives. They agree that antibiotics should never replace proper hygiene practices. The effecti eness of an antibiotic on microorganisms can vary depending on the species or even strain, meaning the antibiotic may work against some spoilage organisms but not others, or it may affect part of the population in a culture but not the entire organism group. Additionally, microorganisms can adapt to increasing concentrations of an antibiotic, leading to the development of resistant strains.

There is also a risk that other organisms, which were not previously significant in food spoilage, may develop resistance to the antibiotic and become problematic. Furthermore, the antibiotic may have effects on the consumer, such as allergic reactions, alterations to the intestinal flora, or the development of antibiotic-resistant pathogens in the body.

However, these risks are likely to be minimized due to the low levels of antibiotics used in foods compared to those used in medical treatments. It has been suggested that antibiotics used for food preservation should not overlap with those used in human medical treatments. Canners believe that, when used in processing, the antibiotic, combined with heat treatment, must effecti ely kill all Clostridium botulinum spores and offer a safety margin, ideally eliminating all spoilage organisms and their spores. If spores survive, the antibiotic must remain in sufficien concentration throughout storage to prevent germination or growth of any surviving cells. This requires that the antibiotic maintain bacteriostatic or sporostatic levels throughout the storage period.

There have been efforts to test the bactericidal effects of edible plant extracts, such as those from carrot, green bean, tomato, and celery, in combination with a milder heat treatment to destroy bacteria and bacterial spores. Using plant extracts in this manner could help avoid many of the problems associated with antibiotic use.

The Food and Drug Administration (FDA) had approved the use of chlortetracycline and oxytetracycline dips for preserving poultry, setting a tolerance level of 7 ppm in uncooked, dressed poultry. This level of antibiotic has been shown to extend the poultry's storage life by two to three times. Approval was granted based on evidence that it (1) provided added protection to consumers, (2) did not replace basic sanitation procedures, and (3) was destroyed during cooking, leaving no harmful by- products. However, this approval has been revoked. Currently, the FDA allows the use of these tetracyclines at a maximum of 5 ppm for fresh fish, shucked scallops, and unpeeled shrimp. The antibiotic may be applied as a dip or in ice.

DEVELOPED PRESERVATIVES

Food fermentations serve two primary purposes- (1) to create new and desired flavors and physical characteristics, transforming the food into a different product, and (2) to aid in preserving the food. The importance of these aims can vary depending on the food and is often difficul to assess. For instance, the first fermented milks and sauerkraut were originally discovered empirically to preserve milk and cabbage over extended storage periods. Over time, people developed a taste for these fermented products, and today, they are made not just for their preservation but also for their appealing flavor

The preservatives produced by microbial action in fermented foods are mainly acids (primarily lactic acid) and alcohol. These naturally occurring preservatives are typically enhanced by additional preservation methods such as low temperatures, heat, anaerobic conditions, sodium chloride, sugar, or added acids.

Acidity plays a significant role in the preservation of foods like sauerkraut, pickles, green olives, fermented milk, cheese, and certain sausages, as well as various plant- based fermented foods. In some products, like pickles and green olives, the fermentation process may be allowed to proceed fully, reaching the maximum acidity. In other products, such as fermented milks and sauerkraut, the fermentation may be halted through chilling or canning before reaching the highest level of acidity. The acidity in these products varies, with sauerkraut reaching approximately 1.7 percent lactic acid, dill pickles and green olives around 0.9 percent, and fermented milks between 0.6 and 0.85 percent. Cheese, on the other hand, is usually measured by its hydrogen: ion concentration, with freshly made cheeses typically having a pH of about 5.0 to 5.2, becoming more alkaline as they cure.

The alcohol produced in beer, ale, fermented fruit juices, and distilled liquors contributes to preservation, though its primary purpose is not preservation but flavor and alcohol content

10 Radiation-Based Preservation Techniques

In their search for new and improved methods of food preservation, researchers have paid particular attention to the possible use of radiation of different frequencies, ranging from low-frequency electric current to gamma rays high frequency. Most of this work has focused on the use of ultraviolet radiation, ionizing radiation and microwave heating.

It is customary to group the entire spectrum of radiation into two categories, one for each side of visible light. Low-frequency, long-wavelength, low-quantum energy radiation extends from radio waves into the infrared. The effect of these radiations on microorganisms is related to their thermal agitation of the food. In contrast, higher frequency, shorter wavelength radiation has high quantum energies and effecti ely excites or destroys organic compounds and microorganisms without heating the product. Microbial destruction without the generation of high temperatures has suggested the term "cold sterilization".

When applied to the food industry, shorter wavelength radiation can be divided into two groups. Low frequency, low energy radiation, for example the ultraviolet part of the spectrum, has enough energy to excite only molecules. This area of the spectrum is used in the food industry and is covered in the ultraviolet radiation section. The higher frequency radiation has a high energy content and is capable of breaking down individual molecules into ions, hence the term ionizing radiation.

ULTRAVIOLET IRRADIATION

The food industry has made extensive use of ultraviolet irradiation out of all the electromagnetic radiations. The most germicidal radiation has wavelengths close to 260 nm because purines and pyrimidines absorb it strongly. Around 200 nm, ultraviolet light is ineffecti e against microorganisms, is strongly absorbed by oxygen, and may produce ozone.

Germicidal Lamps

UV light from quartz-mercury vapor lamps or low-pressure mercury lamps, which emit light at 254 nm, is typically used in the food industry. Both visible and erythemic rays, which irritate skin and mucous membranes, are part of the radiation from these lamps. The lamps come in a range of shapes, sizes, and power levels. The more recent varieties emit very little ozone.

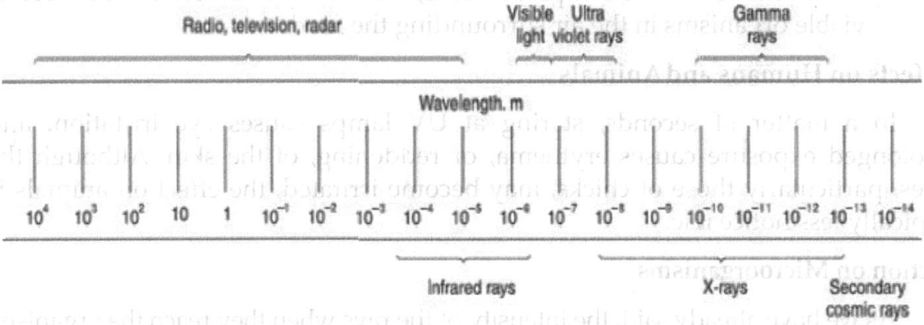

Fig 10.1. Chart of the electromagnetic spectrum, showing the location of various types of radiation. (Courtesy of Westinghouse Electric Corporation, Bloomfield, N.J.

Factors Influencing Effectiveness

It is important to note that only direct rays are effective, and even then, their efficacy is diminished if they originate from specialized reflectors. The following variables affect how effective ultraviolet radiation is:

- **Time:** The longer the time of exposure to a given concentration, the more effective the treatment.
- **Intensity**: The intensity of radiation reaching an object depends on several factors- the power of the lamp, the distance from the lamp to the object, and the type and amount of material in the path of the rays. Naturally, the intensity increases with the lamp's power. Intensity is typically measured in microwatts per square centimeter ($\mu W/cm^2$). The actual dose or amount of irradiation absorbed by an organism or product is calculated by multiplying the time of exposure by the intensity. At shorter distances, such as those used in industrial applications, the intensity of the rays decreases with increasing distance from the lamp. For example, a lamp is about 100 times more effecti e at killing microorganisms when it is 5 inches away than when it is 8 feet away. Most tests are conducted with the lamp placed about 12 inches from the object. The presence of dust in the air or on the lamp reduces effecti eness, as does high atmospheric humidity. Relative humidity above 80% significantly decreases penetration through the air, while humidity levels below 60% have minimal impact.
- **Penetration**: The nature of the object or material being irradiated has an important influence on the effecti eness of the process. Penetration is reduced even by clear water, which also exerts a protective effect on microorganisms. Dissolved mineral salts, especially of iron, and cloudiness greatly reduce the effecti eness of the rays. Even a thin layer of fatty or greasy material cuts off the rays. There is no penetration through opaque material. Therefore, the rays affect only the outer surface of most irradiated foods directly exposed to the lamp and do not penetrate to microorganisms

inside the food. The lamps do serve, however, to reduce the number of viable organisms in the air surrounding the food.

Effects on Humans and Animals

In a matter of seconds, staring at UV lamps causes eye irritation, and prolonged exposure causes erythema, or reddening, of the skin. Although the eyes, particularly those of chicks, may become irritated, the effect on animals is typically less noticeable.

Action on Microorganisms

As we have already said, the intensity of the rays when they reach the organism, the time during which they act and the location of the organism determine the germicidal effect. Each microorganism has a characteristic resistance to ultraviolet rays. This can vary according to the growth stage and physiological state of the cell. It takes up to fi e times more exposure to kill the vegetative cells of some bacteria than others, but in general, the lethal exposure does not vary much between differen species. The amount of ultraviolet radiation required to destroy several differen microorganisms is summarized in Table. The position of the body during the test has a significant impact. For example, 97 to 99 percent of airborne Escherichia coli were killed in 10 seconds at 24 inches with a 15-watt light bulb, but 20 seconds at 11 inches were needed for bacteria on surfaces. of a dish Encapsulation or aggregation of bacteria increases their resistance. Bacterial spores typically experience two to fi e times more exposure than corresponding vegetative cells. Some types of pigmentation also have a protective effect. In general, yeasts are two to fi e times more resistant than bacteria, although some are easily killed.

The resistance of mold is ten to fifty times greater than that of bacteria. Pigmented molds are harder than unpigmented molds and spores are harder than mycelium. The destructive effect of ultraviolet rays is generally explained by the "target theory", which is described in the discussion of ionizing radiation.

Table: Ultraviolet Radiation Doses to Destroy Certain Groups of Microorganisms

Microorganisms	Dose needed for 1 log cycle reduction or 1 D value (μW sec × 10^3)
Gram- negative bacteria	
Facultative anaerobes	0.8–6.4
Aerobes	3.0–5.5
Phototrophic	5.0–6.0
Gram- positive bacteria	
Bacillus	5.0–8.0
Bacillus spores	5.0–8.0
Micrococcus	6.0–20.0
Staphylococcus	2.2–5.0

Microorganisms	Dose needed for 1 log cycle reduction or 1 D value (μW sec × 10^3)
Molds	10.0–200.0
Yeasts	3.0–10.0

Source- Summarized from Ingram and Roberts (1980).

Applications in the Food Industry

The use of ultraviolet irradiation in the food industry will be discussed in connection with the preservation of specific foods. Examples of the successful use of these rays include treatment of water used for beverages; aging of meats; treatment of knives for slicing bread; treatment of bread and cakes; packaging of sliced bacon; sanitizing of eating utensils; prevention of growth of film yeast on pickle, vinegar, and sauerkraut vats; killing of spores on sugar crystals and in sirups; storage and packaging of cheese; prevention of mold growth on walls and shelves; and treatment of air used for, or in, storage and processing rooms.

IONIZING RADIATIONS

Kinds of Ionizing Radiations

Ionizing radiation includes protons, neutrons, alpha particles, cathode or beta rays, x-rays or gamma rays, and more. Protons and alpha particles have limited penetration, while neutrons cause residual radioactivity in food. As a result, these rays will not be discussed because they are impractical for use in food preservation.

When cathode rays are fired at a heavy metal target inside an evacuated tube, penetrating electromagnetic waves known as X-rays are created. At the moment, they are not thought to be cost-effective for use in the food industry.

Gamma rays are like x-rays but are emitted from by- products of atomic fission or from imitations of such by- products. Cobalt 60 and cesium 137 have been used as sources of these rays in most experimental work thus far, with cobalt 60 being the most promising for commercial applications.

Beta rays are streams of electrons (beta particles) emitted from radioactive material. Electrons are small, negatively charged particles of uniform mass that form part of the atom. They are deflected by magnetic and electric fields. Their penetration depends on the speed with which they hit the target. The higher the charge of the electron, the deeper its penetration.

Cathode rays are streams of electrons (beta particles) from the cathode of an evacuated tube. In practice, these electrons are accelerated by artificial means.

Definition of Terms

Before the utilization of ionizing radiations can be discussed, a few terms must be defined.

A roentgen (r) is the quantity of gamma or x- radiation which produces one electrostatic unit of electric charge of either sign in a cubic centimeter of air under standard conditions. A roentgen- equivalent- physical (rep) is the quantity of ionizing energy which produces, per gram of tissue, an amount of ionization equivalent to a roentgen. A megarep is 1 million rep. One r, or 1 rep, is equivalent to the absorption of 83 to 90 erg per gram of tissue.

The rad now is employed chiefly as the unit of radiation dosage, being equivalent to the absorption of 100 erg per gram of irradiated material. A megarad (Mrad) is 1 million rad, and a kilorad (Krad) is 1,000 rad.

- An electronvolt (eV) is the energy gained by an electron in moving through a potential difference of 1 volt. A meV is 1 million electronvolts.
- A meV, then, is a measure of the intensity of the irradiation, and a rep is a measure of the absorbed energy that is effecti e within the food.
- A Gray (Gy) equals 100 rads and is being used as a term to replace rads in some references.
- Radappertization is a term used to define "radiation sterilization" which would imply high dose treatments, with the resulting product being shelf: stable.
- Radurization refers to "radiation pasteurization" low- dose treatments, where the intent is to extend a product's shelf life.
- Radicidation also is a low- dose "radiation pasteurization" treatment, but with the specific intent being the elimination of a particular pathogen.
- Picowaved is a term used to label foods treated with low- level ionizing radiation.

X- Rays

X- rays, gamma rays, and cathode rays are all equally effective for sterilization, given equal amounts of absorbed energy. X- rays and gamma rays have good penetration, while cathode rays have relatively poor penetration. The major current disadvantage of using X- rays for food preservation is the low efficienc and high cost of their production, since only about 3- 5% of the applied electron energy is used in the production of X- rays. Focus on the application of gamma rays and cathode rays.

GAMMA RAYS AND CATHODE RAYS

These two types of rays will be discussed together and compared whenever possible because they are equally effecti e at sterilizing food for equal amounts of energy absorbed and seem to cause comparable changes in the food being treated.

Sources

Chief sources of gamma rays are: (1) radioactive fission products of uranium and cobalt, (2) the coolant circulated in nuclear reactors, and (3) other fuel elements used to operate a nuclear reactor. Cathode rays usually are accelerated by special electrical devices. The greater this acceleration (i.e., the more meV), the deeper the penetration into the food.

Penetration

Gamma rays have good penetration, but their effecti eness decreases exponentially with depth. They have been reported to be effecti e up to 20 cm in most foods, but this depth will depend on the time of exposure. Cathode rays, on the other hand, have poor penetration, being effecti e at only about 0.5 cm per meV when "cross firing", that is, irradiation from opposite sides, is employed. The absorption dose level in a material is not a uniformly decreasing fraction with depth but rather builds up to a maximum at a depth equal to about one- third of the total penetration and then decreases to zero.

Efficiency

Because cathode rays are directional, they can be made to hit the food and therefore are used with greater efficienc than are gamma rays, which are constantly emitted in all directions from the radioactive sources. Various estimates of the maximal efficiency of utilization of cathode rays range between 40 and 80 percent, depending on the shape of the irradiated material, but only a maximum of 10 to 25 percent utilization efficienc is estimated for gamma rays. Radioactive sources of gamma rays decay steadily and hence weaken with time.

Safety

The use of cathode rays presents fewer health problems than the use of gamma rays, since cathode rays are directional and less penetrating, can be turned off for repair or maintenance work, and present no hazard of radioactive materials after a fire, explosion, or other catastrophe. Gamma rays are emitted in all directions, are penetrating, are continuously emitted, and come from radioactive sources. Gamma rays require more shielding to protect workers. Tests thus far on animals and human volunteers have not indicated any ill effects from the eating of irradiated foods.

Effects on Microorganisms

The effectiveness of a specific dose of irradiation in killing microorganisms is influenced by several factors:

- The type and species of the microorganism, as demonstrated by the data in Table.
- **The Initial Number of Microorganisms (or spores) Present:** A higher number of organisms reduces the effecti eness of a given dose.
- **The Composition of the Food Itself:** Certain components, such as proteins, catalase, and reducing substances like nitrites, sulfites, and sulfhydr l compounds, may offer protection. Conversely, compounds that interact with SH groups can make the organisms more sensitive. Ionization byproducts may also harm the microorganisms.
- **The Presence or Absence of Oxygen:** The effect of oxygen varies depending on the organism, with it either having no effect or increasing the organism's sensitivity. Undesirable side reactions are more likely to

occur in the presence of oxygen, whereas they tend to be less frequent in a vacuum or in a nitrogen atmosphere.

Table :Approximate Killing Doses of Ionizing Radiations in Kilograys (KGay)

Organisms	Approximate lethal dose		Approximate lethal dose
Humans	0.0056–0.0075	**Bacteria (cells of saprophytes)**	
Insects	.22–.93	**Gram- negative**	
Viruses	10–20	*Escherichia coli*	1.0–2.3
Yeasts (fermentative)	4–9	*Pseudomonas aeruginosa*	1.6–2.3
Saccharomyces cerevisiae	5	*Pseudomonas fluorescens*	1.2–2.3
Torula cremoris	4.7	*Enterobacter aerogenes*	1.4–1.8
Yeasts (film)	3.7–18	**Gram- positive**	
Hansenula sp.	4.7	*Lactobacilius* spp.	0.23–0.38
Candida krusei	11.6	*Streptococcus faecalis*	1.7–8.8
Molds (with spores)	1.3–11	*Leuconostoc dextranicum**	0.9
Penicillium spp.	1.4–2.5	*Sarcina lutea**	3.7
Aspergillus spp.	1.4–3.7	**Bacterial spores**	
Rhizopus sp.	10	*Bacillus subtillis*	3.1–37
Fusarium sp.	2.5	*Bacillus coagulans*	12–18
Bacteria (cells of pathogen)		*Clostridium botulinum* (A)	10
Mycobacterium tuberculosis	1.4	*C. botulinum* (E)	19–37
Staphylococcus aureus	1.4–7.0	*C. perfringens*	15–18
Corynebacterium diphtheriae	4.2	Putrefactive anaerobe 3679	3.1
Salmonella spp.	3.7–4.8	*Bacillus stearothermophilus*	23–50

- **The Physical State of the Food During Irradiation:** Both moisture content and temperature affect different organisms in differen ays.
- **The Condition of the Organisms**: Age, temperature of growth and sporulation, and state—vegetative or spore—may affect the sensitivity of

the organisms. These factors have been discussed previously in connection with other methods of processing foods. The type of irradiation and, within limits, the pH of the food seem to have little influence on the dose needed to inactivate the organisms.

Some researchers have suggested that a microorganism's resistance to ionizing radiation generally mirrors its resistance to conventional heat processing, though there are notable exceptions. For example, spores of *Clostridium botulinum* have been found to be more resistant to gamma rays than spores of a flat sour bacterium (No.1518) and a thermophilic anaerobe (T.A. No. 3814), even though the latter two are more heat- resistant. Table 10.2 provides data from various sources on the approximate radiation doses required to kill different microorganisms. These values can vary based on the conditions mentioned earlier. However, a few key observations can be made- (1) humans are much more sensitive to radiation than microorganisms; (2) bacterial spores tend to be far more resistant than vegetative cells; (3) gram- negative bacteria are generally less resistant than gram- positive bacteria; and (4) yeasts and molds show considerable variation in resistance, with some being more resistant than most bacteria. For instance, *Candida krusei* (Table 10.2) is as resistant as many bacterial spores. Certain microorganisms, like a radiation- resistant micrococcus similar to *Micrococcus roseus* and *Microbacterium* species in meat, have been found to be particularly resilient. This suggests the potential for the isolation of resistant strains from foods subjected to low- level irradiation. Preliminary gamma irradiation of bacterial spores has been shown to increase their sensitivity to heat, while prior heat shocking does not affect the lethal impact of subsequent gamma radiation.

Additionally, prior ultrasonic treatment can make organisms more susceptible to radiation. The destruction of irradiated microorganisms is thought to occur when an ionizing particle or quantum of energy strikes a sensitive area of the cell, causing ionization in that region and ultimately killing the organism, a process known as the target theory. Furthermore, much of the germicidal effect is believed to result from the ionization of the surrounding environment, especially water, which creates free radicals that can aid in the destruction of the organisms. Irradiation may also cause mutations in the microorganisms present.

Effects on Foods

Radiation doses high enough to achieve sterilization have been shown to cause undesirable "side reactions" or secondary changes in various food types, resulting in unwanted colors, odors, tastes, or even alterations to physical properties. Among the effects of sterilizing radiation on foods are- (1) in meats, an increase in pH, destruction of glutathione, and an elevation in carbonyl compounds, hydrogen sulfide, and methyl mercaptan; (2) in fats and lipids, the destruction of natural antioxidants, oxidation followed by partial polymerization, and an increase in carbonyl compounds; and (3) in vitamins, a decrease in the levels of thiamine, pyridoxine, and vitamins B12, C, D, E, and K in most foods, while riboflavin and niacin remain relatively stable. The likelihood of these undesirable effects is reduced with lower radiation doses. It takes five to ten times the radiation dose needed to kill microorganisms to destroy most food enzymes, and enzyme activity may continue unless a pre- irradiation blanching treatment is applied. The primary concern regarding the healthfulness of irradiated foods is the loss of vitamins. However, the overall nutritional value of irradiated foods is comparable to that of foods processed by other methods to achieve the same level of shelf stability. There is no evidence of radioactivity production when electron beams are used below 11 meV or when gamma rays from cobalt 60 are used.

Applications

Currently food irradiation has been approved only in a very limited way in the United States. Low- level irradiation (1 kiloGray) can be used on fresh fruits and vegetables to kill insects and to inhibit spoilage. Dry or dehydrated vegetables (herbs and spices) can be irradiated at up to 30 kiloGray to kill insects and bacteria. Additionally, processes for irradiating pork (trichinae), wheat (insects), and potatoes (sprout formation) have been approved. However, renewed interest and regulatory proposals will probably result in expanded use in this country. Close to thirty countries now have approved some form of food irradiation. The specific applications of food irradiation are summarized in Table 10.3.

Table: Applications of Food Irradiation

Type of food	Radiation dose (kiloGrays)	Effect of treatment
Meat and Poultry	1 - 3 kGy	Inactivation of pathogens, extended shelf life
Fruits (e.g., mangoes, bananas)	0.5 - 1 kGy	Delayed ripening, reduced spoilage
Vegetables (e.g., potatoes, onions)	0.2 - 0.5 kGy	Prevention of sprouting, extended storage
Seafood	1 - 3 kGy	Inactivation of spoilage microorganisms, longer shelf life
Spices and Herbs	10 - 30 kGy	Microbial reduction, improved safety, extended storage
Grains and Cereals	0.3 - 0.5 kGy	Insect control, increased shelf life
Dried Fruits	1 - 2 kGy	Reduction of microbial load, prevention of mold growth
Eggs (Shell)	0.1 - 0.3 kGy	Inactivation of Salmonella and other pathogens

MICROWAVE PROCESSING

Microwave heating and processing of food has become increasingly popular, especially among consumers. Microwaves are electromagnetic waves between infrared waves and radio waves . Specific frequencies are typically 915 megacycles or 2450 megacycles. The energy or heat produced by microwaves as they pass through food results from the extremely rapid oscillations of food molecules as they attempt to align with the electromagnetic field produced. This rapid oscillation, or intermolecular friction, generates heat. The protective effect of microwaves or the bactericidal effect produced is actually a function of the heat generated. In other words, microwaves themselves do not cause inactivation of microorganisms present in food; rather, it is the heat produced by the excitation of food molecules that actually results in microbial destruction.

CASE STUDY

Preservation of Foods by Irradiation

Irradiated food storage has gained importance, both in terms of advantages and disadvantages. This report provides an illustration of the use of these techniques in food preservation.

Treating food with ionizing radiation can kill most bacteria and parasites that otherwise cause foodborne illness, as reported by the Centers for Disease Control and Prevention (CDC). It works in a similar way to pasteurizing milk and pressure cooking canning.

Radiation can be used in a variety of foods to eliminate pests and replace toxic chemicals currently used to fumigate many foods. It can also slow mold growth, inhibit germination, and extend shelf life.· Gamma rays, electron beams, and X: rays are the three different irradiations used.

Gamma rays have been used routinely for more than 30 years to sterilize medical, dental, and household products. They are also used for radiation treatment of cancer. Gamma rays can penetrate foods to a depth of several feet. They do not make anything around them radioactive.

Electron beams (E- beams) are propelled out of an electron gun that is a larger version of the part of a TV tube that propels electrons into the TV screen, making it light up. They have been used as sterilizers for more than 15 years, according to the CDC. No radioactivity is involved. The electrons can penetrate food only a little over an inch, so the food treated must be no thicker than that. Two opposing beams can treat food twice as thick.

The newest technology is X- ray irradiation. The X- ray machine is a more powerful version of the machines used in many hospitals and dental office to take X- ray pictures. X- rays can pass through thick foods. They require heavy shielding for safety.

When food is irradiated, the high- energy ray is absorbed as it passes through food. The ray gives up its energy, causing the food to be slightly warmed. Irradiation damages the DNA in any microbe, fungus, or parasite present, thus killing the organism.

Pathogenic organisms vary in their sensitivity to radiation. Irradiation is very effecti e at killing parasites and bacteria in food, but it does not work to kill viruses or prions. Parasites and insects have large amounts of DNA; therefore, they are quickly killed by extremely low doses of radiation. Bacteria have smaller amounts of DNA, so more radiation is needed to kill bacteria and bacterial spores, the dormant state of some bacteria. Viruses are the smallest pathogens that have DNA or RNA and are relatively resistant to radiation at levels approved for food. Prions, such as the one that causes "mad cow" disease (bovine spongiform encephalopathy, or BSE), do not have DNA and are not affected by radiation at levels approved for food.

One reason is that the food industry and consumers are reluctant to adopt a process that seems dangerous. Many people associate radiation with nuclear power plants and radioactive contamination.

It takes a large dose of radiation, much larger than is necessary, to make food radioactive. At the low levels of radiation commonly used in food processing, there is no chance that the food will become radioactive. Irradiation must be accompanied by other food safety measures, such as good hygiene, healthy animals, and proper cooking.

The disadvantage is that irradiation does not work on all foods. For example, it will cause vegetables and leafy greens to wilt. And it does not kill all viruses. Some For example, viruses found in raw shellfish appear to be resistant to radiation. Although hepatitis A can be killed by radiation, the virus requires higher doses than are currently used.

Irradiated foods can cost more. But studies have shown that consumers were willing to pay more for irradiated meat because they knew the meat was safer.

Currently, any food that has undergone this process must be labeled with a special red symbol, indicating that it has been irradiated, and must be marked "irradiated" or "irradiated treated." The symbol and words may appear in small print on the back of the label, along with the list of ingredients.

Part-III

Food Contamination, Preservation Techniques, And Spoilage Pattern

Fruits and vegetables are harvested, milk is collected, eggs are gathered, fish and other aquatic products are sourced from natural waters, and animals are slaughtered—all of which carry microorganisms from natural environments (refer to Chapter 4). Once human handling begins, additional contamination is introduced and continues during handling and processing. To minimize contamination, processors strive to clean and sanitize equipment that comes into contact with food and use packaging materials that do not contribute significant contamination. The term "sanitize" is used instead of "sterilize" because, despite efforts to sterilize equipment—eliminating all living organisms—true sterility is rarely achieved.

In Part Three, preservation methods discussed in Chapters 5 to 10 are applied to major food categories, and the primary spoilage mechanisms for these foods are explored.

11 Cereal and Grain Management

Cereal and grain management involves the handling, storage, and preservation of cereal grains to maintain their quality and prevent contamination. Grains, including wheat, rice, corn, and oats, are highly susceptible to microbial spoilage, particularly by fungi, bacteria, and insects. Proper management ensures that these products remain safe, nutritious, and of high quality.

Handling includes careful harvesting, transportation, and processing to avoid physical damage to grains, which can create entry points for microbes. Storage plays a critical role in preventing contamination and spoilage. Grains should be stored in cool, dry environments with controlled humidity to prevent mold growth, especially from fungi like Aspergillus and Penicillium, which can produce harmful mycotoxins.

Quality maintenance involves monitoring moisture content, temperature, and pest control during storage. Proper sanitation practices, including cleaning storage facilities and equipment, are essential in minimizing microbial load. In addition, the use of preservatives or natural methods, such as drying, can further extend the shelf life and maintain the nutritional value of cereals and grains. Effecti e management practices reduce spoilage, improve food safety, and help preserve the integrity of cereal-based products.

Cereal products discussed in this chapter include the grains themselves, meals, flours, alimentary pastes, and breads, cakes, and other bakery products.

CONTAMINATION

The external part of harvested seeds preserves some of the microorganisms that they contain during growth, as well as contamination from the ground, insects and other sources. Freshly harvested grains contain several thousand to millions of bacteria per gram and from zero to several hundred thousand mold spores. Bacteria mainly belong to the families *Pseudomonadaceae, Micrococcaceae, Lactobacillaceae* and *Bacillaceae.* Cleaning and washing the grains removes some of the microorganisms, but most of the microorganisms are removed. with the outer parts of the grain during grinding. Milling processes, especially blanching, reduce the number of organisms, but then there is a risk of contamination during other procedures, such as mixing and packaging.

Bacteria present in wheat flour include *Bacillus* spores, coliform bacteria and some representatives of the genera *Achromobacter**, *Flavobacterium, Sarcina,*

Micrococcus, Alcaligenes and *Serratia*. Mold spores are mainly those of aspergilli and penicillia, and also those of *Alternaria, Cladosporium* and other genera. The number of bacteria varies greatly, from a few hundred per gram to millions. Most commercial samples of white wheat flour contain several hundred to several thousand bacteria per gram, twenty to thirty Bacillus spores per gram, and 50 to 100 mold spores per gram. Patent flours generally give lower counts than pure or clean flours, and their counts decrease as the flour is stored. Prepared flours generally yield higher results, and even higher (8,000 to 12,000 per gram on average) in graham and whole- wheat flours, which also contain the outer parts of the wheat kernel and are not bleached. Table illustrates the normal microflora found in many cereals and cereal products.

Wheat flour and spelt flour contain several hundred to several thousand bacteria and molds per gram. *Fusarium* and *Pencillium* species are the dominant fungi. Due to the incubation in humid conditions, the mountains contain a large number of bacteria, usually millions per gram.

The surface of a fresh loaf of bread is practically free of viable microorganisms, but it is subject to contamination by mold spores present in the air during cooling and before packaging. During cutting, contamination can occur from microorganisms in the air, on the knives or on the packaging. Pastries are also prone to contamination. Spores of bacteria capable of making stringy bread survive the baking process.

Table: Microbiological Profile of Cereal Grains and Cereal Products

Product category	Normal microflora	Quantitative range	Remarks
Raw cereal grains	Molds Yeasts and yeastlike fungi Bacteria Aerobic plate count Coliform group *E. coli* Actinomycetes	10^2–10^4/g 10^2–10^4/g 10^2–10^4/g 10^2–10^4/g 10–10^3/g 10^3–10^6/g	Counts representative of ''normal'' grains in commercial channels; ''mildeward'' or ''musty'' or "spoiled" grain obviously be beyond these ranges Retained to amount of soil incorporated in grain sample
Flour(s)*, cornmeal, corn gifts, semolina	Molds Yeasts and yeastlike fungi Bacteria Aerobic plate count Coliform group ''Rope'' spores	10^2–10^4/g 10–10^2/g 10^2–10^6/g 0–10/g 0–10^2/g	Microbial counts in flour can vary from one storage period to another depending on moisture content and storage; however, increase have also been noted Soy flours sometimes contain salmonellae; other flours rarely do

Breakfast cereals and "snacks"	Molds Yeasts and yeastlike fungi Bacteria Aerobic plate count Coliform group	10^2–10^4/g 10^2–10^4/g 10^2–10^4/g 10^2–10^4/g	
Refrigerated and frozen doughs	Molds Yeasts and yeastlike fungi Bacteria Aerobic plate count Coliform group Psychrotrophs	10^2–10^4/g 10^5–10^6/g 10^2–10^6/g 10–10^2/g 10–10^3/g	Yeasts count reflect inoculums intentionally added as part of the product formulation– do not represent "contamination" The special case of "buttermilk biscuits" which contain 102 – 104 lactic acid producers have been omitted from this compilation.
Baked goods	Molds Yeasts and yeastlike fungi Bacteria Aerobic plate count Coliform group	10–10^3/g 10–10^3/g 10–10^3/g 10–10^2/g	
Soya protein	Bacteria Aerobic plate count Coliform group *E. coli* Psychrotrophs *Cl. perfringens*	10^2–10^5/g 10^2–10^3/g 0–10^2/g 10^2–10^4/g 0–10^2/g	Quantitative rangers reflect both original contamination and growth during storage of intermediate- moisture products
Pasta products	Bacteria Aerobic plate count Coliform group Molds and yeasts	10^3–10^5/g 10–10^3/g 102–10^5/g	Wide rangers in bioloads of these products reflect difference between egg- based and macaroni- type products, which are all included in "pasta" category
Dry cereal mixes	Molds Yeasts and yeastlike fungi Bacteria Aerobic plate count Coliform group	10^2–10^4/g 10^5–10^6/g 10^2–10^6/g 10–10^2/g	

Table based on "routine" quality control tests normally performed on various items of specified category; data represent industrywide experience; data presented as "orders of magnitude" for illustrative purposes only. Source- Condensed from Hobbs and Greene (1984). The potential presence of mycotoxins has made the contamination of grains and cereal products by molds a serious public health concern. The regular isolation of *Aspergillus flavus* and *A. parasiticus*, which can produce aflatoxin, highlights the necessity of minimizing mold contamination and avoiding environments that support their growth. Other commonly isolated molds, such as fusaria and penicillia, are undesirable since certain species of these genera are also capable of producing mycotoxins . The distribution of aflatoxin B_1 in various corn fractions is shown in Table.

PRESERVATION

Most grains and grain products have such a limiting ambient temperature that it is easy to prevent the growth of microorganisms as long as these products are kept dry. These products are stored in bulk or in containers to keep out pests, to resist fire, and to avoid rapid changes in temperature and therefore increased humidity. A storage temperature of about 4.4 to 7.2°C is recommended for dry products. Many bakery products, such as breads, rolls, cakes, pastries, pies, and canned mixes, contain enough moisture to undergo spoilage unless special storage methods are used or circulation is rapid.

Asepsis

Equipment must be properly cleaned and sanitized for hygienic and preservation reasons, just like in other food industries. Rope bacteria and the acid-forming bacteria that give dough its sour taste can be found on improperly sanitized equipment. Mold spore contamination should be prevented in bread, cakes, and other baked products that are susceptible to mold deterioration. Bread protection is particularly crucial. The bread should be immediately cooled in an environment free of live mold spores after leaving the oven, then sliced with spore-free knives and wrapped right away.

Use of Heat

Bakery products may be sold raw, partially baked, or cooked. The complete baking process generally destroys all bacterial cells, yeast spores, and mold spores, but not spores of string- forming bacteria or other bacteria. However, it has been reported that mold spores in the leavening tissues of the oven can develop sufficien heat resistance to survive baking. Raw or partially baked products are usually kept on the retailer's shelves for a short time or kept refrigerated for longer storage. Some specialty breads, e.g. Boston brown bread and walnut bread have been successfully preserved.

USE OF LOW TEMPERATURES

Although ordinary room temperatures may be used by homemakers for short- term storage of baked goods, keeping times could be lengthened and risk of food poisoning lessened if really warm temperatures, like those of hot kitchens or summer weather, were avoided and the foods were stored in a cool place or even in the refrigerator.

Table: Distribution of Aflatoxin B_1 in Various Corn Fractions

				BCMF+	Fluorescence kernels and pieces			Fluorescence visible under seedcoat		Discolored and damaged kernels		Onwards sound kernel		
U.S. No.	Types of corn	Weight of sample examined, kg	Total sample aflatoxin B_i, ppb	Aflatoxin B_i, ppb*	Total %	Aflatoxin B_i, ppb	Total, %	Aflatoxin B_i, ppb*	Total %	Aflatoxin B_i, ppb	Total %	Aflatoxin B_i, ppb	Total, %	Origin
1	W	2.0	88	<1	<1	10	11	59	67	10	11	9	10	Ariz.
3	Y	1.0	144	2	1	7	5	51	35	51	35	33	23	S.C.
3	W	2.0	150	8	5	32	21	38	25	47	31	25	17	Mo.
4	W	2.0	116	7	6	30	26	27	23	16	14	36	31	Tex.
4	W	2.0	132	14	11	27	20	33	25	37	28	21	16	Tex.
4	W	2.0	276	8	3	59	21	95	34	70	25	44	16	Mo.
5	Y	1.0	61	2	3	7	11	15	24	2	3	35	57	Va.
Sample														
Grade	Y	2.0	61	48	79	3	5	5	8	3	5	2	3	S.C.
Grade	W	2.1	145	4	3	32	22	33	23	29	20	47	32	Ala.
Grade	W	2.0	321	10	3	37	12	123	38	31	6	130	40	Mo.
Average					12		16		31		19		25	

*W = White, Y = Yellow: +ppb of total sample weight: #BCFM = broken corn- foreign material:
§ BGY (blue- green- yellow) fluorescence under ultraviolet light (365 nm): Source- Shotwell et al. (1974).

The freezing- storage of bakery goods is on the increase. Unbaked or partially baked products, waffles cheesecake, ice cream pie, and fish, poultry, and meat pies are usually frozen. Bread and rolls can be stored successfully for months in the frozen condition.

Use of Chemical Preservatives

Limited drying facilities or wet weather can result in grain being stored at relatively high moisture content. Grain stored at moisture contents above 20%, for example, is likely to develop mold and possibly form mycotoxins. In addition to insecticides and fumigants, ammonia and propionic acid have been evaluated for their effecti eness in preventing mold growth and mycotoxin production. Ammonia (2%) and propionic acid (1%) reduce mold growth in grain with high moisture content.

Several preservatives are used, particularly as mold inhibitors, in breads, rolls, cakes, and other baked goods. Sodium calcium propionate, sodium diacetate, and sorbates are widely used. Acidification of pulp with acetic acid has been used to combat fibrillation

Use of Irradiation

In bakeries, ultraviolet rays have been used to destroy or reduce numbers of mold spores in dough and proof rooms, on the knives of slicing machines, in the room where the bread is packaged, and on the surface of bread, cakes, and other bakery products. The application of radio- frequency radiations to loaves of bread to reduce the likelihood of mold spoilage has been reported, and ionizing radiations, gamma and cathode rays, have been applied experimentally for the preservation of baked goods. Low- level irradiation can also be used to destroy insects in stored grains.

SPOILAGE

Cereals, flours, and cereal- based foods should not be subject to microbial spoilage if properly prepared and stored because their moisture content is too low to support mold growth. However, if these products are moist beyond the minimum for microbial growth, growth will occur. Mild moisture will only allow mold to grow, but higher moisture will allow yeast and bacteria to grow.

Although the microbial load of cereals, flours, and cereal- based foods is not a spoilage problem per se, the number and types of microorganisms present in these products are of concern, as these products are used in the formulation of many other foods. The microbial contribution of cereals and flours to prepared foods is an important consideration from a public health perspective and as a source of potential spoilage agents.

Cereal Grains and Meals

Since grains and flours are not usually treated to significantly reduce their natural flora of microorganisms, they are likely to contain molds, yeasts, and bacteria that are ready to grow if sufficien moisture is added. In addition to starch, which is not available to many organisms, these grains contain sugars and available nitrogen compounds, minerals, and additional growth substances; amylases will release more sugars and proteinases will produce more food with available nitrogen if the grain is soaked. A little extra moisture will cause molds to grow on the surface, where air is available. A wet grain or flour mash will undergo acid fermentation, primarily by lactic acid and coliform bacteria that are normally found on the surface of the plant. This may be followed by alcoholic fermentation by yeasts once the acidity has increased enough to favor fermentation. Eventually, mold (and possibly a film tip) will grow on the upper surface, however Acetic bacteria, if present, can oxidize the alcohol to acetic acid and inhibit mold.

The main factors involved in mold spoilage of stored grain include microbial content, moisture levels above 12- 13%, physical damage, and temperature. Many different molds can be involved, but the most common are *Aspergillus, Penicillium, Mucor, Rhizopus,* and *Fusarium*. As mentioned, many of these molds can produce mycotoxins. Mold- damaged grains represent a potential risk to human or animal health, as well as significant economic loss

Flours

Dry washing and scouring of grain, as well as milling and cutting of flour, reduce the content of microorganisms, but important species are still represented in wholemeal flour, for example wheat or buckwheat, and the deterioration would be similar to that described for cereals. and grains and flours

White wheat flour, however, is usually bleached by an oxidizing agent, such as nitrogen oxide, chlorine, nitrosyl chloride, or benzoyl peroxide, and this process serves to reduce the number and types of microbes. It has been reported that the moisture content of the flour below 13 percent inhibits the growth of all microorganisms. Other researchers say that 15% allows good mold growth and more than 17% allows mold and bacteria to grow. Therefore, a slight soaking of white flour leads to mold spoilage. Due to variations in the microbial content of different flour lots, the type of spoilage in flour dough is difficul to predict. If acid-forming bacteria are present, a Acid fermentation begins, followed by alcoholic fermentation by yeast if present, then acetic fermentation by Acetobacter species. This pattern of changes would be more likely in freshly milled flour than in flour that has been stored for a long period, resulting in a reduction in the types and numbers of microorganisms. In the absence of lactic acid bacteria and coliforms, micrococci acidify the dough and in their absence *Bacillus* species can grow, producing lactic acid, gas, alcohol, acetoin and small amounts of esters and other aromatic compounds. Most flour pastes have the characteristic of developing an odor of acetic acid and esters.

Bread

Chapter 22 will cover the fermentations that occur in the doughs for different types of bread, noting that some alterations brought about by microbes are preferable and even required in the production of particular types of bread. If too much time is allowed, the lactic and coliform bacteria that normally ferment flour pastes and doughs may cause an excessive amount of acid, which could make the dough and bread made from it too "sour." Overgrowth of proteolytic bacteria during this time may result in a sticky dough by destroying some of the gas-holding capacity that is so important for the dough's rising.

However, sticky doughs are typically caused by overmixing or the breakdown of gluten by reducing agents.

Molds

Molds are the primary and most prevalent cause of spoilage in bread and bakery products. The high temperatures reached during the baking process are typically sufficien to destroy mold spores present on or within the loaf. However, contamination occurs post: baking when molds reach the surface or penetrate the bread. Sources of contamination include exposure to air during cooling, handling, or contact with wrappers. Molds often start growing in the creases of loaves or between slices in sliced bread.

The main molds responsible for bread spoilage are *Rhizopus stolonifer* (commonly known as bread mold) with its white cottony mycelium and black sporangia, *Penicillium expansum* or *P. stoloniferum* with green spores, Aspergillus niger featuring greenish or purplish- brown to black conidial heads and yellow pigments diffusing into the bread, and *Monilla (Neurospora) sitophila,* characterized by its pink conidia that impart a reddish color. Additional molds, such as *Mucor, Geotrichum,* or other genera, may also appear.

Factors promoting mold spoilage include: (1) heavy contamination post- baking, such as air carrying numerous spores, extended cooling periods, significant air circulation, or contaminated slicing machinery; (2) slicing, which introduces more air into the loaf; (3) wrapping warm bread, which leads to moisture condensation; and (4) warm, humid storage conditions. Bread crusts resist mold growth at relative humidity levels below 90%. Bread containing 6% milk solids retains moisture better than milk- free bread, resulting in less condensation between loaf and wrapper, though this effect is of limited practical significance. Molding often starts inside sliced bread, especially in creases where moisture levels are higher than on the surface.

Methods Used to Prevent Bread Mold

Minimizing bread contamination by mold spores as much as possible. This involves keeping the surrounding air low in spores by removing mold breeding grounds like returned bread, cleaning walls and equipment, and filtering or washing air. Spore- laden flour dust is often implicated in mold outbreaks. Air filtration, washing, and ultraviolet irradiation of air and room surfaces significantly reduce contamination.

- Destroying surface molds through electronic heating.
- Adequate and rapid cooling of loaves before wrapping to prevent moisture condensation beneath wrappers.
- Using ultraviolet irradiation on loaf surfaces and slicing knives.
- Storing bread at cool temperatures to slow mold growth or freezing bread to prevent it entirely.

Adding mycostatic chemicals to the bread dough, such as sodium or calcium propionate (0.1–0.3% of flour weight), which also prevents rope spoilage. Sorbic acid (up to 0.1%) and sodium diacetate (up to 0.32%) are alternatives. Historically, vinegar or acetate was added to dough, or loaves were treated externally with vinegar to combat mold growth.

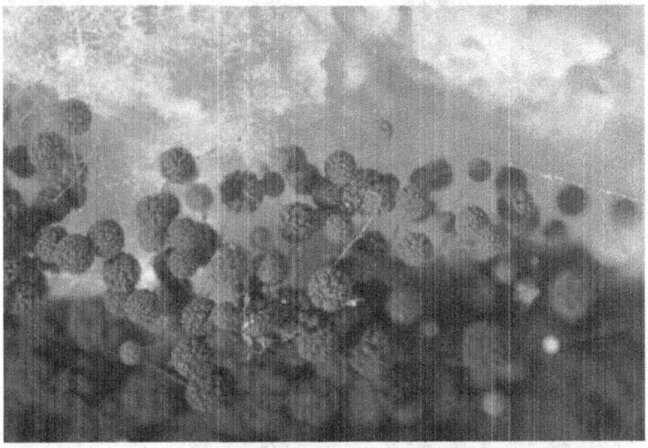

A

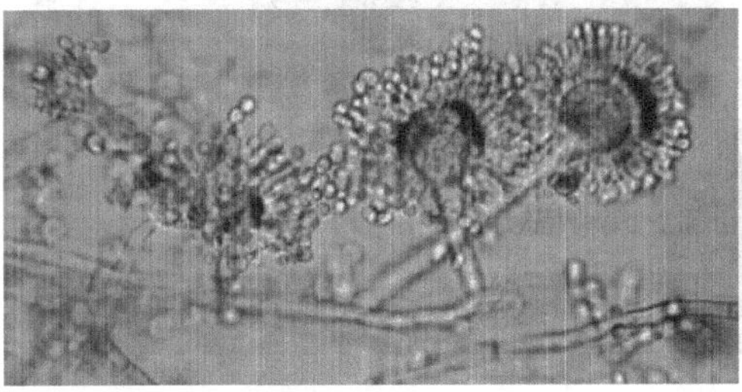

B

Fig 11.1. Aspergillus growing on moldy bread (A) and photomicrograph of conidial heads (vesicles bearing catenate conidia on phialdes)(B).

Ropiness

Ropiness in bread is a common issue in home- baked loaves, particularly in warm weather, but it is rarely seen in commercially baked bread due to effective preventive measures. This condition is caused by a mucoid variant of *Bacillus subtilis* or *B. licheniformis*, previously referred to by other names such as *B. mesentericus* and *B. panis*. The spores of these bacteria can survive the baking process, as bread temperatures do not exceed 100°C, and can germinate and thrive under favorable conditions.

Ropiness results from the bacillus forming a capsule and the organism's proteinases breaking down flour proteins (gluten) along with its amylase hydrolyzing starch into sugars that promote rope formation. Affected areas are soft and sticky, with a yellow to brown discoloration. In advanced stages, the slimy substance can be stretched into long threads when the bread is pulled apart . The condition produces an unpleasant odor, often described as resembling decomposed or overripe melons. Initially, the odor becomes noticeable, followed by discoloration, softening of the crumb, and eventually stickiness and stringiness.

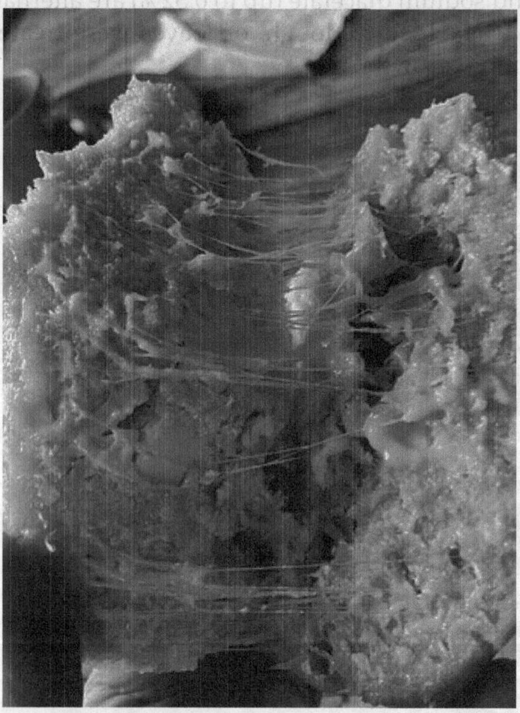

Fig 11.2. Ropy bread showing stringy capsular material stretching between the halves of the loaf.

A complete discussion of factors favoring rope formation and methods of prevention can be found in the second edition of this book (Frazier, 1967).

Red Bread

Red or "bloody" bread, though rare, is visually striking. This coloration is typically caused by the growth of pigmented bacteria, most commonly *Serratia marcescens*, which often produces a brilliant red hue on starchy foods. In ancient times, the unexpected appearance of what seemed like drops of blood on bread was regarded as miraculous. For this phenomenon to occur, the bread must be accidentally contaminated with the red bacteria and stored in unusually moist conditions that promote their growth. Additionally, molds such as *Monilia* (*Neurospora*) sitophila, previously discussed, can impart a pink to red color to bread. In dark bread, a red hue in the crumb has also been linked to *Geotrichum aurantiacum* (syn. *Oidium aurantiacum*).

Chalky Bread

Chalky bread, also uncommon, is so named because of white, chalklike spots. The defect has been blamed on the growth of yeastlike fungi, *Endomycopsis fibuligera* and *Trichosporon variable.*

Cakes and Bakery Products

Molds are the primary contributors to the microbial spoilage of cakes and other bakery items, as the baking process typically eliminates much of the initial microflora. Preventive measures are similar to those used for bread. However, the microbiology of these products becomes more complex when they include toppings like frostings or fruits, or fillings such as custards, imitation creams, or sauces.

These additions are often more susceptible to microbial spoilage than the baked portions. Fillings in pastries frequently provide favorable conditions for microbial growth. Frostings, though relatively stable due to their high sugar content, can still be spoiled by molds or yeast during storage. Meanwhile, the staling of breads, cakes, pies, and similar products is primarily caused by physical changes during storage, rather than microbial activity.

Pasta, Macaroni, and Tapioca

Egg- based pastas, typically made from flour, water, and eggs, are usually delivered and stored in a dry state, making spoilage rare. Macaroni, which generally consists of flour, water, and added nutrients, has occasionally been reported to swell due to gas production by bacteria resembling *Enterobacter cloacae*. In rare cases, molds of the genus *Monilia* have caused purple streaks on macaroni during drying, particularly at points of contact with paper. This issue arises despite the extended drying process. Tapioca, derived from cassava root starch, is prone to spoilage when moistened, with an orange- pigmented, starch-hydrolyzing bacterium identified as the cause

Breakfast Cereals and Other Cereal Snacks

Hobbs and Green (1984) identified three fundamental methods for producing breakfast cereals: flaking, puffing and extrusion. There is a chance of microbial growth during the early stages of these products' manufacturing because of the high moisture content. But in their final form, they typically stand for low-number products (Table).

Prepared Doughs

A wide variety of retail products consist of prepared, refrigerated, or frozen bakery doughs designed for convenience. These items often include inoculums of yeast or lactic acid bacteria. The microbial quality and contamination levels depend heavily on the quality of the ingredients and the sanitary measures taken during production. During refrigerated storage, microbial populations (as shown in Table) may grow until the product undergoes its final "heat treatment" at the consumer's end.

12 Contamination and Preservation Challenges in Sweeteners

Sugars and sweeteners are essential ingredients in food production, providing sweetness, texture, and energy. They are widely used in a variety of products, ranging from candies and baked goods to beverages and processed foods. However, like other food products, sugars and sweeteners are susceptible to microbial contamination, which can compromise their safety, quality, and shelf life. Microorganisms, including bacteria, molds, and yeasts, can proliferate in sugary environments, leading to spoilage, fermentation, and the production of undesirable flavors and odors

Sweeteners, including sugars and artificial sweeteners, are highly prone to microbial contamination due to their high moisture content and, in some cases, nutrient-rich environments. Bacteria, molds, and yeasts can grow on sweeteners, leading to spoilage, fermentation, and the production of off-flavors Contamination typically occurs during processing, storage, or handling, where improper hygiene, temperature, or packaging can provide favorable conditions for microbial growth.

Preservation methods for sweeteners focus on controlling moisture content, temperature, and packaging. Drying and proper storage in sealed containers can help reduce the risk of microbial contamination. Additionally, the use of preservatives like potassium sorbate or sodium benzoate is common in some sweeteners to inhibit microbial growth. Ensuring good manufacturing practices (GMP) and sanitation during production also helps maintain the safety and quality of sweeteners.

This chapter explores the various aspects of microbial contamination in sugars and sweeteners, emphasizing the factors that contribute to their vulnerability. The high moisture content in syrups, the presence of organic compounds, and the warm and humid conditions during processing and storage create an ideal environment for microbial growth. While refined sugars and dry sweeteners are generally resistant to microbial attack, products like syrups, molasses, and liquid sweeteners are more prone to contamination.

The preservation of sugars and sweeteners involves numerous strategies to minimize microbial growth. These include the use of preservatives, controlled storage conditions, and proper handling during manufacturing and packaging. Furthermore, the application of heat treatments such as pasteurization and sterilization can help eliminate harmful microorganisms without compromising the product's quality. Despite these efforts, challenges persist, particularly in natural and minimally processed sweeteners, which may be more vulnerable to microbial spoilage. This chapter will also examine the latest advancements in microbial control techniques to enhance the safety and longevity of these commonly used ingredients.

CONTAMINATION

Sucrose

Raw sugar extracted from sugarcane can become microbially rich if not processed quickly. The microorganisms in question are those of the sugarcane and the soil that contaminates it and therefore include slime producers such as species of *Leuconostoc* and *Bacillus*; representatives of the genera *Micrococcus, Flavobacterium, Alcaligenes, Xanthomonas, Pseudomonas, Erwinia* and *Enterobacter*; a variety of yeasts, mainly of the genera *Saccharomyces, Candida* and *Pichia*; and some molds (Table 12.1). Most contamination can come from debris or fines on the sides or joints of the plant tables. If the organisms grow to a certain level, sucrose inversion or even sugar destruction can occur. The activity of the organisms continues from the cutting of the cane to the extraction and purification of the sugar, a process that kills yeast and vegetative bacterial cells. Bacterial spores are present during this time, by sedimentation, filtration, evaporation, crystallization and centrifugation, but can be reduced in number by these processes, although thermophilic spores can be added by the equipment. Adding raw sugar can also add microorganisms. During the processing of raw sugar, contamination can come from the equipment and organisms are added during bottling

In the production of sugar cane, the refined sugar is cut into thin slices and the sugar is removed by a diffusion process at 60 to 85°C. The sources of contamination are canal water and water from diffusio batteries. In the latter, thermophiles can grow up to 70°C. Contamination can also occur during sugar processing and drying. Granulated sugar currently on the market is very low in microbes for the most part, containing a few to several hundred organisms per gram, mostly bacterial spores.

Maple Syrup

The sap of sugar maple trees in their vascular bundles is sterile or nearly so, but it gets contaminated by external sources in tapholes, spouts, buckets, and other collection vessels. Significant yeast and bacterial growth may occur in the sap if there is an unusually warm period prior to sap collection.

Table: Microbiological Profile of Sugarcane, Cane Juice, Raw Sugar, and Sucros

Product	Microorganisms present	Approximate quantitative range
Sugarcane	Bacteria	10^2–10^8/g
	Enterobacter	

	Leuconostoc	
	Flavobacterium	
	Xanthomonas	
	Bacillus	
	Erwinia	
	Pseudomonas	
	Molds	10^2–10^8/g
	Yeast	10^2–10^4/g
Raw cane juice	Bacteria as above plus	10^4–10^8/ml
	Micrococcus	
	Lactobacillus	
	Actinomyces	
	Molds	
	Aspergillus	
	Cladosporium	
	Monilia	
	Penicillium	
	Yeast	
	Saccharomyces	
	Candida	
	Pichia	
	Torulopsis	
Raw sugar	Bacteria	10^2–10^4/g
	Bacillus	
	Clostridium	
	Desulfotomaculum	
	Osmophilic yeast	
	Aspergilus	
	Penicillium	
	Osmophilic molds	
	Hansenula	
	Pichia	
	Saccharomyces	
Sucrose	Bacteria	10^1–10^2/g
	Mostly sporeformers, if any, and minimal yeast and molds	

Microorganisms that enter the sugar as it flows from the tree until it is boiled and concentrated are mainly gram- negative psychrotrophic rods of *Pseudomonas, Alcaligenes* and *Flavobacterium,* as well as yeast and mold. Paraformaldehyde pellets are inserted into the drilled hole to prevent microbial growth from blocking the flow. In areas where the trees are exposed to unusual dust and air pollution, collecting sap from a series of plastic tubes results in lower bacterial contamination.

However, in a well- controlled sugar mill, the microbial content of the sugar collected from the tubes is not significantly different from that obtained with individual buckets. Liquid collection tanks, usually portable, must be disinfected regularly to prevent the development of large numbers of bacteria in the liquid as it reaches the evaporator. Bacterial counts in fluids are usually less than 10,000 per milliliter, but higher numbers can develop due to warmer late- season temperatures and poor hygiene.

Honey

Nectar from flo ers and honeybees are the main sources of microorganisms in honey. It has been demonstrated that bacteria and yeasts originate from the intestinal contents of bees as well as from the nectar. Enteric bacteria and staphylococci are uncommon in honey. Acidophilic and glycolytic yeasts are common isolates that can harm the final product. It has been discovered that honey contains lysozyme, an enzyme that has both a lytic and bacteriostatic effect on the majority of gram-positive bacteria. Antibiotics like streptomycin and neomycin are frequently used in beekeeping, and honey made from treated bees and larvae has been found to contain these antibiotics.

Traces of these antibiotics in the honey would, of course, have an effect on its microbial flora. Honey is one of the suspected food vehicles for the source of *C. botulinum* spores in cases of infant botulism. About 10 percent of the suspected honey samples contained viable spores.

A study by Ruiz-Argueso and Rodriguez-Navarro (1975) suggested that *Gluconobacter* and *Lactobacillus* are the two main groups of bacteria present during maturation of nectar to honey.

Candy

Retail candies contain anywhere from 0 to 2 million bacteria per piece, but most contain no more than a few hundred. Few coliform bacteria are found here. Contamination of candies comes primarily from their ingredients, although some contamination can be added to unwrapped candies through air, dust, and handling. Thousands of types of pastries and cakes can be divided into two categories for microbiological reasons- (1) cold cakes and (2) cold pastries. Poured chocolate and chocolate coatings for creamy centers are in the first category. Processing temperatures can approach pasteurization temperatures. The second category includes hard candies, jellies, candies, and fudges. The processing temperatures of these products vary, but all are exposed to more severe heat treatment than products in the first category

Candies are rarely linked to food poisoning outbreaks, but chocolate candies have been implicated in salmonellosis cases. The problem appears to be factory cross- contamination between raw and roasted cocoa beans, with raw beans or environmental isolates serving as the source of contamination. Although temperatures of 60°C for 10 hours are not uncommon when processing and mixing milk chocolate, the low moisture content or dryness of the chocolate appears to protect salmonella from the heat.

PRESERVATION

Like grains, sugars generally have such a low aw that microorganisms cannot grow. Only when moisture has been absorbed is there a risk of microbial spoilage. Storage conditions should be such that pests are kept out and the sugar remains dry. The recommended storage temperature is similar to that of cereals.

Sugar cane or sugar beet can be stored in a controlled atmosphere. Fungal growth is inhibited by 6 percent carbon dioxide and 5 percent oxygen.

During the production of raw sugar and the subsequent refining process, the number of microorganisms present, which can be important during extraction from sugar cane or sugar beet, is reduced by most subsequent processes, for example, purification, evaporation, crystallization, centrifugation and filtration. Chemical preservatives are effecti e in reducing the number of microbes during sugar refining. Special treatments to reduce the number and type of organisms may be applied during refining when the sugar is to be used for special purposes, such as for carbonated drinks or canning. Care is taken to avoid aggregation of the organisms and their spores during processing, and their numbers may be reduced by ultraviolet irradiation or by the combined action of heat and hydrogen peroxide.

Because of their high sugar concentration and low aw, most confections are not subject to microbial spoilage, although some chocolate confections contain a small amount of sugar, which can promote the growth of microorganisms. Chocolate explosion is prevented by a uniform and sufficientl thick coating of chocolate and by the use of foundations or other fillings that do not allow the growth of gas generators.

Syrups and molasses are usually heated sufficientl to destroy most microorganisms, but they must be stored at low temperatures to prevent or slow chemical changes and microbial growth. Some molasses may contain sufficien sulfur dioxide to inhibit microorganisms, but most syrups and molasses do not contain added preservatives and inhibit microbial growth due to the high osmotic pressure of the sugar solution. The osmotic pressure increases with the rate of inversion (hydrolysis) of sucrose. Surface mold growth is prevented by filling the container completely and is reduced by periodically topping off the syrup or molasses.

The boiling process of evaporating maple sap into maple syrup kills important spoilage organisms. This syrup, bottled hot and in a tightly sealed container, generally keeps well.

Commercially distributed honey is usually pasteurized at 160 to 180°F (71 to 77°C) for several minutes. A recommended treatment is to rapidly heat to at least 160°F (71°C), hold at this temperature for 5 minutes, and then rapidly cool to 90°F (32°C). 2 to 38°C.

SPOILAGE

The spoilage of sugars or concentrated solutions of sugars is limited to that caused by osmophilic or xerotolerant microorganisms. Certain yeasts, especially those of the genus *Saccharomyces,* and certain molds would be the principal spoilage flora. Some species of bacteria have also been suggested as possible spoilage problems, including species of *Bacillus* and *Leuconostoc.* As the sugar concentrations decrease, increasing numbers of kinds of organisms can grow, so that sap from a maple tree would show types of spoilage that maple sirup could not.

Sucrose

The original cane or beet juice is purified more and more toward sucrose during the sugar-making process, and the concentration of sugar in solution increases until crystalline sugar and high-sugar molasses are eventually achieved. The more concentrated the product, the fewer types of organisms can grow in it; the purer the product, the worse it is as a microorganism culture medium.

Raw Juice

Raw cane or beet juice is not high in sugar and contains a good deal of random food for microorganisms; therefore, it is easily damaged by the many organisms present if given enough time. While waiting for clarification, gum and mucus may form, for example dextran from *Leuconostoc mesenteroides* or *L. dextranicum** and levan from *Bacillus* spp. or, less commonly, from yeast or mold.

Sugar in Storage

Liquid sugar with sugar content as high as 67 to 72 brix will support the growth of yeasts (*Saccharomyces, Candida, Rhodotorula*) and molds which may enter from the air. Dilution by absorption of moisture at the surface may result in growth of microorganisms and hence deterioration of the product. This can be prevented by circulation of filtered sterile air across the top of the storage tank or exposure to ultraviolet lamps.

Molasses and Syrups

Microbial spoilage of molasses is not common, although it is difficul to sterilize by heat because of the protective effect of the sugar. Canned molasses or syrup may be subject to spoilage by osmophilic yeasts that survive the heating process. Molasses or syrup exposed to air will eventually mold on the surface, and this can also occur on the surface of bottled or canned syrup if air has been trapped and contamination has occurred before sealing. Some types of molasses are acidic enough to cause hydrogen expansion during prolonged storage.

Maple Sap and Syrup

English As previously indicated, sugar maple sap is contaminated when extracted. Although moderate growth can improve flavor and color, sugar is often found in conditions that promote excessive growth of microorganisms and therefore spoilage. Five main types of spoilage are recognized- (1) a stringy or stringy liquid, usually caused by *Enterobacter aerogenes*, although *Leuconostoc* spp. may be responsible, (2) a cloudy liquid, sometimes green, resulting from the growth of *Pseudomonas fluorescens*, with *Alcaligenes* and *Flavobacterium* species sometimes contributing to the turbidity, (3) a red fluid, colored by pigments from red bacteria, e.g. , *Micrococcus roseus*, or yeast fungus or yeast, (4) sour liquid, a general group for types of spoilage that do not show visible changes in color but have a sour odor and are caused by a variety of bacteria or yeast, and (5) Moldy juice, spoiled by mold.

Maple syrup may be affected by *Enterobacter aerogenes*, yeast by the growth of *Saccharomyces* species of yeast, pink by the pigment *Micrococcus roseus*, or mold on the surface where *Aspergillus, Penicillium*, or other genera may grow. The syrup may be dark due to the alkalinity produced by the bacteria growing in the sugar and the inversion of the sucrose.

Maple sugar keeps well unless it is damp, in which case mold may develop.

Honey

Honey is of variable composition, but should not exceed 25% moisture. Due to its high sugar content, 70 to 80%, mainly glucose and levulose, and its acidity, pH 3.2 to 4.2, the main cause of its deterioration is due to osmophilic yeasts- species of *Zygosaccharomyces*, such as *Z. mellis, richteri* or *nussbaumeri*, or *Torula* (*Cryptococcus*) *mellis*. Most molds do not grow well in honey, although *Penicillium* and *Mucor* species are known to grow slowly.

Most bees do not grow in the laboratory at sugar concentrations such as those typically found in honey. Therefore, specific theories have been proposed for the initiation of yeast growth in honey- (1) honey, being hygroscopic, is diluted to the surface, where the yeasts begin to multiply and adapt quickly to the high sugar concentration, (2) crystallization of glucose. . hydration from the honey leaves a reduced concentration of sugars in solution, or (3) after a long time, the yeast gradually adapts. to high sugar concentrations. The critical moisture content for the initiation of yeast growth has been established at 21%. The rate of conversion of sucrose to glucose and levulose by bees and the available nitrogen content are also listed as factors determining the likelihood of growth. The fermentation process is generally slow, lasting several months, and the main products are carbon dioxide, alcohol, and non- volatile acids that give the honey an unpleasant taste. Darkening and crystallization usually accompany fermentation.

Candy

Most candies are generally resistant to microbial spoilage due to their high sugar content and low moisture levels. However, there are exceptions, particularly in chocolates with soft fillings such as fondant or inverted sugar. Under specific conditions, these chocolates may experience issues like bursting or exploding. The cause of this spoilage is the growth of yeasts within the candy, which produces gas. This gas buildup can create enough pressure to disrupt the candy, causing the syrup or fondant to leak out, usually through a weak point in the chocolate coating. Such weak points are often found on the bottom of the chocolate, where the coating may be insufficient This issue can be prevented by ensuring the filling does not support the growth of gas- producing microorganisms and by applying a thick, even coating of chocolate that strengthens the candy's structure. The microbial spoilage microorganisms involved in the contamination of various confectionery products.

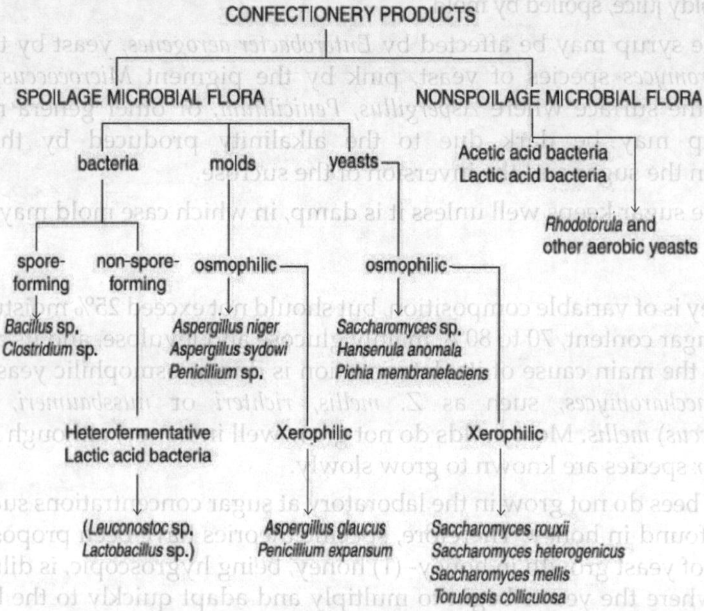

Fig 12.1. Spoilage flora of confectionery products. (From Speck, 197).

13 Contamination and Preservation of Fruits and Vegetables

It is estimated that approximately 25% of all harvested produce spoils before it is consumed (Salunkhe, 1974). The spoilage of fresh fruits and vegetables typically occurs during storage, transport, and while waiting for processing. Unlike many other foods covered in this book, fruits and vegetables remain "alive" for a considerable period after harvest and before processing. The respiration and natural ripening processes of these products make it challenging to discuss their microbiological spoilage independently.

A significant portion of the microbiological spoilage issues are considered "market diseases," which are typically addressed in plant pathology literature. Fruits and vegetables can be consumed in various forms, including fresh, dried, frozen, fermented, pasteurized, or canned, with spoilage of canned products.

CONTAMINATION

After fruits and vegetables are collected in crates, baskets, or trucks at harvest, they are subject to contamination by spoilage organisms from each other and from containers unless they have been properly disinfected. During transport to the market or processing plant, mechanical damage can increase susceptibility to spoilage and growth of microorganisms. Pre- cooling the product and chilling during transport will slow this growth.

Washing of fruits or vegetables may involve pre- soaking or may be accomplished by agitation in water, or preferably by spray treatment. Washing with immersion and agitation tends to disperse spoilage organisms from spoiled foods into the whole food. Recycled or reused water is likely to add organisms, and the washing process can wet the surface sufficientl to allow organisms to grow during storage. Washing with detergents or germicidal solutions will reduce the number of microorganisms in the food.

Sorting spoiled fruits or vegetables or cutting off spoiled parts removes microorganisms, but further processing can lead to mechanical damage and therefore greater susceptibility to spoilage. When these products are sold to the retail market without processing, they are generally not subject to much contamination, except for storage in the market in contaminated bins or other containers, possible contact with decaying products, handling by vendors and customers, and perhaps a spray of water or a pack of crushed ice. This spray keeps the vegetables fresh and delays decomposition, but it also adds organisms, for example.

In the processing plant, the fruit or vegetable is subject to additional contamination and risk of growth of microorganisms, or the number and type of organisms can be reduced by certain processes. Proper washing in the factory results in a reduction in the number of microorganisms in the food, as well as peeling with steam, hot water or sauce and blanching (heating to deactivate enzymes, etc.). Sweat products during processing increase their number. Processes such as mechanical cutting, abrasion or peeling, shearing, coring or grinding, and various disintegration methods can add contaminants from the equipment used. In fact, any equipment that comes into contact with food can be a significant source of microorganisms if not properly cleaned and disinfected. Modern metal equipment with smooth surfaces and no cracks, corners, etc. are designed to facilitate these treatments. Trays, bins, tanks, pipes, channels, tables, conveyor belts and aprons, fillers, bleachers, presses, sieves, and filters are examples of potential sources of food contamination by microorganisms. Wooden surfaces are difficul to clean and disinfect and are therefore particularly likely to be sources of contamination, as are fabric surfaces, such as on conveyor belts. Neglected parts of any food handling system can accumulate large numbers of microorganisms that contaminate food. Hot water blanching, although it reduces the total number of organisms in foods, can cause the accumulation of spores of thermophilic bacteria, leading to spoilage of canned foods. For example, flat, sour spores in peas

The accumulation of microbial populations on equipment due to microbial growth in exudates and fruit and vegetable waste can greatly influence food contamination rates and contaminant growth. Not only is it possible that large numbers of organisms from this source are added, but it is also likely that they are organisms in the logarithmic growth phase and therefore capable of continuing rapid growth. This effect is especially noticeable in vegetables after blanching. This heat treatment significantly reduces the bacterial content, damaging many surviving cells and therefore extending their latency period. On the other hand, active growth of contaminants from equipment can reach large quantities if sufficien time is allowed before freezing, drying or canning; such an increase is usually due to very high levels of bacteria.

The inclusion of broken fruit parts increases the number of microorganisms in fruit juices. The number of microorganisms in orange juice, for example, and the number of coliforms increases significantly. with the inclusion of fruits showing soft rot. Heating the grapes before extraction reduces the number of organisms in the pressed juice, but the press introduces contamination.

The types of microorganisms that come from the equipment will depend on the product being processed, since that product will be the culture medium for the organisms. Thus, pea waste favors bacteria that grow well in a pea medium, and tomato organisms that can grow in tomato juice. As the equipment Used throughout the day, the organisms can continue to grow. However, at the end of the cycle, when the equipment is cleaned and disinfected, the total number of microorganisms present is significantly reduced and, if the operation is effecti e, only the resistant forms survive. Therefore, bacterial spores are likely to survive, and if conditions for growth are suitable while the equipment is idle, these spores can multiply, especially in poorly cleaned rooms. Thermophilic spores, so troublesome to vegetable preservers, accumulate in this way and add to the difficult of subjecting foods to adequate heat treatment. The number of these organisms on poorly cleaned and disinfected equipment may be high at the beginning of a working day and decrease as the day progresses, but usually the opposite is true. A break from work during work allows a further increase in the number of bacteria. It is clear that the number of microorganisms entering food from the equipment depends on the opportunities for growth offered to these organisms and that these opportunities are the result of inadequate cleaning and disinfection combined with favorable conditions of humidity and temperature for a significant period of time. Adding ingredients such as sugar and starch can increase spoilage organisms, especially spores of thermophilic bacteria.

PRESERVATION OF VEGETABLES

Along with the typical surface flora, soil, water, and possibly plant pathogens are among the microorganisms found on the surfaces of recently harvested fruits and vegetables (Table). There may also be a variety of molds and occasionally a few yeasts. Between harvesting and processing or eating the vegetables, some microorganisms may grow if the surfaces are damp or if the outer surface has been damaged. Such growth will be inhibited by proper temperature and humidity control.

Table: General Microbiological Profile of Harvested Fruits and Vegetables

Product	Microorganisms isolated	Approximate quantitative range
Apples	Yeasts, Molds, Bacteria (e.g., *Erwinia* spp., *Pseudomonas* spp.)	10^3 - 10^6 CFU/g
Citrus Fruits	Yeasts, Molds, *Penicillium* spp., *Aspergillus* spp., *Bacillus* spp.	10^2 - 10^4 CFU/g
Tomatoes	*Enterobacteriaceae, Pseudomonas* spp., *Clostridium* spp., *Fusarium* spp.	10^2 - 10^5 CFU/g
Lettuc	*Lactic acid bacteria, Bacillus spp., *Pseudomonas* spp., *Escherichia coli*	10^3 - 10^6 CFU/g
Carrots	*Bacteria (e.g., *Pseudomonas* spp., *Bacillus* spp.), Fungi (e.g., *Fusarium* spp.)	10^2 - 10^5 CFU/g
Strawberries	*Molds (*Botrytis* spp., *Penicillium* spp.), Yeasts	10^2 - 10^4 CFU/g
Potatoes	*Molds (*Fusarium* spp., *Rhizoctonia* spp.), Bacteria (e.g., *Erwinia* spp.)	10^2 - 10^6 CFU/g
Bananas	*Molds (*Fusarium* spp., *Alternaria* spp.), Yeasts	10^2 - 10^5 CFU/g

Product	Microorganisms isolated	Approximate quantitative range
Spinach	*Bacteria (e.g., *Pseudomonas* spp.), Yeasts, Molds	10^2 - 10^5 CFU/g
Grapes	*Molds (*Botrytis* spp., *Penicillium* spp.), Yeasts	10^2 - 10^4 CFU/g

*Note- The values provided are approximate and can vary based on environmental conditions, handling, and storage. The unit CFU/g (colony- forming units per gram) is commonly used to express microbial counts in food products.

Asepsis

Although some contamination of vegetables can occur between harvest and processing or consumption, significant contamination can be prevented. Containers such as boxes, lugs, and baskets must be kept free of microbial growth and should be cleaned and sanitized between uses. For instance, lugs used for transporting peas to processing plants can harbor substantial bacterial growth on their moist interiors, which can transfer high levels of microorganisms to the peas. If vegetables in the process of spoiling come into contact with healthy ones, it can lead to further contamination and potential losses. At the processing plant, contamination from equipment can be minimized with thorough cleaning and sanitization. A particular concern is the buildup of heat- resistant spores from spoilage bacteria, such as those from flat sour bacteria, putrefactive anaerobes, or *Clostridium thermosaccharolyticum*. When fresh vegetables arrive at the processing plant, bacterial counts can range from 10^2 to 10^7 per gram, depending on the vegetable type and its condition.

REMOVAL OF MICROORGANISMS

Washing vegetables thoroughly removes most of the surface contaminants but leaves much of the natural microbial flora intact. If the wash water is not of good bacteriological quality, it can introduce additional organisms, potentially leading to microbial growth on the moist surface. To address this, chlorinated water is sometimes used for washing, and detergents may be added to help remove dirt and microorganisms. For instance, washing strawberries with a nonionic detergent solution can help eliminate some of the mold growth.

Heat

The enzymes in vegetables that are to be dried, frozen, or canned are rendered inactive by scalding or blanching them. At the same time, there is a noticeable decrease in the number of microorganisms, possibly by 1,000–10,000 times (Splittstoesser, 1970). Chapter 6 has covered the topic of heat processing canned vegetables.

Use of Low Temperatures

As has been indicated, a few kinds of vegetables that are relatively stable, such as root crops, potatoes, cabbage, and celery, can be preserved for a limited time by common or cellar storage .

Freezing

The selection and preparation of vegetables, their blanching, freezing, and the changes that occur during these processes were discussed in Chapter 7. Microorganisms from the natural flora, as well as contaminants from soil and water, are found on the surface of vegetables. If the surface is moist, some of these organisms will grow before the vegetables reach the frozen plant. Here, washing reduces the number of some organisms and increases others, and scalding or blanching (86 to 98°C) results in a large reduction in numbers, up to 90 to 99 percent in some cases.

However, during cooling and handling prior to freezing, there is a risk of recontamination from equipment and growth of organisms, as under poor conditions 1 million or more organisms may be present per gram of vegetable at the time of freezing. The freezing process reduces the number of organisms by a percentage that varies depending on the species and the numbers initially present, but on average about half of them are killed. Table illustrates the evolution of the number of organisms in pods during the various operations carried out in a freezing facility. During frozen storage, the number of organisms steadily decreases, but at least some survivors of most organisms remain after the usual storage period. The type of bacteria most likely to grow during thawing depends on the temperature and time elapsed. *Micrococcus** species are Predominant in thawing vegetables such as sweet corn and peas when thawing temperatures are quite low, although *Achromobacter** and *Enterobacter* are also common. Lactobacilli are also common in peas under such conditions. One species of *Micrococcus** may grow first, followed by another species later. At higher temperatures, *Flavobacterium* species can also multiply. Since small packages of frozen vegetables are usually processed at home, where frozen foods are placed directly in boiling water and cooked, there is no longer a chance for microbial growth. During freezing, most vegetables shrink and become soft, and during storage, frozen vegetables may undergo color changes.

Table. Numbers of Organisms Per Gram on Snap Beans after Passing through Unit Operations in a Freezing Plant

Source of sample	Average plate count per gram*
Before cutter	740,000
After cutter and shaker	573,000
After blancher	1,000
After shaker, before sorting belt	188,000
Final package	36,000

*Average of seventeen samples during 9 days. Plates incubated at 32°C.

When thawed vegetables are kept at room temperature for extended periods, there is a risk of food- poisoning bacteria growing and producing toxins. For example, Jones and Lochhead (1939) discovered enterotoxin- forming staphylococci in frozen corn. In their study, sterilized corn inoculated with food-poisoning staphylococci, then frozen and thawed at a room temperature of 20°C for one day, allowed the bacteria to grow and produce enough enterotoxin to cause food poisoning symptoms. This toxin would not be fully destroyed by the usual cooking of the vegetable. Additionally, *Clostridium botulinum* has been detected in frozen vegetables, and while its growth and toxin production require specific conditions, such as a freezer power failure during a flood or hurricane, it remains a concern. Cooking frozen vegetables may not kill all *C. botulinum* spores, and such cooked food should not be left at room temperature for long periods. Bacterial counts in frozen vegetables can range from very low to about 10^2 per gram, with coliforms and enterococci frequently found. The presence of E. coli is rare, but its detection raises concerns about the hygiene practices involved.

Chilling

Most vegetables intended for storage without special processing are quickly cooled and stored at refrigerated temperatures. Cooling is accomplished with cold water, ice, or mechanical or vacuum cooling (wet and evacuated), as for salad. In many cases, pre- cooling, that is, cooling prior to normal cold storage, is accomplished immediately after harvest with a stream of cold water, a practice called hydrocooling. Each type of vegetable has its own optimum temperature and relative humidity for cold storage, as illustrated in Chapter 7 and as recommended in special bulletins and manuals. Cooling leafy vegetables (lettuce, spinach) by spraying with water will cool the product if cold water is used and will contribute to its preservation.

Control of atmospheric composition in vegetable storage has not been used as for fruits. Adding carbon dioxide or ozone to the air has been recommended by some workers. UV rays have not been effecti e because they do not reach all surfaces of the vegetables when they are packed and handled.

Sweet potatoes were mentioned in Chapter 7 as an example of a vegetable that requires special cold storage conditions. Regular potatoes become sweet at temperatures below 2.2 to 4.4°C and are stored at higher temperatures if they are to be used for making French fries. Sweet potatoes and onions undergo special drying treatments before storage.

Drying

As drying methods for vegetables and vegetable products have advanced, public acceptance has grown, leading to a wide market for various dried food items. Dried vegetables are commonly found in dried soups, while dried spices and condiments are widely used for flavoring.Many vegetables are dried using a process called explosive puffing Small pieces of diced, partially dehydrated vegetables are placed in a sealed rotating chamber, where heat is applied, and the chamber is pressurized to a specific level before being rapidly depressurized. This process causes additional water loss, but more importantly, it creates a porous network of capillaries in the product. The increased porosity aids in further drying and enhances reconstitution.

Microbial growth can occur after blanching but before drying, which can contribute to the final microbial count in the dried product. While heat drying kills yeasts and most bacteria, bacterial and mold spores, as well as more heat- resistant vegetative cells, typically survive. Microbial counts in dried vegetables, both after drying and in retail products, tend to be much higher than in dried fruits due to a higher initial microbial load and a greater survival rate during drying. Vegetables are less acidic than fruits, so heat is less effecti e at killing microorganisms. Dried vegetables from retail markets often contain hundreds of thousands or millions of microorganisms per gram, although the number can be much smaller if produced under more stringent conditions.

Sulfuring dried vegetables helps preserve their light color and reduces their microbial content. When dried and stored properly, microbial growth is prevented. Over time, there is a gradual decrease in viable organisms, with the reduction being more rapid in the first few months and slowing thereafter. Spores from bacteria and molds, along with certain micrococci and microbacteria, are more resistant to desiccation and survive longer, making up a larger portion of the microbial population as storage time increases.

Use of Preservatives

Although, some vegetables may receive special treatment on their surfaces, preservatives are not frequently added to vegetables. Turnips and rutabagas are occasionally paraffinate to extend their storage period. On spinach, beets, and lettuce, zinc carbonate has been shown to eradicate the majority of mold growth. Fusarium on potatoes will be managed by biphenyl vapors (McKee and Boyd, 1962). Although, it has been tried experimentally, a controlled atmosphere of ozone or carbon dioxide surrounding chilled vegetables has not proven very useful.

Added Preservative

Sodium chloride is the most commonly used chemical preservative. The amount of salt added to vegetables can range from 2.25 to 2.5 percent for making sauerkraut, to saturation levels for preserving cauliflo er. Lower salt concentrations allow for acid fermentation by bacteria, but as the salt content increases, the rate of acid production slows down until a level is reached where no fermentation or acid production occurs.

Vegetables with high protein content, such as green peas and lima beans, as well as those that soften easily like onions and cauliflo er, are preserved by adding sufficien salt to prevent fermentation. The salt concentration typically ranges from 70 to 80° salometer (18.6 to 21.2 percent salt) up to saturation at 26.5 percent salt (100° salometer). When brine or salt is added to vegetables, water is drawn out, which in turn lowers the salt concentration in the liquid.

The growing popularity of salad bars has led to increased use of sulfites as salad fresheners, preventing enzymatic browning in lettuce, cole slaw, and other salad items. However, sulfite residues in foods have been linked to asthmatic reactions, and the levels of sulfites in restaurant salads ha e been studied (Martin et al., 1986).

Developed Preservatives

At room temperature, acid fermentation is normal for chopped, chopped, or chopped vegetables that contain sugar, but instead of a sharp, sour taste due to the action of lactic acid bacteria, unpleasant odors and changes in the body can result from the growth of coliform bacteria. bacilli, anaerobes, proteolytic bacteria and others. The addition of salt to these materials serves to reduce competition from undesirable organisms and therefore promotes lactic fermentation. Salt is also used to remove juices from vegetables and to ensure a better distribution of lactic acid bacteria. The amount of sugar in the vegetable affects the acidity that can be produced, while the amount of salt and temperature determine the rate of acid production and the types of bacteria involved. In general, as salt content increases, the rate of acid formation slows and the number of bacterial species involved decreases. Some recipes call for a relatively low salt content initially, then increasing as fermentation progresses, and finally enough salt to prevent bacterial growth. This method is used for pickling vegetables such as green beans and corn.

Preservation by Irradiation

After being experimentally treated with gamma rays to inactivate the microorganisms that cause decay, most vegetables have deteriorated, softened, or become discolored. Nonetheless, irradiation has been effecti ely used to stop insects from reproducing on certain vegetables and to postpone the sprouting of potatoes, onions, and garlic.

METHODS OF PRESERVING FRUITS AND FRUIT-BASED PRODUCTS

The preservation of fruits and fruit products generally follows principles similar to those for vegetables and their products. The surface of healthy fruits contains natural flora, as well as contaminating microorganisms from soil and water, which results in a microbial profile comparable to that of vegetables. However, yeasts and molds are typically more prevalent in fruits. Additionally, some fruits may harbor plant pathogens or saprophytic spoilage organisms that can proliferate after harvest. To maintain quality, defective fruits should be sorted, and any spoiled areas should be trimmed. Occasionally, some microorganisms may also be found in the interior of healthy fruits.

Asepsis

As with vegetables, fruits are susceptible to contamination between harvest and processing through contact with containers or spoiled fruits. To minimize contamination, careful handling is crucial. Prior to harvest, fruits are often treated with insecticides and fungicides, which can alter their natural flora.

REMOVAL OF MICROORGANISMS

Washing fruits thoroughly not only removes dirt but also helps eliminate casual contaminating microorganisms and potentially harmful pesticides.

Washing can be done using water, detergent solutions, or bactericidal agents like chlorinated water. Trimming fruits can also help in removing microorganisms, and fruit juices may be sterilized by filtration for clarity.

Use of Heat

Unlike vegetables, fruits are rarely blanched before processing, as blanching can cause excessive damage. The heat processing of canned fruits, as discussed in Chapter 6, involves different methods depending on the pH of the fruit. Fruits are generally categorized into acid foods (e.g., tomatoes, pears, pineapples) and high-acid foods (e.g., berries). Most fruits do not require a steam- pressure sterilizer; heating to around 100°C via steam or boiling water is typically sufficient The higher the fruit's acidity, the less heat is required for preservation. These principles are similarly applied when canning fruit juices.

Use of Low Temperatures

While some fruits, such as apples, can be stored at room temperature for a limited period, most fruits require controlled, lower temperatures for optimal storage.

Chilling

Each fruit has specific temperature and humidity requirements for chilling storage, and even different varieties of the same fruit may have distinct needs. Various chemicals have been applied to fruits before or during storage to enhance preservation. These include hypochlorites, sodium bicarbonate, borax, propionates, and sulfur dioxide, among others. Fruits can also be wrapped in chemically treated materials, such as sulfite paper for grapes or borax paper for oranges. To provide mechanical protection, fruits may be treated with waxed wraps, paraffin oil, or mineral oil.

Controlled Atmosphere and Modified Atmosphere Storage

Extensive research has been conducted on combining chilling storage with controlled atmosphere conditions. This may involve adjusting the oxygen and carbon dioxide concentrations or even introducing or removing gases such as ozone. Controlled- atmosphere (CA) storage involves altering the levels of gases from their normal atmospheric concentrations, typically increasing CO_2 levels and decreasing O_2.

Modified atmosphere (MA) storage refers to similar conditions but with less precise control, or where the atmosphere is initially altered but not continuously regulated. In some cases, a single gas, such as nitrogen, may be used in "gas storage." The specific concentrations of carbon dioxide and oxygen needed for optimal storage vary depending on the type of fruit and sometimes even its variety. The conditions for CA storage are summarized in Table.

Table: Conditions of Controlled- atmosphere Storage for Several Fruits and Vegetables

Fruit/ vegetable	Temperature (°C)	Relative humidity (%)	Oxygen concentration (%)	Carbon dioxide concentration (%)	Storage duration
Apples	0 to 4	85 to 90	2 to 3	2 to 5	3 to 6 months
Pears	0 to 4	90 to 95	2 to 3	2 to 5	2 to 3 months
Grapes	0 to 2	90 to 95	5 to 7	1 to 3	1 to 3 months
Tomatoes	12 to 14	85 to 90	5 to 10	2 to 5	1 to 2 weeks
Strawberries	0 to 2	90 to 95	3 to 5	2 to 5	1 to 2 weeks
Bananas	13 to 15	90 to 95	5 to 7	2 to 4	2 to 4 weeks
Carrots	0 to 2	95 to 100	2 to 3	5 to 8	3 to 6 months
Potatoes	7 to 10	90 to 95	3 to 5	5 to 8	2 to 4 months
Cucumbers	10 to 12	90 to 95	5 to 10	2 to 5	1 to 2 weeks
Lettuc	0 to 2	95 to 100	3 to 5	5 to 8	1 to 2 weeks

Note: The temperature and humidity levels are indicative of the ideal storage conditions: The oxygen and carbon dioxide concentrations are adjusted in controlled atmosphere storage to slow down the ripening process, prevent spoilage, and extend shelf life: The storage duration is an estimate and may vary based on fruit/vegetable variety and storage conditions.

Although carbon dioxide storage is primarily used for apples, it has also been effecti ely applied to pears, bananas, citrus fruits, plums, peaches, grapes, and various other fruits. Ozone concentrations of 2 to 3 ppm in the atmosphere have been found to extend the storage life of lightly packed small fresh fruits, such as strawberries, raspberries, currants, and grapes, as well as delicate apple varieties, by up to twice the usual duration. Ethylene, used in the atmosphere, accelerates ripening or induces specific color changes and is not regarded as a preservative, although a combination of this gas with activated hydrocarbons has been proposed for fruit preservation.

Freezing

The surfaces of fruits harbor both natural surface flora and contaminants from soil and water. Any spoiled areas may introduce molds or yeasts. During fruit preparation for freezing, undesirable changes like darkening, flavor deterioration, and microbial spoilage, especially by molds, can occur. Washing the fruit eliminates most of the soilborne microorganisms, while proper selection and trimming help reduce molds and yeasts involved in spoilage. If handled correctly, microbial growth before freezing should be minimal. Some fruits are frozen in large drums (up to 50 lb), and it's essential to cool the fruit before filling the container to ensure rapid freezing.

The freezing process lowers microorganism counts but can cause tissue damage, leading to flabbiness and juice loss. During storage in a frozen state, physical changes as described in Chapter 7 occur, alongside a gradual but consistent reduction in microorganism numbers. Yeasts (such as *Saccharomyces* and *Cryptococcus*) and molds (e.g., *Aspergillus, Penicillium, Mucor, Rhizopus, Botrytis, Fusarium, Alternaria*) are commonly found in frozen fruits, although a few soil organisms, like *Bacillus, Pseudomonas,* and *Achromobacter* species, may survive the freezing process. Yeasts are more likely to grow during slow thawing. The number of viable microorganisms in frozen fruits is significantly lower than in frozen vegetables. High mold hyphae counts may indicate poor-quality fruit with rotten parts.

The microbial count in frozen fruit juices depends on the fruit's condition, the washing process, filtration method, and the chance for contamination and microbial growth before freezing. At the time of freezing, there may be anywhere from a few hundred to over a million organisms per milliliter in the juice. Including decayed fruit increases the organism count substantially. The washing method, particularly the type of solution used, plays a key role in removing microorganisms, as those on the fruit's surface are difficul to eliminate. Microbial counts can increase in the washing solution, on the washed fruit's moist surfaces, and in the juice itself before freezing.

Contamination from equipment in the processing plant is also possible. Freezing significantly reduces microorganism numbers, but added sugar or higher juice concentrations may protect some organisms from being killed. While microbial numbers decrease slowly during frozen storage, this decline is faster than in most neutral foods. The microorganisms mainly include soil, water, and rotting organisms, along with the natural surface flora of the fruit. Coliforms, enterococci, and lactics such as *Leuconostoc* and *Lactobacillus, Alcaligenes,* and yeasts are commonly found.

Since coliform bacteria, primarily of the *Enterobacter aerogenes* type, are part of the natural flora of fruits, they are present in both fresh and frozen fruit juices. Using decayed fruit in juice production increases the coliform count, though these bacteria decrease during storage. Because coliforms are typically present, the presumptive test for coliforms is not considered suitable for assessing the sanitary quality of the juice. It is suggested that tests for fecal coliforms, such as *Escherichia coli* or *Streptococcus faecalis*, be conducted instead.

Drying

The drying of fruits has been discussed in Chapter 8, where it was noted that the numbers of microorganisms in dried fruits are comparatively low and that spores of bacteria and molds are likely to be the most numerous. An occasional sample may contain high numbers of mold spores, indicating that growth and sporulation of molds has taken place on the fruit before or after dehydration. Alkali treatment, sulfuring, blanching, and pasteurization reduce numbers of microorganisms.

Use of Preservatives

The use of chemical preservatives to extend the shelf life of fruit was discussed in Chapter 9, where it was noted that the chemicals were applied to the fruit primarily as dips or sprays or impregnated into the fruit packaging. The substances that were applied to the external surface of the fruit included wax, hypochlorite, biphenyl, and sodium alkaline o- phenylphenate. The fruit packaging was impregnated with various chemicals, including iodine, sulfite, biphenyl, o- phenylphenol, and hexamine, among others. Carbon dioxide, ozone, and ethylene plus chlorinated hydrocarbons were tested as gases or mists around the fruit. Sulfur dioxide and sodium benzoate are preservatives that are added directly to fruit or fruit products. Most of the chemical preservatives mentioned have primarily an antifungal function.

Green olives are the only fruit that can be preserved on a commercial scale by acid fermentation. However, other fermented fruits are sometimes prepared, such as fermented green tomatoes and preserved Romanian apples. In all of these products, lactic acid fermentation is of great importance.

SPOILAGE

Damage to raw fruits and vegetables may be due to physical factors, the action of their enzymes, microbial action, or a combination of these factors. Mechanical damage resulting from the action of animals, birds, or insects or from bruises, wounds, cracks, cuts, freezing, drying, or other uses may predispose to increased enzymatic action or to the penetration and growth of microorganisms. Previous damage by plant pathogens may render the part of the plant used as food unfit for consumption or may pave the way for the growth and deterioration of saprophytes. Contact with decaying fruits and vegetables may result in the transfer of organisms, causing spoilage and the growth of waste. Improper environmental conditions during harvesting, transportation, storage, and marketing may promote spoilage. Most of the discussion that follows focuses on microbial spoilage, but it should always be remembered that plant enzymes continue their activity in raw plant foods. If oxygen is available, plant cells will respire as long as they are alive, and hydrolytic enzymes can continue their action after the cell has died. As discussed in Chapter 4, the suitability of foods for consumption is judged in part on the basis of their ripeness. If the desired stage of ripeness has been passed, the food may be considered inedible or even spoiled. An example is a ripe banana, with its black skin and soft brown interior.

Diseases of vegetables and fruits it can result from the growth of an organism that takes food from the host and usually damages it or from unfavorable environmental conditions that cause abnormalities in the functions and structures of the vegetable or fruit. Diseases caused by pathogens and decays caused by saprophytic organisms will be of great interest in the following discussion, although a clear distinction between these types of organisms is not possible. However, diseases that are not caused by organisms it should be mentioned as it can sometimes be confused with those caused by organisms that can be quite similar in appearance. Examples of non- pathogenic diseases are brown heart of apples and pears, black heart of potatoes, black leaf of cabbage and red heart of cabbage.

No attempt should be made to treat changes caused by plant pathogens growing on plants, or parts of plants used for food, before harvest; instead we examine the microbial changes that can it occurs during harvesting, sorting, packing, transportation, storage and handling by the wholesaler and retailer, although some of these changes may begin before harvest. The space available will only permit a general treatment of the subject and only from the perspective of the food microbiologist and not the plant pathologist. The reader should consult the references listed at the end of the chapter for further details, particularly the bulletins of the USDA Bureau of Plant Industry.

General Types of Microbial Spoilage

The predominant type of spoilage differs depending on the fruit or vegetable and, in some cases, the variety. Microbial spoilage can result from (1) plant pathogens att cking the stems, leaves, flo ers, or roots of the plant, including fruits or other edible parts such as tubers, or (2) saprophytic organisms that either invade after a plant pathogen or infect healthy fruits and vegetables, causing issues like rots or surface growth, as seen when bacteria thrive on moist, piled vegetables. Sometimes, a saprophyte follows a pathogen, or multiple saprophytes may contribute to spoilage. For example, coliform bacteria can proliferate as secondary invaders and may be found in significant numbers in fruit and vegetable juices if decayed products are included.Although spoilage types and microorganisms vary with each fruit or vegetable, certain general types of microbial spoilage are more commonly observed in both fruits and vegetables. The most frequent types of spoilage include:

- **Anthracnose:** Caused by *Colletotrichum* species like *C. lindemuthianum* and *C. coccodes*, characterized by spots on leaves, fruit, or seedpods.
- ***Alternaria* Rot:** Caused by *Alternaria tenuis* and other species, it starts as greenish- brown spots, later turning brown or black.
- **Blue Mold Rot:** Caused by *Penicillium digitatum* and other species, marked by a bluish- green color from the mold's spore masses.

- **Downy Mildew:** Caused by *Phytophthora, Bremia,* and other genera, characterized by white, woolly mold growth.
- **Bacterial Soft Rot:** Caused by *Erwinia carotovora* and similar species, which ferment pectins. Other bacteria like *Pseudomonas marginalis* and *Clostridium* and *Bacillus* species have also been identified. This results in a water- soaked appearance, mushy texture, and often a foul odor.
- **Gray Mold Rot:** Caused by *Botrytis* species, especially *B. cinerea.* It thrives in high humidity and warm temperatures, with the mold's gray mycelium giving the rot its name.
- ***Rhizopus* Soft Rot**: Caused by *Rhizopus* species, such as *R. stolonifer*, leading to soft, mushy rot with cottony mold growth and black sporangia dots.
- **Watery Soft Rot:** Mainly caused by *Sclerotinia sclerotiorum,* found primarily in vegetables.
- **Stem- End Rots**: Caused by molds like *Diplodia, Alternaria, Phomopsis,* and *Fusarium,* affecting the stem ends of fruits.
- **Black Mold Rot:** Caused by *Aspergillus niger,* resulting in dark brown to black spore masses, often referred to as "smut" in common terms.
- **Black Rot:** Typically caused by *Alternaria* species, but sometimes by *Ceratostomella, Physalospora,* and others.

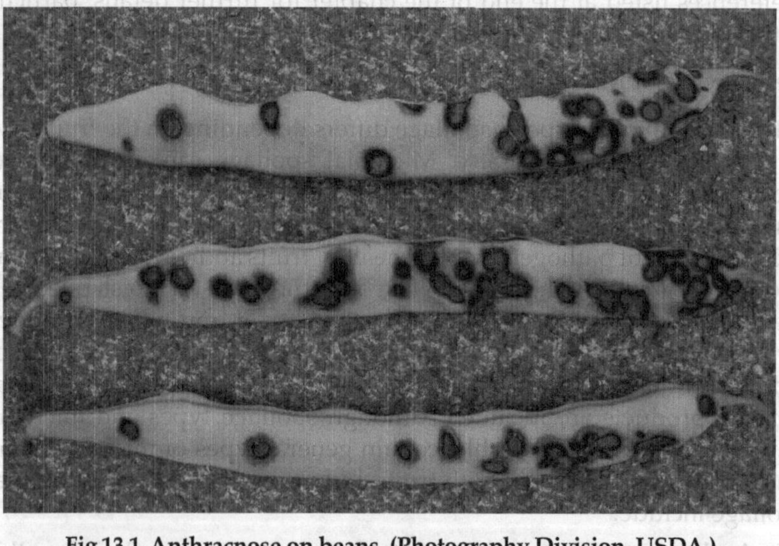

Fig 13.1. Anthracnose on beans. (Photography Division, USDA.)

- **Pink Mold Rot:** Caused by the pink- spored *Trichothecium roseum*.
- ***Fusarium* Rot:** Caused by various *Fusarium* species, resulting in different types of rots.
- **Green Mold Rot:** Usually caused by *Cladosporium* species, but sometimes by other green- spored molds like *Trichoderma.*

- **Brown Rot:** Primarily caused by *Sclerotinia* species (e.g., *Monilinia fructicola*).
- **Sliminess or Souring:** Caused by saprophytic bacteria in wet, piled vegetables that begin to heat up.

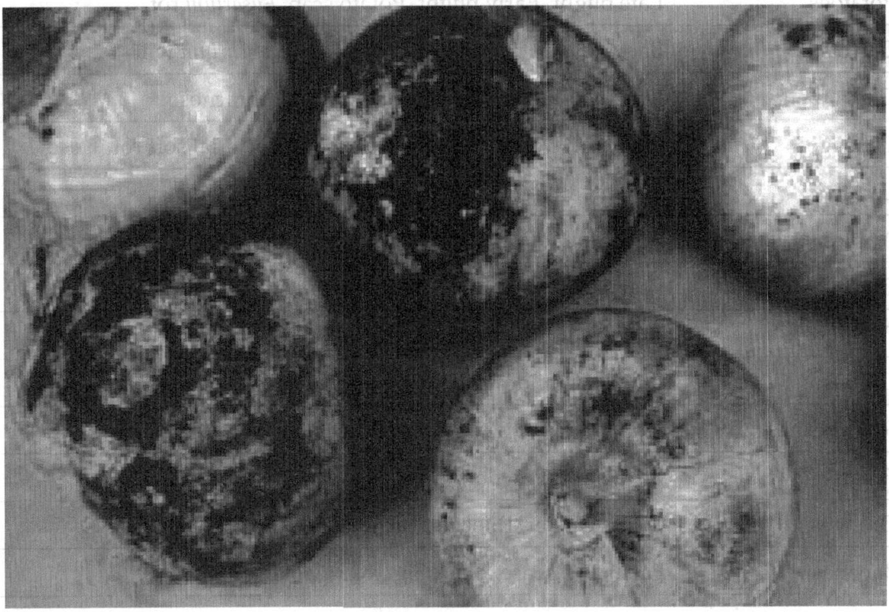

Fig 13.2. Black mold rot of onions by *Asperbillus niger*. (Photography Division, USDA).

Fungal spoilage in vegetables often leads to waterlogged, mushy patches, while fungal rots in fleshy fruits like apples and peaches typically manifest as brown or cream- colored areas where mold mycelia grow beneath the skin, with aerial hyphae and spores potentially appearing later. Some fungal spoilage forms "dry rots," where the infected area becomes dry, hard, and often discolored. Juicy fruits affected by rots may also exhibit leakage.

The likelihood of spoilage is influenced by the composition of the fruit or vegetable. Bacterial soft rot is more common in vegetables with lower acidity and fruits that are also not highly acidic (as shown in Table 13.4). Since most fruits and vegetables are mildly acidic, relatively dry on the surface, and lack significant amounts of B vitamins, molds are the most frequent cause of spoilage. The composition of the produce also determines the specific types of molds that are most likely to thrive, with some fruits and vegetables supporting a wide range of spoilage organisms, while others only support a few.

Table: The Chief Market Diseases of Several Vegetables and Fruits.

Vegetable/Fruit	Diseases
Tomatoes	Late blight, Early blight, *Fusarium* wilt, *Verticillium* wilt
Potatoes	Late blight, Early blight, Potato scab, *Fusarium* rot
Carrots	Bacterial soft rot, *Cercospora* leaf spot, *Fusarium* wilt
Cucumbers	Downy mildew, Powdery mildew, Anthracnose
Cabbage	Black rot, Downy mildew, Clubroot, Bacterial soft rot
Lettuc	Downy mildew, Tip burn, Lettuce mosaic viru
Apples	Apple scab, Powdery mildew, Fire blight, Apple rust
Pears	Pear scab, Fire blight, Brown rot, Powdery mildew
Peaches	Brown rot, Powdery mildew, Peach leaf curl, Bacterial spot
Grapes	Powdery mildew, Downy mildew, Black rot, *Botrytis* bunch rot
Strawberries	Gray mold rot, Powdery mildew, Leaf spot, *Verticillium* wilt
Plums	Brown rot, Powdery mildew, Black knot, Plum curculio
Oranges	Citrus canker, Root rot, Brown spot, Greening disease
Bananas	Panama disease, Black Sigatoka, Moko disease

This table highlights the major diseases that affect various vegetables and fruits in the market, impacting both their appearance and quality.

The possibility of spoilage and the type of spoilage that occurs are influenced by the potential for spoilage organisms to enter the product. Factors such as mechanical damage, plant pathogens, or improper handling can facilitate this entry. The location of the plant part used is also significant; for example, underground parts like roots, tubers, or bulbs in radishes, beets, carrots, and potatoes are exposed to moist soil, making them more susceptible to contamination. Fruits such as strawberries, cucumbers, peppers, and melons may come into direct contact with the soil surface. Leaves, stems, and flo ers, as seen in lettuce, cabbage, asparagus, rhubarb, and broccoli, are particularly vulnerable to contamination by plant pathogens, as well as damage from birds and insects, similar to most fruits.

The nature of the spoilage depends on the specific product and the organism involved. Soft and juicy foods are more likely to experience soft, mushy rots, often accompanied by leakage. However, some spoilage organisms can cause drying effects, leading to dry, leathery rots or discolored spots. In some cases, the mold's mycelial growth occurs beneath the surface, with only a rotten spot visible, as seen in many apples. In other types of spoilage, the mold grows on the surface, often appearing colored due to the spores. Identifying the type of spoilage enables the application of preventive measures to reduce or avoid such decay.

SPOILAGE OF FRUIT AND VEGETABLE JUICES

Juices can be extracted directly from fruits or vegetables, squeezed from mashed or crushed materials to include a significant amount of pulp, or obtained through water extraction, such as prune juice. These juices can be used in their original form or concentrated through evaporation or freezing and preserved by canning, freezing, or drying.

The acidity of fruit juices varies, with a pH range from approximately 2.4 for lemon or cranberry juice to 4.2 for tomato juice. All fruit juices contain sugars, with amounts ranging from about 2 percent in lemon juice to nearly 17 percent in some grape juice samples. While molds can grow on the surface of these juices if exposed to air, the high moisture content supports the rapid growth of yeasts and bacteria. The type of microorganism that predominates in juices low in sugar and acid depends more on temperature than the composition. The extraction and sieving of solids from the juices increase the oxidation- reduction potential, thus promoting the growth of yeasts. The majority of fruit juices are acidic enough and contain enough sugar to favor yeast growth within the temperature range of 15.6 to 35°C. The low levels of B vitamins in these juices also discourage bacterial growth.

At room temperature, the typical process for raw fruit juices is alcoholic fermentation by yeasts, followed by alcohol oxidation and the oxidation of fruit acids by film yeasts or molds on the surface if exposed to air, or the conversion of alcohol to acetic acid if acetic acid bacteria are present. The types of yeasts that grow depend on the prevailing strains in the juice and the temperature. Wild yeasts, such as apiculate strains, often carry out the first fermentation, producing moderate amounts of alcohol and volatile acid. At the higher end of the temperature range (32.2 to 35°C), lactobacilli are more likely to grow, forming lactic and volatile acids since these temperatures are too high for most yeasts. Below 15.6°C, wild yeasts may still grow, but as temperatures approach freezing, bacteria and molds tend to dominate over yeasts. The acidity may be further reduced by the activity of film yeasts and molds on the surface.

Apart from the usual alcoholic fermentation, fruit juices may undergo other microbial changes. These include- (1) lactic acid fermentation of sugars, typically by heterofermentative lactic acid bacteria like *Lactobacillus pastorianus, L. brevis,* and *Leuconostoc mesenteroides* in apple or pear juice, and by homofermentative bacteria such as *Lactobacillus arabinosus, L. leichmanii,* and *Microbacterium,* (2) fermentation of the organic acids present in the juice, such as the conversion of malic acid to lactic and succinic acids, quinic acid to dehydroshikimic acid, and citric acid to lactic and acetic acids by lactic acid bacteria like *Lactobacillus pastorianus,* (3) slime production by *Leuconostoc mesenteroides, Lactobacillus brevis,* and *L. plantarum* in apple juice, and by *L. plantarum* and streptococci in grape juice.

Vegetable juices contain sugars but are less acidic than fruit juices, with pH values typically ranging from 5.0 to 5.8. These juices also provide abundant accessory growth factors for microorganisms, supporting the growth of more demanding lactic acid bacteria. Acid fermentation of raw vegetable juice by these bacteria and other acid- producing microorganisms is a likely cause of spoilage, although yeasts and molds can also grow.

Concentrated fruit and vegetable juices, due to their higher acidity and sugar content, provide an environment conducive to the growth of yeasts and acid- and sugar- tolerant species like *Leuconostoc* and *Lactobacillus*. These concentrates are usually canned and then heat- treated or frozen. The heat treatment kills the microorganisms responsible for spoilage, while freezing prevents their growth.

Meat Products: Contamination, Preservation and Spoilage

14

Meat products are among the most consumed and nutritionally significant food sources worldwide, yet they are highly perishable due to their biochemical composition. Their high protein and water content create an ideal environment for the growth of microorganisms, making them susceptible to contamination and spoilage. Contamination can occur at various stages, from processing and handling to storage and distribution. Microbial contamination, including bacteria like *Salmonella, Escherichia coli,* and *Listeria* poses significant risks to both product quality and public health. Additionally, chemical contaminants and improper hygiene practices exacerbate these concerns.

Preservation techniques are essential to extending the shelf life of meat products while maintaining their nutritional and sensory qualities. Traditional methods like salting, smoking, and drying have been practiced for centuries, while modern approaches such as refrigeration, freezing, vacuum packaging, and the use of chemical preservatives have significantly advanced the industry. Innovative technologies, including high- pressure processing and irradiation, further enhance preservation by minimizing microbial activity without compromising the meat's integrity.

Spoilage dynamics in meat are influenced by microbial activity, enzymatic reactions, and environmental factors. Microbial spoilage can lead to unpleasant odors, discoloration, and the production of slime, while enzymatic reactions may result in texture and flavor deterioration. Understanding the interplay between contamination, preservation, and spoilage is critical for ensuring food safety and minimizing waste. By adopting stringent quality control measures and effecti e preservation strategies, the meat industry strives to meet consumer demands while addressing the challenges posed by perishability.

CONTAMINATION

The inner flesh of healthy meats is generally reported to have few or no microorganisms, though small amounts have been detected in lymph nodes, bone marrow, and even muscle tissue. Bacteria such as Staphylococci, Streptococci, *Clostridium,* and *Salmonella* have been isolated from the lymph nodes of red-meat animals. Standard slaughtering practices typically remove lymph nodes from parts of the animal designated for consumption. However, the primary sources of contamination arise from external factors during the processes of bleeding, handling, and processing. The hide, hooves, hair, and intestinal tract of the animal serve as the main contributors to contamination during skinning, cutting, and bleeding. Although modern "humane" slaughtering methods—mechanical, chemical, or electrical—do not significantly affect contamination levels, the subsequent steps of sticking and bleeding may introduce harmful microorganisms.

Contamination can also occur through the transfer of bacteria from tools such as knives used during processing. Microorganisms present on an animal's exterior, originating from soil, water, feed, and manure, as well as its natural surface flora, can spread to the meat. The intestinal contents further contribute to contamination with intestinal bacteria. Secondary sources of contamination include knives, cloths, air, and the hands or clothing of workers, as well as equipment like carts, boxes, grinders, and sausage stuffers. Psychrotrophic bacteria, introduced from chilled meat or other storage environments, are especially problematic. Ingredients such as fillers and spices used in processed products may also introduce microorganisms. Additionally, microbial growth on equipment or meat surfaces exacerbates contamination, potentially leading to significant increases in bacterial populations.

Table. Average Numbers of Microorganisms Contaminating Beef in Packing- Plant Slaughter Room (Empey and Scott, 1939)

Sample	Bacteria	Yeasts	Molds
Beef, dressed, on floo	6,400–83,000/cm2		
Soil from animals (dry)	110,000,00/g	50,000/g	120,000/g
Animal feces (fresh)	90,000,000/g	200,000/g	60,000/g
Rumen content	2,000,000,000/g	180,000/g	1,600/g
Room air	140/cm2 of plate		2/cm2
Water, washing beef	20- 10,000/ml		
Water, washing floo	1,000- 16,000/ml		

Table : Frequently Isolated Microorganisms from Meats

Category	Microorganisms	Sources	Effects
Gram- Positive Bacteria	*Staphylococcus aureus, Streptococcus* spp., *Listeria monocytogenes, Clostridium perfringens*	Human handling, processing equipment, environment	Foodborne illness, spoilage
Gram- Negative Bacteria	*Salmonella* spp., *Escherichia coli* (*E. coli* O157-H7), *Pseudomonas* spp., *Campylobacter jejuni*	Animal intestines, external surfaces, contaminated water	Foodborne illness, off-odor formation
Anaerobic Bacteria	*Clostridium botulinum, Clostridium sporogenes*	Soil, intestinal contents	Toxin production, spoilage
Psychrotrophic Bacteria	*Pseudomonas fluorescens, Lactobacillus* spp., *Brochothrix thermosphacta*	Chilled storage, cross-contamination	Slime formation, discoloration

Category	Microorganisms	Sources	Effects
Fungi (Molds)	*Penicillium* spp., *Aspergillus* spp., *Mucor* spp., *Cladosporium* spp.	Air, improperly cleaned equipment, storage environments	Spoilage, toxin production (mycotoxins)
Yeasts	*Candida* spp., *Saccharomyces* spp., *Rhodotorula* spp.	Air, processing equipment, brine solutions	Off- flavors discoloration
Spoilage Microorganisms	Lactic acid bacteria (*Lactobacillus, Leuconostoc*), *Shewanella putrefaciens*	Animal surfaces, processing equipment	Sour odors, gas production
Pathogens	*Listeria monocytogenes*, *Salmonella* spp., *E. coli* O157-H7, *Campylobacter jejuni*	Cross-contamination, improper hygiene practices	Severe foodborne illness

Note: This table highlights the key microorganisms frequently found in meats, their sources, and the effects they can have on meat safety and quality.

Meats can become contaminated by a wide variety of microorganisms due to their diverse sources (Table). Meat surfaces can become infected with molds of various genera. *Cladosporium, Sporotrichum, Geotrichum, Thamnidium, Mucor, Penicillium, Alternaria,* and *Monilia* species are particularly significant. There are frequently yeasts present, primarily asporogenous ones. *Pseudomonas, Acinetobacter, Moraxella, Alcaligenes, Micrococcus, Streptococcus, Sarcina, Leuconostoc, Lactobacillus, Proteus, Flavobacterium, Bacillus, Clostridium, Escherichia, Campylobacter, Salmonella,* and *Streptomyces* are some of the more significant bacteria among the numerous genera that are present. Chilling temperatures are ideal for the growth of many of these bacteria. Additionally, human pathogens, particularly those of the intestinal type, could contaminate meat and meat products.

In the retail market and in the home additional contamination usually takes place. In the market knives, saws, cleavers, slicers, grinders, chopping blocks, scales, sawdust, and containers as well as the market operators may be sources of organisms. In the home refrigerator containers used previously to store meats can serve as sources of spoilage organisms.

PRESERVATION

The preservation of meats, like other perishable foods, typically relies on a combination of preservation techniques. Meats present a unique challenge due to their suitability as an excellent growth medium, characterized by high moisture content, a nearly neutral pH, and rich nutrient availability.

Furthermore, the presence of microorganisms in lymph nodes, bones, and muscle, combined with unavoidable contamination by spoilage organisms, makes meat preservation more complex than most other foods. If cooling is not initiated quickly and effecti ely after slaughter, meats can experience undesirable changes in appearance and flavor and may facilitate microbial growth before preservation processes are applied. Additionally, prolonged storage at chilling temperatures can still permit some microbial growth over time.

Asepsis

Asepsis, or keeping meat free of microorganisms during slaughter and handling, allows for easier preservation by any method. Refrigerated storage time can be extended, aging to soften meat becomes less hazardous, curing and smoking methods are safer, and heating processes are more efficien.

Asepsis begins by avoiding, as much as possible, external contamination of the animal. It is recommended that the animal be sprinkled with water before slaughter to remove as much coarse soil as possible from the hair and skin, and a footbath may be used to remove soil from the hooves. Despite this, the animal's skin and hair are important sources of contamination of the surface of the carcass during skinning. The knife used to bleed the animal after slaughter can contribute to blood contamination and introduce organisms by penetrating the skin. During scalding, organisms can be added to the pig's skin and lungs. Contamination comes not only from the skin during skinning, but also from the knives and workers and their clothing. During evisceration, contamination can come from the animal's intestines, the air, water from washing and rinsing the carcass, rags and brushes used on the carcass, various knives, saws, etc. used, as well as the hands and clothing of the workers. Some organisms may come from walls affected by the dead body or from splashes or mist from the floor. Meat in the cold room can be contaminated by the air, walls, floor, and workers. Sawdust scattered on the floor is a particularly good source of mold spores. Additional contamination during cutting and slicing comes from knives, saws, conveyors, tables, air, water, and workers.

The fact that microorganisms added from these sources usually include almost all the organisms involved in meat spoilage, many of them in significant numbers, emphasizes the importance of aseptic methods.

When meat is contaminated with microorganisms, its removal is difficult Coarse soil can be removed from the surface, but washing water can add organisms. The use of hot water or pressurized disinfectant sprays is an effecti e way to reduce the overall number of bacteria on the surface of the carcass and possibly extend its shelf life in the refrigerator. Moldy or damaged surfaces of large pieces of meat, especially "sluggish" or aged meat, can be trimmed off, but this should not be considered an effecti e method of preservation.

The films used to wrap the rubber prevent the entry of bacteria and affect the growth of those already present. These films differ significantly in their permeability to water, oxygen and carbon dioxide. Meat has been reported to have a shorter shelf life in films that are less permeable to water. Fresh meats retain their red color better in a non- evacuated oxygen- permeable film. With an oxygen- impermeable film, more carbon dioxide is retained by the bacteria, resulting in a poorer color, but favoring the lactic acid bacteria, *Lactobacillaceae* and *Brochothrix thermosphacta*. Dried meat is preferably packaged in vacuum-sealed oxygen- permeable films. Evacuation helps limit the growth of aerobic bacteria, especially molds, reduces the growth of *staphylococcus*, and promotes the growth of lactic acid bacteria, but apparently does not promote the growth of *Clostridium botulinum*, any more than simple overpacking.

Use of Heat

Meat preservation is a highly specialized technique in that the procedure varies greatly depending on the meat product being preserved. Most meat products are low-acid foods that provide a good growth environment for surviving bacteria. The rate of heat penetration varies from fairly fast in meat broths to very slow in well- packaged meats and meat products. Chemicals added to the meat, such as spices, salt, or nitrates and nitrites in the curing process, also affect the heat treatment, making it generally more tender. effecti e. The nitrates in the meat help kill anaerobic bacterial spores with heat and prevent the germination of surviving spores.

Commercially canned meats can be divided into two groups based on the heat treatment used- (1) meats that are heat- treated in an attempt to render the contents of the can sterile or at least "commercially sterile," as with milk for storage in retail stores, and (2) meats that are heated sufficientl to kill some of the spoilage organisms but must be refrigerated to prevent spoilage. Preserved hams and breads are treated in this manner.

Group 1 meats are called shelf- stable preserved meats, and Group 2 meats are called "non- refrigerator- safe" or "non- stable" preserved meats. Dried preserved meats owe their microbial stability to heat processing and various curing salts. The processing temperature for shelf- stable meats is 98°C and the container size is usually less than 1 lb. Unstable dried gums are packaged in containers that can hold up to 22 lbs and are processed at a temperature of approximately 65°C.

Heat can be applied to meat products in ways other than canning. Treating the surfaces of meat with hot water has been suggested to extend shelf life, although it may reduce nutrients and damage color. Cooking sausages in the packing plant with steam or hot water reduces the number of microorganisms and promotes preservation. The heat applied when smoking meat and meat products helps reduce the number of microbes. Pre- cooking or tenderizing bacon reduces the number of bacteria somewhat, but does not sterilize them. These products should be refrigerated because they spoil and can support the growth of toxic organisms if stored at room temperature. Similar considerations apply to cooked sausages such as frankfurters and liverwurst, which are also spicy but should be refrigerated. Cooking meat intended for direct consumption significantly reduces the microbial content and therefore extends shelf life. Pre- cooked frozen meat should contain few viable microorganisms.

Use of Low Temperatures

More meat is preserved by the use of low temperatures than by any other method, and much more by chilling than by freezing.

Chilling

Meat is quickly and efficientl chilled to temperatures close to freezing using modern packing-house techniques, and storage is kept just a little bit above freezing. There will be fewer opportunities for mesophilic microorganisms to grow the faster and more quickly this cooling occurs. Meats and other foods are covered by the chilling storage principles covered in Chapter 7. The ideal storage temperature is between 1.4 and 2.2 degrees Celsius, but lower temperatures are preferred. Depending on the temperature, relative humidity, and the number of microorganisms present, the chilling storage period for beef is approximately 30 days; for pork, lamb, and mutton, it is 1 to 2 weeks; and for veal, it is even shorter.

Uncooked sausage, like uncured pork sausage in bulk or in links, must be preserved by refrigeration. It was emphasized in Chapter 7 that the relative humidity usually is lowered with an increase in storage temperature. Storage time can be lengthened by storage of meats in an atmosphere containing added carbon dioxide or ozone, or the temperature and relative humidity can be raised without shortening storage time.

Although considerable experimental work has been done on the gas storage of meats, this method has not been used extensively. Ships equipped for storage of meat in a controlled atmosphere of carbon dioxide have been employed successfully. Increasing amounts of carbon dioxide in the atmosphere inhibit microorganisms but also hasten the formation of metmyoglobin and hence the loss of "bloom," or natural color . The storage life of meat has been doubled, according to reports, by such gas storage. Experts do not agree on the optimal concentration of carbon dioxide, with recommendations varying from 10 to 30 percent for most meats and up to 100 percent for bacon.

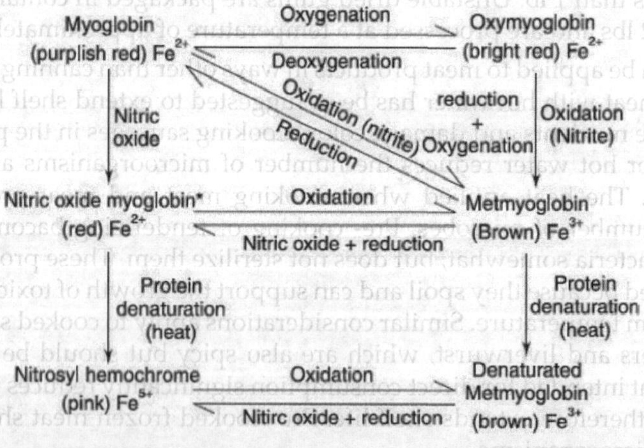

Fig 14.1. Chemical changes of myoglobin during meat processing and curing. (From John C. Forrest et al., Principles of Meat Science. W. H. Freman and Company. Copyright © 1975.)

Storage time also can be increased by the presence of 2.5 to 3 ppm ozone in the atmosphere. Storage up to 60 days at 2.2°C and 92 percent relative humidity without development of molds or slime has been reported. Ozone is an active oxidizing agent, however, that may give an oxidized or tallowy flavo to fats. It has been observed that while the levels of ozone cited will inhibit microorganisms, much higher concentrations are necessary to stop growth that already has begun.

The microorganisms that give trouble in the chilling storage of meats are the psychrotrophic bacteria, chiefly those of the genus *Pseudomonas,* although bacteria of the genera *Acinetobacter, Moraxella, Alcaligenes, Micrococcus, Lactobacillus, Streptococcus, Leuconostoc, Pediococcus, Flavobacterium,* and *Proteus* and yeasts and molds can grow in meats at low temperatures.

Freezing

Most meats sold in retail stores are not frozen, but freezing is often used to preserve meat during long- distance transport or to preserve it until times of scarcity. Of course, significant quantities of meat are now frozen in home freezers. Larger cuts of meat, such as halves and quarters, are frozen, while hamburgers and smaller, thinner cuts can be frozen in prepackaged packages. The preservation of frozen meat becomes more and more effecti e as the storage temperature decreases. - 12°C to approximately - 28.9°C.

Meat intended for freezing is subject to the same risks of contamination and growth of microorganisms as meat intended for any other use. The freezing process kills about half of the bacteria and their numbers slowly decrease during storage. The low- temperature bacteria that grow in meat during refrigeration, *Pseudomonas, Acinetobacter, Moraxella, Alcaligenes, Micrococcus, Lactobacillus, Flavobacterium* and Proteus species, can resume growth during thawing of meat if it is. carried out slowly. If the directions are followed, frozen packaged meat will thaw too quickly to allow significant growth of microorganisms.

Use of Irradiation

Irradiation with ultraviolet rays has been used in conjunction with chilling storage to lengthen the keeping time. It has been employed chiefly on large, hung pieces of meat in plant storage rooms. The rays serve to reduce numbers of microorganisms in the air and to inhibit or kill them on the surfaces of the meat reached directly by the rays. To be affected, the microorganisms must be on the immediate surface, unprotected by fatty or opaque materials.

Irradiation has been used in the rapid aging of meats that are "hung" at higher than the usual chilling temperatures to reduce the growth of microorganisms, especially molds, on the surface. The aging, or hanging, process tenderizes the meat by its own proteolytic enzymes and is used especially for obtaining tender steaks and other fancy cuts. Ordinary aging is for several weeks at 2.2 to 3.3 C with the relative humidity between 80 and 90 percent and an air movement of 10 to 30 fpm, but with exposure to ultraviolet rays the time is reduced to 2 to 3 days at 18 C in a relative humidity of 85 to 90 percent. Some oxidation, favored by ultraviolet rays, and hydrolysis of fats may take place during aging.

Gamma irradiation of meats still is limited and in the experimental stage. When sterilization is effected, doses of 20 to 70 KiloGrays are applied and undesirable changes in color and flavor may appear

Preservation by Drying

Drying meat for preservation is a practice that has been around for centuries. Jerky, or strips of beef dried in the sun, was a staple of American pioneers. Some types of sausage are preserved primarily by drying. In beef, made primarily from smoked and cured pork, microorganisms can grow before processing and in the "pickle" during curing, but the number of organisms is reduced by the smoking and drying process. The organisms can contaminate cured ham during storage and slices during cutting and packaging

Meat products such as dry sausages, dry sausages, and dry cervelas are primarily preserved due to their low moisture content, as some varieties are not smoked. A dry outer surface on the casing of any sausage is protective.

Older methods of curing meat usually combined salting and smoking. During World War II, fresh cuts of beef and pork were dried in heat. Another method of curing pork is to cook it briefly in nitrate- nitrite before drying and add lecithin as an antioxidant and stabilizer. Drying can be done in a vacuum, in trays or by other methods. The final product can be stored without refrigeration

Freeze- drying of meat is growing, with more success for processed products such as meatballs, patties and stews than for fresh meat. The efficienc of the process has improved enough to reduce costs to the point that retail production has become possible for specialty markets, for example. , hikers, campers and backpackers.

Meat to be dried must be of good bacteriological quality, without prior development of a significant number of microorganisms or undesirable flavors

Use of Preservatives

The utilization of a controlled atmosphere containing added carbon dioxide or ozone in the chilling storage of meats has been discussed. Preservation by heavy salting is an old method that usually results in an inferior product. Ordinarily salting is combined with curing and smoking in order to be effecti e.

Curing

The curing of meats is primarily applied to beef and pork, including both ground meat and specific cuts such as hams, briskets, loins, and bellies of hogs, as well as leg muscles of beef. Historically, curing was used as a preservation method relying solely on salting without refrigeration. However, modern cured meats typically include additional ingredients, are refrigerated, and are often smoked to enhance flavor and extend shelf life. Permitted curing agents include sodium chloride, sugar, sodium nitrite, and vinegar, although the first three are most commonly used.

Sodium chloride serves as a preservative and flavor enhancer, reducing water activity (aw) in the meat. Sugar, usually sucrose or glucose, adds flavor and provides an energy source for nitrate- reducing bacteria during curing. Sodium nitrite, essential for fixing the meat's color, produces nitric oxide, which reacts with muscle myoglobin and hemoglobin under acidic and reducing conditions to create the characteristic red color. Sodium nitrate acts as a reservoir for nitrite during longer curing processes and has bacteriostatic properties, particularly against anaerobic bacteria.

Curing agents can be introduced into meat using four methods- dry curing, where dry ingredients are rubbed onto the meat; pickle curing, involving immersion in a curing solution; injection curing, where the solution is injected into the meat; and direct addition for finely ground meats like sausage. Traditional curing methods required months, but modern "quick cure" techniques, such as pumping the solution into the meat, have significantly reduced processing times

Smoking often follows curing to further aid preservation, though some products like corned beef are cured but not smoked. Certain sausages, including salami and summer sausages, undergo lactic acid fermentation during curing, enhancing both preservation and flavor. Many processors now use pure bacterial cultures like Pediococcus cerevisiae for better control and faster fermentation, as detailed in studies of bacteria used in fermented and cured meats.

Vinegar is added to the pickling solution in the preservation of foods such as pickled pigs' feet, pickled spiced beef, and souses. Pigs' feet are cured in a solution of salt, sodium nitrate, and sodium nitrite, cooked, and then held in a brine of salt and

Table: Microorganisms Reported in Cured Meats

Meats	Microorganisms
Sausages Salami Big bologna Smoked links Frankfurters Fresh pork	Homofermentative lactobacilli *Leuconostoc* mesenteroides, heterofermentative lactobacilli. Leuconostoc mesenteroides, heterofermentative lactobacilli Streptococci, pediococci, leuconostocs, lactobacilli, micrococci*, sporeformers, yeasts. Leuconostocs, microbacteria, lactobacilli, pseudomonads.
Bacon Sliced, packaged Wiltshire Vacuum- wrapped	Mostly lactobacilli; also micrococci*, enterococci. Micrococci*, lactobacilli, Streptococci, leuconostocs, pediococci, lactobacilli.
Ham Raw Sliced, packaged Pressed, spiced Canned Irradiated Heated, irradiated	Lactobacilli, micrococci*, microbacteria, enterococci, leuconostocs, *Streptococcus faecium, Microbacterium* spp. Heterofermentative lactobacilli, leuconostocs Enterococci, bacilli, micrococci *Enterococci Bacilli, Clostridia.

After curing, meats are packed into jars or containers and covered with a fresh salt- vinegar brine before sealing. Proper acidity prevents spoilage. The microorganisms present in curing brines and on submerged meats depend on the meat's initial condition and the curing method. While the salt itself carries microorganisms, their impact is minimal, except for halophilic bacteria that may cause red surface colonies on salted meats after brining or dry salting.

In modern American curing methods, such as ham curing, bacteria in the brine have minimal influence as their growth is limited, and smoking post-curing eliminates most of them. These brines primarily harbor lactic acid bacteria, including lactobacilli and pediococci, while micrococci and yeasts may develop on the surface. Traditional long curing methods relied on bacteria, particularly micrococci, to reduce nitrates to nitrites, fixing the meat's red color

Foreign curing methods, such as those used for bacon, often involve prolonged immersion in concentrated brines. These brines support the growth of halotolerant or halophilic microorganisms, including cocci and both gram- positive and gram-negative rods, many of which reduce nitrates to nitrites. In dry- cured hog bellies compressed in boxes, salt- tolerant, nitrate- reducing psychrotrophs thrive. Similarly, beef- curing brines have been found to contain micrococci, lactobacilli, streptococci, *Achromobacter*, vibrios, pediococci, and other bacteria in smaller numbers. Species of *Micrococcus*, particularly in high- salt pickling solutions, play a significant role in curing British and Canadian bacon.

Smoking

In Chapter 9, the use of wood smoke as a preservative was covered. It was noted that smoking serves two primary functions: it helps with preservation and adds desired flavors. It was found that the heat from smoking and the preservatives added to the meat have a germicidal effect, and that the drying process and the chemicals from the smoke prevent the growth of microorganisms while the meat is being stored.

Older methods of curing and smoking, where high salt concentrations were used in curing and greater drying and incorporation of preservative chemicals was accomplished in smoking, produced hams, dried beef, etc., that would keep without refrigeration. Many of the newer methods, however, yield a perishable product that must be refrigerated. Precooked or tenderized hams and sausages of high moisture content are examples.

Spices

Spices and condiments added to meat products such as meat loaves and sausages are not in concentrations high enough to be preservative, but they may add their effec to those of the other preservative factors. Certainly products such as bologna, Polish, and frankfurter and other sausages owe their keeping quality to the combined effec of spicing, curing, smoking (drying), cooking, and refrigerating.

Antibiotics

Although, in this country the only use of antibiotics in meat products is for fish (chlortetracycline at 7 ppm in ice), experiments have shown that antibiotics can be used successfully in meat to extend its shelf life in cold storage or at cooler temperatures. The most recommended antibiotics are chlortetracycline, oxytetracycline, nisin, and chloramphenicol. Antibiotics can be applied to meat in several ways- (1) the antibiotic can be administered to the animal over a long period of time. period, (2) it can be administered more intensively for a short period before slaughter, (3) it can be introduced into the carcass or part of it, or (4) it can be applied to superficial cuts of meat or mixed with ground meat. The administration of an antibiotic results in a selection of microorganisms in the intestinal tract of the animal, which is likely to reduce the number of spoilage bacteria found there and therefore the number of bacteria that can reach the meat from this source during slaughter and dressing. It has been suggested that injection of antibiotics before slaughter can be used to extend the shelf life of carcasses at room temperature before they reach refrigeration or to briefly store beef at a temperature that promotes tenderization of particular cuts and extend the shelf life of meat stored at refrigerated temperatures. Infusion of an antibiotic into the carcass immediately after slaughter or into separate parts can serve similar purposes. The shelf life of meat can be extended by an antibiotic bath or by incorporating an antibiotic into the ground meat.

SPOILAGE

Both microbial activity and the meat's own enzymes can alter raw meat, and its fat can undergo chemical oxidation. When hanging or aging beef and game, a moderate amount of autolysis is desired; however, this is not recommended for the majority of other raw meats. A small amount of fat hydrolysis and some proteolytic activity on muscle and connective tissues are examples of autolytic alterations. The defect resulting from excessive autolysis has been referred to as "souring," an imprecise term used to describe a wide range of food spoilage types and, in fact, nearly any type that imparts a sour smell. It can be challenging to differentiate autolysis-induced sourness from microbially-induced defects, particularly from simple proteolysis.

However, this preliminary hydrolysis of proteins by the meat enzymes undoubtedly helps microorganisms start growing in the meat by furnishing the simpler nitrogen compounds needed by many microorganisms that cannot attack complete native proteins.

General Principles Underlying Meat Spoilage

It has been pointed out that during slaughter, dressing, and cutting, microorganisms come chiefly from the exterior of the animal and its intestinal tract but that more are added from knives, cloths, air, workers, carts, boxes, and equipment in general.

A great variety of kinds of organisms are added, and so it can be assumed that under ordinary conditions most kinds of potential spoilage organisms are present and will be able to grow if favorable conditions present themselves.

Invasion of Tissues by Microorganisms

- **Physiological Condition Before Slaughter:** Animals that are stressed, feverish, or fatigued before slaughter are more susceptible to bacterial invasion. Incomplete bleeding can further aid microbial spread, while chemical changes in tissues, such as higher pH and earlier protein denaturation, enhance bacterial growth. Fatigue depletes glycogen, preventing the pH from dropping from 7.2 to around 5.7, as it would under normal conditions.
- **After the Animal's Death:** tissues are invaded by contaminating microorganisms. Several factors influence this in asion.
- **Gut Microbial Load:** A higher microbial load in the animal's gut increases tissue invasion, which is why a 24- hour starvation period prior to slaughter is often recommended.
- **Killing and Bleeding Methods:** Proper and hygienic bleeding enhances meat preservation. Although humane slaughter methods' effects on meat quality are not well- documented, some studies claim more "greening" in pork and bacon from electrically stunned animals compared to those killed with carbon dioxide.
- **Cooling Rate:** Rapid cooling slows microbial invasion of tissues.
- **Microorganisms spread through the meat:** via blood, lymph vessels, connective tissue spaces, and grinding processes.

GROWTH OF MICROORGANISMS IN MEAT

Meat provides an ideal medium for microbial growth due to its high moisture content, nitrogen- rich nutrients, mineral availability, and accessory growth factors. Its glycogen content and favorable pH also promote microbial proliferation. Factors influencing microbial growth and spoilage include

Microbial Contamination and Spread: The type and quantity of contaminating organisms play a critical role. For instance, meat with a high proportion of psychrotrophic organisms spoils faster at chilling temperatures compared to meat with fewer such organisms.

Physical Properties of Meat: The surface area significantly affects spoilage rates. Exposed surfaces have higher microbial loads and provide oxygen for aerobic organisms. Fat can shield some areas but is itself susceptible to enzymatic and chemical spoilage. Grinding meat increases exposed surface area, releases moisture, and disperses bacteria, accelerating spoilage. The skin protects internal meat, although microorganisms grow on its surface.

Chemical Properties of Meat: The moisture content of meat determines microbial growth types, especially at the surface where drying can occur. Dry surfaces inhibit growth, slightly moist areas favor molds, wetter surfaces encourage yeasts, and very moist surfaces support bacterial growth. The relative humidity of the storage environment impacts this dynamic. High protein and low carbohydrate levels in meat favor nonfermenting microorganisms that use proteins and their byproducts. The pH, varying from 5.7 to over 7.2 depending on glycogen levels at slaughter, influences microbial growth rates and types, with higher pH favoring faster growth.

Oxygen Availability: Surface areas with aerobic conditions promote molds, yeasts, and aerobic bacteria. Within solid meat, anaerobic conditions persist, although oxygen can diffuse into ground meat unless packaging is oxygen- impermeable. Anaerobic conditions favor putrefaction.

Temperature: Meat should be stored just above freezing to limit microbial growth. At these low temperatures, psychrotrophic bacteria, molds, and yeasts grow slowly, causing specific spoilage defects.

True putrefaction is rare at low temperatures but more common at room temperature. Temperature largely determines the type of organisms that dominate and the resulting spoilage. For instance, psychrophiles dominate at chilling temperatures, leading to proteolysis, while mesophiles thrive at higher temperatures, producing acids through limited carbohydrate fermentation.

GENERAL TYPES OF SPOILAGE OF MEATS

The common types of spoilage of meats can be classifi d on the basis of whether they occur under aerobic or anaerobic conditions and whether they are caused by bacteria, yeasts, or molds.

Spoilage under Aerobic Conditions: Under aerobic conditions bacteria may cause the following:

- Surface slime, which may be caused by species of *Pseudomonas, Acinetobacter, Moraxella, Alcaligenes, Streptococcus, Leuconostoc, Bacillus,* and *Micrococcus*. Some species of *Lactobacillus* can produce slime. The temperature and the availability of moisture influence the kind of microorganisms causing surface slime. At chilling temperatures, high moisture will favor the *Pseudomonas- Alcaligenes* group; with less moisture, as on frankfurters, micrococci and yeasts will be encouraged; and with still less moisture, molds may grow. At higher temperatures, up to that of the room, micrococci* and other mesophiles compete well with the pseudomonads and related bacteria. The numbers of microorganisms necessary before detection of off- odor or slime in meats and other proteinaceous foods are shown in Table 14.4. Numbers in the millions per square centimeter or gram are required.

- Changes in color of meat pigments. The red color of meat, called its "bloom," may be changed to shades of green, brown, or gray as a result of the production of oxidizing compounds, e.g., peroxides, or of hydrogen sulfide, by bacteria. Species of *Lactobacillus* (mostly heterofermentative) and *Leuconostoc* are reported to cause the greening of sausage.

Table: Numbers of Microorganisms at Time of Appearance of Odor and Slime in Proteinaceous Foods

Food	Numbers	
	When odor evident	When slime evident
Poultry meat	2.5- 100 ′ 10^6/cm2	10- 60 ′ 10^6/cm2
Beef	1.2- 100 ′ 10^6/cm2	3- 300 ′ 10^6/cm2
Frankfurters	100- 130 ′ 10^6/cm2	130 ′ 10^6/cm2
Processed meats		10- 100 ′ 10^6/cm2
Wiltshire bacon		1.5- 100 ′ 10^6/cm2
Fish	1- 130 ′ 10^6/cm2	
Shell or liquid eggs	10 ′ 10^6/g	

- **Changes in fats:** The oxidation of unsaturated fats in meats takes place chemically in air and may be catalyzed by light and copper. Lipolytic bacteria may cause some lipolysis and also may accelerate the oxidation of the fats. Some fats, such as butterfat, become tallowy on oxidation and rancid on hydrolysis, but most animal fats develop oxidative rancidity when oxidized, with off- odors due to aldehydes and acids. Hydrolysis adds the flavor of the released fatty acids. Rancidity of fats may be caused by lipolytic species of *Pseudomonas* and *Achromobacter** or by yeasts.
- **Phosphorescence:** This rather uncommon defect is caused by phosphorescent or luminous bacteria, e.g., *Photobacterium* spp., growing on the surface of the meat.
- **Various surface colors due to pigmented bacteria:** Thus "red spot" may be caused by Serratia marcescens or other bacteria with red pigments. Pseudomonas syncyanea* can impart a blue color to the surface. Yellow discolorations are caused by bacteria with yellow pigments, usually species of *Micrococcus** or *Flavobacterium*. *Chromobacterium lividum* and other bacteria give greenish- blue to brownish- black spots on stored beef. The purple "stamping- ink" discoloration of surface fat is caused by yellow-pigmented cocci and rods. When the fat becomes rancid and peroxides appear, the yellow color changes to a greenish shade and later becomes purplish to blue.
- **Off- odors and off- tastes:** "Taints," or undesirable odors and tastes, that appear in meat as a result of the growth of bacteria on the surface often are evident before other signs of spoilage. "Souring" is the term applied to almost any defect that gives a sour odor that may be due to volatile acids, e.g., formic, acetic, butyric, and propionic, or even to growth of yeasts. "Cold- storage flavor" or taint is an indefinite term for a stale flavor Actinomycetes may be responsible for a musty or earthy flavor

Under aerobic conditions yeasts may grow on the surface of meats, causing sliminess, lipolysis, off- odors and tastes, and discoloratins—white, cream, pink, or brown—due to pigments in the yeasts. Aerobic growth of molds may cause the following:

- **White Spot:** *Sporotrichum carnis* is the most common cause of white spot, although any mold with wet, yeastlike colonies, e.g., *Geotrichum*, can cause white spot.
- **Green patches**: These are caused for the most part by the green conidia of species of *Penicillium* such as *P. expansum, P. asperulum*, and *P. oxalicum*.
- **Stickiness:** Incipient growth of molds makes the surface of the meat sticky to touch.
- **Whiskers:** When meat is stored at temperatures near freezing, a limited amount of mycelial growth may take place without sporulation. Such white, fuzzy growth can be caused by a number of molds, including *Thamnidium* chaetocladioides, or *T. elegans*; *Mucor mucedo, M. lusitanicus*, or *M. racemosus*; *Rhizopus*; and others. Controlled growth of a special strain of *Thamnidium* has been recommended for improvement in flavor during aging of beef.
- **Black Spot:** This usually is caused by *Cladosporium herbarum*, but other molds with dark pigments may be responsible.
- **Decomposition of Fats:** Many molds have lipases and hence cause hydrolysis of fats. Molds also aid in the oxidation of fats.
- **Off- odors and off- tastes**. Molds give a musty flavor to meat in the vicinity of their growth. Sometimes the defect is given a name indicating the cause, e.g., "thamnidium taint." Spots of surface spoilage by yeasts and molds usually are localized to a great extent and can be trimmed off without harm to the rest of the meat. The time that has been allowed for diffusion of the products of decomposition into the meat and the rate of that diffusion will determine the depth to which the defect will appear. Extensive bacterial growth over the surface may bring fairly deep penetration. Then, too, facultative bacteria may grow inward slowly.

SPOILAGE UNDER ANAEROBIC CONDITIONS

Facultative and anaerobic bacteria can thrive in meat under anaerobic conditions, leading to spoilage. The terminology associated with this spoilage is often unclear. Terms like "souring," "putrefaction," and "taint" are commonly used, but they seem to have different meanings for different peopl

- **Souring**: This term refers to a sour odor, and possibly taste, caused by organic acids such as formic, acetic, butyric, propionic, and higher fatty acids, or other acids like lactic or succinic. Souring can occur due to (a) the meat's own enzymes during aging or ripening, (b) anaerobic bacterial production of fatty acids or lactic acid, or (c) proteolysis without putrefaction, often called "stinking sour fermentation." Acid and gas formation occur due to the action of "butyric" *Clostridium* species and coliform bacteria on carbohydrates. Vacuum- packed meats, particularly in airtight packaging, often promote lactic acid bacteria growth.

- **Putrefaction:** True putrefaction refers to the anaerobic breakdown of proteins, producing foul- smelling compounds such as hydrogen sulfide mercaptans, indole, skatole, ammonia, and amines. It is primarily caused by *Clostridium* species, although facultative bacteria may assist in or cause putrefaction, as seen in species with names like putrefaciens, putrificum, and putida, typically within the genera *Pseudomonas* and *Alcaligenes*. Some *Proteus* species also contribute to putrefaction. The term "putrefaction" is often misused, as spoilage with foul odors from either the anaerobic breakdown of proteins or other compounds, even non- nitrogenous ones, may incorrectly be labeled as putrefaction. For example, trimethylamine in fish and isovaleric acid in butter are described as putrid odors. Gas formation, including hydrogen and carbon dioxide, accompanies *Clostridium*- induced putrefaction.
- **Taint**: The word "taint" is even more vague, applied to any off- taste or off-odor. "Bone taint" in meats refers to either souring or putrefaction near the bones, particularly in hams, though it usually indicates putrefaction.

Both air and temperature significantly affect the type of spoilage in meat. When meat is stored at near 0°C, as recommended, microbial growth is limited to molds, yeasts, and bacteria that grow at low temperatures. These microorganisms, such as *Pseudomonas, Acinetobacter, Moraxella, Alcaligenes, Lactobacillus, Leuconostoc, Streptococcus,* and *Flavobacterium* species, produce sliminess, discoloration, and spots on the surface and may cause souring. True putrefiers, like those in the genus *Clostridium,* generally require temperatures higher than those found in refrigerators.

Spoilage of Various Meats

Meats processed through methods like curing, smoking, drying, or canning often undergo changes that modify both the meat itself and its microbial flora, leading to spoilage types not typically found in fresh meats.

Spoilage of Fresh Meats

Fresh meat spoilage was covered earlier under general spoilage types. Typically, during extended refrigeration, fresh meats spoil due to the growth of species such as *Pseudomonas, Acinetobacter,* and *Moraxella*. Lactic acid bacteria, including *Lactobacillus, Leuconostoc, Streptococcus, Brevibacterium,* and *Pediococcus,* are present in most meats, whether fresh or cured, and grow even in refrigerator temperatures. While their growth is typically minimal and does not affect meat quality, certain sausages like salami, Lebanon, and Thuringer benefit from their lactic fermentation. However, lactic acid bacteria can cause three types of spoilage- (1) slime formation on or inside the meat, especially in the presence of sucrose, (2) green discoloration, and (3) souring due to the accumulation of excessive lactic and other acids.

Hamburger

Hamburger left at room temperature typically undergoes putrefaction, but when kept near freezing, it develops a stale, sour odor. This sourness at low temperatures is mainly caused by *Pseudomonas, Acinetobacter,* and *Moraxella,* with assistance from lactic acid bacteria. Other *jenera* like *Alcaligenes, Micrococcus,* and *Flavobacterium* may also grow in certain samples. Numerous microorganisms have been found in hamburger stored at higher temperatures, though there's no clear distinction between their mere presence and actual growth. Bacteria such as *Bacillus, Clostridium, Escherichia, Enterobacter, Proteus, Pseudomonas, Alcaligenes, Lactobacillus, Leuconostoc, Streptococcus, Micrococcus,* and *Sarcina,* as well as molds like *Penicillium* and *Mucor,* are commonly present. Some yeasts have also been identified.

Fresh Pork Sausage

Fresh sausage, primarily composed of ground fresh pork with added salt and spices, can be sold in bulk or in casings. This product is highly perishable and must be refrigerated, where it spoils quickly. Souring, the most common spoilage type at temperatures of 0-11°C, is caused by the growth and acid production of lactobacilli and leuconostocs, though *Microbacterium* and *Micrococcus* can grow at higher temperatures. Cased pork sausages, especially the "little- pig" variety, are prone to slime formation on the casing surface or to mold- induced color spots. For example, *Alternaria* causes dark spots on refrigerated sausages.

Spoilage of Cured Meats

Cured meats, mostly pork but sometimes beef, are preserved with nitrites that inhibit anaerobes. Nitrite is said to promote lactic acid bacteria growth in sausages such as Thuringer and Essex, where lactic fermentation is encouraged. Curing salts make meats more favorable to gram- positive bacteria, yeasts, and molds, compared to the gram- negative bacteria typically responsible for spoilage. These salts also reduce the thermal processing needed to stabilize heated meat products like pork luncheon meats. Meats like bulk- chipped beef are preserved by their high sodium chloride content. The microorganism load on the meat and any prior deterioration can affect the success of curing. This can result in discolored cured products, inferior appearance and flavor due to incipient spoilage, or problems with the curing process due to spoilage bacteria.

Fresh Beef

Fresh beef undergoes various color changes- (1) the loss of bloom and the formation of reddish- brown methemoglobin and metmyoglobin due to the oxidation of hemoglobin and myoglobin, resulting in green- gray- brown pigments caused by oxygen and microbial action, (2) spots of various colors such as white, green, yellow, and purple, caused by pigmented microorganisms, (3) phosphorescence, and (4) spots resulting from various bacteria, yeasts, and molds. Beef can also become slimy from bacterial or yeast growth, sticky due to molds, and develop whiskers from mold mycelial growth. Additionally, souring and putrefaction may occur. At 10°C or lower, *Pseudomonas* predominates, but at 15°C or above, *Micrococcus* and *Pseudomonas* grow in nearly equal numbers.

Dried Beef or Beef Hams

Beef hams are made spongy by *Bacillus* species, sour by various bacteria, red by *Halobacterium salinarium* or a red *Bacillus* species, and blue by *Pseudomonas syncyanea, Penicillium spinulosum* (purplish), and *Rhodotorula* yeasts. Water content and relative humidity are crucial factors. As humidity rises and the product absorbs water, shelf life decreases. Gas formation in jars of chipped dried beef is caused by denitrifying aerobic organisms similar to *Pseudomonas fluorescens,* producing oxides of nitrogen, while *Bacillus* species can generate carbon dioxide.

Sausage

In boxed sausages, spoilage microorganisms can grow outside the casing, between the casing and the meat, or inside.

Organisms can only grow outside the outer layer if there is enough moisture. If moisture is present, the microcaps* and yeast can form a slimy coating, as often happens in frankfurters that have become moldy after being removed from the refrigerator at warmer temperatures. With less moisture, mold can produce a fuzzy, blotchy appearance. Carbon dioxide, produced mainly by the heterofermentation of lactic acid bacteria, can cause packages of frankfurter or breakfast sausage to swell when wrapped in flexible gas- proof fil

Growth between the intestine and the meat is favored by the accumulation of moisture in this area during cooking if the casing is permeable to water; When two tubes are used, the inner tube can be wetted before the outer tube is placed, trapping water between them. Mucus on the surface of the meat or between the intestines is formed mainly by acidifying micrococci*. The permeability of the inner layer to soluble nutrients promotes bacterial growth.

Various species of bacteria have been reported to be able to grow in sausages during prolonged cold storage or at storage temperatures above 10.5°C. Acidifying micrococci*, such as *Micrococcus candidus**, can be grown in liver sausage and mortadella, and *Bacillus* species have been found to grow in liver sausage. Leuconostocs and psychotrophic lactobacilli can also develop and cause a sourness that is not favored in most sausages, but is favored in some varieties, such as Lebanese, Thuringian and Essex sausages. The fading of red sausages to a chalky gray has been attributed to oxygen and light and may be accelerated by bacteria. Several causes for "cooling rings" have been suggested, including oxidation, production of organic acid or reducing substances by bacteria, excess water and cooking.

Green sausage casing appears as a green ring not far from the casing, a green core or a green surface. The cause of greening is probably the production of peroxides, e.g. hydrogen peroxide, by heterofermentative *Lactobacillus* species and by *Leuconostoc* or other catalase- negative bacteria, according to Niven (1961). Jensen (1954) stated that hydrogen sulfide may also be involved. Greening is favored by a slightly acidic pH and the presence of small amounts of oxygen. The green ring under the large surface sausage or the green heart of small sausage develops in 12 to 36 hours after processing the sausage, even in the refrigerator; it is evident as soon as the sausage is cut and is usually not accompanied by surface dross. Bacterial growth and heat- stable peroxide production occurred before smoking and cooking, and the peroxide continues to act to produce green after processing. Green hearts of large sausages, for example. large mortadella, they usually develop after 4 or more days of storage and in 1 to 12 hours after cutting, as a large number of causative bacteria develop due to insuffi ent processing and inadequate cooling. Green discoloration of a cut surface indicates contamination and growth by salt-tolerant, peroxide- forming bacteria (probably lactic acid bacteria) that can grow at low temperatures. Viscosity of the surface often accompanies the green color. The defect can spread from one sausage to another.

Production of nitric oxide gas in sausages by nitrate- reducing bacteria has been reported. Unless the casing or packaging material allows the passage of carbon dioxide, it can accumulate under the action of heterofermentative lactic acid bacteria and cause bloating. It can also appear in dried and packaged minced meats, sandwiches, and similar products packaged in plastic bags or boxes.

Bacon

The types of spoilage and the organisms involved vary depending on the part of the pig used to make bacon and the curing methods used in different parts of the world. The wings used in the American method are typically not altered and come out of the smoker with a low bacterial count and a comparatively mold and yeast-free appearance. Because *Streptococcus faecalis* can grow at low temperatures and tolerate salt, it is frequently found. The ham's surface flora may also include staphylococci and micrococci*.

Molds are the primary spoilage organisms in cured ham, especially ham that is sliced and packaged (breathed) when stored in a home refrigerator. Most problems occur in late summer and early fall with *Aspergillus, Alternaria, Monilia, Oidium, Fusarium, Mucor, Rhizopus, Botrytis* and *Penicillium* species. Few microbiological problems are encountered with cured ham and Oxford-style ham. Any problems that do occur are usually due to chemical changes. Sliced ham can be spoiled by oxidizing and lipolytic bacteria during prolonged storage, although chemical oxidation can also occur. Oxidizing and sulfide-forming bacteria can also be responsible for the poor color of ham, although this is more often due to low nitrite concentrations, and chromogenic bacteria can cause areas to discolor. A yellow- brown stain, indicating the presence of tyrosine, has been attributed to proteolytic bacteria. The thinness of the small and the sides, now rare, results from the formation of gum by one of several types of bacteria and yeast.

A thorough study of the bacteriology of Wiltshire pork was carried out in Canada. To make this hazard, the pork loins are salted in a highly concentrated brine for a short time (6 to 8 days) at a low temperature (3.3 to 4.5 days). 5 C), which allows the growth of only salt- tolerant psychrotrophic bacteria. Little growth occurs in the brine, but noticeable bacterial growth occurs on the sides of the meat, sometimes enough to make the surface slippery. Visible growth or drooling usually occurs when the count is greater than 71.5 million per square centimeter. Micrococci are most common in brine, but other organisms, unable to grow in cold brine, may grow before brining or during storage of the salted sides after embalming.

Unopened and packaged cured ham (eric) is spoiled primarily by lactobacilli, but fecal micrococci* and streptococci may develop, especially if the packaging is slightly permeable to oxygen. Opened ham may be spoiled by mold.

The Wisconsin process has been proposed as a means of reducing nitrite levels in bacon (Tanaka et al., 1985). Bacon prepared with 40 or 80 ppm sodium nitrite, 0. Sucrose at 7% and *Lactobacillus plantarum* had a greater antibotulinum effect than bacon prepared with only 120 ppm sodium nitrite.

Ham

The term "acidification", used to define the spoilage of hams, covers all important types of spoilage, from relatively odorless proteolysis to true putrefaction with its very unpleasant odors of mercaptans, hydrogen sulfide, amines, indoles, etc., which can be caused by a wide variety of salt- tolerant psychrotrophic bacteria. Jensen (1954) listed a number of genera whose species can cause acidification- *Alcaligenes, Bacillus, Pseudomonas, Lactobacillus, Proteus, Serratia, Bacterium**, *Micrococcus, Clostridium,* and others, as well as several unnamed hydrogen sulfide- producing streptobacilli that cause the sourness of ham meat. The types of sourness are classified according to their location- sourness of the marrow or tibia, body or meat, coccyx bone, stifle joint, body or meat of the femur bone, and arch. "Blows," or gassed hams, are not encountered in the market, but they do occasionally occur when curing is done without expertise.

The common or rapid drying method of hams, in which the curing solution is pumped into the ham through veins, has greatly reduced the incidence of drying out. Reducing contamination and bacterial growth by proper slaughter and bleeding of pigs, proper cooling, closing of marrows with locks in appropriate places, prompt handling, use of bacteriologically satisfactory saline solution, and good general hygiene help reduce the amount of sourness.

Cured hams are actually precooked and lightly seasoned. These hams are perishable and must be protected from contamination and refrigerated during storage to prevent spoilage by microorganisms. Mishandled cured hams can be spoiled by any of the common spoilage bacteria, including *Escherichia coli, Proteus* spp. , and staphylococci that cause food poisoning (*Staphylococcus aureus*) have been reported.

Refrigerated Packaged Meats

Packaging films that allow for good oxygen and carbon dioxide penetration encourage the growth of more aerobic bacteria, including *Moraxella, Acinetobacter,* and *Pseudomonas,* which can produce slime, putrefaction, and off-flavors The unwrapped meat's spoiling is similar to this. Lactic acid bacteria are encouraged by films with poor gas penetration, particularly when vacuum packing is used. Over time, these bacteria produce atypical flavors, slime, and souring. Chapter 19 discusses canned meat spoilage.

Curing Solutions or Pickles

Spoilage of the pickle or curing solution for ham and other cured meats is more likely when sugar is available and the pH is above 6.0. Multiuse brines typically experience putrefaction caused by *Vibrio, Alcaligenes,* or *Spirillum.* Souring can result from *Lactobacillus* and *Micrococcus,* while slime formation is linked to *Leuconostoc* or *Micrococcus lipolyticus.*

Turbid and ropy vinegar found in pickled pigs' feet or sausages is primarily caused by lactic acid bacteria from the meats, although yeasts may contribute to the cloudiness. Black spots on pickled pigs' feet could be due to hydrogen sulfide–producing bacteria, and gas in vacuum- sealed pickles may originate from heterofermentative lactic acid bacteria or yeasts.

15 Contaminants and Preservation in Fish and Seafood

Fish and seafood are highly perishable products due to their high moisture content, delicate texture, and nutrient- rich composition, making them susceptible to contamination, spoilage, and deterioration. Understanding the various types of contaminants, preservation techniques, and spoilage processes is crucial for maintaining the quality, safety, and shelf life of these marine foods. Contaminants in fish and seafood can be biological, chemical, or physical, with bacteria, parasites, and viruses being the primary biological threats. Pathogenic microorganisms like Vibrio, Salmonella, and Listeria can pose significant health risks, making proper handling and sanitation essential during processing. Chemical contaminants, including heavy metals like mercury and environmental pollutants, can also accumulate in marine organisms, affecting their safety for human consumption. Effecti e preservation methods are vital for extending the freshness of fish and seafood. These methods, such as freezing, refrigeration, salting, smoking, and canning, help slow down the natural spoilage processes by inhibiting microbial growth and enzymatic activity. Additionally, the use of antioxidants and antimicrobial agents can further enhance the preservation of these products. Spoilage in fish and seafood can occur rapidly due to enzymatic activity and microbial growth. The common signs of spoilage include off- odors, discoloration, sliminess, and texture changes. The breakdown of proteins and lipids by bacteria and enzymes leads to the production of compounds such as ammonia, hydrogen sulfide, and fatty acids, which are responsible for unpleasant odors and taste. This chapter explores the various factors influencing the contamination, preservation, and spoilage of fish and seafood, emphasizing the importance of proper handling and storage practices to ensure food safety.

CONTAMINATION

The flora of living fish depends on the microbial content of the water in which it lives. The slime covering the external surface of the fish was found to contain bacteria of the genera *Pseudomonas, Acinetobacter, Moraxella, Alcaligenes, Micrococcus**, *Flavobacterium, Corynebacterium, Sarcina, Serratia, Vibrio* and *Bacillus*. The bacteria found in fish from northern waters are mainly psychrophilic, while fish from tropical waters contain more mesophilic bacteria. Freshwater fish carry freshwater bacteria, which include members of most genera found in saltwater, as well as species of *Aeromonas, Lactobacillus, Brevibacterium, Alcaligenes* and *Streptococcus*. In the intestines of fish from both sources there are bacteria of the genera *Alcaligenes, Pseudomonas,* F*lavobacterium, Vibrio, Bacillus, Clostridium* and *Escherichia.* Boats, crates, tanks, fish shelters, and fishermen quickly become heavily contaminated with these bacteria and pass them on to the fish during cleaning. The number of bacteria in saliva and so The skin of freshly caught saltwater fish can contain 100 to several million per square centimeter, and the intestinal fluid can contain 1,000 to 100 million per milliliter. Gill tissue can contain 1,000 to 1 million per gram. Washing reduces the number of surface bacteria.

Clams and other molluscs pass large amounts of water through their bodies, so they pick up microorganisms from the soil and water, including pathogens if present. There are *Alcaligenes, Flavobacterium, Moraxella, Acinetobacter* and some gram- positive bacteria.

Shrimp, crab, lobster and similar shellfish have a slimy, bacterially loaded coating on their surface that probably resembles that of fish. *Bacillus, Micrococcus, Pseudomonas, Acinetobacter, Moraxella, Flavobacterium, Alcaligenes* and *Proteus* species have been found on shrimp.

The number of microorganisms on the skin of fish can be affected by the method of capture. For example, casting fishing nets along the bottom for Long periods of time results in the exposure of fish to high levels of bacteria in disturbed bottom sediments, which may be reflected in the initial microbial load of fi

Fish cakes and fish sticks or similar products account for a significant percentage of seafood consumed in the United States. These products represent additional sources of contamination. When fish cakes are made, various other products, including potatoes, spices, and flavorings, are mixed with the fish and then The product is formed, coated with batter and breaded, packaged, and usually frozen if not used immediately. Fish sticks are mechanically cut from frozen blocks of fish, coated with batter and breaded, packaged, and frozen for distribution. Many fish sticks are pre- cooked in hot oil at temperatures of 204 to 232°C. The cooking process is short (2 minutes or less) and the interior of the product remains frozen. The microbial content of these products would, of course, be very different from that of fresh fish due to contamination of ingredients, increased handling, contact with machinery and packaging.

PRESERVATION

Of all meat foods, fish is most susceptible to autolysis, fat oxidation and hydrolysis, and microbial spoilage. Therefore, its preservation requires rapid treatment with preservation methods and these methods are often more rigorous than those used for meat. When fish are harvested from the processing plant, preservation methods must also be applied on the fishing boat. Evisceration must be done quickly to stop the digestive enzymes active in the intestine. The benefits obtained from evisceration may be offset by a possible delay in the rapid cooling of the fish

Rigor mortis is particularly important in fish preservation because it delays postmortem autolysis and bacterial decomposition. Therefore, any procedure that prolongs rigor mortis prolongs life. It is longer if the fish had less muscle activity before death and was not roughly handled and bruised during capture and subsequent processing, and it is longer in some fish species than in others. The final pH of postmortem flesh is related to the amount of glycogen available at the time of death. The more glycogen present, the lower the pH. The less muscle activity before death, the higher the glycogen level or the lower the final pH. Lowering the storage temperature extends the period.

Aseptic methods to reduce contamination of seafood are difficul to implement, but some serious contamination before processing can be avoided by general cleaning and disinfection of seafood. boats, decks, holds, drums or other containers and processing equipment in the factory and by using ice of good bacteriological quality. Removing soil from the encrusted surface and the fish with appropriate cleaning methods, including effecti e detergent solutions, goes a long way in reducing the microbial load of fish

The elimination of organisms is difficult but the fact that most contamination is on the external surface of fish and other seafood allows for much to be eliminated. microorganisms remove mud and soil.

Use of Heat

Live crabs are cooked in autoclaves at 121°C to facilitate removal of the meat from the shell. Manual harvesting and packaging of the meat is common. Processing times and temperatures for canned crab meat range from 85.6 to 87.2°C for 92 to 150 minutes (Dickerson and Berry, 1974). These processes are considered pasteurization and canned foods are stored in the refrigerator. Some seafood, such as oysters, are "canned" by packing them in cans or jars and are not heat- treated, but stored in the refrigerator.

However, most canned seafood is heat- treated to be sterile, or at least "commercially sterile". "Like meat, seafood is a low- acid food and, for the most part, has a slow rate of heat penetration and is therefore difficul to reheat. In addition, some types of seafood will shrink significantly or even burst when you try to sterilize them in a can.

The process varies depending on the product being canned and the size and shape of the container. IN In general, thermal processes are more severe than those used for meats, but some special products are easily handled. Preservation practices carried out in accordance with the FAO Code of Practice (FAO, 1973) minimize the health hazards associated with canned seafood.

Use of Low Temperatures

Only after the fish or other sea animal has died does autolysis begin, resulting in softening and the production of an off-taste, and microbial growth becomes unchecked; as previously mentioned, rigor mortis delays these changes. For instance, oysters in their shells will not break down as long as they are alive, and storing them in a cold environment prolongs their shelf life. By being transported in tanks to the New York market, carp seined from midwestern lakes have been kept alive and are therefore in good condition. Fish that are "feedy," or packed with food, appear to decompose more quickly than regular fish

Chilling

Since fish flesh autolyzes and fats oxidize at temperatures above freezing (rapidly in summer and more slowly as temperatures drop toward freezing), refrigerated storage is temporary at best. When fish or other seafood is caught at a distance from the receiving dock, the need for on- board refrigeration depends on the type of fish, whether or not it is prepared there, and the ambient temperature. In general, smaller fish are more susceptible to spoilage than larger fish, and prepared fish autolyzes more slowly than whole fish, but spoils more easily by bacteria. When outside temperatures are warm and shipping distances are long, it is necessary to cool fish and related foods on fishing boats, packing them in crushed ice or by mechanical cooling to slow autolysis and microbial growth until the products are marketed or processed for a longer shelf life. life. The inclusion of preservatives in ice used for freezing fish will be discussed later. The shelf life of ice or cold storage varies greatly depending on the type of fish or other seafood, but it will not last long in most cases. In general, cold storage on land is only useful when retail markets are nearby and turnover is fast. Otherwise, another preservation method is applied, such as freezing, salting, drying, smoking, canning, or a combination of these methods.

Freezing

Many modern freezing techniques were initially developed for preserving fish. In the past, ice combined with salt was used, but with the development of mechanical refrigeration, rapid freezing methods were introduced, and fish were "glazed" by freezing a layer of ice around them. Larger fish, in particular, are often frozen quickly in air or salt brine. Quick freezing is also applied to wrapped fillets or steaks, and smaller whole fish can undergo the same process. Similar to meats, fish frozen quickly generally retain their original quality better than those frozen slowly. However, during storage, the fats in frozen fish undergo hydrolysis and oxidation, with fatty fish deteriorating faster than lean ones, likely due to more rapid hydrolysis.

Raw, decapitated shrimp are typically frozen and glazed, and some cooked shrimp are also preserved through freezing. Other frozen seafood products include scallops, clams, oysters, lobster tails, and cooked crab and lobster meat, most of which are packaged before freezing.

While freezing does kill some microorganisms, it doesn't eliminate all of them. Microbial growth can resume after thawing if conditions allow. Fish typically carry psychrotrophic bacteria, such as *Pseudomonas, Acinetobacter, Moraxella, Alcaligenes,* and *Flavobacterium,* which can survive freezing and multiply upon thawing. Spores of *Clostridium botulinum* type E can also endure freezing and may grow and produce toxins if the temperature exceeds 3.3°C. Frozen raw seafood usually contains few enterococci, coliforms, or staphylococci, but these bacteria may increase during processing, especially when cutting, breading, or battering. Precooking mainly reduces coliform le els.

Use of Irradiation

Preservation of fish by ultraviolet rays has been tried but not put into practice. Experiments have indicated that gamma or cathode irradiation of some kinds of fish may be successful.

Preservation by Drying

Fish can be dried by dry-salting it or by submerging it in brine, which removes or ties up moisture. Fish oil oxidation is not slowed down and can lead to degradation. Fish salting is still a common practice worldwide, though it is less common in the United States. Salting and air drying are two methods used to prepare salt cod. After that, the flesh is extracted from the skin and bones.

In the United States, it is not common practice to sun-dry fish, either small fish or strips of flesh.

Smoking causes the fish to dry out, which contributes to the preservative effect

Use of Preservatives

The salting or marination of fish by dry salt or in brine is effecti e not only because of the drying effect mentioned in the preceding section but also because of the effect of the sodium chloride as a chemical preservative. This method is used to a considerable extent in many countries. The chemical and bacteriological qualities of the salt are important, for impurities such as calcium and magnesium salts may hinder the penetration of the sodium chloride, and halophilic or salt-tolerant bacteria that are introduced may cause discolorations of the fish.

Because of the great perishability of fish, investigators have tried numerous chemicals as preservatives, either applied directly to the fish or incorporated in the ice used in chilling them.

Preservatives Used on Fish

In the intensive search for chemical preservatives that can be applied directly or as a dip to fish or fillets, a large number of chemicals have been tested, ranging from those that most regulatory agencies would approve to those whose use would be controversial. Sodium chloride, an acceptable preservative, is being discussed.

Fish can be dry- salted to contain 4 to 5 percent salt. Salt introduces halophiles that can discolor the fish (e.g. , a red color that comes from *Serratia salinaria**). *Micrococcus* species* generally increase in fish and there is a reduction in *Flavobacterium, Alcaligenes, Pseudomonas* and others. Processing of the fish can be "soft", i.e. lightly salted, or it can be done in a thick or hard brine and can be followed by smoking. Benzoic acid and benzoates have had moderate success as preservatives. Sodium and potassium nitrites and nitrates have been reported to extend shelf life and are permitted in some countries. Sorbic acid has been found to slow the spoilage of smoked or salted fish. Boric acid has been used in Europe with some improvement in preservation quality, but its use is illegal in the United States. Other chemicals for which there have been claims of success but whose use is contraindicated include formaldehyde, hypochlorite, hydrogen peroxide, sulfur dioxide, undielenic acid, capric acid, epoxybenzoic acid, and chloroform.

Antibiotics have also been tested experimentally, usually in a bath or on ice. Of those tested, chlortetracycline and oxytetracycline appear to be the best, and their use is now authorized. Chloramphenicol is quite effecti e, while penicillin, streptomycin, and subtilin are weak or useless.

Storing fish in an atmosphere containing increased levels of carbon dioxide has been shown to extend shelf life. The normal spoilage flora is replaced by lactobacilli and others, and the product "crumbles" as it begins to spoil.

Burst of fish can mean salting or acidification with vinegar, wine or sour cream. Herring is processed in various ways- salted, pickled and sour. Various combinations of these treatments, combined with an airtight container, allow the preservation of the fish, although refrigeration must also be used for some products.

In the past, fish was smoked mainly for preservation and smoking was intensive, but now that preservation, refrigeration and freezing are available to extend shelf life, most fish smoking is mainly for flavor and therefore light. The smoking treatment and other related preservation methods vary depending on the type of fish, the size of the pieces and the desired length of storage. Fish for drinking are usually gutted and decapitated, but may be cut or cut into pieces. In general, salting, light or heavy, precedes smoking and serves not only to give flavor to the fish, but also to improve its keeping quality by reducing its moisture content. Drying may be assisted by air currents. Smoking can be carried out at relatively low temperatures (26.7 to 37.1 °C). 8°C) or high temperatures such as 63 to 92°C which result in partial cooking of the fish

Microbiology of Fish Brines

The number of bacteria in fish- cured brines varies depending on the salt concentration, the temperature of the brine, the type and amount of contamination from the introduced fish, and the length of time the brine has been used. It is between 10,000 and 10 million bacteria per milliliter. Salinity concentrations are usually between 18% and saturation, but can be lower, especially after the introduction of fish. The higher the salting temperature, the more salt is needed to prevent spoilage. Contamination comes from fish, which usually contains *Pseudomonas, Acinetobacter, Moraxella, Alcaligenes,* and *Flavobacterium* species; ice, which contains genera such as *Corynebacterium* and cocci; and mechanically introduced sources, e.g. , dust, which adds cocci. With continued use of the brine, the number of organisms increases, due to the addition of successive batches of fish and the growth of salt- tolerant bacteria, such as micrococci*. As the brine ages, a decrease in the number and an increase mainly of corynebacteria in low- salt brine and of micrococci* in highly saline brine are observed.

Preservatives Incorporated in Ice

Before freezing, a chemical preservative is added to water to create so-called germicidal ices. When the added chemical is evenly distributed throughout, as with sodium chloride, these ices are eutectic; when it is not uniformly distributed, as with sodium benzoate, they are noneutectic. When applied to fish, noneutectic ice is finely crushed to ensure that the chemical is distributed uniformly.

Many investigators have sought the ideal chemical to be incorporated in ice for icing fish and have tested with some success a large number of chemicals, including hypochlorites, chloramines, benzoic acid and benzoates, colloidal silver, hydrogen peroxide, ozone, sodium nitrite, sulfonamides, antibiotics, propionates, levulinic acid, and many others. Both the American and Canadian governments and those of other nations now permit the incorporation of the tetracyclines at up to 7 ppm in ice to be used by fishers to preserve fish on trawlers and during transportation.

The purpose of the application of preservative chemicals to fish either directly or as dips or germicidal ices is to kill or inhibit microorganisms on the surfaces of the fish, where at first they are most numerous and act e.

Antioxidants

Fats and oils of many kinds of fish, especially the fatter ones such as herring, mackerel, mullet, and salmon, are composed to a great extent of unsaturated fatty acids and hence are subject to oxidative changes producing oxidative rancidity and sometimes undesirable alterations in color. To counteract these undesirable changes, antioxidants may be applied as dips, coatings, glazes, or gases. Good results have been reported with nordihydroguaiaretic acid, ethyl gallate, ascorbic acid, and other compounds and with storage in carbon dioxide.

SPOILAGE

Like meat, fish and other seafood may be spoiled by autolysis, oxidation, or bacterial activity or most commonly by combinations of these. Most fish flesh, however, is considered more perishable than meat because of more rapid autolysis by the fish enzymes and because of the less acid reaction of fish flesh that favors microbial growth. Also, many of the unsaturated fish oils seem to be more susceptible to oxidative deterioration than are most animal fats. The experts agree that the bacterial spoilage of fish does not begin until after rigor mortis, when juices are released from the flesh fibers

Therefore, the more this is delayed or protracted, the longer the keeping time of the fish. Rigor mortis is hastened by struggling of the fish, lack of oxygen, and warm temperature and is delayed by a low pH and adequate cooling of the fish. The pH of the fish flesh has an important influence on its perishability, not only because of its effect on rigor mortis but also because of its influence on the growth of bacteria. The lower the pH of the fish flesh, the slower in general bacterial decomposition will be. Lowering of the pH of the fish flesh results from the conversion of muscle glycogen to lactic acid.

The type and rate of spoilage in fish are influenced by s eral factors:

Species of Fish: Different fish species have varying degrees of perishability. For example, flatfis tend to spoil faster than roundfish because they undergo rigor mortis more quickly. However, certain flatfis like halibut last longer due to the low pH (5.5) of their flesh. Fatty fish, which contain unsaturated fats, deteriorate quickly due to oxidation, and those with high levels of trimethylamine oxide soon release trimethylamine, creating a "stale- fishy" odor.

Condition at Capture: Fish that are stressed from struggling, low oxygen levels, or rough handling spoil faster. This is likely because their glycogen stores are depleted, resulting in a smaller pH drop in the flesh. Fish that are "feedy," meaning they are full when caught, are also more perishable than those with an empty stomach.

Bacterial Contamination: Fish can be contaminated with bacteria from mud, water, handlers, and their external slime or intestinal contents. These bacteria enter through the gills or the intestinal tract and spread through the vascular system to the flesh. Contamination increases spoilage, especially if it occurs during handling in the net, on the boat, at the docks, or in processing plants. Fish that are not gutted have less contamination in the flesh, but decay from the gut can still cause odors. Gutting fish on the boat can spread bacteria, although proper washing and chilling will help minimize their growth.

Temperature: Chilling is the most common method for slowing bacterial growth and spoilage. The fish should be cooled rapidly to 0 to - 1°C and kept at this low temperature. Warmer temperatures shorten the fish's shelf life, while prompt freezing enhances preservation.

Use of Antibiotic Ice or Dip: This can also help in reducing spoilage by limiting bacterial growth.

Evidences of Spoilage

It is hard to pinpoint or agree upon when spoiling first appears because the change is gradual, going from a fresh state to staleness and finally to inedibility. For many years, there has been a search for a practical test to assess fish quality, but none of them have been completely successful. While some support alternative methods, such as an estimate of volatile acids or volatile bases or a test for pH, hydrogen sulfide, ammonia, etc., most experts support a chemical test for trimethylamine for use on saltwater fish. Tests for bacteria are too slow to be of any use.

According to Reay and Shewan (1949), a fish undergoes a series of external changes as it deteriorates and eventually turns putrid. The fish's distinctively vivid colors gradually disappear, giving way to discolorations that are dirty, yellow, or brown. The fish's skin becomes more slimy, particularly around the gills and flaps. The pupil gets hazy and the cornea gets opaque as the eyes progressively droop and shrink. The gills first become pale pink, then turn grayish-yellow. The most noticeable change is the softening of the flesh, which makes it easier for the fingers to indent and releases juice when squeezed. The oxidation of hemoglobin causes a reddish-brown discoloration that spreads toward the tail, making it easy to remove the flesh from the backbone.

Meanwhile a sequence of odors is evolved; first the normal, fresh, seaweedy odor, then a sickly sweet one, then a stale- fishy odor due to trimethylamine followed by ammoniacal and final putrid odors due to hydrogen sulfide, indole, and other malodorous compounds. Fatty fish also may show rancid odors. Cooking will bring out the odors more strongly.

Spoilage by bacteria

The bacteria most commonly implicated in fish spoilage are part of the natural flora of the external mucus of the fish and its intestinal contents. The predominant species of bacteria responsible for spoilage vary depending on the temperature at which the fish is stored, but at commonly used refrigeration temperatures, *Pseudomonas* species predominate, followed by *Acinetobacter*, *Moraxella* and *Flavobacterium* species. Bacteria of the genera *Micrococcus* and *Bacillus* appear less frequently and at higher temperatures. Reports in the literature cite other genera as species implicated in fish spoilage, such as *Esherichia, Proteus, Serratia, Sarcina* and *Clostridium*. Most of these grow only at ordinary atmospheric temperatures and would probably not do much at refrigeration temperatures.

Normally, the number of pseudomonads increases in cold fish during storage, achromobacteria* decreases and flavobacteria temporarily increases and then. are in decline. The bacteria first grow on the surface and then penetrate the flesh. Fish have a high content of non- protein nitrogen, and the autolytic changes caused by their enzymes increase the supply of nitrogenous nutrients (e.g. amino acids and amines) and glucose for bacterial growth. From these compounds, bacteria produce trimethylamine, ammonia, amines (for example, putrescine and cadaverine), fatty acids and lower aldehydes, and eventually hydrogen and other sulphides, mercaptans and indoles, which are products that show decay. A musty or muddy smell and fishy taste has been attributed to the growth of *Streptomyces* species in the mud at the bottom of the water body and the absorption of the smell by the fish.

As noted, discoloration of fish flesh can occur during spoilage; yellow to green- yellow colors caused by *Pseudomonas fluorescens*, yellow micrococcus and others; red or pink colors due to the growth of *Sarcina, Micrococcus* or *Bacillus* species or from mold or yeast; and a chocolate brown color due to an asporogenous yeast. Pathogens that parasitize fish can cause spots or lesions.

DEGRADATION OF SPECIFIC FISH AND SEAFOOD VARIETIES

The preceding discussion has been largely limited to the spoilage of refrigerated fish. Salted fish is spoiled by halophilic or salt- tolerant bacteria of the genera *Serratia, Micrococcus, Bacillus, Alcaligenes, Pseudomonas,* and others which often cause stains, the most common of which is a red color. Molds are the main spoilage organisms of smoked fish. Marinated fish (pickled in acid) should not have problems with spoilage unless the acid content is low enough to allow the growth of lactic acid bacteria or the entry of air allows mold. Frozen fish should also not have bacteriological problems after freezing, but of course its quality depends on what happened to the fish before freezing. The spoilage of canned fish and other seafood will be discussed in Chapter 19. Japanese fish sausages are prone to rancidity caused by the production of volatile acids by bacteria or by putrefaction, despite the addition of nitrites and authorized preservatives.

In general, shellfish are subject to similar types of microbial spoilage as fish. However, in chilled shrimp, *Acinetobacter, Moraxella,* and *Vibrio* are primarily responsible for spoilage, although there may be a temporary increase in *Pseudomonas* and a decrease in *Flavobacterium, Micrococcus**, and *Bacillus*. Crab meat is spoiled by *Pseudomonas, Acinetobacter,* and *Moraxella* at refrigeration temperatures and primarily by *Proteus* at higher temperatures. *Pseudomonas, Alcaligenes, Flavobacterium,* and *Bacillus* species have been implicated in the spoilage of raw lobster. Crabs and oysters may contain *Vibrio* species, including *V. parahaemolyticus*. Levels in these products fluctuate with seasonal temperature changes.

Pearls remain in good condition as long as they are kept alive in their shells at refrigeration temperatures, but they decompose rapidly when they die, as in the case of oysters. The type of spoilage in sealed oysters depends on the temperature at which they are stored. Oysters are not only rich in protein, but they also contain sugars, which come from the hydrolysis of glycogen. At temperatures near freezing, *Pseudomonas, Acinetobacter* and *Moraxella* species are the most important spoilage bacteria, but *Flavobacterium* and *Micrococcus* species* can also grow. The change is called "acidification", although the changes are mainly proteolytic. At higher temperatures, acidification can result from the fermentation of sugars by coliform bacteria, streptococcus, lactobacilli, and yeast, producing acid and a sour odor. Initial growth of *Serratia, Pseudomonas, Proteus,* and *Clostridium* may occur. A rare type of spoilage by asporogenous yeast causes pink oysters.

16 Contamination, Preservation, and Spoilage of Eggs

Eggs are highly susceptible to microbial contamination, particularly from bacteria like Salmonella, which can cause foodborne illnesses. Contamination typically occurs through cracks in the eggshell or during handling and processing. The interior of eggs is sterile when intact, but bacteria can enter through pores in the shell, leading to spoilage. Preservation methods for eggs include refrigeration, which slows down bacterial growth and extends shelf life. Coating eggs with mineral oils or using controlled atmosphere storage can also help maintain quality by reducing moisture loss and protecting against microbial invasion.

Spoilage in eggs is characterized by off-odors, changes in texture, and bacterial growth, leading to an unpleasant taste. Proper handling, including washing eggs carefully, maintaining clean storage conditions, and following strict hygiene practices, are crucial in minimizing contamination risks. Effecti e preservation techniques ensure eggs remain safe for consumption and retain their nutritional value.

Eggs are a highly perishable food product, and their contamination, preservation, and spoilage are crucial concerns in food safety and quality control. Eggs can be contaminated by a variety of microorganisms, including bacteria, fungi, and viruses, which can enter through the porous shell or from improper handling during the collection, storage, and transportation processes. The primary pathogen of concern in eggs is *Salmonella*, which can lead to foodborne illnesses if eggs are not properly cooked or stored. Other bacteria, such as *Escherichia coli* and *Listeria monocytogenes*, can also pose risks to egg safety.To prevent spoilage, various preservation methods are employed, such as refrigeration, coating the eggs with mineral oil, or even pasteurization.

These methods help slow down bacterial growth and enzymatic activity, which are the main contributors to spoilage. Refrigeration is the most common preservation technique and significantly extends the shelf life of eggs by inhibiting the growth of spoilage microorganisms and preventing the breakdown of proteins and fats.However, despite these preservation techniques, eggs will eventually spoil. Spoilage can manifest in several forms, including changes in appearance, odor, and texture. Spoiled eggs may emit a sulfurous or rotten odor due to the breakdown of proteins by bacteria. The texture may become watery or slimy, and the yolk may lose its firmness. Understanding the factors influencing contamination, preservation methods, and spoilage of eggs is essential for ensuring food safety and minimizing waste in the egg industry.

CONTAMINATION

The majority of recently laid eggs are sterile, at least on the inside, but the shells quickly get contaminated by the hen's excrement, the cage or nest, the water used to wash the eggs, handling, and possibly the packing material. According to reports, there are between 10^2 and 10^7 microorganisms overall per hen's egg shell, with a mean of roughly 10^5. Numerous kinds of microorganisms were found within the shell.

A comparison of the flora of the shell (Table 16.1) and the flora isolated from spoiled eggs (Table 16.2) suggest a high number of gram- positive organisms in the former but a low number in the latter. Therefore, those organisms which frequently spoil or "rot" the egg are in relatively low numbers initially on the shell.

Table. Incidence of Microorganisms on the Shell of Hens' Eggs

Type	Percent of flour		
	Farms	**Egg- breaking plants***	**Packaging station***
Streptococcus		8(5)	
Staphylococcus	5	30	9(16)
*Micrococcus**	18	23(20)	37(94)
Sarcina	2	20	
Arthrobacter			5(23)
Bacillus	30	18	(2.5)
Pseudomonas	6		22.5(36.5)
*Achromabacter**	19		1.5(3)
Alcaligenes			(2)
Flavobacterium	3		
Cytophaga			(1)
Coli- aerogenes	5	19(20)	10.5(11.5)
Aeromonas		20(20)	1
Proteus	1	20(50)	
Serraita		10(20)	
Molds	7		
Unclassified			12(11)

*Numbers represent data from clean eggs; numbers in parentheses, data from soiled or cracked eggs. Source- Condensed From Board (1969).

Salmonella spp. may be on the shell or in the egg as laid, build up during processing, and appear in significant numbers in frozen or dried eggs.

Table. Types of Organisms Isolated from Spoiled Eggs

Organism	Halnes (1939)	Alford et al. (1950)	Florian and Trussell (1957)	Board (1965)	Board and Board (1968)
Gram- positive	–	–	±	±	±
Coli- aerogenes	+	+	+	+	+
Proteus	+	+	+	+	+
Aeromonas	–	–	+	+	+
Pseudomonas	+	+	+	+	+
Alcaligenes	+	+	+	+	+
*Achromobacter**	+	+	+	+	+

+ = Isolated on many occasions; ± = isolated occasionally; – = not isolated.
Source- Condensed From Board (1969).

PRESERVATION

Methods of preserving eggs have received much attention because of their perishability. "What manufacturer would be so reckless as to attempt to package a perishable product in a semi- permeable membrane in a fragile, porous shell and distribute and market it under uncontrolled conditions?" Bordi (1969) continues- "That is what the chicken seems to have done."

The egg has several ways of protecting itself from microbial invasion. Shells and A thin surface layer of proteinaceous material known as the cuticle or bloom is the first line of defense and serves to delay entry. However, the shell is porous for gas exchange during embryonic development. The membranes in the shell also tend to serve as a mechanical barrier. This barrier is likely to be only temporary and does not provide protection against the infiltration of fungal hyphae through the pores of the shell and membrane. This fact highlights the need to store eggs in a manner that avoids the accumulation of moisture on the shell surface. A rapid change in storage temperature can allow bacteria to overcome the physical barrier of their shell and membrane. For example, if a warm egg is placed in a cold environment, microorganisms on the surface of the shell can be removed from the pores as the egg contents shrink. Changes in the membranes occur with aging and promote faster bacterial growth. The rate of physical and chemical changes in the egg depends on the storage time and the temperature, relative humidity, and composition of the atmosphere around the egg.

In addition to the physical barrier of the shell and its membranes, numerous studies have shown that the albumen is an inadequate growth medium for many microorganisms. The characteristics of albumen that hinder microbial growth include a pH of 9 to 10 that may be reached during storage; low levels of simple nitrogenous compounds; apoprotein, which ties up riboflavin; avidin, which ties up biotin; antiproteolytic factors, which might prevent bacterial proteinases from releasing nitrogenous compounds necessary for growth; conalbumin (ovotransferrin), which chelates iron; and lysozyme, an enzyme which degrades the cell walls of gram- positive bacteria.

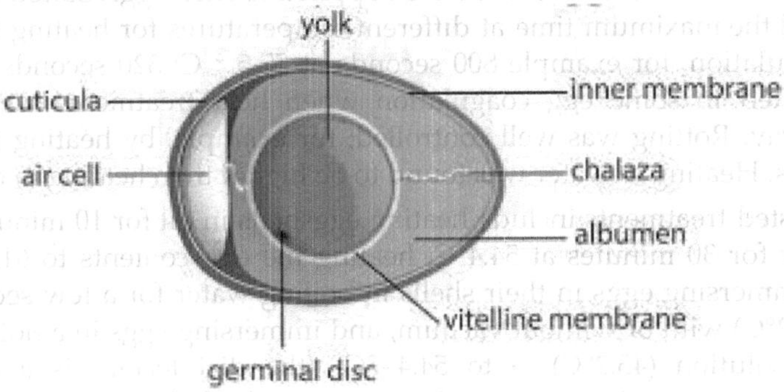

Fig 16.1. Internal structure of an egg

Asepsis

Great care is taken to reduce the contamination of the outside of the shell by hen feces and dirt from the nests. When eggs are broken for drying or freezing, care is taken to discard those in which microbial growth has taken place and to reduce contamination from equipment by cleaning and sanitizing it.

Removal of Microorganisms

Since dirty eggs are cheaper than clean eggs, several methods have been tried to remove impurities. Chemical cleaning, such as sandblasting, removes dirt and mucus. Washing with hot water removes dirt, mucus, and some microorganisms, but promotes the penetration of bacteria into the egg through the pores of the shell. If precautions are not taken, the wash water will accumulate a lot of spoilage bacteria, increasing contamination during washing. Experiments have shown that hand- washed eggs are more prone to rotting than unwashed eggs, and that machine- washed eggs show more rotting than those washed by hand. The rate of decay that results varies with the type of washing machine and the type of wash solution. Attempts to reduce contamination with spoilage bacteria by washing the machine and disinfecting with a 1% hypochlorite solution have not always been successful, but the use of this disinfectant solution as a water wash has reduced the percentage of spoilage in washed eggs. The use of 1- 3% acetic acid was effective in eliminating the flora, but resulted in a decrease in shell thickness and egg quality (Heath and Wallace, 1978). Dyes, acids, formalin hypochlorite, quaternary ammonium compounds, various detergents and detergent- disinfectant combinations have been tested in wash solutions. These solutions are used at temperatures ranging from 32 to 40°C to 60°C, depending on the chemicals used. A washing solution Heating is essential to prevent liquid absorption into the cold egg. A properly functioning mechanical egg washer will remove almost all flora from the shell.

Use of Heat

The thermal coagulability of egg white largely determines the maximum thermal treatment that can be applied to shell eggs. Salton et al. (1951) determined the maximum time at different temperatures for heating in water to avoid coagulation, for example 800 seconds at 57.5 ° C; 320 seconds at 60°C or more resulted in some egg coagulation when heat treatments were used to control decay. Rotting was well controlled, for example, by heating to 60°C for 320 seconds. Heating in water was found to be higher than heating in oil.

Suggested treatments include heating eggshells in oil for 10 minutes at 60°C or in water for 30 minutes at 54.4°C; heating the egg contents to 61.7°C for 30 minutes; immersing eggs in their shells in boiling water for a few seconds or in hot oil (57.2°C) with or without vacuum; and immersing eggs in a hot detergent-sanitizing solution (43.2°C). 3 to 54.4 °C) (the disinfectant is a quaternary ammonium compound). A heat stabilization method that involves immersing eggs in hot water reduces the evaporation of moisture from the egg by slightly coagulating the outermost part of the egg white.

The heat treatments used in the United States to eliminate salmonella are- (1) liquid whole egg, 60 °C for at least 3.5 minutes, (2) liquid egg yolk, 61. 1 °C for at least 3.5 min or 60 °C for at least 6.2 min, (3) yellow carbohydrates, 63.3 °C for at least 3.5 min, or 62. 2 °C for at least 6.2 min, (4) egg whites with salt, 63.3 °C for at least 3.5 min or 62.2 °C for at least 6.2 min. 2 min. Treatments used in other countries are similar but vary slightly.

Pasteurization is required for most egg products. An exception is salted egg yolk used in salad dressings. This product is exempt if it contains at least 1. 4% acetic acid (pH 4.1 or less). Due to the thermal coagulation of eggs, a stabilization process is required before pasteurization. This includes the addition of aluminum salts and adjusting the pH.

Use of Low Temperatures

The most common method of preservation of eggs is the use of low temperatures including chilling temperatures for shell eggs and freezing for egg "meats." Oiling, gas storage, or treatment with chemical preservatives may be combined with the chilling of shell eggs.

Chilling

Most shell eggs are refrigerated. They are selected for storage on the basis of their general appearance and the result of the candle. To hatch an egg, it is held and turned in front of a light to examine for defects such as cracks, decay, mold, blood, a developing embryo, a crusted or lopsided yolk, a small white cell or large air. Eggs must be cooled as soon as possible after production and stored at a temperature and relative humidity that depends on the expected storage time. The minimum relative humidity is below 99. English The higher the relative humidity, the faster the egg loses moisture and therefore weight, and the larger the air chamber becomes. The higher the relative humidity, the greater the risk of microbial spoilage of the egg. The higher the temperature, above - 1.67 ° C, the faster the penetration of microorganisms into the egg and their growth, and the greater the physical and chemical changes, e.g. , white shrinkage and weakened yolk membrane. For commercial storage of 6 months or more, a temperature of - 1.7 to - 0.55°C and a relative humidity of 70 to 80% are recommended. Air circulation in the storage room is important to maintain the desired relative humidity around the eggs, and a constant storage temperature is essential to prevent moisture condensation on the eggshells.

Special treatments improve the keeping quality of eggs during cold storage. Impregnation of the egg with colorless and odorless mineral oil is a common method that prevents moisture from entering, slows drying and air penetration, retains carbon dioxide, and delays physical and chemical changes in the egg. Eggs are easily sprayed with oil, especially eggs intended for long- term commercial storage, with little apparent effect on the rate of microbial change in the eg

Freezing

The selection and preparation of the egg contents for freezing are the primary bacteriological issues that arise when "meat" or "pulp" eggs are frozen. Frozen eggs are no better than their pre-frozen counterparts, just like other frozen foods. Many eggs that have been frozen or dried have flaws that lower their quality as shell eggs but do not impact the quality of the contents. These flaws include eggs with weak shells, dirt, cracks, or irregular cuts.

Eggs are first selected with a candle, then mechanically washed with a final rinse of chlorine at 200 to 500 ppm (iodine is also effecti e) and then broken in circuit breakers. The use of automatic egg breakers requires strict quality control of whole eggs and inspection of broken eggs before mixing or "pooling" large quantities. The eggs are broken and their contents fall into inspection cups. During inspection, the yolks and whites are separated by the action of the cup.

The careful disposal of broken eggs has a very important impact on the types and numbers of bacteria present in the frozen product, as well as hygiene throughout the breaking process. All equipment that comes into contact with shell eggs or their contents should be cleaned and disinfected daily or more frequently. Whole or split eggs are strained to remove shell fragments and stringy material (chalaza), blended or blended, standardized for solids content, and frozen in 30- or 50- pound cans. or other containers, usually by a quick- freezing process. Separately frozen eggs and stored frozen form a gelatin that does not become liquid when thawed. This difficul is avoided by including 5 percent or more of sugar, salt, or glycerin before freezing. Frozen eggs are stored at - 17°C. 8 to - 20.5 °C.

If proper precautions are not taken, frozen eggs can contain large numbers of bacteria, up to millions per gram. These large numbers can result from the use of highly concentrated egg pulps. contaminated, from contamination from shell parts and equipment in the cracking chamber, and from growth prior to freezing. Egg- spoiling bacteria stored at low temperatures, particularly *Pseudomonas* organisms, are likely to be abundant, as are bacteria of the genera *Alcaligenes*,

Proteus, and *Flavobacterium.* Gram- positive cocci and eggshell bacilli and coliforms are present in smaller numbers, and it is possible that anaerobes and other bacteria are incidental contaminants. *Salmonella* may be present in eggs from infected or contaminated hens. The freezing process reduces the numbers, but some of each type of organism present is likely to survive. Numbers decline slowly during frozen storage. If thawing is done at too high a temperature or if thawed eggs are stored too long before use, bacterial numbers will increase due to the growth of dominant psychrotrophic bacteria. Thawing at temperatures above 2 to 3 °C should be as short as possible. Some suggested time and temperature combinations (for 30 lb boxes) are 10- 15 °C for 8- 15 hours or 2-3 °C for 48- 72 hours.

Preservation by Drying

In the preparation of whole pulp, egg white, or grape seed for drying, the principles involved are similar to those discussed earlier for the preparation of these materials for freezing. Egg white requires additional processing before drying to maintain its whipping properties. Removal of glucose, one of the reactants in the Browning or Maillard reaction, must be accomplished before drying. Several methods of glucose removal have been suggested, including fermentation by group D streptococci, *Enterobacter aerogenes* or *Saccharomyces cerevisiae,* and an enzymatic process using glucose oxidase. In the latter case, glucose is converted to gluconic acid, with the addition of hydrogen peroxide serving as an oxygen donor. The cold desugarization process with glucose oxidase at 10°C has the advantage of producing a product with a low bacterial count.

Most egg drying operations in the United States use spray drying, where the liquid is sprayed into a stream of hot, dry air. Another method is the roller or drum process, in which the liquid egg is passed over a heated drum, with or without vacuum. Air drying is accomplished by means of open trays, such as those used by the Chinese, or by the belt system, where the liquid from the egg is on a belt that passes through a heated tunnel (60 to 71.1°C). Spray drying or pan drying combined with tunnel drying is used for egg whites. Historically, eggs have been dried to a moisture content of about 5%, but the keeping quality of dried egg whites or whole eggs improves as the moisture content increases. has fallen to 1%, and the trend is in that direction.

The most commonly used drying equipment is similar to the spray drying equipment used in the dairy industry for drying milk, and similar problems are evident. A major concern in both processes is the bacteriological quality of the air to which the product is exposed during the drying operation. The use of absolute filters and air preheating has had significant effects. Furthermore, heat applied during drying cannot be used to completely reduce the number of bacteria in the final product or even as a pasteurization technique. Therefore, monitoring or pre-pasteurization of the original product is a necessary protective measure. Whole eggs and egg products can be pasteurized before drying, while a secondary heat treatment is usually applied to the egg white after drying. Bulk packages of egg whites are exposed to temperatures of 52 to 54 °C for 7 to 10 days, depending on the moisture content of the egg whites. the final product

Dried eggs can contain from a few hundred microorganisms per gram to more than 100 million, depending on the broken eggs and the processing methods used. The same reasons explain the presence of many microbes as in frozen eggs. The drying process can reduce the microbial content by ten to a hundred times compared to liquid eggs, while still allowing a large number of microbes to survive. Several organisms have been found in dried eggs, including micrococci*, streptococci (enterococci), coliform bacteria, *Salmonella* species, bacterial spores, and fungi. Gram-positive rods and sticks are likely to be present due to contamination from the shell during breaking or from holders or equipment rather than from damaged eggs. *Salmonella* can come from infected hens; however, these are usually not present and most buyers specify products as "salmonella- free". When egg white has been pretreated through a fermentation process, the dried product may have a high microbial content. Properly dried egg products contain too little moisture for microbial growth. In fact, during storage, the number of organisms in dried eggs will decrease, rapidly at first, then gradually. Desiccation- resistant organisms such as micrococci* and bacterial spores and molds will constitute an increasing proportion of survivors as storage continues. The more the moisture content of the dried egg is reduced by 5%, the more rapid the bacterial death will be.

Use of Preservatives

Preservatives can be used on egg shells, in the atmosphere around them, or in egg packaging or containers. A large number of different substances have been applied to the surface of the eggshells or used as wrapping material around the eggs to help preserve them. Some of these substances are mainly used to keep the shell dry and reduce the penetration of oxygen into the egg and the passage of carbon dioxide and moisture from the outside; Examples include wax, shell oil and other sealing methods. Other materials inhibit the growth of microorganisms and some are microorganisms. Materials used for dry packing eggs at home include salt, lime, sand, sawdust and ash. Immersing the sodium silicate solution in a glass of water has long been an effecti e method of home preservation. The solution is inhibitory because of its alkalinity. Other chemical inhibitors have been tested, including borates, permanganates, benzoates, salicylates, formates and a host of other compounds. The use of hot or warm microbicidal solutions to wash eggs, such as hypochlorite solutions, saline, acids, formalin, quaternary ammonium compounds and detergent- disinfectant combinations, has been mentioned. Coating the shell with a dimethylolurea solution has been shown to be effecti e in inhibiting the growth of mold.

Several attempts have been made to reduce the spoilage of eggs by mold during storage by treating the storage trays and crates with a mycostatic or chemical mold inhibitor. Sodium pentachlorophenate and related compounds have been used successfully.

Fumigating eggs with ethylene oxide gas before storage protects them from bacterial spoilage.

The only two gases added to the atmosphere around eggs to improve their keeping quality are carbon dioxide and ozone, although nitrogen has been used experimentally. Recommendations vary as to the optimum concentration of carbon dioxide in the air for this purpose. A low concentration, say 2.5 percent, slows down the physical and chemical changes in the egg that accompany the rise in pH as carbon dioxide leaves the egg, but has little effect on microbial growth, especially mold. Concentrations up to 60 percent significantly delay microbial spoilage, especially if the temperature is near freezing, although as the relative humidity approaches saturation, the white becomes thinner and an unpleasant taste appears. Therefore, Recommendations range from 0.5 to 0. 6 percent at -1°C and 2.5 to 5 percent at 0°C up to a maximum of 15 percent. There is some disagreement about the effecti eness of ozone. It has been stated that from 0.6 ppm ozone (for clean eggs) to 1.5 ppm ozone (for clean eggs), the maximum allowable concentration is 15 percent. 5 ppm (for dirty eggs) at - 0.55°C and 90% relative humidity will keep eggs fresh for 8 months and 3.5 ppm will not harm them, but some workers say that 0.5 to 1. 5 ppm has little effect on microorganisms. It has been shown to be low The concentration of ozone improves the taste of stored eggs due to the deodorizing effect of the gas

Use of Irradiation

Experiments have indicated that pathogens (e.g., *Salmonella*) in liquid, frozen, and dried eggs can be inactivated by means of ionizing radiation. However, damage by relatively light dosages has also been observed.

SPOILAGE

Some of the defects of eggs are obvious from their general appearance, others are shown by candling with transmitted light, and some show up only in the broken egg.

Defects in the Fresh Egg

Fresh eggs may have cracks, leaks, loss of luster or color, spots or contamination on the outside, as well as "meat spots" (blood clots), general blood discoloration, or translucent yellow spots. Among these items, any broken shell or dirt inside the egg will promote deterioration during storage.

Changes During Storage

The changes that take place in eggs while they are being held or stored may be divided into those due to nonmicrobial causes and those resulting from the growth of microorganisms.

Changes not Caused by Microorganisms

Untreated eggs lose moisture during storage and therefore lose weight. The degree of shrinkage can be seen by observing the size of the air space or cell at the open end of the egg, a large cell showing considerable shrinkage. The change in the physical state of the egg contents, as indicated by the ignition or cracking of the egg, is more important. The white of the egg becomes thinner and more watery as the egg ages and the yolk membrane weakens. The poorer the egg, the more the yolk moves and the closer it is to the shell when the egg is turned during firing. When an old egg is cracked on a plate, the thinness of the white is more apparent and the weakness of the yolk membrane allows the yolk to flatte or even break. In contrast, a freshly cracked egg has a thick white and a yolk that remains firm in the shape of a hemisphere. During storage, the alkalinity of the egg white increases from a normal pH of about 7.6 to about 9.5. Any marked growth of chicken embryos in fertilized eggs also serves to condemn the eggs.

Changes Caused by Microorganisms

To cause spoilage of an intact shell egg, the causative organisms must do the following- (1) contaminate the shell, (2) penetrate the pores of the shell to the shell membranes (usually the shell must be moist for this to occur), (3) grow through the shell membranes to reach the albumen (or reach the yolk if it touches the membrane), (4) grow in the egg white, despite the previously mentioned unfavorable conditions, to reach the yolk, where they can easily develop and completely spoil the egg. Bacteria that cannot grow in the albumen can reach the yolk and grow there only when the yolk touches the inner cell membrane.

The time it takes for bacteria to penetrate the shell membranes varies between organisms and temperatures, but can take several weeks at refrigerator temperatures. The special set of environmental conditions, the selective medium of egg white and the low storage temperature of around 0°C combine to limit the number of bacterial and mould species that can cause spoilage, especially those mentioned below.

The time it takes for bacteria to penetrate the shell membranes varies between organisms and temperature, but can take several weeks at refrigerator temperatures. The particular set of environmental conditions, the selective environment of the egg white and the low storage temperature of around 0°C combine to limit the number of types of bacteria and moulds that can cause spoilage, mainly those mentioned.

In general, Bacteria are more responsible for spoilage of eggs than moulds. The types of bacterial spoilage or "rot" in eggs have different names. Alford et al. (1950) list five groups of rots found in Australian eggs intended for export. Among the three main ones is green rot, mainly caused by *Pseudomonas fluorescens,* a bacterium that grows at 0°C. The rot is so named because of the bright green color of the egg white during the early stages of development. This stage is difficult to observe with a candle, but is clearly visible when the egg is broken. Later, the yolk may disintegrate and mix with the egg white to mask the green. The odor is absent or fruity or "sweet". The contents of broken eggs fluoresce strongly under ultraviolet light. A second important group of rots are colorless rots, which can be caused by *Pseudomonas, Acinetobacter, Alcaligenes,* some coliform bacteria, or other types of bacteria. These rots are easily detected by candlelight, because the yolk is usually involved, except in the early stages, and it disintegrates or at least has a white clot. The odor ranges from barely noticeable to fruity or "very bad". The third important group of rots is black rot, where the eggs are almost dark under candlelight, because the yolks blacken and then decompose to turn the contents of the whole egg a muddy brown color. The odor is *putrid*, with visible hydrogen sulfide, and gas pressure may develop in the egg. *Proteus* species are most commonly the cause of these rots, although some species of *Pseudomonas* and *Aeromonas* can cause black rot. *Proteus melanovogenes** causes a distinctively black color of the yolk and a dark color of the white. The development of black rot and red rot generally means that the egg has at some point been kept at temperatures higher than those normally used for storage. Pink rots are less common and red rots are even rarer. Pink rot is caused by strains of *Pseudomonas* and can sometimes be a later stage of some green rots. It resembles colorless rot except for a pink to yellow precipitate and a pink to white color. Red sores, caused by *Serratia* species, have a mild odor and are not unpleasant.

Florian and Trussell (1957) listed rots caused by ten different species of the genera *Pseudomonas, Alcaligenes, Proteus, Flavobacterium* and *Paracolobactrum**. These decays were characterized by fluorescent, green and yellow, cream, black, red, rust red, colorless and mixed. These authors also list secondary invaders of the genera *Enterobacter, Alcaligenes, Escherichia, Flavobacterium* and *Paracolobactrum**. These bacteria can grow on the eggs, but can not initiate penetration.

Fungal spoilage of eggs occurs through stages of mold growth that give the defects their name. Very early mold growth is called spot mold because of the small, compact colonies of mold that appear and are usually confined to the shell. The color of these spots varies depending on the type of mold; *Penicillium* species cause yellow, blue, or green spots on the shell, *Cladosporium* species give dark green or black spots, and *Sporotrichum* species produce pink spots. In high- humidity storage environments, various molds can cause superficial fungal spoilage, initially as a haze or "whiskers" covering the shell and later as a more luxuriant growth. When eggs are stored at a temperature close to freezing, As is generally the case, the temperature is high enough to slow the mycelial growth of some molds, but too low for sporulation, while other molds can produce asexual spores. Molds responsible for egg spoilage include species of *Penicillium, Cladosporium, Sporotrichum, Mucor, Thamnidium, Botrytis, Alternaria* and other genera. The final stage of mold decay is mold rot, as mold mycelium has grown through the pores or cracks of the egg. This can result in white gel and color can be, for example, red fungal rot caused by *Sporotrichum* and a black color caused by *Cladosporium*, the cause of black spots on eggs, and also other foods. Fungal hyphae can weaken the yolk membrane enough to cause it to rupture, after which mold growth is strongly stimulated by the food released by the yolk.

17 Microbial Contamination and Preservation of Poultry Products

Microbial contamination of poultry products is a significant concern for both food safety and quality, as it can lead to spoilage and the potential growth of pathogenic microorganisms. Poultry, due to its high moisture content, nutrient- rich nature, and vulnerability to environmental conditions, provides an ideal medium for microbial growth. Common contaminants include bacteria such as *Salmonella, Campylobacter, Escherichia coli,* and *Listeria,* which pose serious health risks. These pathogens can enter poultry through various stages of production, from the farm to slaughterhouses, and during handling or processing in packing and distribution centers.

Preservation methods are essential to mitigate the risks associated with microbial contamination. Effective preservation strategies such as refrigeration, freezing, and chemical treatments are crucial to prolong the shelf life of poultry products while maintaining safety and quality. Refrigeration slows down microbial growth, whereas freezing halts it entirely, though careful management of thawing processes is vital. Additionally, methods like vacuum sealing, irradiation, and the use of antimicrobial agents can help control microbial loads, ensuring that poultry products reach consumers without compromising their health or taste.

Understanding the factors that contribute to microbial contamination and spoilage, such as the condition of the poultry when harvested, environmental conditions, and the specific processing techniques employed, is critical. This chapter will explore these key aspects, focusing on both the risks of microbial contamination and the various preservation techniques that can be implemented to ensure the safety and longevity of poultry products.

CONTAMINATION

The sources of contamination mentioned for meat also apply to poultry. The skin of live birds can contain an average of 1,500 bacteria per square centimeter. These numbers probably reflect the natural flora of the skin, as well as other organisms that may come from feet, feathers, and feces. Contamination of the skin lining and body cavity occurs during washing, skinning, and evisceration. Table 1 shows the number of microbes obtained during the different stages of processing. Of course, processing processes have changed since 1956. Chickens are currently processed by a fully automated conveyor or vacuum evisceration production line.

The number of bacteria varies greatly on the surface of chickens. However, this variation is greater between birds than between different areas of the same bird.

The types of organisms isolated depend on where the samples are collected and the stage of processing. Isolates from poultry and poultry products include members of several genera Offal (giblets, hearts and livers) are processed separately and the number and types of microorganisms present may differ from those in the carcass.

Table. Number of Microorganisms on Poultry and in Processing Waters

Point of sampling	Usual range ($\times 10^3$)*
Skin of live bird	0.6–8.1
Scald water (58.3–60°C)	5.9–17
Fresh chill water	50–210
Aerated chill water	34–240
Skin, after rough pick	8.1–45
After neck pick	3.3–32
After pinning	10–84
After singe	13–210
After evisceration	11–93
Cavity after evisceration	1.4–12
In chill tank	50–600
After aeration	3.4–240
Final product	4–330

*Counts on waters are per milliliter, on surfaces per square centimeter: Source- Walker and Ayres (1956).

Table. Geometric Means ($\log_{ig}$) of Aerobic Plate Counts Per Gram of Neck Skin at Different Stages of Processing*

Stage	Plant 1†	Plant 2‡
After picking	5.24	4.60
After eviseration	5.42	4.92
After spray washing	5.15	4.64
After immersion chilling	4.51	–
After air chilling	–	4.54
After packaging	4.72	4.52

*The report summarizes many plants; only two are presented for illustrative purposes: † This plant was using a countercurrent immersion chiller: ‡ This plant was using tunnel air chilling. Source: Commission of European Communities (1976).

Table. Microbiological Profile of Poultry

Micro-organisms	Commonly found locations	Potential hazards	Typical contamination source
Salmonella spp.	Internal organs, skin, feathers, and feces	Foodborne illness, gastroenteritis	Contamination from feces, improper handling
Campylobacter spp.	Intestinal tract, skin, and feathers	Gastroenteritis, fever, abdominal cramps	Contaminated water, improper slaughtering, handling
Escherichia coli	Gut, skin, and meat	Diarrhea, kidney failure, food poisoning	Contaminated water, improper handling, fecal contamination
Staphylococcus aureus	Skin, respiratory tract, gastrointestinal tract	Food poisoning, nausea, vomiting	Poor handling, improper refrigeration, infected workers
Clostridium perfringens	Gut and skin	Food poisoning, diarrhea, abdominal cramps	Improper cooking or storage, undercooking
Listeria monocytogenes	Meat and gastrointestinal tract	Listeriosis (serious infections)	Contaminated environment, improper handling or storage
Pseudomonas spp.	Skin, meat, and feathers	Spoilage, off- odor	Poor hygiene, improper storage
Yersinia enterocolitica	Gut and lymph nodes	Diarrhea, abdominal pain	Contaminated water, undercooking

The incidence of salmonellae on poultry carcasses and the role of poultry processing in transmitting salmonellosis have received considerable attention. The incidence of *Salmonella*-positive birds has been reported to range from 0 to 50 percent. There is also a high incidence of *Campylobacter jejuni* in poultry processing plants and on the processed bird.

PRESERVATION

Most of the principles of preservation discussed for meat in Chapter 14 also apply to poultry, although the harvesting and processing of poultry presents different problems. As with the slaughter of animals for meat, the methods of killing and bleeding poultry have a significant effect on the quality of the product. Modern methods involve slicing the jugular veins while the bird is suspended by its legs and draining the blood.

If the trachea is left intact, it is called an external incision; a kosher cut cuts the trachea. When birds are scalded, they may gasp, sucking the scalding water into their air sacs. Apparently, the kosher cut minimizes the absorption of boiling water because the cut end of the breathing tube is pulled under the skin. The method of harvesting or harvesting has some influence on the keeping quality of the bird. Dry- skinned birds are more resistant to decay than those that are half- burned or charred because the skin is less likely to break, but more feathers remain. In most cases, harvesting is done by the semi- scalding method, in which the birds are immersed in water at about 55°C for 2 minutes. Experiments have shown that water from the semi- boiled method is not a significant source of contaminating microorganisms if reasonable precautions are taken to change the water. Although the total number of bacteria may increase in the scalding water during processing, contamination of the birds is minimized by (1) the temperature of the scalding water, (2) the low initial bacterial count in some birds, and (3) a dilution effect due to the addition of fresh water to the scalding tank (Brune and Cunningham, 1971). The USDA requires a minimum of 1 quart per bird per minute.

Steam scalding of poultry is more effective than hot water in reducing bacteria, including coliforms and *salmonella*.

Asepsis

Comparatively little can be done to keep microorganisms from contaminating the dressed poultry. The sanitation of the housing of the birds before killing has some influence on the numbers of microorganisms on the skin at dressing, but even under the best conditions enough spoilage organisms contaminate the skin to permit microbial deterioration if conditions of handling and storage are not good. Contamination of the lining of the body cavity of the bird can be prevented if the fowl is not eviscerated until sold in the retail market, but visceral taints may develop unless the birds are adequately refrigerated. The shackles holding the feet and head of the fowl may be a source of heavy contamination. Contamination can be reduced if equipment is adequately cleaned and sanitized at intervals.

Use of Heat

Dressed chickens and other fowls may be canned, whole or dissected, in their own juices or in jelly. Heat processes are analogous to those for canned meats (Chapter 14). The chicken or other fowl may be salted in a weak brine before being packed into the glass jars or cans.

USE OF LOW TEMPERATURES

Most poultry is chilled or frozen. In both cases, it is essential to perform a rapid chilling immediately after hatching and remove the birds (if this has been done). Several commercial methods are used to immerse the birds in cold water, ice water, or crushed ice. Variations include a counterflow cooler, a counterflow drum cooler, and a rotating tank cooler, agitation of ice and water, jets of cold air or CO_2, or sprays of coolant or solid O_2. Cooling tanks can serve as a source of contamination if not properly controlled. A backflow system would be more effecti e in preventing the accumulation of germs because the fresh drinking water added to the cooler flows against the movement of the carcasses. Chlorine can be added to the water in the chilling tank to reduce the number of organisms. However, the effect of chlorine on carcass longevity is a matter of debate. Chilling with cold air jets will leave the birds relatively dry compared to those coming from chilling tanks. Increased moisture in the carcasses can not only favor the spread of organisms, but also promote their growth.

Freezing

Poultry can be kept in good condition for months if the freezing is rapid and the storage temperature is low enough. Rapid freezing is desirable because it produces a clear bird due to the formation of fine ice crystals in the fibers. Slow freezing, on the other hand, causes large crystals to form on the outside of the fibers and makes the meat appear darker. A bird quickly frozen while fresh will have smaller crystals than a bird frozen after a short time. Most commercially frozen chickens are packed ten to a paper box, sealed from moisture and air, and most are coated but not detailed.

Poultry must be frozen quickly enough to retain most of the natural color or appearance of the freshly prepared poultry. Storage temperatures should be below - 17.8°C and relative humidity above 95% to reduce surface drying. Most birds are frozen at about - 29°C or lower in circulating air or on a conveyor belt in a freezing tunnel. Quick freezing requires a smaller package, usually a whole bird, a cut bird, or a boneless bird, packed in a special waterproof and nearly airtight container. In fact, a large chicken would not freeze fast enough to meet the definition of quick freezing in Chapter 7

Although some bacteria are killed by the freezing process and their numbers slowly decrease during storage, enough remains to cause spoilage when the bird is thawed. . Bacterial growth can occur at the time of collection, dressing, removal, chilling, and even during the freezing process until the temperature of the poultry falls below 0°C. Spoilage that has developed due to bacterial growth, the diffusion of contaminants from internal organs, and the activity of poultry enzymes before freezing will be reflected in the frozen product. Even if bacterial growth is stopped, some enzymatic action will continue if the storage temperature is not too low.

If proper health precautions are not taken, A notable increase in bacteria occurs when bones are removed from cooked poultry for canning or quick freezing. Low-temperature bacteria of the genera *Proteus* and *Alcaligenes*, as well as coliform bacteria, have been found in significant numbers. Canning will destroy them, but quick freezing allows many to survive.

Chilling

Chilling storage of poultry is for only a short period, usually less than a month; birds to be stored longer should be frozen. Packing the dressed birds in ice has been used for short periods of holding and where mechanical refrigeration is not available. The lower the temperature of storage, the longer the birds can be stored without undesirable changes. In tests on cut- up chicken, Ayres (1959) found that compared with room temperature, storage life was extended 2 days at 10°C, 6 days at 4.4°C, and 14 days at 0°C.

Use of Preservatives

Feeding antibiotics to birds may lead to increased percentages of resistant microorganisms in the fecal matter and hence on the birds, although low levels of antibiotic may be deposited in the flesh. Low levels of antibiotic in the meat of treated birds are mostly destroyed by cooking.
Soaking cut- up poultry in solutions of organic acids (acetic, adipic, succinic, etc.) at pH 2.5 has also been reported to lengthen shelf life.

Turkey sometimes is cured in a solution of salt, sugar, and sodium nitrate for several weeks at about 3.3 °C, washed, dried, and then smoked. Usually a light smoking process is used, more for flavor than for preservation. Recommended temperatures during smoking range from 43.3 to 60 °C, and the time ranges from a few hours to several days.

Carbon Dioxide Atmosphere

Increasing carbon dioxide concentrations (10 to 20 percent) in the atmosphere of stored chickens inhibits the growth of psychrotrophs. Dry ice packed with the carcasses may serve as the source of the carbon dioxide. The use of films of both high and low gas permeability in combination with a carbon dioxide atmosphere is the significant factor in reducing microbial counts.

Use of Irradiation

Irradiation of poultry with cathode or gamma rays could be a successful preservation method since the rays apparently produce less objectionable change in appearance and flavor than in some other foods, but to date the method has not been practiced commercially. Radiation doses of 1 to 10 kilograys would reduce the microbial flora and extend the product's refrigerated shelf life. Chicken carcasses have been treated with 2.5 kilograys to effecti ely destroy salmonellae (Mulder et al., 1977).

SPOILAGE

Although poultry enzymes contribute to the spoilage of prepared poultry, bacteria are the primary cause of spoilage, with the intestines being the main source of these organisms. Work on bacterial spoilage of poultry has shown that most bacteria grow on the surface, i.e. on the skin, in the lining of the body cavity, and on any cut surface, and that the decomposition products are slowly distributed throughout the meat. Surface odor was noted when the number of bacteria on the skin was about 2. 5 million per square centimeter. This lasted about 4 weeks at 0° C and 5 weeks at 1.1°C in a series of experiments. Poultry excreta preserved at 10°C or below are spoiled mainly by Pseudomonas and, to a lesser extent, by yeast, for example. , *Torulopsis* and *Rhodotorula*. Above 10°C, micrococci generally predominate and growth of *Alcaligenes* and *Flavobacterium* is also observed. Over time, the surface of the meat usually becomes slippery. Small amounts (1 to 5 ppm) of iron in the bath water can induce bacterial growth on the surface and production of the fluorescent pigment pyoverdine by pseudomonads; higher amounts of iron will reduce pigmentation. Approximately 100 ppm of magnesium is optimal for pigment production by *P. fluorescens*.

Iced, cut- up poultry often develops a slime that is accompanied by an odor described as "tainted," "acid," "sour," or "dishraggy." This defect is caused chiefly by species of *Pseudomonas*, although *Alcaligenes* also may be concerned. Similar bacteria grow whether the temperature is as low as 0 °C or as high as 10 °C, and enormous numbers must be present, about 10^8 per square centimeter, before the odor becomes evident. The major species involved in spoilage are summarized in Table.

Table Major Bacteria Involved in the Spoilage of Refrigerated Poultry

Product	Bacteria	Reference
Raw eviserated carcasses	*Pseudomonas fluorecens*, *P. putida. Acinetobacter*, *Moraxella*	
Dark meat, pH 6.4 – 6.7	*Acinetobacter, Alteromonas, Pseudomonas*	Barnes and Impey (1968)
White meat, pH 5.7 – 5.9	*Pseudomonas* and others	Barnes and Impey (1968)
Chicken wrapped inoxygen impermeablefilm	Microaerophilic bacteria, lactic acid bacteria, and others	
Vacuum–packed chicken	*Enterobacter* and othes	Arafa and Chen (1975)

It should be kept in mind that chemical changes in poultry meat other than those caused by microorganisms occur during refrigerated storage and will in time reduce the quality.

18

Microbial Contamination and Preservation in Dairy Products

Milk and dairy products are highly nutritious and perishable foods that provide essential nutrients, including proteins, vitamins, and minerals. However, their high moisture content and rich nutrient composition make them ideal mediums for microbial growth. The microbial contamination of milk and its products is a significant concern, as it can lead to spoilage, reduced shelf life, and even pose health risks. Contaminants can be introduced at various stages, including during milking, handling, processing, and storage. Pathogenic microorganisms such as *Salmonella, Listeria,* and *Escherichia coli* can contaminate milk and cause foodborne illnesses. Additionally, spoilage bacteria like *Pseudomonas* and *Lactobacillus* can lead to undesirable changes, including souring, curdling, and off- flavors.

To prevent microbial contamination and spoilage, various preservation methods are employed, such as pasteurization, refrigeration, and fermentation. Pasteurization effecti ely kills harmful pathogens and extends the shelf life of milk, while refrigeration slows down microbial growth. Fermentation, which is used in the production of products like yogurt, cheese, and buttermilk, encourages the growth of beneficial bacteria that inhibit spoilage and enhance product safety. Understanding the types of microorganisms involved in contamination, the mechanisms behind spoilage, and the preservation methods available is essential for ensuring the safety and quality of milk and dairy products. This chapter will explore these aspects, providing insights into effecti e microbial control strategies in dairy production.

CONTAMINATION

On the Farm

Milk contains few bacteria when it leaves the udder of a healthy cow, and these bacteria do not usually grow in milk under normal processing conditions. However, micrococci and streptococci have been found in aseptic milk. However, during normal milking, milk is subject to contamination from the animal, especially from the outside of the udder and surrounding areas. Bacteria found in manure, soil, and water can enter this source. This contamination is reduced by clipping the cow's hair, especially on the arms and udder, grooming, and washing the udder with water or a microbial solution before milking. Contamination of cows from soil, water, and manure is reduced by lining and draining pens, preventing cows from wading in pools of standing water, and by cleaning manure from stalls or milking parlors.

Perhaps the two most important sources of contamination are milk containers and milk contact surfaces, including milk pails or milking machines, as appropriate, milk filters, cans or lines, and bulk milk coolers. If milk containers or milk contact surfaces are not cleaned, disinfected, and dried, bacteria can grow in large numbers in the diluted- like residue of milk and enter other milk that touches these surfaces. Unwanted bacteria from these sources include lactic acid streptococci, coliform bacteria, gram: negative psychrotrophic bacilli, and thermophilic bacteria, such as those that survive pasteurization. , micrococci*, enterococci, bacilli and brevibacteria*. In general, these bacteria grow well in milk and therefore compromise its storage quality. When properly cleaned and disinfected, milk contact containers and surfaces contribute few bacteria per milliliter of milk, but under very poor conditions these sources can increase the bacterial content of milk by millions per milliliter. The application of quaternary ammonium compounds as disinfectants tends to increase the percentage of gram-negative bacilli in the dishes. (psychrotrophs, coliforms), while hypochlorites favor gram- positive bacteria (micrococci*, bacilli). Modern milk contact containers and surfaces, especially milking machines, bulk milk lines and coolers, are designed to provide easy access for cleaning, disinfection and drying. The farm's bulk milk coolers are also equipped with excellent cooling and mixing capabilities to ensure adequate milk cooling.

Other possible sources of contamination are the hands and arms of the milker or dairy workers, the air of the barn or milking parlor, and flies. Normally these sources would contribute very few bacteria, but they might be a source of pathogens or spoilage microorganisms. The quality of the farm water supply used in the milking parlor for cleaning, rinsing, etc., will have some effect on the quality of the milk.

The numbers of bacteria per milliliter of milk added from the various sources depends on the care taken to avoid contamination. For example, the exterior of the cow contributes comparatively few organisms if precautions are taken and a milking machine is used, but under very poor conditions thousands per milliliter could enter the milk. Table 18.1 lists the approximate range of microorganisms usually found in milk at different points of sampling.

Table. Estimated Numbers of Microorganisms in Milk*

Point of sampling	Usual range (Microorganisms/ml)
Raw milk (from farm)	100,000 - 1,000,000
After milking (farm bulk tank)	10,000 - 100,000
After pasteurization (if not contaminated)	1 - 10,000
Milk stored in refrigerator	100 - 10,000
Milk at room temperature (unrefrigerated)	10,000 - 100,000
Milk from retail or packaging station	10 - 1,000
Raw milk from retail or processing plant	10,000 - 1,000,000

*This table provides general estimates of microbial counts at different points of milk handling and processing, which can vary based on factors like milk hygiene, handling practices, and storage conditions.

In Transit and at the Manufacturing Level

After milk leaves the farm, additional contamination can occur through sources such as the tanker truck, transfer pipes, sampling tools, and equipment at the market- milk plant, cheese factory, condensing plant, or other processing facilities. The primary culprits of contamination are the milk- contact surfaces. These include pipelines, vats, tanks, pumps, valves, separators, clarifiers, homogenizers, coolers, strainers, stirrers, and fillers, all of which can harbor bacteria. The extent of contamination from these sources is influenced by the cleaning and sanitizing procedures in place. Moreover, employees, especially their hands and arms, can also contribute to contamination. The paper packaging used for fluid milk is another significant source. It's important to remember that the number and types of microorganisms in milk or dairy products may increase due to either contamination or the growth of existing organisms. Production, handling, storage, and manufacturing methods are implemented to prevent both.

PRESERVATION

Milk is a highly perishable and subtly flavored food, making it difficult to preserve without causing undesirable changes or, at best, altering it into a different product. In fact, many milk or cream- based products were developed primarily to improve their shelf life. For example, nomadic tribes discovered that milk fermented through lactic acid could be stored for extended periods, though today we produce fermented milks for their unique texture and flavor. Similarly, various methods of processing milk curds were found to enhance their longevity, leading to the creation of various cheeses, each with its distinct qualities. Milk and its products, which serve as prime examples of food preservation and spoilage, have been extensively studied, with more research conducted on them than most other foods. Many texts and reference books have been published on the subject, and readers should consult these for more detailed information than what is covered here.

Asepsis

Preventing contamination of milk is important for its preservation. The keeping quality is generally improved when the number of microorganisms present is lower, especially those that grow readily in the milk. Although the type of microorganisms present is very important, in general, the lower the initial total microbial load, the better the storage quality of the milk. For example, a low microbial load, especially the number of spores present, is an important consideration to be taken into account in the case of milk to be treated with ultra-high temperature or commercial sterilization processes.

Since the number of bacteria in milk is indicative of the sanitary precautions and proper handling used during production, the bacterial content of milk is used to measure its sanitary quality and, historically, milk has been classified based on a method of estimating the number of bacteria in the milk. The exterior of the cow and the surfaces in contact with the milk have been highlighted as potential sources of a large number of undesirable microorganisms. Particular undesirable bacteria in commercial milk are bacteria that grow well in milk, for example lactic acid bacteria and coliforms; psychrotrophic bacteria, those that grow well at the refrigeration temperatures at which milk is usually stored; thermoactive bacteria, those that survive the pasteurization treatment of milk; and, of course, human pathogens. When milk is to be used as a substrate for microbial fermentation, as in the production of fermented milk or cheese, microorganisms capable of competing with the starter bacteria and producing defects in the product are very important. Thus, coliform, anaerobic and yeast bacteria can cause off- gassing and off- flavors in these products. Other organisms can inhibit the desired starter culture or cause defects in body, texture or taste. The presence of heat- resistant microorganisms or spores can be a potential source of spoilage in highly heat- treated milk, such as evaporated milk and condensed milk.

Packaging is used to protect packaged milk, fermented milk, packaged butter, canned milk, powdered milk and packaged cheese from microorganisms, as well as plastic, wax or other protective coatings on finished cheeses. The bacteriological quality of paper used in the production of paper milk cartons was examined. Normally, the packaging material contributes very little to the total microbial load of the finished product

Removal of Microorganisms

It is challenging to successfully eradicate microorganisms from milk once they have entered. Similar to clarifying or separating, centrifugation will eliminate some microorganisms from milk. About 99 percent of the spores and more than half of the bacterial vegetative cells, along with some protein, are eliminated by high-speed centrifugation (at 10,000 g). However, —a centrifugal process used to remove bacteria from milk—is not widely employed in the commercial sector. Some types of cheese can have molds physically removed from their surface during the curing process by scraping or washing the cheese occasionally, but other than these rare situations, physical removal is challenging.

Use of Heat

Pasteurization and Ultrapasteurization

Because milk and cream are easily spoiled by heat, a mild heat treatment called pasteurization is used to preserve them. Historically, milk was initially treated with heat to increase its shelf life. When it became clear that milk could be a source of foodborne illness, pasteurization became a necessary protective measure. The purposes of liquid milk pasteurization are (1) to kill any pathogens that may enter the milk and be transmitted to humans and (2) to improve the keeping quality of the milk. Ideally, this thermal treatment should be carried out without affecting the taste, appearance, nutritional properties or creaminess of the milk. When milk is pasteurized to make cheese or cream is pasteurized to make butter, a third purpose is to destroy microorganisms that might interfere with the activity of desired organisms, such as starter cultures, or cause inferiority or spoilage of the product. Cheese also ensures that the heat treatment does not damage the curd properties of the milk. Heat treatment of cream also destroys lipases that can cause spoilage of butter during storage

The first widely used milk pasteurization process involved heating the milk in large containers or vats to 60°C for at least 20 minutes. This storage method was later modified to 61.7 °C for 30 min and finally at 62.8 °C for 30 min to eliminate *Coxiella burnetii*, a rickettsia responsible for Q fever that can be transmitted in milk. This was not a continuous process and was called vat pasteurization. The use of plate heat exchangers and continuous operation involves the high- temperature short- time pasteurization (HTST) process at a temperature of at least 72 °C for at least 15 seconds. The HTST system is the most widely used commercial pasteurization process today. However, most processors heat their product beyond the minimum temperature and time. For example, many pasteurize milk at temperatures close to 79°C for 20 to 25 seconds. The primary goal is to reduce the total microbial load and thus increase the shelf life of the product. Recent outbreaks of illness attributed to milk and other dairy products have implicated *Listeria monocytogenes* as the causative agent . It has been questioned whether the minimum temperatures and times of HTST pasteurization are sufficient to eliminate *L. monocytogenes* from milk and other dairy products.

Heat treatment processes beyond pasteurization for milk and dairy products are defined as very high temperature (VHT) and ultra high temperature (UHT) systems. There does not appear to be a precise definition for a VHT system. According to the International Milk Federation, UHT processes generally refer to pasteurization techniques with temperatures of at least 130°C in continuous flow, with holding times of approximately 1 second or more. States for liquid milk. Current federal standards for identification state that a product must be heated to

137.8°C or higher and held at that temperature for at least 2 seconds to be labeled "ultrapasteurized." Products such as whipped cream, coffee cream, and half- and- half are processed by UHT systems. The current disadvantage of UHT systems is that the intense heat required can affect or change the nutritional and organoleptic properties of the product. The most popular UHT systems are direct heating methods, specifically a method of injecting the stick into the milk and a method of injecting the milk into the steam, respectively called the steam injection technique and the steam infusion technique. In both systems, the added steam or excess water is removed after heat treatment in a sterile vacuum chamber. The combination of this type of heat treatment with aseptic packaging results in a product category generally referred to as "sterilized milk" or "sterilized cream". This designation does not imply absolute sterility but a sterile product in the commercial sense. These products have an extremely long shelf life. Sterilized fluid milk or milk product must be packaged in containers that maintain the "sterility" of the product and its shelf life. In the United States, some processors guarantee that their sterilized milk products have a shelf life of more than 6 weeks. With a convenient combination of effecti e sterilization, aseptic packaging, and refrigeration, it would not be unusual for these types of products to last more than 90 days.

The effecti eness of milk pasteurization, or the reduction in microorganism numbers during the process, depends on several factors- (1) the pasteurization temperature, (2) the holding time, (3) the initial bacterial count, and (4) the proportion of spore- formers or thermoduric organisms within the total microbial load. Generally, the conventional HTST (High- Temperature Short- Time) system reduces microbial counts by 90 to 99 percent. After pasteurization, milk is rapidly cooled to 7.2°C or lower. The shelf life of pasteurized milk is influenced by the storage temperature and the types and numbers of microorganisms that survive the process.

Cream for butter- making undergoes a more intense heat treatment than market cream, typically heated to 71.1°C for 30 minutes using the holding method or 87.7 to 93.3°C for a few seconds via HTST. Cream is more protective of microorganisms than milk, and thus, cream for butter- making may have a higher microbial load. Rapid heating is achieved by injecting steam or through vacreation, a process combining steam injection and evacuation.

The pasteurization process for sweetened condensed milk involves forewarming at 71–100°C for 10–30 minutes, followed by evaporation at 48.9–57.2°C, which eliminates pathogens and spoilage organisms. Similarly, high-temperature pasteurization is applied to bulk condensed milk with preheating at 65.6–76.7°C before evaporation and superheating at 82.2–93.3°C.

Processed cheese production involves cooking at 65.6°C or higher, effecti ely pasteurizing the cheese. Conventional pasteurization eliminates yeasts, molds, and most vegetative bacterial cells, leaving behind thermoduric bacteria. These bacteria belong to various groups, with spore- forming thermodurics, such as *Bacillus* and *Clostridium* species, being of particular concern as pasteurization temperatures increase to extend shelf life.

Steam under Pressure

Evaporated milk is canned and then heat- processed by steam under pressure, often with accompanying rolling or agitation. The forewarming of the milk at about 93 to 100 °C or higher before evaporation kills all but the more resistant bacterial spores. Sealed cans of evaporated milk are processed at about 115 to 118 °C for 14 to 18 min, which results in a commercially sterile product. Some of the heat- cool- fill methods, e.g., the Martin process mentioned in Chapter 6, have been applied to the processing of canned whole milk cream, and whole milk concentrate.

Use of Low Temperatures

With the exception of canned milk and dry milk, most dairy products require the use of low temperatures as one factor in their preservation; often this is the most important factor.

Refrigerated Storage

For the production of milk of good quality it is essential that it be cooled promptly after it is withdrawn from the cow. The Grade A Pasteurized Milk Ordinance of the United States Public Health Service stipulates that Grade A raw milk for pasteurization shall be cooled to 10°C or less within 2 hr after being drawn and kept that cold until processed. Newly pasteurized milk is to be cooled to 7.2°C or less and maintained there. It is preferable, of course, to cool it to temperatures well below 7.2°C. For example, the bulk- milk coolers on farms can rapidly cool milk to 3.0 to 4.5°C or lower and hold that temperature, except for short periods when fresh milk is entering, and then the temperature usually does not exceed 7.2°C. Also, it is not unusual to find the temperature of milk as it is being filled into milk cartons or bottles approaching 2 to 3°C.

Table. Storage Conditions and Shelf Life of Various Dairy Products

Product	Temperature, °C	RH, %	Approximate storage period
Chesse			
Blue	0- 1.1	70	3- 6 months
Cheddar	0- 1.1	70	12 months
Cream	0- 1.1	70	4 week
Pasteurized processed	0.4.4		6- 10 months
Swiss	0- 4.4	70	8- 12 months
Milk			
Evaporated and condensed	0		+1 year
	4.4		6- 12 months
	10		Few months
	21.1		Few weeks
HTST	1.6- 4.4		2- 3 weeks
	4.4- 7.2		1- 2 weeks
	1.6- 4.4		+1 months
UHT	4.4	60	10 months
Nonfat dry milk	21.1	60	5 months
	37.7	60	2 months

Milk is held at refrigeration temperatures during storage on the farm, in the truck or tank during transportation to the plant or receiving station, and during storage there. Refrigeration temperatures are recommended for the milk or related products during storage in the plant or in the retail market and during delivery and in the home or restaurant until consumption. Fermented milks and unrip- ened cheeses are chilled after their manufacture and kept chilled until they reach the consumer. Most kinds of ripened cheese also are stored at chilling temperatures after their ripening is complete. Table 18.2 lists some recommended storage temperatures for various dairy products.

Freezing

Ice cream and other frozen dairy desserts undergo freezing during production and are stored at low temperatures, which prevent microbial growth. The microbial content of the ingredients—such as milk, cream, sugar, eggs, stabilizers, and flavorings—along with any contamination introduced during processing, determines the type and quantity of microorganisms in the mix. While pasteurization reduces microbial numbers and types, freezing does not eliminate many microorganisms, and storage at freezing temperatures allows most microorganisms to survive for extended periods.Butter is stored at temperatures between −17°C and −18°C, which inhibits microbial growth. Similarly, frozen cream is kept at these temperatures. Milk that is concentrated to one- third of its volume can be frozen at −17°C to −18°C and stored at −23°C to −24°C or lower, remaining stable for weeks without quality loss. Frozen milk can also be concentrated using freeze- drying techniques. Pasteurized whole milk has been frozen at approximately −28°C to −29°C for shipping and storage while maintaining its frozen state.

Drying

Various milk products are made by removing different percentages of water from whole or skim milk. Only in the manufacture of dry products is enough moisture removed to prevent the growth of microorganisms. The reduction in moisture and consequent increase in the concentration of dissolved substances in liquid condensed- milk products inhibits the growth of some kinds of bacteria.

Condensed Products

Evaporated milk is produced by removing approximately 60 percent of the water from whole milk, resulting in a product with about 11.5 percent lactose in solution, along with twice the amount of soluble inorganic salts compared to whole milk. This high sugar concentration inhibits the growth of certain bacteria, potentially preventing the growth of survivors from previous heat treatments. Bulk condensed milk, being more concentrated than evaporated milk, serves as an even less favorable environment for microorganisms that cannot tolerate high sugar levels. Similarly, condensed whey, known as whey semisolids, and condensed buttermilk, or semisolid buttermilk, are concentrated dairy products, with higher concentrations of acid and other solutes due to the condensation process.

In the production of sweetened condensed milk, sugar (mainly sucrose, occasionally glucose) is added to whole milk before evaporation, resulting in a sugar content of around 54 percent, with over 64 percent in the liquid part. Sweetened condensed milk made from skim milk contains about 58 percent total sugar and 66 percent in the liquid part. The very high sugar concentration, combined with increased soluble inorganic salts, binds moisture, making it inaccessible to all but osmophilic microorganisms. Therefore, drying—through water removal and binding—is a primary preservation method. The sealed can also provides an aseptic environment, ensuring the product remains stable and has a good shelf life.

Dry Products

Dairy products that are prepared in dry form include milk, skim milk, cream, whey, butter ilk, ice cream mix, and malted milk. While similar principles apply to most of these products, dry skim milk or nonfat dry milk solids serve as a typical example. Most dry milk is produced using the roller process, with or without vacuum, or the spray process discussed in Chapter 8. Before the final drying, the milk is concentrated by three to fi e times for the roller process and two to three times for the spray process. The milk is typically preheated before drying to 65–85°C for the roller process and 68.8–93.3°C for the spray process. This preheating serves as pasteurization, killing less heat- resistant microorganisms. Modern methods for manufacturing nonfat dry milk optimize conditions for better solubility and flavor. Some drying processes include an instantization step, where the dry powder is wetted and redried. In this process, the product is exposed to air at nine stages. A salmonellosis outbreak linked to powdered milk occurred due to air contamination during this process.

The microbial content of heat- dried dairy products depends on the liquid product's initial content, preheating time and temperature, evaporation, contamination during storage, the drying method, and air contamination. Preheating pasteurizes the milk, killing most microorganisms except thermodurics. Evaporation can increase thermoduric and thermophilic bacteria. If the evaporated product is stored, microorganisms may increase. The roller process, with its high temperature, destroys nearly all organisms except bacterial spores. However, spray- drying alone cannot guarantee the elimination of microorganisms, especially thermoduric bacteria, like heat- resistant streptococci, micrococci, aerobic and anaerobic sporeformers, and microbacteria. Outbreaks of food poisoning from milk powder, including those caused by *Salmonella* and *Staphylococcus*, show that these pathogens sometimes survive in the final product.

Use of Preservatives

Added Preservatives

The addition of preservatives to dairy products is permitted only to a limited extent. The use of sorbic or propionic acid or one of their salts is permitted in cottage cheese, yoghurt and certain hard and processed cheeses. The main purpose of adding a preservative to hard or preserved cheeses is to prevent the growth of mould on the surface of the product. Similarly, the addition of preservatives to cottage cheese and yoghurt is done to prevent the growth of mould on the surface of the product and to extend its shelf life.

Added sugar acts as a preservative in sweetened condensed milk; it reduces aw, making moisture unavailable to microorganisms. Sodium chloride or common salt is added to the production of various types of cheese, but it is generally used more for flavor or to control the growth of microorganisms during production and ripening than to preserve the finished product

Sodium chloride in salted butter is present in the liquid phase at a concentration sufficien to inhibit the growth of many bacteria and to cause a reduction in the number of those that do not tolerate salt. In butter containing 16.34 percent moisture and 2.35 percent salt, the water phase would be about 12. 6% brine salt.

The cheese is smoked primarily for flavor, although drying, especially of the rind, and chemical preservatives from smoking can improve its preservation. Deterioration of cheese by mold is generally delayed or prevented when sorbic acid, sorbates, propionic acid, or propionates are added or incorporated into the shell.

The addition of hydrogen peroxide combined with a mild heat treatment has been used to pasteurize milk for some types of cheese (e.g. , Swiss and Cheddar). Excess peroxide is usually destroyed by the addition of catalase.

Developed Preservatives

Most fermented products are microbiologically more stable or have a longer shelf life than the initial substrate. Fermented milks and cheese are preserved partly by the developed acidity produced by the bacterial culture and therefore have a longer shelf life than fluid milk.

Other Methods

Although an effect equal to pasteurization can be obtained by treating milk with ultraviolet rays, this method is not used for milk preservation because only a thin layer of milk can be successfully irradiated and, unless great precautions are taken, it will result in "burning." "taste. . Other uses of ultraviolet light in the dairy industry include ambient irradiation to reduce the number of microorganisms in the air of processing rooms where sweetened condensed milk is prepared. where sliced cheese is packaged and in cheese ripening rooms. The rays prevent mold growth on the sides of ripened cheese that are directly exposed to them, but are not effecti e on the shaded side. Ultraviolet light is also used in storage tanks containing liquid sugar or corn syrup (an ingredient in ice cream) to prevent mold from growing on the surface.

Several preservation factors are included in the storage of milk and its products. Milk intended for sale on the market or for the production of dairy products is produced as aseptically as possible, cooled rapidly and kept fresh. It is pasteurized, then packaged to prevent the penetration of microorganisms. Cream is processed in the same way. Fermented milks owe most of their keeping qualities to the acid formed during fermentation, but they require refrigeration and storage conditions. Butter is mainly stored at low temperatures, in the refrigerator for short-term storage or frozen for long- term storage. Low moisture and salt content also aid in preservation, as does packaging or sealing to prevent contamination. Cheese is preserved by the acidity produced during its production, by refrigeration, and by rind or impermeable packaging. Powdered milk, if properly prepared, contains very little moisture for microbial growth, but requires packaging to prevent contamination. Evaporated milk is boiled to kill all or most microorganisms and sealed in cans to keep out contaminants. Sweetened condensed milk is pasteurized during its preparation, contains a high concentration of sugars, and is protected by a sealed can.

SPOILAGE

As has been indicated, milk and products made from it are preserved in a number of different ways, some of which involve killing only part of the microorganisms present and inhibiting the growth of the remainder. Some products therefore have a limited keeping time, and many spoil readily if the methods of preservation are inadequate.

Milk and Cream

Milk is an excellent medium for the growth of many types of microorganisms because it is high in moisture, has an almost neutral pH, and is rich in microbial nutrients. An abundant food source for energy is present in the form of milk sugar (lactose), butter fat, citrates and nitrogenous compounds in many forms (proteins, amino acids, ammonia, urea and other compounds), as well as supplementary foods necessary minerals. for microorganisms are available. Some inhibitory substances (lactoperoxidase and agglutinin) are present in freshly expressed milk, but they quickly become relatively ineffecti e. Because of the fermentable sugar, acid fermentation by bacteria is more likely under ordinary conditions in raw milk, but other changes can occur if the conditions are unfavorable for acidifiers or if they are absent. With the trend towards higher pasteurization temperatures, the spoilage flora of pasteurized milk more often become heat- resistant bacilli, which form spores that can be psychotrophic.

When milk turns sour, it is generally considered spoiled, especially if curdled. Signs of acid formation are fir t a sour taste, then curdling of the milk to produce a firm, gelatinous curd or a weaker curd that exudes clear whey. Lactic acid fermentation is most likely to occur in raw milk stored at room temperature.

In raw milk at temperatures between 10 and 37 °C, Streptococcus lactis is most likely to cause sourness, with possibly an increase in coliform bacteria, enterococci, lactobacilli and micrococci*. At higher temperatures, e.g. For example, at 37 to 50°C, *S. thermophilus* and *S. faecalis* can produce about 1 percent acid and are followed by lactobacilli, such as *Lactobacillus bulgaricus**, which produce more acid. Some lactobacilli can grow at temperatures above 50°C, but produce less acid there. Thermophilic bacteria can grow at even higher temperatures, for example *L. thermophilus**. Some forms of acid in milk stored at temperatures near freezing, but proteolysis can occur. Pasteurization of milk kills most active acid-forming bacteria, but may allow the survival of heat- resistant lactic acid bacteria (e.g., enterococci, *Streptococcus thermophilus*, and lactobacilli), which will cause lactic acid fermentation if the subsequent storage temperature is high enough.

Many bacteria other than those called lactic acid bacteria can cause acid fermentation in milk, especially if conditions are unfavorable for lactic acid bacteria. Coliform bacteria produce lactic acid and significant amounts of volatile products, such as hydrogen, carbon dioxide, acetic acid, formic acid, alcohol, etc. *Micrococcus**, *Microbacterium*, and *Bacillus* species can produce acid in milk, primarily lactic acid, but they generally cannot compete with lactic acids.

Butyric acid can be produced in milk by the action of *Clostridium* spp. under conditions that prevent or inhibit the normal formation of lactic acid. Thus, after a heat treatment that destroys all vegetative bacterial cells but allows the survival of *Clostridium* spores, milk can undergo butyric fermentation with the production of hydrogen and carbon dioxide.

Gas Production

Gas production by bacteria is usually accompanied by acid formation and, with few exceptions, is undesirable in milk and milk products. The main gas generators are coliform bacteria, *Clostridium* spp. , *Bacillus* species that form gas producing hydrogen and carbon dioxide, and heterofermenting yeasts, propionic and lactic acid, which produce only carbon dioxide. Gas production in milk is evidenced by foam on the surface if the milk is runny and supersaturated with gas, by gas bubbles trapped in the curd or emptying, by floating curds containing gas bubbles, or by rupture of the curd by rapid production. . of gas, causing what is known as stormy milk fermentation.

The possibility of gas formation and the type of microorganisms that cause it depends on the pretreatment of the milk and the storage temperature. In raw milk, coliform bacteria are more likely to be the main gas generators. Heterofermentative lactic acid bacteria can also produce gas, but are usually not as visible in the milk. Yeasts (lactose fermenters) are usually absent or in small quantities in milk and do not compete well with the bacteria.

Gas- forming Clostridia and Bacilli do not compete well with acid- forming bacteria at higher temperatures, but can function if the acid- forming bacteria are absent or relatively inactive. Thus, in milk heated to pasteurization temperatures or higher, the main acid generators will be killed, spores of *Clostridium* and *Bacillus* species will survive, and gas formation by sporogenous bacteria may occur. Propionic acid- forming bacteria are not active in milk, but they do form gas (carbon dioxide) in cheese, as we will see later.

Proteolysis

Hydrolysis of milk proteins by microorganisms is generally associated with the production of a bitter taste caused by some of the released peptides. Proteolysis is favored by low- temperature storage, by the destruction of lactic acid and other acidifiers by heat, and by the destruction of acid formed in milk by molds and yeasts on the skin or by the neutralization of acid by products of other organisms.

The types of changes produced by proteolytic microorganisms include (1) acid proteolysis, in which acid production and proteolysis occur together, (2) proteolysis at low acidity or even alkalinity, (3) sugar scavenging, which is caused by bacterial renin- like enzymes at an early stage of proteolysis, (4) slow intracellular proteolysis. enzymes of bacteria after their autolysis, and (5) residual proteolytic activity of thermostable proteinases. For example, *Pseudomonas fluorescens* produces a proteinase that survives pasteurization even though it is not a bacterium.

Acid proteolysis results in the production of curdled curds and the expression of a large amount of whey. The curd undergoes slow digestion, changing its appearance from dark to translucent, and can be completely digested by some types of bacteria. Sometimes separate curd particles are formed, which are so small that they are barely visible in the large mass of milk. Acid proteolysis can be caused by several species of *Micrococcus**, some of which grow in the udder of cows and cause acid proteolysis of aseptically expressed milk. One of the intestinal streptococci or enterococci, *Streptococcus faecalis* var. *liquefaciens**, is a lactic acid organism that is also actively proteolytic. It is thermostable, like other enterococci, and can cause acid proteolysis in pasteurized milk. Spores of proteolytic strains of lactose fermenting bacteria of some *Bacillus* species can survive pasteurization or more rigorous heat treatment of milk and cause acid proteolysis.

Proteolysis by bacteria incapable of fermenting lactose varies depending on the bacteria involved, from apparent digestion of casein to slight proteolysis that can only be detected by chemical testing. Most of these bacteria produce little or no acidity; in fact, milk generally becomes alkaline over time from protein products. Many of these bacteria gently "skim" the milk (coagulate but slightly acidic) before digesting the casein, but others hydrolyze the protein so rapidly that it does not curdle. visible and ultimately a fairly clear liquid remains without any sign of casein or curd. Active proteolytic bacteria are found among the species of *Micrococcus**, *Alcaligenes*, *Pseudomonas*, *Proteus*, *Flavobacterium*, and *Serratia*, all of which are nonsporulating bacterial genera, and the genera Bacillus and *Clostridium* of spore- forming bacteria. Some species of the genera *Micrococcus**, *Pseudomonas*, *Alcaligenes**, *Flavobacterium*, and *Bacillus* can grow at low temperatures and are therefore likely to cause some proteolysis and/or bitterness in milk stored at refrigerated temperatures. *Bacillus cereus* is included in the sweet curd of pasteurized milk. This spoilage state has become more common in milk due to (1) higher pasteurization temperatures, (2) the psychrotrophic capacity of some bacilli, and (3) longer storage or holding times. Coagulation or curd formation generally begins at the bottom of the carton and may not even be visible to the consumer in its early stages.

Slow proteolysis by intracellular enzymes of bacteria after their autolysis is not important in milk under ordinary circumstances, but is important when a lot of time is allowed to act, as in cheese processing or in long- life products.

Ropiness

Ropiness and sliminess can occur in milk, cream, or whey, though they are most significant in market milk and cream. Nonbacterial ropiness or sliminess may result from (1) stringiness caused by mastitis, particularly from fibrin and leukocytes from the cow's blood (unlike bacterial ropiness, it is present when the milk is drawn and not developed during storage), (2) sliminess due to the thickness of cream, such as at the top of a bottle, and (3) stringiness caused by thin films of casein or lactalbumin during cooling, sometimes seen on surface coolers. This effect is usually temporary

Bacterial ropiness is caused by slimy capsular material from the cells, usually gums or mucins, and tends to develop most effectively at low storage temperatures. The ropiness generally decreases as the acidity of the milk or cream rises. There are two primary types of bacterial ropiness- one where the milk is most ropy at the top, and the other where the milk becomes uniformly ropy throughout. Surface ropiness is most commonly caused by *Alcaligenes viscolactis,* an organism typically found in water or soil, which can grow effectively at temperatures around 10°C. Some thermoduric micrococci, such as *Micrococcus freudenreichii,* can also lead to surface ropiness. Ropiness throughout the milk may be caused by a variety of bacteria, including: *Enterobacter aerogenes, E. cloacae, Klebsiella oxytoca,* and occasionally *Escherichia coli.* Ropiness from *Enterobacter* is typically worse near the top of the milk.

Certain strains of common species of lactic acid bacteria. *Streptococcus lactis* var. *hollandicus* causes ropiness in milk and is used in the production of Scandinavian fermented milk. *Lactobacillus casei, L. bulgaricus,* and *L. plantarum* occasionally cause ropiness, as do strains of *Streptococcus cremoris*. Many of these lactic bacteria grow in long chains, a feature believed to contribute to the stringy nature of the milk.

Other miscellaneous bacteria among alkali formers, micrococci, streptococci, and bacilli. Typically, these bacteria would be suppressed by acid- forming organisms.

As the bacteria causing ropiness typically come from water, manure, utensils, and feed, reducing or eliminating contamination from these sources is essential to preventing ropiness. Proper pasteurization of milk effecti ely destroys most of these bacteria.

Changes in Milkfat

Milkfat may be decomposed by various bacteria, yeasts, and molds that do not constitute distinct groups on the basis of other characteristics. The bacteria are for the most part aerobic or facultative, proteolytic, and non- acid- forming. The following changes in the milkfat take place:

- Oxidation of the unsaturated fatty acids, which, coupled with other decomposition, yields aldehydes, acids, and ketones and results in tallowy odors and tastes. The reaction is favored by metals, sunlight, and oxidizing microorganisms.

- Hydrolysis of the butterfat to fatty acids and glycerol by the enzyme lipase. The lipase may have been in the original milk or may be microbial.
- Combined oxidation and hydrolysis to produce rancidity.

Species of lipase- forming bacteria are found in many of the bacterial genera e. g., *Pseudomonas, Proteus, Alcaligenes, Bacillus, Micrococcus**, *Clostridium*, and others. Many of the molds and some species of yeasts are lipolytic. *Pseudomonas fragi* and *Staphylococcus aureus* produce fairly heat- resistant lipases which may survive pasteurization if present in the raw milk.

Flavor changes

The flavor of milk as drawn is low, delicate, and easily altered. Since individuals differ in their ability to detect flavors and disagree in their description of them, a number of more or less- descriptive terms have been suggested to name the off- flavors. As drawn from the cow, milk may be abnormal in flavor because of the individual cow, mastitis, the stage of lactation of the cow, or feed.

Off- flavors caused by microorganisms

Sour or Acid Flavor: The acidity may be described as "clean," as produced by *Streptococcus lactis* and other lactics; as "aromatic," when lactic streptococci and aroma- forming *Leuconostoc* species are growing together; and as "sharp," when appreciable amounts of volatile fatty acids (formic, acetic, or butyric) are produced by coliform bacteria, *Clostridium* spp., and other organisms. Clean and aromatic flavors are desired in fermented milk products, but sharp flavors are undesirable.

Bitter Flavors: Bitterness usually results from proteolysis but may follow lipolysis or even fermentation of lactose. Milk from cows late in their lactation period sometimes is slightly bitter. Microorganisms causing proteolysis and hence bitterness have been mentioned in a previous paragraph. Other organisms causing bitterness are certain strains of coliform bacteria and of asporogenous yeasts. Some cocci cause very bitter milk, and actinomycetes sometimes give bitter- musty flavors.

Burnt or Caramel Flavor: Certain strains of *Streptococcus* lactis var. *maltigenes* produce this flavor, which resembles the cooked flavor of overheated milk.

Miscellaneous Other Flavors: Other flavors that are found less commonly make up a long list, only part of which will be mentioned- a barny flavor by *Enterobacter oxytocum**; soapiness by ammonia formers like *Pseudomonas sapolactica**; a turniplike flavor by *Escherichia coli* and *P. fluorescens*; a malty flavor by yellow micrococci from the udder; fruity flavor by *P. fragi*; a potatolike flavor by *P. muci- dolens*, fishiness by *Aeromonas hydrophila* or various cocci that produce trimeth- ylamine from lecithin; earthy or musty flavors by actinomycetes; fruity, esterlike, and alcoholic flavors by yeasts; an amyl alcohol flavor by white and orange micrococci; and putrefaction by species of *Clostridium*, *P. putrefaciens**, and other putrefactive bacteria. Other flavors have ben termed unclean, stale, astringent, oily, weedy, carroty, etc.

Inadequately cooled raw milk that has been held in a tightly covered can so that volatile products of bacterial metabolism have collected above the milk has an undesirable odor that varies in nature. Milk in this condition is termed smothered.

Alkali Production

The group of alkali formers includes bacteria which cause an alkaline reaction in milk without any evidence of proteolysis. The alkaline reaction may result from the formation of ammonia, as from urea, or of carbonates, as from organic acids such as citric acid. Most of these bacteria grow from moderate to low temperatures, and many can survive pasteurization. Examples of alkali formers are *Pseudomonas fluorescens* and *A. viscolactis**.

Color Changes

The color of milk or cream is affected by its physical and chemical composition, e.g., by the amount and yellowness of the butterfat, the thinness of the milk, the content of blood and pus, and the feed of the animal. Color changes caused by microorganisms may occur along with other changes previously discussed, but some special changes in color should be mentioned. The color may be due to the surface growth of pigmented bacteria or molds in the form of a scum or ring or may be present throughout the milk.

- **Blue Milk:** *Pseudomonas syncyanea** produces a bluish- gray to brownish color in milk in pure culture but when growing with an acid former like *Streptococcus lactis* causes a deep- blue color. This defect and the blue color produced by actinomycetes or species of the mold *Geotrichum* are rare.
- **Yellow Milk:** *Pseudomonas synxantha** may cause a yellow color in the cream layer of milk, coincident to lipolysis and proteolysis. Species of Flavobacterium can also give yellowness.
- **Red Milk:** Red milk usually is caused by species of Serratia, e.g., S. marcescens, but is rare because other bacteria ordinarily outgrow the red-pigmented species. *Brevibacterium erythrogenes** produces a red layer at the top of the milk, followed by proteolysis. *Micrococcus roseus* may grow and produce a red sediment, and yeast may produce pink or red colonies on the surface of sour milk or cream. Blood in milk will give it a red color. The red blood cells settle out or can be centrifuged out.
- **Brown Milk:** A brown color may result from *Pseudomonas putrefaciens** or by the enzymic oxidation of tyrosine by *P. fluorescens.*

Spoilage of Milk at DifferentTemperatures

At any given storage temperature, most raw milk samples undergo a series of changes due to a succession of microorganisms. At refrigeration temperatures, proteolysis may begin with psychrotrophic bacteria like *Pseudomonas*, followed by the appearance of molds. At room temperature, an acid fermentation is most likely to occur, initially by lactic streptococci and coliform bacteria, followed by acid- tolerant lactobacilli. Molds or film yeasts on the surface lower the acidity, allowing more acid to form. Eventually, when most of the acid is consumed, proteolytic or putrefactive bacteria complete the decomposition.

Commercial pasteurization using HTST systems eliminates yeasts, molds, most psychrotrophic bacteria, coliforms, and rapid acid producers like *Streptococcus lactis*. The spoilage of pasteurized milk thereafter depends on:

- The surviving bacteria, known as "thermodurics" and sporeformers.
- Bacteria that enter the milk after pasteurization due to postpasteurization contamination from equipment, the filling process, or the packaging
- The potential presence of heat- resistant microbial enzymes.
- The storage temperature.

Once pasteurized milk is sealed in a carton, the microbial population is established unless the carton is compromised. Therefore, storage temperature determines which organisms will dominate and the rate of spoilage. The initial number and types of microorganisms present after pasteurization also affect spoilage rates, given a fixed storage temperature. Since milk is refrigerated, spoilage is typically caused by psychrotrophic organisms. While growth at low temperatures is slow, it can still be significant. For example, assuming an 8- hour generation time at 7°C, one cell could grow into a population of 1 million in about 6 to 7 days, or 2 million in 7 to 8 days, and 1 billion in 10 days.

Given the high- quality refrigeration milk (both raw and pasteurized) is exposed to and the increasing use of higher pasteurization temperatures, it is reasonable to expect highly heat- resistant psychrotrophic organisms to be a challenge in pasteurized milk. The current spoilage issues with pasteurized milk are largely associated with spore- forming psychrotrophic bacilli.

Condensed and Dry Milk Products

This category includes evaporated milk (unsweetened), bulk condensed milk, frozen milk, sweetened condensed milk, condensed whey or buttermilk, and condensed sour skim milk, as well as dry milk. The quality of these products is directly linked to the quality of the raw materials used for drying or condensation, as any defects in the raw materials will be carried over into the final product. All condensed products have a relatively high concentration of solutes, which helps inhibit the growth of certain bacteria. Dry milk, being extremely low in moisture, does not present microbial spoilage issues when handled correctly. However, if the moisture content exceeds 8 percent, mold growth may occur. The spoilage of condensed buttermilk and sour skim milk is mainly caused by mold growth when exposed to air, as the high concentration of acid and solutes prevents the growth of bacteria or yeasts.

Evaporated Milk

Unsweetened evaporated milk is canned and heat- processed under steam pressure to eliminate microorganisms. Spoilage can occur if the heat process is insufficien or if the can is compromised, allowing organisms to enter. Bacterial spores that survive the heat treatment can lead to can swelling, milk coagulation, or the development of a bitter taste.Can swelling is typically caused by gas- forming anaerobic sporeformers like *Clostridium,* though overfilling with cold milk can also cause swelling. The reaction of milk's acid components with the iron of the can can produce hydrogen gas, leading to bulging during prolonged storage.

Coagulation in the can can range from small flakes to a solid curd, usually due to species of *Bacillus,* such as *B. cereus, B. subtilis, B. megaterium, B. coagulans,* or B. calidolactis. The degree of curd formation is influenced by the amount of air in the can. Thermophilic spoilage should not be an issue if the milk is cooled quickly and kept cool, but can be problematic in tropical regions.Bitterness is often a result of proteolysis by *Bacillus* species, and less frequently by *Clostridium.* Some *Clostridium* species may also cause putrefaction in rare cases. Spoilage caused by leakage, evident through the presence of nonsporeformers, can lead to gas and swelling from coliform bacteria or yeasts, coagulation by streptococci, or bitterness caused by cocci.

Sweetened Condensed Milk

Sweetened condensed milk has been subjected to a fairly high temperature (71.1 to 100°C) during forewarming and to a milder heat treatment (48.9 to 54.4°C) during condensing, so that the yeasts, molds, and most of the vegetative cells of bacteria are destroyed. In addition, there is a high concentration of sugar, about 55 to 60 percent of total sugar (lactose plus added sugar). Also, the can is evacuated and sealed. Spoilage, then, is due primarily to organisms that have entered after the heat treatments, especially if air is present. The chief types of spoilage are (1) gas formation by sucrose- fermenting yeasts or, more rarely, by coliform bacteria, (2) thickening caused by micrococci, which probably produce renninlike enzymes, and (3) "buttons," which are mold colonies growing on the milk surface. The size of these buttons is determined by the amount of air in the can. Species of *Aspergillus,* e.g., *A. repens,* and of *Penicillium* have been incriminated.

Bulk Condensed Milk

The forewarming temperatures employed in the making of plain condensed milk are equivalent to no more than pasteurization, and the evaporating process is at a temperature low enough to permit the growth of thermophiles. Therefore, although refrigerated, this product has only a short storage life and is subject to spoilage by thermoduric bacteria that tolerate the increases concentration of solutes in the condensed product. In superheated condensed milk the temperature of the milk is raised to 65.6 to 76.7°C during the introduction of steam, a process that probably destroys most of the vegetative cells of bacteria but not the spores. This product, too, has a short storage life.

Frozen Desserts

Frozen desserts, such as ice cream, ice milk, frozen custards, sherbets, and ices, are made from various combinations of ingredients like milk, cream, evaporated milk, condensed milk, dried milk, coloring materials, flavors, fruits, nuts, sweeteners, eggs, egg products, and stabilizers. These ingredients may introduce microorganisms into the product, influencing its bacterial content or the presence of specific bacteria, such as coliforms. However, these desserts typically do not spoil as long as they are kept frozen. Spoilage is primarily a concern before the ingredients are mixed or within the mix itself prior to freezing. Since the mix is pasteurized before freezing, spoilage is unlikely unless the mix is stored above freezing temperatures for an extended period, allowing acid- forming bacteria to cause souring.

Butter

Many defects in butter arise from the cream used to make it, particularly when the cream is stored for several days on the farm before being collected by the creamery. During this time, lactic acid bacteria, gas producers, and other spoilage organisms may grow, often followed by molds like *Geotrichum candidum.* Occasionally, lactose- fermenting yeasts can develop high gas pressures in the cream cans. In fact, most types of spoilage described earlier for milk can also affect the cream and, consequently, the butter produced from it

The likelihood and type of spoilage depend on the type of butter and the conditions under which it is stored. Salted butter, with its high salt concentration and minimal moisture, is less prone to microbial growth than unsalted butter. Sweet- cream butter generally has a longer shelf life compared to sour- cream butter. Nowadays, most butter is made from pasteurized cream, which eliminates most spoilage organisms. Additionally, butter is often kept refrigerated, typically at about −17.8°C during commercial storage, where microbial growth is prevented. As a result, bacterial growth in butter is rare, and even when it does occur, it is not extensive. However, since the flavor of butter is very delicate, even small amounts of bacterial growth can lead to noticeable flavor deterioration

Flavor Defects

Undesirable flavors in butter can arise from several sources, including the cream itself, which may pick up flavors from the cow's feed, absorb odors from the atmosphere, or develop undesirable tastes during microbial growth. Feeds such as onions, garlic, French weed, peppergrass, and poor silage can impart off- flavors to the cream. Volatile compounds from the air, such as barn odors or chemicals like kerosene, gasoline, fly sprays, and disinfectants, can also affect flavor. Microbial growth in the cream or milk can lead to various bad flavors, including

- **Cheesiness :** caused by lactobacilli
- **Metallic flavors** due to dissolved metals in highly acidic cream
- **Flat lavor :** caused by *Pseudomonas* species destroying diacetyl
- **Highly acidic flavor :** due to excessive acidity in the cream
- **Rancidity :** resulting from lipolytic bacteria, molds, or lipase in the cream
- **Barny lavor :** produced by *Enterobacter* species

- **Malty flavor :** caused by *Streptococcus lactis* var. *maltigenes*
- **Yeasty flavor :** produced by yeasts
- **Musty flavors :** caused by molds and actinobacteria
- **Unclean flavor :** caused by coliform bacteria

Processing errors can lead to additional flavor defects, such as a cooked flavor from over- pasteurization or a "neutralizer" flavor if too much neutralizing compound is used or unevenly distributed.

Butter can also absorb volatile substances from the air, and microorganisms in butter can cause the following defects

- **Surface taint (rabbito or putridity) :** caused by *Pseudomonas putrefaciens*, typically introduced by wash water or equipment. This is more common in unsalted or low- salt butter
- **Fishiness :** caused by *Aeromonas hydrophila*
- **Esterlike flavors :** due to *P. fragi*
- **Skunklike flavors :** caused by *P. mephitica*
- **Roquefortlike flavors** produced by molds

Chemically produced flavors include

- **Rancidity :** due to lipase in the cream
- **Tallowiness :** caused by oxidation of unsaturated fats, influenced by copper, bacterial enzymes, low pH, low- temperature pasteurization, salt, air, and ozone
- **Fishiness :** where trimethylamine is produced from lecithin, especially when the butter has high acidity, is o erworked, or contains copper.

Color Defects

Some color defects in butter are not caused by microorganisms and include issues such as mottling due to improper working, a pink hue resulting from the sulfur dioxide used as a refrigerant, surface darkening caused by water loss from the surface layers, and bleaching that occurs alongside tallowiness.Discolorations, primarily on the surface, may be caused by molds, yeasts, or bacteria originating from various sources such as churns, wrappers, liners, tubs, the air, or unpasteurized cream.

Molds can cause colored growths that lead to smudged or *Alternaria*- type discoloration, characterized by dark, smoky, or occasionally greenish areas where fungi like *Alternaria* or *Cladosporium* have grown, or small black spots caused by *Stemphylium*. *Penicillium* molds produce green hues, while *Phoma* or *Alternaria* molds cause brown discolorations, and *Geotrichum* (also known as *Oospora*) species result in orange or yellow spots. *Fusarium culmorum* is known to cause bright reddish- pink patches. Yeasts can sometimes form pink colonies, and *Pseudomonas nigrifaciens* causes the reddish: brown "black smudge" in mildly salted butter.

19 Microbial and Chemical Changes in Canned Foods

Canned foods can undergo microbial and chemical changes if preservation methods are compromised. Improper sealing or processing may allow spore-forming bacteria like *Clostridium botulinum* to survive, leading to spoilage and toxin production. Chemical changes, such as oxidation, can alter flavor, color, and nutritional quality, especially if cans are damaged or improperly stored. Acidic foods may react with the metal lining, causing discoloration and off-flavors To prevent these changes, cans must be processed at appropriate temperatures, sealed properly, and stored under cool, dry conditions to maintain safety and quality.

Canned foods are designed to offer long shelf lives by using heat processing techniques to destroy harmful microorganisms and inactivate enzymes that could lead to spoilage. However, despite the careful processing methods, microbial and chemical changes can still occur in canned foods, which may affect their quality and safety. These changes can be the result of improper canning techniques, insufficien heating, or post-processing contamination. One of the most common microbial causes of spoilage in canned foods is the survival of heat-resistant spores, particularly those of *Clostridium* and *Bacillus* species. These bacteria are capable of surviving the canning process and can lead to gas production, souring, or putrefaction of the food.

Molds and yeasts can also contribute to spoilage, especially in cans with compromised seals. While microorganisms are a major contributor to spoilage, chemical reactions also play a significant role. Oxidation is one of the most common chemical changes, particularly in canned fruits, vegetables, and meats, which leads to flavor alterations, color changes, and loss of nutrients. Furthermore, enzymatic activity may continue to affect the food even after the canning process, especially if the food was not heated sufficientl or the temperature was not properly controlled. This chapter explores the complex interaction between microorganisms and chemical reactions in canned foods, examining the processes that lead to spoilage and quality degradation. Understanding these changes is crucial for improving canning methods, ensuring food safety, and extending the shelf life of these products.

As discussed in Chapter 6, the heat treatments applied to foods for preservation can range from a gentle pasteurization process, like that used for milk or fruit juice, to full commercial sterilization through pressurized steam, as seen with canned vegetables or soups. Clearly, the less intense the heat treatment, the more heat-resistant the microorganisms must be to survive, and the greater the variety and quantity of organisms that may persist. There is always the potential for a surviving microorganism to proliferate and lead to spoilage if the conditions allow.

CAUSES OF SPOILAGE

Spoilage of heated foods can be caused by either chemical, biological, or a combination of both factors. The most significant type of chemical spoilage in canned foods is hydrogen swelling, which occurs due to the pressure of hydrogen gas produced by the reaction between the food's acid and the iron of the can. Hydrogen swelling is more likely with (1) increased food acidity, (2) higher storage temperatures, (3) flaws in the can's tinning or lacquering, (4) inadequate exhaust, and (5) the presence of soluble sulfur and phosphorus compounds. Other issues related to the interaction between the can's steel base and its contents include (1) discoloration of the can's interior, (2) discoloration of the food, (3) off-flavor in the food, (4) cloudiness in the syrup or liquids, (5) corrosion or perforation of the metal, and (6) a decrease in nutritional value.

Biological spoilage of canned foods by microorganisms can occur due to two primary causes: (1) organisms surviving the heat treatment, and (2) leakage of the container post-heat process, allowing microorganisms to enter. Mild heat treatments may only be sufficien for short-term storage with the aid of additional preservation methods, such as refrigeration. Surviving microorganisms can include several types, even vegetative cells. Acid foods processed at temperatures near 100°C kill all vegetative cells and most bacterial spores, leaving only heat-resistant bacterial spores. Container leaks may allow various microorganisms to enter, potentially causing spoilage. Leakage may stem from mechanical damage, rough handling, or contamination during the cooling process.

APPEARANCE OF THE UNOPENED CONTAINER

The ends of a food can are typically referred to as flat, though they are actually slightly concave, with a partial vacuum inside. When pressure builds up within the can, it undergoes several stages of distortion due to the increasing pressure, and the can is classified as a flipper, springer, soft swell, or hard swell. A flipper can have flat ends, but one end becomes convex when the can is struck sharply or when the contents are heated. A springer features bulging ends, and while both ends may remain concave if pressed, one end will pop out if a swollen end is pushed in. The terms "flipper" and "springer" are sometimes used to describe slight pressure changes caused by factors like poor exhaust, overfilling, dents, or temperature fluctuations, but similar outward signs can appear when gas is produced by either microbial or chemical causes, or a combination of both. A soft swell shows bulging ends, but the gas pressure is low enough that the ends can be dented manually. A hard swell is marked by high internal pressure, making the can too firm to dent by hand, often leading to distortion or buckling of the ends or side seam. The final stage is the can bursting, usually at the side seam, though sometimes at the end seals. A breather is a can with a tiny leak, allowing air to move in and out without necessarily letting microorganisms enter

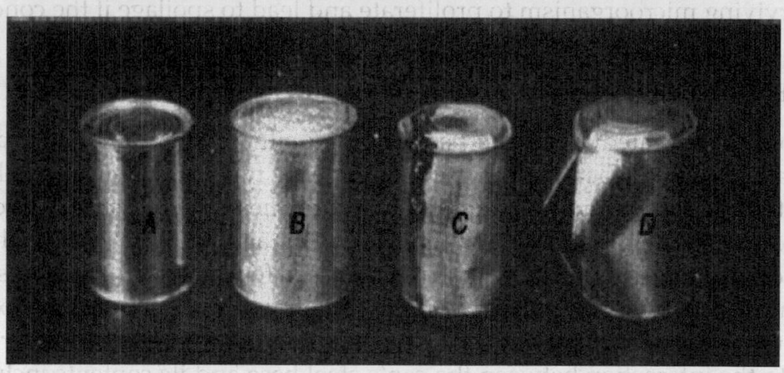

Fig. 19.1. Normal can of food and swells- (A) normal can with concave ends, (B) swollen can with ends bulged out, (C) swollen can with leakage where seams are breaking, (D) a burst can. (In Microbiology- General and Applied, 2d ed., by William Bowen Saiies, William Carroll Frazier, Joe Bransfield ilson, and Stanley Glenn Knight. Copyright © 1951, 1956 by Harper & Row, Publishers, Inc. By permission of the publisher.)

Other defects in the general appearance of the can are noted before and after it is opened- dents, which may be responsible for a flipper; rust; perforations; defective side seam or end seals; and corrosion.

The glass container of food under gas pressure may have its cover bulged or popped off or may show leakage of food through the broken seal. Of course, it is possible to see evidence of microbial growth through the glass sides, such as gas bubbles, cloudiness, and films of growth.

FORMS OF MICROBIAL SPOILAGE IN CANNED FOODS

The spoilage of canned foods by microorganisms is typically categorized into two main types- those caused by thermophilic bacteria and those caused by mesophilic microorganisms. Additionally, spoilage can be classified based on the specific changes it causes in the food, such as putrefaction, acid production, gas formation, and discoloration. Another way to categorize spoilage is by the type of food affected. The three most significant types of biological spoilage in commercially canned foods are flat sour spoilage, TA spoilage, and putrefaction. A fourth notable type of spoilage occurs due to the interaction between food acids and the iron of the can, leading to hydrogen swell.

Types of Spoilage by Thermophilic Spore-forming Bacteria

Most spoilage of commercially heat processed canned foods resulting from under-processing is caused by thermophilic bacteria because their spores are more heatre-sistant than those of most mesophilic bacteria. The three chief types of spoilage by thermophiles are flat sour spoilage, TA spoilage, and sulfide spoilage, or "sulfide stinker."

Flat Sour Spoilage

This kind of spoilage derives its name from the fact that the ends of the can of food remain flat during souring, or the development of lactic acid in the food by the flat sour bacteria. Because the can retains a normal outward appearance, this type of spoilage cannot be detected by examination of the unopened can but must be detected by cultural methods. The spoilage occurs chiefly in low-acid foods, such as peas and corn (group I), and is caused by species of *Bacillus*. Flat sour spoilage of acid foods, e.g., tomatoes or tomato juice, is caused by a special facultatively thermophilic species, *B. coagulans*. The various species of *Bacillus* that are able to form acid without gas in food may be mesophiles, facultative thermophiles, or obligate thermophiles. The spores of the mesophiles are the least heat-resistant and are usually killed by the heat processing and hence are rarely concerned with flat sour spoilage of low-acid foods. The spores of the thermophiles, on the other hand, are considerably more heat-resistant and may survive the heat process to cause flat sour spoilage. Surviving thermophiles, such as *B. stearothermophilus*, would not cause spoilage unless the food were held hot for a while, as in slow cooling or storage in the tropics, but facultative thermophiles could grow at ordinary temperatures. The immediate source of the flat sour bacteria is usually the plant equipment, e.g., the blanchers, but they may come originally from sugar, starch, or soil.

The ability of *B. coagulans* to grow in tomato juice depends on the number of spores present, the availability of oxygen, and the pH of the juice. The organism, which is homofermentative under almost anaerobic conditions and heterofermentative under aerobic conditions, can grow in low concentrations of oxygen.

TA Spoilage

The bacterium that causes this kind of spoiling has been dubbed *Clostridium thermosaccharolyticum*, or *TA* for short, which stands for "thermophilic anaerobe not producing hydrogen sulfide." Acid and gas are produced in food by this thermophilic spore-forming anaerobe. If held at a high temperature for an extended period of time, the gas—a mixture of hydrogen and carbon dioxide—swells the can and may eventually cause bursting. The spoiled food typically smells sour or "cheesy." The same sources as for flat sour bacteria are used.

Sulfide, or "Sulfur Stinker," Spoilage

This spoilage, caused by *Desulfotomaculum nigrificans*, is found, and then uncommonly, in low-acid foods such as peas and corn. The spores of this bacterium have considerably less heat resistance than those of flat sour and TA bacteria; hence their appearance in canned foods is indicative of gross underprocessing. The organism is an obligate thermophile and therefore also requires poor cooling of the heat-processed foods or hot storage for its development. It is detected by means of the black (FeS) colonies it forms in an iron sulfite agar at 55 C. Hydrogen sulfide, formed in the canned peas or corn, is evident by odor when the can is opened. In corn, a bluish-gray liquid is evident in which blackened germs and gray kernels of corn float. Peas usually give the H_2S odor but without any marked discoloration.

Sources of the spores are similar to those for flat sour and TA bacteria, but manure can also be an original source.

Types of Spoilage by Mesophilic Spore-Forming Bacteria

Most spoilage by mesophilic microorganisms that results from underprocessing is caused by spore-forming bacteria of the genera *Bacillus* and *Clostridium*, but lightly heated foods, e.g., some acid ones, may permit the survival of, and spoilage by, non-spore-forming bacteria or even yeasts or molds.

Spoilage by Mesophilic *Bacillus* Species

The heat resistance of spores from different *Bacillus* species varies significantly, with mesophilic spores generally being less heat-resistant than thermophilic ones. While most mesophilic spores are destroyed in a short time at temperatures of 100°C or lower, some can survive the heat treatments used in steam-pressure processing. However, the surviving spores do not always lead to spoilage, as the conditions inside the can may not be conducive to germination and growth. Many *Bacillus* species are aerobic, meaning they cannot thrive in a well-evacuated container. Additionally, the food's acidity or other environmental factors might hinder bacterial growth. Despite this, there have been instances of *Bacillus* species such as *B. subtilis* and *B. mesentericus* growing in low-acid, home-canned foods processed at 100°C. *Bacillus* species have been known to spoil commercially canned foods, especially when the cans are poorly evacuated. These spoilage cases have primarily been in canned seafood, meats, and evaporated milk. Gas-forming Bacillus species, such as B. polymyxa and B. macerans, have been linked to spoilage in canned vegetables like peas, asparagus, and tomatoes, though it's uncertain if they survived the heat treatment, with leakage from the container being a potential source of contamination. The heat resistance of these spores is similar to that of *Clostridium pasteurianum*.

Spoilage by Mesophilic *Clostridium* Species

Species of *Clostridium* may be sugar-fermenting, e.g., *C. butyricum* and *C. pasteurianum*, and cause the butyric acid type of fermentation in acid or medium-acid foods, with swelling of the container by the carbon dioxide and hydrogen gas produced. Other species, such as *C. sporogenes*, *C. putrefaciens*, and *C. botulinum*, are proteolytic or putrefactive, decomposing proteins with the production of malodorous compounds such as hydrogen sulfide, mercaptans, ammonia, indole and skatole. The putrefactive anaerobes also produce carbon dioxide and hydrogen, causing the can to swell. The spores of some of the putrefactive anaerobes are very heat resistant; therefore, putrefaction joins flat sour and TA spoilage in constituting the chief types of biological spoilage of canned foods resulting from underprocessing.

Because the spores of the saccharolytic clostridia, sometimes called "butyrics," have a comparatively low heat resistance, spoilage by these anaerobes takes place most commonly in canned foods which have been processed at 100°C or less, as are many of the commercially canned acid foods and home-canned foods processed by the hot-water, flowing-stream, or oven methods. Thus, canned acid foods such as pineapple, tomatoes, and pears have been found spoiled by *C. pasteurianum*. Such spoilage is more likely when the pH of the food is above 4.5. Home-canned foods heated to about 100°C may be spoiled by the saccharolytic bacteria with the production of butyric acid, carbon dioxide, and hydrogen.

The putrefactive anaerobes grow best in the low-acid canned foods, such as peas, corn, meats, fish, and poultry, but on rare occasions may spoil other foods. One of the putrefiers, *C, botulinum,* is a cause of food poisoning and will be discussed in Chapter 24.

Spoilage by Non-spore-forming Bacteria

If viable, non-sporulating bacteria are found in canned foods, or a very mild heat treatment has been used for bacteria that have entered the container through a leak. The vegetative cells of some types of bacteria are sufficiently heat-resistant to withstand pasteurization. Among these thermoregulatory bacteria are enterococci, *Streptococcus thermophilus,* some species of *Micrococcus,* and *Lactobacillus* and *Microbacterium**. Acidifying strains of *Lactobacillus* and *Leuconostoc* have been found to grow in canned tomato products, pears, and other fruits. Heterofermenting species can release enough CO_2 gas to cause the skin to swell.

Micrococci* have been reported in meatballs and similar products with very low heat penetration, and *S. faecalis* or *S. faecium* are often present in canned jams that are only partially sterilized and may be responsible for spoilage during storage.

In general, however, the presence of viable, non-sporulating bacteria in heat-treated canned foods indicates a leak in the container. Since cooling water is most often the source of contamination, the types of bacteria found in water generally cause spoilage of leaking cans. Some of them, such as coliform bacteria, produce gas that causes the milk to swell.

The small hole through which the bacteria enter is apparently blocked by a food particle, allowing gas pressure to build up in the can. It is worth noting that sporulated bacteria can also get into the can through a leak, so that aerobacilli (*B. macerans* and *B. polymyxa*) or clostridia may be responsible for the gas formation. Non-spore-forming bacteria often grow in food in leaky milk, along with spore-forming bacteria or alone. It is certainly possible that only one type of bacteria can enter the food, to grow an apparently pure culture. Spore-forming and non-spore-forming bacteria that can enter food include those of the genera *Pseudomonas, Alcaligenes, Micrococcus, Flavobacterium, Proteus,* and others. Agents that are not common spores, other than those present in water, can enter through leaks in cans and cause spoilage.

Spoilage by Yeasts

Because yeast and its spores are easily killed by most pasteurization treatments, their presence in canned foods is the result of mishandling or leakage. Canned fruits, jams, jellies, fruit juices, syrups, and sweetened condensed milk are spoiled by yeast fermentation, where the milk is blown by the CO_2 produced. Skin yeast may grow on the surface of pickled pork, pickles, or repackaged olives and similar products, but its presence indicates recontamination. or lack of heat treatment, as well as poor evacuation.

Spoilage by Molds

Mold is probably the most common cause of spoilage in home canned foods because it enters the container through a leak. Jams, jellies, marmalades, and fruit preserves allow mold to grow when the sugar concentration reaches 70% and acidity is usually present in these products. It has been reported that adding soluble extract of jam to 70-72% sugar in the presence of 0.8-1.0% normal acid virtually eliminates the risk of mold spoilage. Species of *Aspergillus, Penicillium,* and *Citromyces,* found in jelly and candied fruit, are capable of growing in sugar concentrations up to 67.5%. Acidification to pH 3 inhibited the growth of the first two molds, and heating the food to 90°C for 1 min killed all strains. Some fungi are quite resistant to heat, especially those that form tight masses of mycelium called sclerotia. *Byssochlamys fulva,* a pectin-fermenting mold, has ascospores that are resistant to heat treatment of bottled and canned fruits and has caused their spoilage. The high sugar content of fruit syrups helps protect microorganisms from heat, and this protective effect is enhanced if the sugar and fruit are added separately to the can, thus localizing the sugar during processing.

Spoilage of Canned Foods of Different Acidities

The previous discussion has indicated that the grouping of commercially canned foods on the basis of pH divides them also on the basis of the chief types of spoilage to be expected. Thus, the low-acid foods with a pH above 5.3 are especially subject to flat sour spoilage and putrefaction. Foods with a pH between 5.3 and 4.5 are likely to undergo TA spoilage. High-acid foods with a pH between 4.5 and 3.7 usually are spoiled by a special flat sour bacterium or by a saccharolytic anaerobe. High-acid foods with a pH below 3.7 ordinarily do not undergo spoilage by microorganisms, but in cans may become hydrogen swells (as may other high-acid foods).

Spoilage of Canned Meats and Fish

Canned meats and fish generally experience two primary types of spoilage- (1) spoilage by *Bacillus* species, leading to softening and souring, and (2) spoilage by *Clostridium* species (such as *C. sporogenes*), resulting in putrid swells. In rarer instances, *Bacillus* species may generate acid and gas, causing the cans to swell. Even non-spore-forming bacteria have been found in some canned products. In addition to spoilage caused by spore-forming organisms that survive the heat process, spoilage can also occur from organisms that enter through leaks. Canned cured meats, such as ham or luncheon meats, which undergo heat processing insufficient for sterilization, may be susceptible to the production of gases like carbon dioxide, nitrogen oxides, or nitrogen gas by *Bacillus* species (e.g., *B. licheniformis, B. coagulans, B. cereus,* or *B. subtilis*) from the interaction of nitrates, sugars, and meat. Alternatively, they can undergo putrefaction, with gas production by *Clostridium* species. This type of spoilage is typically prevented by proper refrigeration. Gas production can also be caused by heterofermentative lactic acid bacteria (e.g., *Leuconostoc* species) but only after inadequate processing. Spoilage without gas production but accompanied by souring and changes in color and texture may be due to *Bacillus* species or homofermentative lactic acid bacteria (e.g., *Streptococcus faecium* or *faecalis*).

Unusual Types of Spoilage of Canned Foods

Certain types of spoilage seem to be limited to one or two kinds of food. Sulfide spoilage has been reported only for peas and sweet corn. Black beets are caused by the mesophilic *Bacillus betanigrificans** in the presence of a high content of soluble iron. This is distinct from the darkening resulting from a deficiency of boron in the soil. *Bacillus* species can cause bitterness, acidity, and curdling in canned milk, cream, and evaporated milk. The only important alkaline canned vegetable, hominy (pH 6.8 to 7.8), undergoes flat sour spoilage which is characterized by a sweetish taste. Canned poultry is more often spoiled by putrefactive than by saccharolytic clostridia, chiefly because of the lower heat resistance of spores of the latter.

Canned sweetened condensed milk may becomes gassy because of growth of yeasts or coliform bacteria, may become thickened by a *Micrococcus** species, or may exhibit buttons, which consist of small masses of mold mycelium and coagulated milk usually on the surface of the milk. The size of the buttons is limited by the quantity of free oxygen in the head space of the can.

Food cans that have clearly experienced biological spoilage may occasionally contain no living organisms due to autosterilization. Every vegetative cell, including sporeformer cells that did not sporulate, has perished.

Figure describes a method for determining the reason behind a canned food's spoilage. Only common types of spoilage are covered by this scheme.

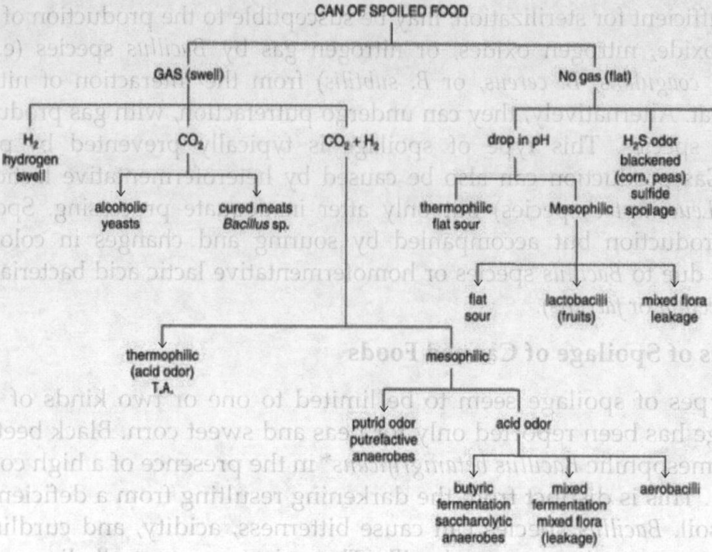

Fig 19.2. Scheme for diagnosis of cause of spoilage of a canned food.

Diverse Food Categories

20

This chapter includes foods that do not fall into the previously discussed categories, such as fatty foods, salad dressings, essential oils, bottled soft drinks, spices and other condiments, salt, and nutmeats. Food products created by combining various food groups may combine their microbial contents, which could provide a favorable environment for microorganisms that otherwise had limited growth opportunities. For example, yeast from sugar added to bottled soft drinks may lead to spoilage. Bottlers of carbonated beverages maintain bacteriological standards for sugar, limiting mesophilic bacteria to no more than 200 per 10 grams and restricting yeast or mold counts to under 10. Water and flavoring materials can also be potential contamination sources. Spices and condiments, while sometimes treated with propylene oxide gas or irradiated to reduce microbial content, can still be significant sources of microorganisms. Ingredients like spices, condiments, eggs, and pickles contribute to microbial presence in salad dressings. Salt, particularly solar salt, can introduce halophilic and salt-tolerant bacteria into salted fish and other salted or brined products

FATTY FOODS

Salad Dressings

Salad dressings contain oil, which can be oxidized or hydrolyzed, and sufficien moisture to permit microbial growth. However, in most cases, their acidity (approximately pH 3 to 4) is too high for most bacteria, but favorable for yeast or mold. Eggs or egg products, pickles, relishes, chilies, sugar, starch, meats, gelatin, spices, and other ingredients can add microorganisms, sometimes in significant numbers, and can make the salad dressing more conducive to microbial growth. The three types of spoilage of mayonnaise and similar salad dressings are (1) separation of oil or water from the emulsion, (2) oxidation and hydrolysis of oils by chemical or biological action, and (3) growth of microorganisms that produce gas. - off-flavor, or other defects. Darkening is often foun

Decomposition of salad and similar products can be caused by bacteria, yeast or mold. The acidity, linked to the sugar content, averages about 4.5% in the aqueous phase of mayonnaise, it is particularly favorable for yeasts, which are responsible for gas. *Zygosaccharomyces* and *Saccharomyces* strains have spoiled mayonnaise, salad dressing and French vinaigrette. The bacteria must be acid tolerant to break down most types of sauces. So it is not surprising to learn that a heterofermenting lactobacillus resembling *Lactobacillus brevis* causes gas in a salad dressing. More surprising is the ratio of *Bacillus* species, for example *B. subtilis* and *B. megaterium,* as organisms that cause gas, spoilage, and decomposition because they are not acid tolerant. Yeasts that grow with *B. megaterium* may be responsible for the gas. Darkening and separation of the Thousand Island habit with a pH of 4.2 to 4. 4 *B. vulgatus** molds originating from pepper and paprika have been reported. The mold can grow in salad dressings if air is present and is encouraged by the addition of starch or pectin to the dressing. A comprehensive study on the microbiology of mayonnaise and salad dressing by Smittle (1977) should be consulted for further details.

Fats and Oils

The fatty portions of foods, foods consisting primarily of fats and oils, and the fats and oils themselves are more often subject to chemical than microbial spoilage. In addition to fatty glycerides, natural fats and oils usually contain small amounts of fatty acids, glycerol or other liquid alcohols, sterols, hydrocarbons, proteins and other nitrogenous compounds, phosphatides, and carotenoid pigments. The main types of change result from hydrolysis, oxidation, or a combination of the two. the process. The terms applied to the various types of spoilage are often used quite broadly, although when applied to the spoilage of a specific type of fat or oil they may have a precise meaning. The term rancidity is sometimes used to refer to any change in fats or oils that is accompanied by an undesirable taste, regardless of the cause. Deterioration by oxidation, whether chemical or microbial, is called oxidative rancidity, as opposed to changes resulting from hydrolysis, e.g., lipases originally present or those originating from microorganisms, causing hydrolytic degradation. Significant oxidation, usually after hydrolysis and release of fatty acids, may result in ketone breakdown. Off-flavo is defined as the appearance of off-flavor due to less oxidation than that required to produce spoilage. Oils containing linolenic acid, fish oil, and vegetable oils, for example, are subject to flavor in ersion.

The oxidation of fats and oils can be catalyzed by various metals and rays and by moisture and even by microorganisms; such oxidation is prevented or delayed by natural or added antioxidants. Lipase hydrolysis produces fatty acids and glycerol or other alcohols. Fats that undergo one or both of these types of changes may contain oxyfatty acids and hydroxy acids, glycerol and other alcohols, aldehydes, ketones and lactones; in the presence of lecithin, they may contain trimethylamine, with its fishy odor

Butter and meat fats become "rancid" after oxidation, but butterfat is said to be spoiled when only hydrolysis to fatty acids and glycerol has occurred

Some of the pigments produced by microorganisms are fat-soluble and therefore can dissolve in fat, producing stains ranging from yellow to red, purple and brown. The best known is the fat stain of meat due to marking dye, which Jenson (1937) and others have shown to be caused by micrococci* and yellow pigmented bacilli. The fat-soluble pigment is an O-R indicator that changes from yellow to green, blue, and finally purple as the fat is further oxidized by peroxides formed by bacteria. Yellow, pink, and red fat-soluble pigments can be produced by many bacteria, yeast, and molds.

Bacteriostatic and bactericidal properties have been claimed for many fixed vegetable and animal oils, but most of them, like fats, can be hydrolyzed and oxidized by microorganisms. These fats are usually too low in moisture, a condition that favors mold more than other microorganisms. Molds cause oxidative and hydrolytic decomposition that leads to spoilage. The bacteria that cause butter to spoil cause a similar defect in olive oil. Bacteria capable of breaking down fats include *Pseudomonas, Micrococcus**, *Bacillus, Serratia, Achromobacter**, and *Proteus* species; and among molds, *Geotrichum, Penicillium, Aspergillus, Cladosporium,* and *Monilia* species. Some yeasts, especially pellicle yeasts, are lipolytic. Dill and cocoa butter can be spoiled by mold.

ESSENTIAL OILS

The plant kingdom is the source of essential oils, also known as volatile oils, which are products with concentrated flavoring and odorous properties. As food ingredients, such as mustard, cinnamon, garlic, and onion oils, these don't cause spoiling but, on the contrary, may have some preservative effects. The majority of them have no effect on microorganisms' ability to withstand heat

Bottled Beverages

The spoilage of alcoholic beverages will be discussed in Chapter 22. How easily soft drinks spoil and the type of spoilage depends on the composition of the soft drinks. Carbonation is inhibitory, even germicidal, to some microorganisms, and the acidity resulting from carbonation and the addition of acids, such as citric, lactic, phosphoric, tartaric, and malic, inhibit the growth of acid-intolerant organisms. Benzoic acid (75 mg/kg) may also be added as a preservative. Non-acidic beverages, such as root beer, are better culture media for spoilage organisms than acidic beverages, such as cola, ginger ale, and fruit-flavored beverages. Beverage ingredients not only affect the ability of microbes to grow, but can also influence the types and numbers of microorganisms present and therefore the likelihood of spoilage organisms being added. In addition, bottles and closures are potential sources of contamination. The water in beverages is carbonated and mineral-free and filtered. The filtration process can remove microorganisms or, if the filter is heavily contaminated, add them. Ultraviolet radiation is sometimes used to destroy microorganisms in water. Water discoloration and a flaky precipitate can be caused by algae growth. Chlorine or chlorine dioxide treatment is recommended to kill algae and filtration is recommended, for example. , through diatomaceous earth, to remove dead wrinkled cells.

Yeasts, mainly *Torulopsis* and *Candida,* are the most likely cause of spoilage in soft drinks, since most of these drinks are acidic and contain sugar. One worker found that 85 percent of 1,500 samples of spoiled carbonated drinks were spoiled by yeast. Since sugars are a potential source of yeast, American soft drink bottles have set a standard of no more than ten yeasts per 10 g of dry sugar. Fruit concentrates are another possible source of yeast.

Turbidity and viscosity are types of spoilage of carbonated beverages. Turbidity results from the marked growth of various yeasts or bacteria, and viscosity from the development of encapsulated bacteria, most of which appear to belong to the genus *Bacillus*. The bacteria can enter beverages through ingredients, bottles, or closures. Occasionally, *Gluconobacter, Lactobacillus*, or *Leuconostoc* can be isolated from spoiled carbonated beverages. A species of *Achromobacter** has been identified as responsible for the musty aroma and taste of root beer.

Since mold must contain air, it cannot grow in carbonated beverages, but it can grow on the surface of non-carbonated beverages that contain air above the liquid. They can come from sugar, coloring or flavoring materials, air, or bottles or caps.

SPICES AND OTHER CONDIMENTS

Dry spices are typically not prone to spoilage, although mold growth during the drying process can lead to a significant accumulation of mold spores. Chip dips that are flavored with vegetables or spices generally have much higher levels of total bacteria, coliforms, and molds compared to those flavored with cheese. As previously noted, treating spices with propylene oxide significantly decreases their microbial content. Other methods to reduce the initial microbial load include irradiation, steam, hot ethanol vapors, and acid treatments followed by neutralization. Spices can also be purchased with guaranteed low microorganism counts.

SALT

Three types of salt are used in food: (1) solar salt, which is made from surface salt water evaporating; (2) rock or mined salt; and (3) welled salt, which is made from salt dissolved from underground salt deposits. Halophiles, like *Halobacterium salinarium*, are found in solar salt. *Bacillus* organisms make up around three-fourths of the bacteria, with *Micrococcus** and *Sarcina* accounting for the majority of the remaining bacteria. Approximately 70% of mined salt has been found to contain *Micrococcus**, 20% coryneforms, and 4% *Bacillus*; putrefactive anaerobes have also been detected. On average, there are between 10 and 1,000 organisms per gram of wet salt used on fish. However, the majority of purified salts don't add many organisms to food.

NUTMEATS

Nutmeats still in their shells are typically sterile or almost entirely so. However, shelled nuts, which are often used as ingredients in foods like frozen desserts, can be contaminated with bacteria, yeasts, and molds. Coliform bacteria tests are commonly used to detect potential contamination from fecal matter during handling. Roasting and heating in oil or sugar solutions help to reduce the microbial load. Additionally, molds on nuts can produce mycotoxins, such as aflatoxin in peanuts

OTHER FOODS

The number of different food items displayed on a supermarket shelf is proof of the great diversity of commodity items, convenience foods, and prepared foods available. The microbiology of each of these is also varied. Add to this list the numerous foods which are prepared commercially and vended or distributed locally or regionally and it is evident that the microbial spoilage of each cannot be discussed. Table 20.1 provides an indication of the various miscellaneous foods which have been studies. This listing is surely not complete, but it represents a variety of items not covered in the chapters on various commodities.

Table. Summary of Studies Conducted on Various Categories of Food Globally

Item	Comments	Reference
Cream-filled pastries	History of food-borne illnesses	Bryan (1975)
Health foods	Microbial comparison to traditional foods	Appledorf et al. (1973
Barbecued foods	Public health implications	Todd and Pivnick (1972)
Spices and herbs	Microbiological quality Microbiological profile Microbiology	Seligmann and Frankblum (1974) Julseth and Deibel (1974) Powers et al. (1975)
Big game meat (Wyoming)	Microbiological quality	Smith et al. (1973)
Delicatessen foods	Bacteriological quality	Pace (1975) Harris et al. (1975)
Delicatessen salads	Microbiological quality	Flower Clark (1975)
Vended hamburgers	Microbiological quality	Mueller (1975)
Pecans	Salmonellae	Beuchat and Heaton (1975)
Tortillas, maize	Microflor	Capparelli and Mata (1975)
Mushrooms, fresh	Growth of *Clostridium* botulinum	Sugiyama and Yang (1975)
Coleslaw	Microbial shelf life	King et al. (1976)
Breaded fis	Microbiological quality	Baer et al. (1976)
Breaded onion rings	Microbiological quality	Wentz et al. (1984
Soul food	Bacteriological populations	Stewart (1983)
Vegetable salads	Gram-negative isolates	Wright et al. (1976)
Salads, commercially prepared	Microbiological profile	Terry and Overcast (1976)
Salads, fresh	Microbiological survey	Fowler and Foster (1976)
Tofu	Microbiological quality	Rehberger et al. (1984)
Pasta products	Death kinetics of pathogens	Hsieh et al. (1976)

Coconut products	Microbiological profile	Kajs et al. (1976) Kinderler (1984)
Meat loaf	Fate of contaminants	Maxcy (1976)
Dry soup mixes	Microbiological quality	Komarik et al. (1974)
Dry soup and sauces	*Clostridium perfringens*	Nakamura and Kelly (1968)
Cocoa powder	Microbial profile	Gabis et al. (1970)
Imitation cheese	*Clostridium botulinum*	Kautter et al. (1981
Enteral nutrient solutions	Bacterial growth	Fagerman et al. (1984)
Precooked frozen foods	Microbiological quality	Peterson and Gunnerson (1974)
Frog legs	Salmonellae	Rao et al. (1978)
Natural mineral water	Microbiological quality	Schmidt-Lorenz (1976)
Instant coffe	Microbiological profile	Vanos and Bindschedler (1985)
Beef-soy blends	Microbial stability	Bell and Shelef (1978)
Beef-soy pattie	Total and coliform counts	Craven and Mercuri (1977)
Soy-ground beef	Spoilage bacteria	Harrison et al. (1983)
Soy-protein extenders	Microbiological quality	Swartzentruber (1984

Part-IV

Microbial-Driven Food and Enzyme Production

Microorganisms can be utilized as food or feed themselves, or they can be used to create specific nutrients such as organic acids, flavor enhancers, and vitamins for incorporation into food products. They are also employed in the production of specialized foods through fermentation or as sources of enzyme mixtures or individual enzymes that aid in food processing. To serve these purposes effecti ely, the required cultures must be kept in pure and stable conditions, remaining active and growing to large volumes for use in mass or bulk cultures for specific processes

21 Cultivation of Microbial Cultures for Food Fermentation

Microorganisms required for food fermentation can be introduced as pure or mixed cultures, or in some cases, no cultures are needed if the raw material already contains enough of the desired microorganisms in the right quantities. For fermentations discussed in Chapter 22, such as the production of sauerkraut, fermented pickles, green olives, and the processing of cocoa, coffee, poi, and citron, the raw product itself contains sufficien numbers of the necessary organisms, which will develop in the correct sequence if optimal environmental conditions are provided.

Therefore, adding pure or mixed cultures is generally unnecessary, although it can be beneficial in certain fermentations, like pickles and green olives. Conversely, controlled "starter" cultures, whether pure or mixed, are commonly used in producing dairy products like fermented milks, some types of butter, and most cheeses, as well as in other food fermentations such as bread, malt beverages, wines, distilled spirits, and vinegar.

FUNDAMENTALS OF CULTURE MAINTENANCE AND PREPARATION

Selection of Cultures

Cultures used in food fermentations are chosen primarily for their stability and efficienc in producing the desired products or changes. These cultures may be sourced from established laboratories or selected after evaluating numerous strains. Stability is a key factor, as consistent yields and predictable rates of change are essential. While some cultures, such as sporogenous yeasts, can be improved through breeding, strain improvement is most commonly achieved through selection. Cultures with desirable traits may be selected from newly isolated strains, existing ones, or those that have undergone mutations through various methods.

Advancements in plasmid transfer systems in lactic acid bacteria enable gene cloning or amplification of beneficial traits like lactic acid production. For example, since the gene responsible for lactose fermentation in certain lactic streptococci is plasmid-based, it can be easily lost. However, stabilizing these crucial industrial traits has proven feasible. Research by McKay and colleagues (Harlander et al., 1984) demonstrated the successful cloning of lac+ genes from S. lactis and their incorporation into S. sanguis. By integrating the lac+ genes into the host cell's chromosome via a vector plasmid and transformation, the genes became significantly more stable compared to their plasmid-borne state

Maintenance of Activity of Cultures

Once a satisfactory culture has been obtained, it must be kept pure and active. Usually this objective is attained by periodic transfer of the culture into the proper culture medium, incubation until the culture reaches the maximal stationary phase of growth, and then storage at temperatures low enough to prevent further growth. Too frequent transfer of an unstable culture may lead to undesirable changes in its characteristics.

Stock cultures should be prepared for storage of cultures over long periods without transfer. Such cultures tend to remain stable and serve as a source of culture if the active culture deteriorates or is lost. Lyophilization (freeze drying) and freezing in liquid nitrogen (−196 °C) are now frequently used to prepare stock cultures, although some use still is made of a paraffin-oil seal over ordinary tube cultures. Bacterial cultures have been preserved for months to years at room temperature on slants of agar in which 1 percent NaCl had been incorporated. A dry spore stock on sterilized soil can be used to preserve spores of bacteria or molds for long periods.

Maintenance of Purity of Cultures

Cultures should either be routinely checked for purity or periodically obtained from a culture laboratory to guarantee their purity. Depending on the type of culture being tested, different techniques are used to determine its purity.

Microscopic analysis will only reveal contamination if the contaminant is abundant and looks different from the target organism. Placing the culture on an agar medium that will grow contaminants but not the desired organism is an additional technique. It is possible to test for the presence of substances that are not produced by the desired organism. For example, catalase in a culture of lactic acid bacteria that do not produce catalase can be used as a marker for the presence of contaminants that do produce catalase.

Preparation of Cultures

A mother culture is typically prepared daily from a previous mother culture, which originally originates from the stock culture. These mother cultures are used to inoculate a larger volume of culture medium to produce the bulk or mass culture required for fermentation. In large-scale fermentation, however, several intermediate cultures of increasing volume may need to be developed between the mother culture and the final bulk culture.Culture makers aim to create and maintain cultures that- (1) contain only the desired microorganism(s), (2) are consistent in microbial numbers, proportions (for mixed cultures), and activity, (3) actively produce the desired products, and (4) have sufficien resistance to unfavorable conditions, such as heat resistance for use in cheese curds. They ensure uniformity by standardizing the preparation and sterilization of the culture medium, inoculation methods, and incubation temperature and duration.

The growth phase of the culture depends on its intended purpose. For prompt and rapid growth, cultures in the late logarithmic growth phase are used. For greater resistance to heat or other adverse conditions, cultures in the early stationary phase are preferred. Incubation temperatures are generally close to the organism's optimal temperature but may vary depending on specific needs. Temperature and incubation duration are often adjusted to ensure the culture is ready when required, or the culture may be cooled to halt further development.

Activity of Culture

The activity of a culture is judged by its rate of growth and production of products. It should be good if the mother or the intermediate culture is satisfactory and culture medium, incubation time, and temperature are optimal. Deterioration of cultures may result from improper handling and cultivation, frequent transfer over long periods in an inadequate culture medium, selection, variation or mutation, or attack of bacteria by a bacteriophage.

Mixed Cultures

Mixtures of pure cultures may sometimes be prepared either by growing them together continuously or by growing them separately and combining them at the time of use. For instance, the butter or lactic culture used in the dairy industry is a blend of multiple bacterial species, often including several strains of individual species. When different species or strains of the same species are cultivated together, they must be compatible, meaning they can coexist and grow without one suppressing or eliminating the others. Maintaining the proper balance of organisms within these mixed cultures can be challenging.

In some cases, unknown mixtures of microorganisms are used as starters in food production. Examples include the dough carried over from one batch of specialty French bread to the next and the blend of yeasts and bacteria transferred from the surface smear of one Limburger cheese to another.

BACTERIAL CULTURES

Most of the bacterial cultures employed as starters for dairy products, sausage, and bread are pure or mixed cultures of lactic acid bacteria, exceptions being the propionic acid bacteria added to Swiss cheese. Acetic acid bacteria are used in vinegar making, and various bacteria are used for the manufacture of certain enzymes.

Lactic Acid Cultures

Although some dairies still maintain their own cultures that they have been using successfully for years, most operators periodically obtain new cultures or use frozen culture concentrates prepared by commercial culture laboratories. Most commercially available cultures are now liquid nitrogen frozen culture concentrates prepared by growing the cultures in a suitable medium, then harvesting and concentrating by centrifugation. The harvested cell meals are standardized for their activity, then packaged in sealed boxes and flash frozen in liquid nitrogen. The transportation, distribution and storage of frozen culture concentrates are feasible and several advantages are evident. The purchase of such cultures eliminates the need for routine maintenance and transfers involved in a company-maintained culture collection. The problems of culture contamination during transfer and routine maintenance are eliminated. Using different types of commercially available culture can be alternated to provide broader protection against bacteriophage infection. The cell count is so high in many of these culture concentrates that a 16 oz. dish (containing 11 oz. of concentrate) can be used to directly inoculate a cheese vat containing up to 5,000 pounds of milk. This procedure eliminates the old practice of preparing starter inocula in larger and larger batches over several days. Making a starter with enough mass for a large jar of cheese previously required several days of transfer to increasingly larger volumes, all coming from the parent culture.

The most common dairy starter is the lactic starter, which usually consists of a mixture of strains of *Streptococcus lactis* subsp. *lactis** and *S. mesenteroides* subsp. *cremoris** for lactic acid production and *Leuconostoc** *cremoris* or *Streptococcus lactis* subsp. *diacetlactis** for flavor and aroma production. Some strains of lactic acid streptococci with different susceptibilities to bacteriophages are usually included in the same concentrated culture as an insurance against phage problems.

Typically, the lactic acid culture is incubated at 21.1 to 22.2°C, although 23.9 to 26.7°C has been used in the production of lactic acid starters. A culture is matured to the desired titratable acidity to be suitable for the purpose for which the culture is to be used.

A mixed lactic acid culture used in the production of cultured dairy products, yogurt, and certain types of cheese. Flavor bacteria are particularly important in the production of flavor in cultured dairy products. The typical yogurt starter is a mixture of *Streptococcus thermophilus* and *Lactobacillus delbrueckii* subsp. *bulgaricus*. Transfer and handling of mixed cultures should consider the temperature and incubation time that best maintain the desired mixed population and thus prevent dominance of one type or species over another. The use of frozen concentrated cultures eliminates many of these concerns. In addition, cultures from commercial culture laboratories offer the advantage of purchasing compatible strains that have been previously defined and tested.

As mentioned in Chapter 22, the "sourdough" used by rye bread makers is a mixture of various lactic acid bacteria usually grown in mixed, impure culture in flour dough, pasta, or other medium. It is stated that *L. delbrueckii* subsp. *bulgaricus* must be grown to produce sufficient acid and that heterofermentative lactic acids are desirable from the point of view of flavor production. Some bread makers use pure cultures of *Streptococcus lactis* subsp. *lactis**, *Leuconostoc* spp. , *Lactobacillus plantarum*, *L. casei*, *L. brevis*, *L. delbrueckii* subsp. *bulgaricus* and *Streptococcus thermophilus* to inoculate the bread. Other bakers also add yeast.

Lactobacilli cultures and *Pediococcus acidilactici* or *P. pentosaceus* can be used as starters for fermented sausages, Thuringian sausages and the like. Cultures, dry cultures and frozen culture concentrates have been prepared.

Cheese Smear Organisms

Most cheese makers inoculate the surfaces of smear-ripened cheese from previous cheeses, shelves, cloths, brine tank, hands, and other sources in the plant. The micrococci, *Brevibacterium linens,* and film yeasts important in the smear have been isolated and used in pure or mixed cultures to wash cheese surfaces, thereby inoculating them.

Propionic Culture

Spray-dried or lypohilized cultures of *Propionibacterium freudenreichii* are added to milk used in the manufacture of Swiss cheese to improve the flavor and assist eye formation.

Acetic Acid Bacteria

Pure cultures of *Gluconobacter* or *Acetobacter* are not efficient in the production of acetic acid. Therefore, in vinegar making, impure mixed cultures are allowed to develop naturally, are added by means of raw vinegar from a previous run, or are transferred from a vinegar cask or generator.

YEAST CULTURES

Most yeasts of industrial importance are of the genus *Saccharomyces* and mostly of the species *S. cerevisiae.* These ascospore-forming yeasts are readily bred for desired characteristics. A yeast for a given purpose may be improved for that use but must also be guarded against possible undesirable changes.

Bakers' Yeast

Strains of *Saccharomyces cerevisiae* used for producing bakers' yeast are typically single-cell isolates selected specifically for their suitability. These strains should yield a high number of cells in the chosen cultivation medium, remain stable, retain viability in cake or dried forms for extended periods, and rapidly produce carbon dioxide in bread dough during leavening.

Like other large-scale cultures, this strain is developed from the original mother culture through multiple intermediate cultures of increasing size to the final "seed" culture. Cells from the seed culture are concentrated into a "cream" using centrifugation. This dense suspension is then added to the large mash volume, with approximately 3 to 5 pounds of yeast introduced per 100 gallons of medium.

The most common medium for culture buildup and bakers' yeast production is a molasses-mineral-salts mash, which includes molasses, nitrogen sources like ammonium salts or urea, inorganic salts such as phosphates, and accessory growth factors from vegetable or grain extracts, yeast extracts, or vitamins. The pH is adjusted to 4.3–4.5, and the medium is aerated at high rates while being maintained at about 30°C. Molasses is added gradually to keep the sugar level between 0.5–1.5 percent. After four or five budding cycles, the yeast is centrifuged into a "cream," which is filtered to remove excess liquid, then formed into cakes of various sizes with small amounts of vegetable oil.

Active dry yeast is produced by drying yeast cells to below 8 percent moisture. These cells are specially grown for this purpose and dried at low temperatures to preserve their viability and leavening ability for several months. Bakers' yeast can also be made from grain mashes, waste sulfite liquor from paper mills, wood hydrolysate, and similar materials.

Wine Yeasts

For wine making, a special strain of *Saccharomyces cerevisiae* var. *ellipsoideus*, adapted to the making of the specific type of wine, is selected. Famous types are the Burgundy, Tokay, and champagne cultures so widely used. The cultures are grown and built up in volume in must (juice of the grape or other fruit) like that to be used in the main fermentation.

Distillers' Yeast

Distillers' yeast ordinarily is a high-alcohol-yielding strain of *S. cerevisiae* var. *ellipsoideus*, usually one adapted to growing in the medium or mash to be employed. The medium or mash would be malted grain, usually corn or rye for whiskey, molasses for rum, or juices or mashes of fruits for brandy. The liquors are distillates of the fermented mashes.

Yeasts for Malt Beverages

Yeasts used for malt beverage production are either maintained in pure culture within brewery laboratories or sourced as needed from specialized laboratories. The strain chosen depends on the product- specific bottom yeasts for beer, typically top yeasts for ale (though bottom yeasts may occasionally be used), and top yeasts for stout and porter. Top yeasts are strains of *Saccharomyces cerevisiae*, while the bottom yeast commonly used is *S. uvarum* (*carlsbergensis*).

When starting from a pure culture, the yeast must be gradually scaled up in wort from a laboratory culture to a large seed or "pitching" culture. However, in practice, pitching yeast is almost always derived from yeast recovered from a prior fermentation. This recovered yeast is concentrated and may be washed or left untreated. Inevitably, such a culture becomes contaminated with other organisms, including bacteria and wild yeasts that accumulate over successive fermentation and recovery cycles.

Fortunately, most contaminants that grow in the yeast culture are inhibited by the hops and low pH of the wort, minimizing their impact on the malt beverage. However, certain organisms responsible for "beer diseases" can occasionally proliferate in the pitching yeast.

MOLD CULTURES

Stock cultures of molds are typically maintained on slants of an appropriate agar medium, such as malt-extract agar, and can be preserved for extended periods in the spore state through methods like lyophilization (freeze-drying) or as soil stocks. Various techniques are used to prepare spore or mycelial cultures for large-scale industrial use. These include- (1) growing on the surface of liquid or agar medium in flasks or similar containers, (2) surface growth in shallow layers on trays, (3) growth on loose, moistened wheat bran, sometimes acidified or supplemented with liquid nutrients like corn-steep liquor, (4) growth on sterilized and moistened bread or crackers, and (5) submerged growth in aerated liquid medium, often resulting in pellets made of mycelium, with or without spores. The spores are harvested differently depending on the production method, such as washing or scraping from dry surfaces, grinding dried material into a powder, or incorporating spores into dry powders like flour. Pellets, on the other hand, are used as they are.

Spores of *Penicillium roqueforti,* used for blue cheeses like Roquefort, Stilton, and Gorgonzola, are usually cultivated on sterilized, moistened, and often acidified bread cubes. After sporulation, the bread and culture are dried, powdered, and packaged, typically in cans. For *P. camemberti,* spores are produced by growing the mold on moistened, sterilized crackers. A spore suspension is then prepared for surface inoculation of cheeses such as Camembert and Brie.

In industrial submerged fermentations, mold starters are usually prepared as pellets or masses of mycelium, grown during submerged, actively shaken cultivation. When surface growth on liquid, agar medium, or bran is required, spores produced using the earlier-mentioned methods often serve as inoculum.

For soy sauce production, the koji starter—discussed in the next chapter—is typically a mixed culture carried over from a previous batch. However, pure cultures of *Aspergillus oryzae* are also used, often in combination with a yeast and *Lactobacillus delbrueckii*. The mold culture is cultivated on cooked, sterilized rice.

Microbial Transformations in Food Production

22

The lactic acid fermentation of cabbage, cucumbers, and green olives serves a dual purpose- preserving the food while creating unique and flavorful products. In many cases, the primary goal of fermentation is to produce desired new products, with preservation as a secondary benefit. These processes involve yeasts, bacteria, molds, or a combination of these microorganisms. In products like bread, beer, wine, and distilled spirits, yeast-driven fermentation plays a central role. Both yeasts and bacteria contribute to vinegar production from sugar-rich materials, while bacteria are predominantly involved in producing fermented dairy products. Molds are especially significant in crafting certain cheeses and traditional Oriental foods.

BREAD

Microorganisms play two primary roles in breadmaking- (1) generating gas to leaven the dough, resulting in the desired light and porous texture, and (2) producing flavor-enhancing compounds. Additionally, they may contribute to improving the dough's overall condition.

Leavening

Typically, bread yeasts (Chapter 21) leaven dough by fermenting its sugars, primarily producing alcohol and carbon dioxide. However, in place of bread yeasts, other actively gas-forming microorganisms have been used for leavening, including heterofermentative lactic acid bacteria, coliform bacteria, saccharolytic *Clostridium* species, wild yeasts, and various naturally occurring mixtures of these organisms. The direct addition of gas (CO_2) to the dough is another method of leavening.

Leavening by Bread Yeasts

During the initial two hours after yeast is added to dough, little to no growth occurs. Some growth may occur between two and four hours, depending on the time before baking, with a decline observed after four to six hours. Fermentation begins immediately after mixing the dough or sponge and continues until yeast enzymes are inactivated by oven heat. Professional bakers often use a large amount of yeast for a shorter fermentation process, while modern home baking trends similarly favor excess yeast to reduce fermentation time. This short-time approach limits yeast growth during fermentation. Traditional home methods, with less or less effecti e yeast, allowed longer fermentation times, enabling more yeast and bacterial growth.

During fermentation, dough undergoes "conditioning," where flour proteins (gluten) become elastic and springy, enabling them to retain the carbon dioxide produced by yeast. Conditioning results from proteolytic enzymes (present in flour, yeast, malt, or additives) and pH reduction due to added and formed acids. Dough conditioners, such as ammonium salts and various chemical salts (e.g., $KBrO_3$, KIO_3, CaO_2, $(NH_4)_2S_2O_8$), are often added to enhance dough characteristics.

While the natural sugar in flour, along with that produced by flour amylase, may suffic for yeast fermentation, most recipes include added sugar or amylase-bearing malt to increase the gas production rate. Factors influencing this rate include (1) more yeast, (2) sugar or malt, and (3) yeast food, but excessive amounts of yeast food, salt, or improper temperatures can reduce gas production. The baker aims to ensure sufficien gas production and optimal dough condition to retain the gas at the right time.

In the sponge method, some ingredients are mixed at 23–24°C for fermentation until maturity, followed by the addition of remaining ingredients and further fermentation. In the straight-dough method, all ingredients are mixed at 26–28°C. The fermentation room is typically maintained at 27°C for the leavening process.

Leavening can also involve other microorganisms besides bread yeasts. Dough from previous batches can leaven certain breads, such as sourdough, with heterofermentative lactic acid bacteria and saccharolytic anaerobes participating in the process. Salt-rising bread uses "salt-rising yeast" and other microorganisms from the ingredients, sometimes alongside bakers' yeast. Some products, like soda crackers, involve a sequence of organisms for leavening, flavoring, and dough modification. For example, a 3–4 hour fermentation by yeast may be followed by lactic acid bacteria activity, contributing to the final product

Leavening by Chemicals

Dough can be leavened using chemical agents instead of microorganisms, but such products cannot be classified as bread according to identity standards that require yeast leavening. Carbon dioxide gas can be directly incorporated into the dough, or baking powders, which are chemical mixtures that release gas when combined with the dough, can be used for leavening. Ammonium bicarbonate is another option, as the heat from baking causes the release of carbon dioxide and ammonium gas. Self-rising flour contains both the acid and alkaline components of baking powder, which react when moistened.

Continuous Breadmaking

Continuous breadmaking processes usually involve growth and fermentation by the yeast in part of the ingredients to get a large yield of active yeast—or at least the addition of more yeast than usual—before the final dough is formed. Leavening may take place in the pans just before baking.

Flavor Production

Yeasts are believed to contribute to the flavor of bread through the products they release during sugar fermentation, although many experts argue that yeasts have little to no impact on flavor, especially with modern rapid baking methods. Alcohol, acids, esters, and aldehydes are some of the byproducts that may enhance the flavor. However, bacteria growing in the dough are generally seen as the primary contributors to flavor. In typical industrial processes, insufficient time is allowed for bacteria to grow enough to influence flavor significantly. In contrast, older home baking methods provide enough time for bacterial growth, which leads to a greater production of desirable flavors. Dough made from a previous batch can introduce a healthy population of flavor-producing bacteria, resulting in bread with distinctive flavors. Ultimately, most of the flavor in baker's bread comes from the ingredients and chemical reactions, like Maillard browning, that occur during baking. If there is enough time for bacterial growth before baking, both bacteria and yeasts can contribute to the flavor, producing compounds like alcohol, diacetyl, aldehydes, acetoin, isoalcohols, and various acids and esters.

The Baking Process

Although the interior of the loaf does not quite reach 100°C during baking, the heat serves to kill the yeasts, inactivate their enzymes and those of the flour and malt, expand the gas present, and set the structure of the loaf. Baking, besides producing the appearance of the loaf, also contributes desirable flavors. The heat also drives off most of the alcohol and other volatile substances formed by the yeasts but contributes substances such as furfural, pyruvic and other aldehydes, and other compounds that add to the flavor. The most important change in bread during baking is gelatinization of starch. "Set" of bread results from this process, in which gluten gives structural support in the dough, but starch support the structure of baked bread.

Rye Bread

Yeasts are believed to contribute to the flavor of bread through the products they release during sugar fermentation, although many experts argue that yeasts have little to no impact on flavor, especially with modern rapid baking methods. Alcohol, acids, esters, and aldehydes are some of the byproducts that may enhance the flavor. However, bacteria growing in the dough are generally seen as the primary contributors to flavor. In typical industrial processes, insufficien time is allowed for bacteria to grow enough to influence flavor significantly. In contrast, older home baking methods provide enough time for bacterial growth, which leads to a greater production of desirable flavors

Dough made from a previous batch can introduce a healthy population of flavor-producing bacteria, resulting in bread with distinctive flavors. Ultimately, most of the flavor in baker's bread comes from the ingredients and chemical reactions, like Maillard browning, that occur during baking. If there is enough time for bacterial growth before baking, both bacteria and yeasts can contribute to the flavor, producing compounds like alcohol, diacetyl, aldehydes, acetoin, isoalcohols, and various acids and esters.

San Francisco Dough Bread

The leavening of this type of bread results from the action of *Torulopsis holmii*, the asporogenous form of *Saccharomyces exiguus*. The second principal organism involved, responsible for the acid development, has been identified as a heterofermentative lactobacillus, *Lactobacillus sanfrancisco*.

TRADITIONAL INDIAN FERMENTED FOODS

Dahi (Sanskrit- dadhi) is a popular Indian fermented milk product, quite analogous to plain yogurt in appearance and consistency. It is popular with consumers due to its distinctive flavor and because it is believed to have good nutritional and therapeutic value. It is utilized in various forms in many Indian culinary preparations.

Idli

The Indians discovered bacterial fermentation methods and yeast to raise dough made from grains and legumes. People in the Middle East discovered that sour milk combined with wheat made dry soup ingredients with superior nutritional value and excellent keeping quality. Mixed fermented products made from grains and legumes have additional nutritional value.

Idli and dosa, the staple foods of South India, are prepared from rice and legumes and each has a long cooking time. history, although not all the details can be clearly traced. Idli is mentioned frequently in 1025 AD; The poet Chavundaraya describes it unambiguously as urad dal (black mung beans) soaked in buttermilk, ground into a fine paste, mixed with pure curd water, cumin, coriander, pepper and 'asafoetida, then shaped. The Manasollasa of about 1130 AD, written in Sanskrit, describes idli as being made of fine urad flour, formed into small balls, fried in ghee and then seasoned with chili powder, cumin powder and asafoetida.

Dhokla

The use of pulses to make dhokla, a steam-cooked fermented spicy cake, has its first mention in 1066 AD. In northern India, dried spicy hollow balls, called warries, have been made for more than 100 years. They are prepared from black-gram paste fermented for 3 to 10 days.

Nan, bhatura, and kulcha are types of staple foods made from fermented wheat dough and shaped as flattene breads in India, Pakistan, Afghanistan, and Iran.

Dosa

Dosa is a pancake made from the batter of rice and black gram, and its first mention can be noted in the Tamita Sangam literature about the sixth century AD.

Fermented Leafy Vegetables

Ziang sang/Ziang dui

The people of Nagaland and Manipur use fermented leafy vegetables.

Ziang-sang is traditionally prepared in the winter. The process begins by crushing two- to three-day-old withered hangam leaves (*Brassica* sp.) using a wooden mortar and pestle. The crushed leaves are then soaked in warm water, squeezed to remove excess moisture, and placed in an airtight container to undergo a semi-solid fermentation for 7-10 days at room temperature (20-30°C). After fermentation, the juice is extracted by hand-squeezing, and the remaining paste is dried in the sun for 4 to 5 days. This dried paste, known as ziang-sang, can be stored for over a year. The liquid is concentrated by boiling and stored in bamboo containers, where it can also last for more than a year. This concentrated liquid is called ziang-dui. Ziang-sang is typically consumed as a soup with boiled rice, while ziang-dui is used as a condiment with meals (Jeyaram et al., 2009; Tamang and Tamang, 2009).

Sinki

This is a fermented radish (*Raphanus sativus* L.) product consumed by the Nepalese people in Darjeeling, Sikkim, and Nepal. It is prepared in the winter months when the weather is less humid and the vegetable is abundantly available. The fermentation is associated with microbes like *Lactobacillus plantarum, L. brevis*, and *L. fermentum* (Tamang and Sarkar, 1993). To prepare it, fresh radish taproots are cleaned, sun-dried for 1-2 days until soft, then shredded and dipped in lukewarm water, squeezed, and tightly packed into an earthen jar using a wooden pestle. The jar is sealed with an earthen lid and covered with radish leaves, then kept in a warm, dry place for 15-30 days (Tamang and Sarkar, 1993). Alternatively, a pit about 1 meter deep and wide is dug, cleaned, and heated with a fire. After removing the ashes, the sides are plastered with hot mud, and the pit is lined with dried leaves of bamboo, banana, or radish. The shredded radish roots are tightly packed into the pit, covered with dried leaves, and weighed down with heavy stones or wooden planks. The top is sealed with mud or cow dung, and the mixture is left to ferment for 30-40 days. After fermentation, the product is removed, cut into small pieces, and sun-dried for 3-5 days. This fermented product, called sinki, can be stored for over two years at room temperature if exposed to sunlight periodically. It has a highly acidic flavor with a pH of 4.4, a protein content of 14.6 g, and a fat content of 2.5 g per dry weight, and is commonly used as a base for soups and pickles. Sinki is believed to be a good appetizer and serves as a remedy for indigestion.

Gundruk

Gundruk, a fermented vegetable product native to the Nepalese people of the Himalayan region, is commonly sold by Nepalese women in the Darjeeling hills and Sikkim. It is typically prepared during the winter months, from October to December, when fresh leafy vegetables are abundant. The vegetables used include mustard leaves (*Brassica juncea*), rayo-sag (*Brassica rapa*), cauliflower (*Brassica oleracea*), radish (*Raphanus sativus*), and other locally grown varieties. The main microorganisms found in gundruk fermentation are *Lactobacillus brevis, L. plantarum, L. paracasei, Pediococcus pentosaceus, P. acidilactici,* and *Leuconostoc fallax* (Tamang et al., 2005). To prepare gundruk, fresh leaves of the selected vegetables are first wilted and shredded using a sickle or knife, then gently crushed and pressed into an earthen pot. The pot is sealed to make it airtight, and the mixture is left to ferment naturally at room temperature for 7 to 10 days. Once fermentation is complete, indicated by a mild acidic taste, the gundruk is removed and sun-dried for 3 to 4 days to aid in preservation. It is typically consumed as a soup or pickle, with the soup prepared by mixing gundruk with various ingredients, making for a flavorful appetizer.

Goyang

The Sherpa tribe of the Sikkim and Darjeeling hills prepare a fermented product from leaves of the wild plant magane-saag (*Cardamine macrophylla* wild). The product is known to contain the species *Lactobacillus plantarum, L. brevis, Lactococcus lactis, Enterococcus faecium,* and *Pediococcus pentosaceus* (Tamang and Tamang, 2007). During the rainy season, the leaves of the plant magane-saag are found in plenty, which are collected, washed, chopped into pieces, and squeezed to remove the excess water. The leaves are then tightly pressed into a bamboo basket lined with 2-3 layers of fig (*Ficus carica*) leaves. The top of the basket is also covered with fig leaves and is left to ferment at room temperature (15–25°C) for a period of one month. Then the goyang may be transferred to an airtight container where it can be stored for a period of 2-3 months. The product may also be made into balls and sundried, which generally increases its shelf life. Locally, goyang is boiled with beef or yak meat and noodles and made into a thick soup-like dish called thupka.

Anishi

It is native to the state of Nagaland and this product is prepared mainly by the Ao tribe. Leaves of edible yam (*Colocasia* sp.) are used for this preparation. The fresh mature green leaves are collected and washed properly. They are then piled one upon another and finally wrapped with a banana leaf. They are left for about 6 to 7 days till the leaves turn yellow. The yellow leaves are then mixed with salt, chilies, and ginger and ground into a paste. This paste is then made into cakes and kept over the fireplace in the kitchen. After 2 to 3 days of drying, they become ready for consumption. It is used as a condiment and usually cooked with dry meat, especially pork (Mao and Odyuo, 2007).

Khalpi

Khalpi is a product from the state of Sikkim and Darjeeling hills. It is generally prepared for home consumption by the Nepalese Brahmins belonging to the Bahun and Chettri castes. Microbes identified in this product of cucumber include

Lactobacillus plantarum, L. brevis, and *Lecuonostoc fallax*. For this preparation of khalpi, mature and ripened cucumbers are cut into definite sizes and sundried for 2 days. They are then put into bamboo vessels called dhungroo and sealed. Fermentation is allowed to take place for 4 to 7 days at room temperature. The product can be stored for about a week in airtight containers. It is taken as a pickle after mixing with mustard oil, chilies, and salt (Tamang and Tamang, 2009a).

Fermented Fish Products

Ngari

Fermented fish called ngari is an integral part of the diet of the people of Manipur. Traditional methods of preservation are used. The type of fish used for its preparation is P*untius sophore*, and it is used in a sun-dried form called poubu (Jeyaram et al., 2009). Lactic acid bacteria are the main fermenting organisms found in the samples of auto. The identified species are *Lactococcus plantarum* and *Lactobacillus plantarum*. *Bacillus subtilis, B. pumilus* and *Mycoplasma* sp. have also been isolated from the cold. The fungal isolates have been identified as *Candida* sp. (Thapa et al., 2004). Guava preparation is mainly reserved for families in small villages. The fish are generally washed and the intact fish are selected. They are then dried in the sun for 3 to 4 days. When the fish are semi-dried, they are rubbed with essential oils such as mustard or fish oil, and a little salt is added to help the fish's body absorb the oils. Dried fish is then directly used for fermentation or stored in jute bags for later use. When preserved fish are used for fermentation, they are first washed with water in a porous bamboo basket and the water is allowed to drain overnight. The fish are then placed in gunny bags and squeezed to remove excess water and break off the heads and bones. They are then placed in clay pots called chaphus, which are first kept in a jar with mustard oil to be dismembered. For new pots, 8 to 10 coats of oil should be applied at intervals of 7 to 8 days, while for old pots, a single coat is sufficient The layer of oil can serve to create an anaerobic condition in the pot. After packing the fish tightly in the pots, these are sealed with polythene sheets, fish scales, oil, mud and cow dung. The holes in the kapus are filled with kapus paste and finally covered with kapus leaves. The pots are then stored in the dark at room temperature for about 4 to 6 months. At this point, the fermented fish is ready to eat and is also known locally as chaphu kaiba. It has a characteristic odor and a shelf life of 12 to 18 months (Jeyaram et al., 2009; Singh et al., 2010). Most of the LAB strains isolated from the vehicle showed a high degree of hydrophobicity, indicating their probiotic characteristics (Thapa et al. , 2004). It is used to prepare various specialties such as eromba, where it is added either after frying or after steaming. It is also eaten as an accompaniment to rice (Singh et al. 2010).

Tungtap

Tungtap is a traditional food of the Khasi tribe in Meghalaya, prepared at the household and village level and commonly sold at weekly markets throughout the district (Sekar and Mariappan, 2007; Agrahar-Murungkar and Subbulakshmi,

2006). The fermentation process of tungtap involves microorganisms such as *Lactobacillus coriniformis, L. lactis, L. fructosus, Bacillus cereus, B. subtilis, Candida* sp., and *Saccharomycopsis* sp. (Thapa et al., 2004). The fish species used in making tungtap is *Puntius sophore*. To prepare it, the fish are first washed, scaled, and degutted. Salt is then applied both inside and outside the fish. The fish are placed in a clay pot, which is filled with a mixture of salt and either fish or pork fat. The pot is sealed with a banana leaf and tightly bound with a jute cord before being stored at room temperature for 6-7 months. After the fermentation period, the pot is opened, and the fish are removed, with any excess salt and fat scraped off using a sharp knife (Agrahar-Murungkar and Subbulakshmi, 2006). The final product contains 40.6% protein and 19.6% fat on a dry-weight basis. The fermentation process enhances the flavor and texture of the fish by softening the bones and improving the meat. The resulting product has a soft, spongy texture and is typically served as chutney with green leaves, onions, and chilies (Agrahar-Murungkar and Subbulakshmi, 2006). Tungtap is also consumed as a side dish in the form of a pickle (Sekar and Mariappan, 2007).

Hentak

It is another fermented-fish product from the state of Manipur. It comes in the form of paste (Jeyaram et al., 2009). The microorganisms associated with hentak have been identified as *Lactobacillus fructosus, L. amylophilus, Enterococcus faecium, Bacillus cereus, B. subtilis, Staphylococcus aureus, Enterococcus faecium* along with fungus *Candida* sp. (Thapa et al., 2004). For preparing hentak, fishes of the species *Esomus danricus* are first dried in the sun. They are then crushed to powder in a mortar-pestle. On the other hand, petioles of the aroid plant (*Alocasia macrorrhiza*) are cut into small pieces, washed with water, and exposed to sunlight for about an hour. Now equal weights of both the fish powder and the plant material are mixed and crushed together in order to make a paste. These are then made into small balls and transferred into earthen pots. These pots are then left at room temperature for fermentation to take place. The process takes about two weeks after which the product becomes ready to be eaten. These balls become hardened on being stored for a few months, which can then be propounded to paste with a little water and stored as balls for reserved food (Jeyaram et al., 2009). Hentak is consumed as a curry as well as a supplement with boiled rice. Sometimes it is given to women in the final stages of pregnancy or patients recovering from sickness or injury (Sarojnalini and Singh, 1988).

Gnuchi

Gnuchi is a smoked and dried fish product commonly enjoyed by the Lepcha community of Sikkim. The term "gnuchi" translates to smoked fish in the Lepcha language. It is an essential source of protein in the local diet and is prepared using traditional methods passed down by the rural people. The fish species used for making gnuchi include *Schizothorax richardsonii* Gray, *Labeo dero* Hamilton, *Acrossocheilus* spp., *Channa* sp., and others. The microorganisms involved in the fermentation process of gnuchi have been identified as *Enterococcus faecium,*

Pediococcus pentosaceus, Bacillus subtilis, and *Micrococcus* sp. (Thapa et al., 2006). To prepare gnuchi, the fish are first placed on a large bamboo tray, called a sarhang, to drain excess water. They are then degutted and mixed with salt and turmeric powder. The fish are hung on a bamboo strip above an earthen oven and smoked for 7-10 days. After smoking, the product is ready to be consumed. It can be stored at room temperature for 2-3 months. Gnuchi is often made into curry with vegetables and served with boiled rice. It has a protein content of 21.3 g% on a dry-weight basis (Thapa et al., 2006).

Fermented Beans

Kinema

It is a fermented food made from soybeans. The soybeans (*Glycine max*) are locally known as bhatmas and the varieties used are 'yellow cultivar' and 'dark brown cultivar'. It is widely prepared by Nepalese belonging to the Limboo and Rai castes of Sikkim. The product is sticky in nature and has an ammonia-like odor. The knowledge of how to make this delicacy has been protected as a hereditary right and has been passed down from one generation to the next (Tamang et al. , 2009). It is produced by natural fermentation of bacterial species, namely *Bacillus subtilis* and *Enterococcus faecium*. The fungal species *Candida parapsilosis* and *Geotrichum candidum* have also been isolated from commercially available kinema (Sarkar et al., 1994). To prepare kinema, soybeans are soaked overnight and then boiled to soften. The excess water is drained and the cotyledons are separated by lightly grinding in a wooden mortar (okhli) and pestle. This allows for increased surface area for rapid fermentation. Subsequently, about 1% wood ash is added to maintain an alkaline condition. The beans are then placed in a bamboo basket decorated with fresh fern (*Glaphylopteriolopsis erubescens*). The basket is then covered with a jute bag and allowed to ferment naturally at room temperature (which is around 20-35°C in Sikkim). The whole thing is placed in an earth oven and left to rest for 1 to 2 days after the end of fermentation is indicated by the appearance. of a white viscous mass in the soy and the emission of an ammoniacal smell. Its shelf life is 2 to 3 days in summer and 5 to 7 days in winter (Tamang et al., 2009).

Indigenous knowledge in microbiology is related to the practice of not cleaning the mortar and pestle to preserve and supplement microorganisms for spontaneous fermentation without the use of starter cultures (Tamang, 2003). Nitrogen soluble in water, formal nitrogen in relation to the total concentration of nitrogen and ammonia (up to 200 mg/100g) kinema grows rapidly during fermentation due to the high proteolytic activity of *Bacillus subtilis*. This leads to the release of free amino acids followed by deamination. The final pH of the product can reach 8.6 (Tamang and Nikkuni, 1998; Sarkar et al., 1993; Sekar and Mariappan, 2007). It constitutes a major source of protein in the diet of the inhabitants of this region. Kinema contains about 48% (dry weight) of crude protein and free amino acids represent about 26% of the total amino acid content (Sarkar et al., 1994; 1997). Kinema is eaten as a curry with boiled rice. The curry is prepared by frying the quinoa in vegetable oil and then mixing it with chopped onions, tomatoes and turmeric powder. They are then fried for about 2 minutes. Then add salt and chopped green chillies and fry for 3 to 5 minutes. Add some water to make a thick sauce and cook for 5 to 7 minutes (Tamang et al., 2009).

Hawaiijar

Hawaiijar is a sticky fermented soybean product from Manipur, and its name is derived from "hawai," meaning pulses, and "jar," short for achar, meaning pickle (Jeyaram et al., 2009; Premarani and Chhetry, 2010). It has been a staple food for the Meitei people for many decades, with the Brahmin community believed to have initiated its production and consumption. Soybean, known as nung hawai in Manipur, comes in two varieties- small-seeded and large, round-seeded. The final product is brown and covered with a slimy white substance (Jeyaram et al., 2009). The fermentation of hawaijar involves microorganisms such as *Bacillus subtilis, B. licheniformis, B. cereus, Staphylococcus aureus, S. sciuri, Alkaligenes* sp., and *Providencia rettger* (Jeyaram et al., 2008a). To prepare, soybeans are soaked overnight, washed, and boiled until soft. After being washed with hot water, the beans are packed tightly in a bamboo basket with fig or banana leaves at the base. The basket is then covered with jute cloth and placed in the sun or near a stove for fermentation. After 3-5 days, the fermented product is ready, emitting an ammonia-like odor. It is typically wrapped in banana leaves for storage (Jeyaram et al., 2009; Premarani and Chhetry, 2010; Tamang et al., 2009). Hawaijar has a short shelf life of 3-4 days, but it can be dried for long-term storage. It is used in a variety of dishes, such as the Manipuri delicacy chagempomba, and eaten as ametpa with chilies and salt. It is also used in vegetable curries (Premarani and Chhetry, 2010).

Ankhone/Bekang/Peruyyan

Ankhone, Bekang, and Peruyyan are fermented soybean products known by different names among various tribes. The product is prepared from soybeans (*Glycine max*) and is fermented using *Bacillus subtilis* and other *Bacillus* species. The beans are soaked, washed, boiled, and then wrapped in banana or other local leaves before being kept over a fireplace for optimal fermentation. The fermentation process takes about a week, after which the product is ready. It is known as aaknone in Nagaland, bekang in Mizoram, and peruyyan among the Apatanis of Arunachal Pradesh. For long-term storage, it is sometimes molded into pastes or cakes, or individual beans are dried and stored in containers. The fermented product has a characteristic odor and is used in chutney or cooked with meat to enhance flavor (Mao and Odyuo, 2007; amang et al., 2009).

Tungrumbai

Tungrumbai is a fermented soybean-based food from the Khasi tribe of Meghalaya. It is sticky and serves as a cheap source of protein in the diet. The fermentation process involves *Bacillus subtilis* and *Enterococcus faecium*, while fungal strains such as *Candida parapsilosis, Saccharomyces bayanus,*

Saccharomycopsis fibuligera, and *Geotrichum candidum* have been identified (Sohliya et al., 2009; Sarkar et al., 1994). Tungrumbai production remains a traditional practice carried out at the household level by local Khasis in Meghalaya (Agrahar-Murungkar and Subbulakshmi, 2006). To prepare, the soybean seeds are soaked for 4-6 hours, the skins removed by rubbing, and the beans cooked in the soaking water until absorbed. After cooling, the beans are placed in a bamboo basket lined with leaves of *Clinogyne dichotoma* (locally known as lamet), covered with leaves or jute bags, and fermented either at ambient temperature or near a fireplace. The fermentation takes 3-4 days, resulting in a brown mass with a characteristic odor (Agrahar-Murungkar and Subbulakshmi, 2006; Sohliya et al., 2009; Tamang et al., 2009). The fermentation microorganisms are provided by the water source and the raw soybeans and lamet leaves. Tungrumbai contains 45.9% protein on a dry-weight basis, along with 30.2% fiber and 5.5% ash (Agrahar-Murungkar and Subbulakshmi, 2006). It is typically eaten as a side dish with rice or cooked into curry with ginger, garlic, chili, black sesame, and salt (Tamang et al., 2009).

Fermented Bamboo Shoots

Mesu

Mesu is a fermented bamboo-shoot product indigenous to the people of Himalayan regions of Darjeeling hills and Sikkim. It is prepared only during the months of June to September when bamboo shoots sprout. The species of bamboo used are the locally available choya bans (*Dendrocalamus hamiltonii* Nees and Arnott), bhalu bans (*D. sikkimensis* Gamble) and karati bans (*Bambusa tulda* Roxb). Its chief producers are the Limboo women belonging to the Nepalese community (Tamang and Sarkar, 1996; Tamang and Tamang, 2009a; Sekar and Mariappan, 2007). Microbial analysis of young bamboo shoots demonstrated the presence of *Lactobacillus plantarum, L. brevis* and *L. pentosaceus*. It was found that *L. pentosaceus* was the initiator of fermentation, followed by L. brevis and finally dominated by *L. plantarum* (Tamang and Sarkar, 1996). In order to carry out the fermentation of mesu, young edible shoots of the bamboo plant are defoliated, chopped finely, and pressed tightly into green hollow bamboo stems. The opening of such a stem is covered tightly with leaves of bamboo or other wild plants.

This is then left to ferment at room temperature (water is then poured upon the mixture and the brew that drips at the end is collected. The first draw is called tokti, which has the strongest flavor, and the subsequent blackish brew is called ennog (Tiwari and Mahanta, 2007). Fresh mesu has a shelf life of only about a week. However, mesu is commonly used as a pickle by mixing it with salt, chilies, and mustard oil, which can be stored for more than a year without refrigeration. Mesu is also used for preparing curry by frying and mixing with cooked meat (Tamang and Sarkar, 1996; Tamang and Tamang, 2009a).

Lung-Seij

This ethnic fermented bamboo-shoot product belongs to the state of Meghalaya and is produced mainly by the Khasi women. It is prepared from

Dendrocalamus hamiltonii species of bamboo, available locally in Meghalaya. To prepare lung-seij, tender bamboo shoots of about 0.5 meters in length are selected and cut from bamboo groves. The bracts and sheaths are removed, and then they are washed thoroughly with water, cleaned, and the shoots are sliced into small pieces. These are then pressed either into bamboo cylinders or glass bottles. Lactic acid bacteria have been found to be present in the fermented product (Tamang and Tamang, 2009a). The bamboo cylinders used for fermentation are made by cutting one side open and keeping the other side closed with the node. They are filled with the sliced shoots to full capacity and the open side is closed with dried leaves and sealed by tying the rim with thread or grass. Care is taken to prevent the accidental seepage of water into the cylinder, which makes the product black and unfit for consumption. These cylinders are then immersed in streams for a period of 1-2 months for fermentation to take place. The water in which the cylinders are kept should be cold; otherwise, it is believed proper fermentation does not take place. This process is preferred more by farmers and rural people. This product can be stored for up to 1 to 2 months. In case glass bottles are used, the sliced bamboo shoots are filled inside the bottle and water is added till all the shoots are submerged. The bottle is then capped and kept at room temperature or near the fireplace for fermentation. The shoots in the bottle can be kept for up to one year. This process is more preferred by urban people. The protein content of the fermented product has been found to be 8.5 g %, more than unfermented bamboo shoots. It is consumed as a curry by mixing with meat or fish (Agrahar-Murungkar and Subbulakshmi, 2006; Tamang and Tamang, 2009a).

Soibum/Soidon

These are products made from fermented bamboo shoots, a food indigenous to the state of Manipur. They are eaten as an essential part of the Manipuri diet, a social custom known to the people. Soibumi is produced only from the delicious bamboo shoots of the species *Dendrocalamus hamiltonii, D. sikkimensis, D. giganteus, Melocana bambusoide, Bambusa tulda* and *B. balcony*. The fermentation process is carried out from June to September, when the bamboo shoots grow. Relatively known for soybean production in Manipur are mainly located in the hills and are subject to availability and abundance of raw materials (Jeyaram et al., 2009; Bhatt et al., 2003). The organization and structure of the fermentation can be identified as *Lactobacillus plantarum, L. brevis, L. coryniformis, L. delbrueckii, L. lactis, Leuconostoc phallax, L. mesentroides, Enterococcus durans, Streptococcus lactis, Bacillus subtilis, B. licheniformis, B. coagulans* and the yeasts *Candida* sp., *Saccharomyces* sp., *Torulopsis* sp. (Tamang and Tamang, 2009a; Tamang et al., 2008).

Two types of fermentation procedures are followed for the preparation of soyabean, namely noney/kwatha type and andro type. In both methods, the inedible and tough outer part of the tasty bamboo shoots is peeled and the soft parts are cut and pressed tightly in wooden or clay containers and left to ferment for 6 to 12 months. The noney/kwatha type is the most numerous Preferably, it is a batch fermentation which results in a more acidic product with a sourer taste and is carried out in a traditional bamboo chamber lined with wild plant leaves or polythene sheets. Slices of delicious and tender bamboo shoots are squeezed into this bamboo chamber. After it is filled to its maximum capacity, the top opening of the bin is closed with a polythene sheet and weights are placed on it to make the seal intact. The bottom of this basket is perforated to allow the penetration of the acidic juices produced during fermentation. The setup is left like this for 6 to 12 months so that the solid fermentation takes place properly. The product after fermentation can be stored for more than a year.

The Andro type of fermentation is practiced only in the Andro village of Manipur. In this process, batch fermentation is carried out in large clay pots. First, a portion of the pot is filled with bamboo shoots and allowed to ferment. After the volume of the mash is reduced due to fermentation, additional bamboo shoots are added and pressure is applied from above to compact the mass. This process continues until the pot is filled to the top, after which it is stored for a period of 6 to 12 months. Here, fluids cannot flow (Jeyaram et al., 2008a). The product is white in color with a light aroma and sour taste. Prepared soibumi is usually sold in local vegetable markets, only by Maitei women. It is usually eaten with steamed rice as a side dish. It is also cooked with *Colocasia* sp bulbs, peas, pumpkin, potatoes, etc., in various recipes such as chutney. Some people also fry it with fish (Jeyaram et al., 2009; Tamang and Tamang, 2009a).

When the apical meristems of succulent bamboo shoots are fermented, the product is known as soidon. The species used are *Teinostachyum wightii*, a shrub Roxb Hill. , 1999. *Dendrocalamus giganteus* Munro, *Melocana bambooid* Trin. (Jeyaram et al., 2009; Tamang and Tamang, 2009a). Strains of *Lactobacillus brevis*, *Leuconostoc fallax* and *L. lactis* are associated with its fermentation (Tamang et al., 2008). To prepare soidon, mature bamboo shoots are harvested and the tender, delicious meristems are extracted by removing the outer, spiky parts and the lower parts. The shoots are cut crosswise into pieces and immersed in water. a clay pot. The fermented milk (soyjim) from the previous batch is added to this mixture at a 1-1 dilution as a starter culture. The leaves of the locally available heibung plant (*Garcinia pedunculata*) can be added to the fermentation mixture as an acidifier and also to improve the taste. Washed rice water, called chenghi, can sometimes be added at a 1-10 dilution to improve the color. The pot is covered and allowed to ferment for a period of 3 to 7 days. Then, the soydon is ready to be consumed. It can be stored for up to a year if stored in plastic containers at room temperature (Jeyaram et al., 2009; Tamang and Tamang, 2009a). Soidon is also consumed as a pickle. The liquid part can also be used as a spice to add a sour flavor to curries (Tamang and Tamang, 2009a).

Miya Mikhri

It is used by the Dimasa tribe of Assam. Bamboo shoots are collected, cleaned, and cut into small pieces for preparation. They are then wrapped in banana leaves and kept inside an earthen pot. This pot is left at room temperature for 4-5 days.

After the emission of a distinct smell, the shoots are shifted to a glass container. This can be stored for about a year. Miya mikhri can be taken as a pickle or even mixed with curry (Chakrabarty et al., 2009).

Ekung/Hirring

This is an ethnic fermented bamboo-shoot product of Arunachal Pradesh. It is called ekung by the Nyishing tribe and hirring by the Apatani tribe of Arunachal Pradesh. It is prepared from mid-April to early September when young bamboo shoots sprout. The species of bamboo used are *Dendrocalamus hamiltonii* Nees. et Arn. ex Munro, *D. giganteus* Munro, *Bambusa balcooa* Roxb., *B. tulda* Roxb, and *Phyllostachys assamica* Gamble ex Brandis (Tamang and Tamang, 2009a; Tamang and Tamang, 2009b).

The microbes generally associated with its fermentation are *Lactobacillus plantarum, L. lactis, L. brevis, L. casei,* and *Tetragenococcus halophilus* (Tamang and Tamang, 2009a; Tamang and Tamang, 2009b). The young and tender bamboo shoots are collected, the outer sheaths removed, and the edible part is chopped into very small pieces. A pit is dug in the ground and a bamboo basket is laid on it and lined with leaves. The basket is filled with chopped shoots, covered with leaves, and then sealed. Heavy stones are laid upon the basket to drain off the excess water. They are then fermented for 1-3 months. The product can be stored for a year in airtight containers. It is consumed raw or cooked with meat, fish, or vegetables. Sometimes this product is again cut into small pieces and dried in the sun for 5-10 days until the color changes from whitish to chocolate brown. This can be stored for up to two years at ambient temperature (Tamang and Tamang, 2009a).

Bas-tenga

Bas-tenga, meaning "sour bamboo," is a fermented bamboo shoot product made by the Nagas of Nagaland. The fermentation occurs between May and June, when new bamboo shoots emerge. Fresh, tender bamboo shoots are harvested, and the sheaths are removed. They are then cut into small pieces or pounded. A conical bamboo basket is used, with a hole at the bottom, through which a bamboo stick, slightly longer than the basket, is inserted vertically.

The basket's inner walls are lined with bamboo leaves, and the bamboo shoots are placed inside. The basket is tied to a post, covered with banana leaves, and weighted down with stones. The bamboo stick is twisted regularly to allow the sap to drain, and the juices collect at the basket's base. The shoots and juices ferment separately over a week (Mao and Odyuo, 2007). The shoots can be stored in bamboo internodes sealed with leaves or in a wooden vat, covered with banana leaves. The juice is sometimes stored in a gourd jar, a traditional Nagaland container. The shoots can also be sun-dried for a distinct aroma and extended shelf life. These fermented products are used in preparing meat, fish, and vegetable dishes. The juice, with properties similar to vinegar, acts as a preservative and extends the shelf life of cooked dishes (Mao and Odyuo, 2007).

Fermented Alcoholic Beverages

Ennog/Sai Mod

It is a form of black rice beer which is prepared and consumed by the tribal people of Arunachal Pradesh and the Mishings of Assam (Tiwari and Mahanta, 2007). Rice is first boiled and spread on a bamboo mat to cool. Simultaneously, paddy husk is filled into a large tin sheet or drum and allowed to burn slowly and evenly till it becomes black. The burnt husk, while still hot, is mixed with the boiled rice and allowed to cool. After cooling, the mixture is again mixed with crumbled ipoh cakes. They are then transferred to a conical bamboo basket lined with leaves of ekkam (*Phryium capitulum* wild). The whole basket is then covered with leaves and left to ferment for a period of 3 days when strong alcoholic smell is emitted. Then the mixture is transferred to another U-shaped bamboo basket called perop, lined with ekkam leaves. The basket is covered with more leaves and a piece of wood is placed on its top and a stone upon it for proper sealing.

Fermentation is allowed to take place for a period of 10 days after which the beer becomes ready for filtration. For filtration, about 2 kilograms of the mixture is loaded into a cylindrical bamboo tube called petok, fitte with a small opening at one end. To this, water is added and a paste is made by mixing. It is then made into small round cakes, which are kept on clean and dry paddy straws, called kher, spread on a round bamboo utensil, called kula, and again covered with kher. The kula is then kept on a rectangular frame made of bamboo, called dhuasang, above the fireplace. Upon drying, the mod pithas become hard and can be stored for 2 to 3 months. For brewing sujen, 4 to 5 kg of saol is mixed with rice husk, called tuh, and water and cooked with stirring. Cooked saol is poured on a round bamboo utensil, called dola, covered with clean banana leaves. Two to three powdered mod pithas are added to the warm saol and mixed thoroughly. The mixture is gathered into a round mount and on top of it, three jalokias (chilies) and three pieces of burning koila (charcoal) are kept.

Fronds of *Pteridium aquilinum*, called bihlongoni, are spread over the mount and covered with kolpat (banana leaves), above which a dola is placed. A big earthen pot, called koloh, is sterilized by washing with ashes and then drying above a smoking fireplace. The mixture is transferred to this pot and the mouth of the pot is sealed with bihlongoni and kolpat, and wrapped tightly with a cloth. This is allowed to ferment for 3 to 4 days in summer and 7 days in winter. After fermentation, the mass is filtered and sujen is obtained as the filtrate. This can be stored for a month in winter and 2-3 weeks in summer. It can be further diluted according to the requirement (Deori et al., 2007).

Apong

Apong is an alcoholic beverage prepared in Arunachal Pradesh and is known to almost all the tribes of the state. It is also prepared by the Mishings of Assam. It holds a very important place in the tradition of the people of this region. The starter culture used for its preparation is called ipoh, which contains yeast to carry out the fermentation (Tiwari and Mahanta, 2007). The related yeasts are *Saccharomyces cerevisiae, Hanseniaspora* sp. , *Kloeckera* sp. , *Pischia* sp. and *Candida* sp. , *S. cerevisiae* is the dominant strain (Tanti et al. , 2010). To prepare ipoh, rice is first dried and ground into a fine powder. This is then mixed with the powdered seeds and bark of the local plants *Veronia cinerea* Less and *Clerodendron viscosum* Vent. This mixture is poured into a container called Dekchi and made into a paste with water from the previously prepared apong. This paste is poured and spread on bamboo mats and made into small disc-shaped cakes. They are then carefully dried over a fire or left in a cool place for 3 to 4 days. After drying, they can be stored for up to a year (Tiwari and Mahanta, 2007). To prepare aponga, the rice is first washed and boiled in a wide-bottomed aluminum pot. Be careful not to overcook the rice so that it does not become mushy. Ipoh is then mixed with the rice in the right amount. Then transfer everything to another container with a lid and add some water. It is then left to ferment at room temperature for a period of 3 to 5 days after which it emits a strong smell of alcohol. The soup is diluted with water before consumption (Tiwari and Mahanta, 2007).

Kodo ko Jaanr

The tribes of Sikkim prepare a fermented product called kodo ko jaanr from the dried seeds of millet (*Eleusine coracana*), locally called kodo. It is an integral part of the food culture and religious beliefs of the ethnic groups of Sikkim (Tamang et al., 1996; Sekar and Mariappan, 2007). A traditionally prepared mixed inoculum or starter, called murcha, is used for its preparation. The microbes associated with murcha and kodo ko jaanr have been identified as *Mucor cicinelloides, Rhizopus chinensis, R. stolonifer var. lyococcus, Saccharomyces cerevisiae, S. bayanus, Hansenula anomala, Pediococcus pentosaceus, Lactobacillus* sp., *Candida glabrata, Saccharomycopsis capsularis, S. fibuligera, Pichia burtonii, P. anomalie, Cryptococcus* sp. , *Trichosporon* sp. , *Debaryomyces* sp. , *Kluyveromyces* sp. , *Myxozyma* sp. , *Bullera* sp. , *Rhodotorula* sp. , and *Tremella* sp. (Tamang and Sarkar, 1995; Tsuyoshi et al., 2005; Tiwari et al. , 2007; Sekar and Mariappan, 2007).

To prepare morcha, glutinous rice is soaked in water for 6 to 8 hours and pounded in a heavy wooden mortar and pestle. For 1 kg of ground rice, add the roots of *Plumbago zeylanica* L. (2.5 g), the leaves of *Buddleja asiatica* Lour (1.2 g). 2 g), *Vernonia cinerea* Less flowers (1.2 g), *Gingiber officinale* (5.0 g), dried red pepper (1.2 g) and previously prepared marcha (10.0 g) are added. The mixture is mixed into flat cakes placed on a bamboo stove lined with fresh fern leaves [*Glaphylopteriolopsis erubescens* (Wall ex Hook.) Ching] and covered with bags of dried fern and jute. The whole thing is placed on the stove and allowed to ferment for 1 to 3 days. They are then dried in the sun for 2 to 3 days. The product is called murcha and can be stored in a dry place for over a year (Tsuyoshi et al. , 2005).

To prepare kodo ko jaanr, millet grains are cleaned, washed and boiled for about 30 minutes. The excess water is drained and the boiled millet is spread on a bamboo stove called mandro to cool. About 1-2% marcha powder is sprinkled on the cooked grains, mixed well and packed in a bamboo basket decorated with fresh ferns (*Thelypteris erubescens*), locally called thadre unioon or banana leaves, then covered with jute cloth and stored for 2 to 4 days at room temperature. After this, the mass is transferred to an earthen pot or a specially designed bamboo basket called septu and air-dried. The whole is then fermented for 3 to 4 days in summer and 5 to 7 days in winter at room temperature. About 200 to 500 g of the fermented mass is placed in a vessel called a toongbaa and warm water is added to the brim. After about 10 to 15 minutes, the milky white extract of Jaanr is drunk through a narrow bamboo straw, called a pipsing, which has a hole in one side near the bottom to prevent the grains from passing through. Water may be added again 2 to 3 times after drinking the extract (Singh and Jain, 1995; Tamang et al., 1996).

Xaj-pani

The Ahoms of Assam prepare a kind of rice beer which they locally call xaj-pani. It is the most important drink, often used in religious rites and rituals practiced by the Ahoms. They also use it during the Bihu festivals as a refreshing drink and also take it after hard work. To prepare xaj pani, first the starter culture called vekur pitha must be prepared (Saikia et al., 2007). To prepare vekr pitha, the leaves of *Lygodium flaxuosum* Linn. , *Leucas aspera* Spring, C*issampelos pareira, Scoparia dulsis* Linn. , *Cinnamomum glanduliferum* Meissn. , and *Piper betle* Linn. harvested and dried in the sun for 1 to 2 days. These are then ground into a powder and mixed with powdered rice in a container containing a little water. To this mixture is added pre-prepared pita, called ghai pitha, which serves as a source of leavening agent. The mixture is then made into disc-shaped cakes and wrapped in banana leaves (*Musa paradisiaca* Linn.) and kept in an airtight place over a fire for 4 to 5 days. Once dried, the sweets are known as vekur pitha, which serves as a source of *Saccharomyces cerevisiae* and can be stored for later use. For the preparation of rice beer, the main variety of rice used by Ahoms is Bora rice which belongs to the Sali variety. The rice is first boiled and placed on a flat surface and then left uncovered for an hour. Then the cooled and dried rice is mixed with pitha paste. This mixture is then transferred to a clay pot, called kalah, which is kept in a dark place in a corner of the house for a period of 4 to 5 days away from air. After this period, the concentrated alcoholic liquid is recovered from the mash by a filtration process. This is achieved by placing a suitably sized container over the mouth of the pot to act as a lid or by placing rice straw to prevent the semi-solid rice from escaping. The filtrate is known as xaj pani which is highly aromatic, alcoholic and has a sweet taste (Saikia et al., 2007).

Zutho

This rice beer is produced from sprouted rice grains by the Angami tribe of Nagaland. *Saccharomyces cerevisiae* is the most prevalent microorganism in the fermentation process (Teramoto et al., 2002; Sekar and Mariappan, 2007). To prepare zutho, unhulled glutinous rice grains are soaked for 3 days, after which the water is drained and the rice is left to germinate for 3-4 days in summer and 7 days in winter. The germinated rice grains, along with the hulls, are then pounded in a wooden mortar to create the grist. Rice powder is added, followed by boiling water (5 liters for 3 kg), and mixed thoroughly. After cooling, a portion of the grist is added: one handful in summer and two handfuls in winter. Fermentation occurs in a wooden vessel for 2-3 days in summer and 7 days in winter. Water is added to the fermented mash, which is then strained through a bamboo basket to produce jutho, a milky slurry with 5.0% alcohol content, pH 3.6, and an acidity of 5.1 (Teramoto et al., 2002). Similarly, the Zeme Naga tribe of Assam also prepares a rice beer called dekuijao (Chakrabarty et al., 2009).

Judima

Judima is a rice beer made by the Dimasa tribe of Assam, using a starter culture known as humao. To prepare humao, brown rice is soaked for 10-12 hours at room temperature, then crushed with *Glycyrrhiza glabra* L. barks. Water is added to form a paste, which is shaped into flat cakes, dried in the sun, and called humao (Chakrabarty et al., 2009). To make judima, washed rice is cooked, dewatered, and cooled. The rice is then mixed with the humao cakes in appropriate amounts. The mixture is spread overnight on a banana leaf and placed in an earthen pot, which is sealed partially. Fermentation occurs for 3-4 days during summer. The resulting juice is called judima (Chakrabarty et al., 2009).

Antingba

In Manipur, the locals prepare an alcoholic beverage known as Antingba from glutinous rice. The starter culture used is called hamei, and its preparation method is a closely guarded secret passed down through generations (Jeyaram et al., 2008b). To make hamei, raw rice is crushed with yangli plant bark powder (*Albizzia myriophylla*) (0.25 kg per kg of rice) and water to form a dough-like mass. This is mixed with powdered hamei from the previous batch and shaped into flat cakes. The cakes are left over rice husks or in bamboo baskets for 2-3 days at room temperature. After fermentation, the cakes swell, take on an alcoholic flavor, and develop a yellowish hue. These cakes are dried and can be stored for up to a year (Tamang et al., 2007; Jeyaram et al., 2008b; Jeyaram et al., 2009). Lactic acid bacteria like *Lactobacillus plantarum* and *Pediococcus pentosaceus* and fungal agents such as *Saccharomyces cerevisiae* and *Candida tropicalis* are involved in the fermentation (Jeyaram et al., 2008b). For Antingba, glutinous rice is cooked, cooled, and mixed with crushed hamei (5 cakes for 10 kg). This mixture ferments in mud pots, covered with hangla (Alocasia sp.) leaves, for 3-4 days in summer and 6-7 days in winter. The fermentation continues submerged in earthen pots for another 2-3 days. The final be erage is called Antingba (Jeyaram et al., 2009).

Kiad

Kiad is a local liquor popular among the Jaintia tribe of Meghalaya, with significant cultural importance during religious festivals. Its preparation is done in two stages- the creation of natural yeast, thiat, and brewing the liquor itself (Jaiswal, 2010; Samati and Begum, 2007). To make thiat, cleaned leaves of the khawiang plant (*Amomum aromaticum*) are dried and powdered. Local rice called kho-so is soaked and ground into powder. These powders are mixed in a cone-shaped basket, then water is added to form a paste. Small cakes are shaped from the paste, dried in the sun, and are called thiat, which acts as yeast. For brewing kiad, kho-so rice is cooked with spring water, stirred continuously, then cooled and dried. Crushed thiat cakes are mixed into the cooled rice. The mixture is placed in a cone-shaped basket called shang, covered with cloth, and left to ferment for 2-3 days. The fermented mash, known as jyndem, is distilled using a set of vessels called shetkiad. The resulting liquor is kiad (Jaiswal, 2010; Samati and Begum, 2007).

Sujen

Sujen, a rice beer, is popular among the Deori tribe of Assam. It is considered pure and used as holy water by priests during various ceremonies. The preparation of sujen involves two stages- making the starter called mod pitha and then brewing the beer itself (Deori et al., 2007). Mod pitha is made using about 32 plant species, including Artocarpus heterophyllus, *Cinnamomum bejolghota, Costus speciosus,* and *Melastoma malabathricum.* The leaves, barks, roots, and bulbs of these plants are cleaned, sundried, and then ground with soaked rice in a wooden grinder, called dheki. The ground mixture is sieved and left to ferment for 7-15 days, producing a characteristic aroma when complete.

MALT BEVERAGES

Beer and ale are the primary malt beverages produced and consumed in this country, and these will be the focus here. They are made from malt, hops, yeasts, water, and malt adjuncts. The malt is derived from barley grains that are germinated, dried, and have their sprouts or germs removed. Hops are the dried flo ers of the hop plant. Malt adjuncts are additional starch- or sugar-containing ingredients included alongside the carbohydrates in the malt. Starch adjuncts can include corn and its derivatives, rice, wheat, barley, sorghum, soybeans, cassava, and potatoes, with corn and rice being the most commonly used. Sweet adjuncts include sugars and syrups.

Brewing of Beer

The manufacture of beer will be outlined briefly as an example of the brewing process.

Malting

In the preparation of malt, barley grains are soaked, or "steeped," at 10 to 15.6 °C, germinated at 16 to 21 °C for 5 to 7 days, and kiln-dried. Most of the sprouts or germs are removed, and the malt remains. The malt, a source of amylases and proteinases, is crushed before use.

Mashing

The mashing process aims to extract as much as possible from the malt and malt adjuncts, particularly focusing on hydrolyzing starches, polysaccharides, proteins, and their hydrolysis products. To begin, the ground malt is mixed with water at temperatures between 38 to 50°C to prepare the main malt mash. Cooked starchy malt adjuncts, which are at around 100°C after boiling or cooking under steam pressure, are then added. This brings the temperature of the mash to about 65 to 70°C, which allows for saccharification (conversion of starch to sugars) to occur quickly. The temperature is then raised to about 75°C, which deactivates the enzymes. Insoluble materials settle at the bottom of the container, acting as a filter to ensure the liquid, called wort, is clear. A special "lauter" tub may be used for filtration, with rinses from the filtering material added to the wort. Afterward, hops are added to the wort to form the liquid that will be used for fermentation. In more advanced methods, some mashing steps and ingredients may be replaced with partially hydrolyzed syrups derived from corn or barley.

Fermentation

A specific bottom-fermenting beer yeast strain, *Saccharomyces carlsbergensis*, is used to inoculate or "pitch" the cooled wort. This yeast is typically sourced from a previous fermentation. A relatively heavy inoculum, around 1 lb per barrel (31.5 gal) of beer, is added. The fermentation temperature varies across breweries, generally ranging from 3.3 to 14°C. Some brewers maintain temperatures between 3.3 to 4.4°C, while others begin at a lower temperature and gradually increase it. The fermentation process typically takes 8 to 14 days, usually completing in 8 to 10 days.During fermentation, the yeast primarily converts the sugars in the wort into alcohol and carbon dioxide, along with minor amounts of glycerol and acetic acid. Proteins and fat derivatives produce small quantities of higher alcohols and acids, and organic acids and alcohols combine to form aromatic esters. As carbon dioxide is released, foaming increases, eventually decreasing when fermentation concludes. In later stages, the bottom yeast "breaks," meaning it flocculates and settles. Bacterial growth is undesirable during fermentation and the subsequent aging process of the beer.

Aging, or Maturing

The young, or "green," beer is stored, or "lagered," in vats at about 0 °C for from several weeks to several months, during which period precipitation of proteins, yeast, resin, and other undesirable substances takes place and the beer becomes clear and mellowed or matured. Esters and other compounds are produced to add to the taste and aroma, and the body changes from harsh to smooth.

Finishing

After aging, the lager beer is carbonated to a CO_2 content of about 0.45 to 0.52 percent, mostly by means of gas collected during the fermentation. Then the beer is cooled, clarified, or filtered and packaged in bottles, cans, or barrels. The alcohol content is about 3.8 percent by weight. The beer for cans or smaller bottles is pasteurized briefly at about 60 to 61 °C or filtered through membranes or other materials to remove all yeasts.

Continuous Processes

Continuous malting to shorten germination time of the barley involves application of aerated water to the grain as a finely divided spray after the barley has been wetted and washed. Continuous brewing employs nonstop mashing and boiling of wort as well as flow-through fermentation. The beer may be bottled without aging.

Boiling the Wort with Hops

The wort, containing hops, is boiled for approximately 2.5 hours and then filtered through the hop residues to remove hop solids and precipitated proteins. The precipitate is washed with hot water to extract most of the soluble material, and the washings are combined with the original filtrate. This process results in a mash or wort that is ready for fermentation.

Boiling the wort with hops serves several purposes- (1) concentration of the wort, (2) sterilization, (3) inactivation of enzymes, (4) extraction of soluble substances from the hops, (5) coagulation and precipitation of proteins and other compounds, (6) slight caramelization of sugars, and (7) the addition of antiseptic substances such as humulone, cohumulone, and adhumulone, which are effecti e against gram-positive bacteria. Additionally, the boiling extracts bitter acids and resins from the hops, contributing to the beer's flavor, stability, and head retention. Essential oils from the hops add flavor, while tannins are minimized due to their potential to cause off-flavor and haziness. Recent advancements include the use of concentrated hop extracts or vacuum-packed milled hops as substitutes for whole dried hop flowers.

Microbiology

The procedures followed during brewing significantly affect the ability of microorganisms to survive or grow. Although little is known about microbial growth during malting, the main malt mash, or the cereal-malt mash, growth likely occurs in the first two stages. However, boiling the wort and hops for 2.5 hours generates enough heat to destroy most microorganisms, except for highly resistant bacterial spores, such as those from *Bacillus* or *Clostridium* species. The combination of heat and hop-derived antiseptics typically eliminates most of these spores and inhibits any surviving microorganisms. The yeast used for pitching should be a pure culture (though it often is not), ensuring that no contaminating organisms are introduced. The wort is unfavorable to some microorganisms due to its low pH (3.7 to 4.5) and the antiseptics derived from hops. Additionally, fermentation and aging occur at low temperatures, and the anaerobic conditions are also unfavorable for many microorganisms. The alcohol produced further inhibits microbial growth.

Beer is designed to suppress microorganism growth due to its low pH, the presence of antiseptic substances like alcohol and hop extracts (mainly resins or humulones), and its low storage temperature. Anaerobic conditions persist throughout brewing and storage, and much of the beer sold is pasteurized or filtered. Despite these protective factors, beer can still be affected by microorganisms, leading to defects and "diseases." Since the microorganisms that most often cause beer spoilage are easily killed by temperatures below boiling, they typically enter the beer after the wort has been boiled with hops.

Beer Defects and "Diseases"

The term defects will be used here for undesirable characteristics that are not caused by microbes, such as (1) turbidity due to unstable proteins, protein-tannin complexes, starch, and resin. (2) unpleasant odors caused by poor quality ingredients or contact with metals. and (3) poor physical characteristics. This discussion will be limited to disorders caused by microorganisms and therefore called beer infections or beer diseases. St. John's wort in brewing can cause butyric fermentation by *Clostridium* spp. or lactic fermentation by lactic acids if the wort is kept too long at temperatures that favor these bacteria. Off-flavors produced in this way can be found in beer. It was pointed out in Chapter 21 that brewer's yeast is usually contaminated with bacteria and wild yeast and can be a source of spoilage organisms. Yeast and bacteria produce turbidity when grown in beer, and yeast from fermentation can be responsible for turbidity. Similarly, wild yeasts, such as *Saccharomyces pastorianus*, can cause brain fog. Yeast can be inhibited or eliminated by preventing air from entering, fermenting most of the sugar in the wort to produce a "dry" beer, using the right brewer's yeast cultures, and properly disinfecting the brewhouse. Yeast can also be responsible for off-flavors and unpleasant odors. Thus, for example, bitterness can be caused by *S. pastorianus* and ester flavor by *Hansenula anomala*. Most yeasts produce fruity aromas and some produce hydrogen sulfide from hop extract found in beer. Yeasts capable of utilizing beer dextrins (e.g., *Saccharomyces diastaticus*) are potential spoilage organisms.

The bacteria responsible for beer taint mainly belong to the genera *Pediococcus, Lactobacillus, Flavobacterium,* and *Acetobacter*."Sarcina's taint", characterized by sourness, cloudiness, and pungency of beer, is caused by *Pediococcus cerevisiae*. Since the shells often cluster in fours or tetrads, they were originally thought to be sarcinae.Certain lactobacilli, tolerant to acid antiseptics and LUPO, can grow in beer. *Lactobacillus pastorianus** and *L. diastaticus** cause silky acidity and cloudiness. These bacteria produce lactic, acetic, and formic acids, alcohol, and carbon dioxide from sugars, and are particularly harmful in high fermentations, such as those used for beer.

Zymomonas anaerobium, when grown in beer, causes a silky turbidity and produces an odor reminiscent of hydrogen sulfide and apple. Carbon dioxide and alcohol are formed. It is easily destroyed by heat and is rarely found in pasteurized beer. *Obesumbacterium proteus* is responsible for the aroma and taste of moldy parsley and beer. It produces alcohol and acid and does not tolerate pH down to 4.2. It has been discovered as a common contaminant of fermenting yeast. *Acetobacter* and *Gluconobacter* species, which are tolerant to acidic and hop-based antiseptics, can cause sourness in the mill or beer under aerobic conditions. Exposure to oxygen can be found in over-stored musts, empty beer barrels, and brewer's yeast. A number of species can cause sourness; *Gluconobacter oxydans* subsp. *suboxydans** and *G. oxydans* subsp. *industrious** can produce a noble character; and *A. pasteurianus* was blamed for turbidity and acidity.

Other unidentified and incompletely described bacteria have been blamed for beer-related illnesses. The species *Micrococcus**, *Streptococcus* and *Bacillus* were blamed for the cause of the problems, but in some cases they were probably only present. *Streptococcus mucilaginosus**, which is probably a *Pediococcus*, has been reported to cause a noble character.It should also be noted that all yeasts and bacteria that cause infections or diseases in the wort and beer are killed by boiling the wort and hops and must have entered the facility through equipment, air, water or seed yeast and that aseptic and sanitary precautions will help prevent these problems.

Other Malt Beverages and Beer Types

Variations in malt beverages or beer types are usually related to (1) alcohol content, (2) concentration of malt and hops used, (3) length of aging, (4) initial total solids (related to fermentable carbohydrate present and remaining after fermentation), and (5) temperature of fermentation.

- Malt liquor may have a higher alcohol content than does regular beer.
- Bock beer is a very dark beer with a high alcohol content. Brewing involves the addition of higher concentrations of malt and hops followed by longer aging.
- Pilsener is a lager-type beer, light in color, containing little remaining fermentable carbohydrate.
- Low-calorie, light, or no-carbohydrate beers are made from prehydrolyzed wort. Fungal enzymes (glucoamylases and amylases) are used to hydrolyze the dextrin to maltose and glucose, which can be completely fermented to alcohol; the net result is a lower concentration of remaining carbohydrate.

Ale usually is made with a top yeast, a strain of *Saccharomyces cerevisiae*, instead of the bottom yeast employed for beer, although a bottom yeast sometimes is used. The primary fermentation takes place at 12.2 to 24.4 °C, a higher temperature than for beer, and therefore the fermentation is more rapid, taking 5 to 7 days. The top yeast forms clumps which collect carbon dioxide gas and are carried to the top of the wort. At intervals the yeast scum is skimmed off. More hops are used in ale than in beer, and some ales have a higher alcohol content. Ale usually is pale in color and tart in taste.

Weiss beer, porter, and stout are ales in that top yeasts are employed in their manufacture. Weiss beer is a light, tart ale made chiefly from wheat. Porter and stout are dark, heavy, sweet ales.

Related Beverages

Sake is a traditional Japanese alcoholic beverage, often categorized as a yellow rice beer or wine, with an alcohol content of around 14 to 17 percent.

The brewing process begins with the creation of a starter, known as koji, where *Aspergillus oryzae* is cultivated on a soaked and steamed rice mash to maximize enzyme production. This koji contains amylases that break down rice starch into fermentable sugars, along with other enzymes like proteinases. The koji is then combined with more rice mash, converting starch into sugar, and fermentation is carried out by various *Saccharomyces* yeast species. After 10 to 14 days, the liquid is filtered, resulting in sake.

Sonti, an Indian rice beer or wine, involves fermentation by the mold *Rhizopus sonti* and yeasts. Pulque, a Latin American beverage, is another beer-like drink with an alcohol content of about 6 percent, made by naturally fermenting the juice of the agave plant using yeast. Ginger beer, a mildly alcoholic and acidic beverage, is created by fermenting a sugar solution flavored with ginger. The fermentation process involves the "ginger-beer plant," a combination of the yeast *Saccharomyces pyriformis* and the bacterium *Lactobacillus vermiformis,* both encased in the bacterium's gelatinous capsule.

WINES

Unless otherwise specified, the term wine is applied here to the product made by the alcoholic fermentation of grapes or grape juice by yeasts and a subsequent aging process. Wines, however, can be produced by the fermentation of the juices of fruits, berries, rhubarb, dandelions honey, etc.

Grape Wine

Grape wines are for the most part either red or white. The red wines, fermented on the skins, contain the red pigment from the skins of purple or red varieties of grapes, whereas white wines are made from white grapes or the expressed juice of other grapes, fermented free of the skins. The manufacture of red wine will be outlined briefly as an example of the wine-making process.

Preparation of Juice

Grapes of a variety especially adapted to wine making are harvested at a stage when they have the desired sugar content. The concentration of sugar may range from 15 to 25 percent, depending on the grape variety and its degree of ripeness. They are stemmed and crushed by machine and then treated with sulfur dioxide (75 to 200 ppm) or potassium metabisulfite in equivalent amounts to inhibit the growth of undesirable competitors of the wine yeast.

Fermentation

A "natural inoculum" (yeast present on the grapes) or more commonly 2 to 5 percent of a special wine yeast, a strain of *Saccharomyces cerevisiae* var. *ellipsoideus,* is added to the crushed grapes, or must. At first the contents of the tank are mixed twice a day by punching the "cap" of floating skins, stems, etc., pumping juice over the skins, or mixing in some other way to aerate and hence encourage growth of the yeast and aid in the extraction of color from the skins (for red wines). Alternatively, the red pigments may be extracted from the skins by heat and added back to the juice. Later the mixing is discontinued, for anaerobic conditions are most favorable to the alcoholic fermentation. It is very important that the temperature be maintained within an optimal range, i.e., between 24 and 27°C for red wines, during the active fermentation, which takes about 3 to 5 days, and at 10 to 21°C for white wines (active fermentation takes 7 to 14 days). An excessively high temperature inhibits the wine yeasts and permits competing organisms, e.g., the lactobacilli to grow and cause defects; too low a temperature slows action of the wine yeasts and permits wild yeasts, lactic acid bacteria, and other organisms to grow. Heat is liberated during the fermentation, and this, coupled with high atmospheric temperatures, may necessitate artificial cooling of the must.

After the primary or active fermentation has advanced sufficiently the fermented juice is drawn off from the residues (pomace) and placed in a storage tank under a light pressure of carbon dioxide for the secondary fermentation for 7 to 11 days at about 21 to 29°C. Here the remaining sugar is fermented if a dry wine is desired. Clear wine is drawn off, or "racked," from the sediment at the bottom of the tank.

Storing and Aging

The wine may be flash-pasteurized before aging (but usually is not) to precipitate proteins. It is cooled, held for a few days, filtered, and transferred into wooden tanks (usually of white oak or redwood) or plastic-coated concrete tanks for aging. The tanks are filled completely and sealed to keep out air. Periodically the wine is racked from bottom sediment. Final aging may be in the bottle. Aging for months or years results in desirable changes in body and flavor of the wine, giving it the aroma or bouquet that should be one of its characteristics. Esters and alcohols are considered important contributors to bouquet and taste. During aging some fermentation of the malic acid of grape juice by lactobacilli or micrococci* (malolactic fermentation) may take place with the production of lactic acid and carbon dioxide and reduction in acidity.

After aging, the wine is filtered or otherwise clarified, barreled or bottled, and stored. Some wines are pasteurized after aging, usually in the bottle. The final alcohol content varies widely but usually is between 6 and 9 percent by weight or 8 and 13 percent by volume.

Volatile Acidity of Wines

A high content of volatile acid in wines is indicative of a faulty fermentation. In the United States the legal limit for volatile acid content is 0.14 g per 100 ml, expressed as acetic acid, for red wine and 0.12 g for white wine.

Microbiology

The grapes when crushed have a variety of microorganisms on their surfaces, including yeasts and bacteria. Not only is the surface flora of the grape present, but also an array of contaminants from the soil. To suppress these organisms the wine maker adds sulfur dioxide or sulfite or less commonly pasteurizes the must (expressed juice). During the primary fermentation the added wine yeast predominates. During early stages, growth of the yeast is favored by aeration of the must; later, anaerobic conditions favor the alcoholic fermentation by the yeasts, liberating carbon dioxide and ethyl alcohol, both of which help inhibit organisms other than the wine yeasts. The atmosphere of carbon dioxide above the wine during the secondary fermentation prevents the growth of aerobic contaminants, such as the acetic acid bacteria. The pasteurization that follows, although not for that purpose, reduces the numbers of microorganisms that later might cause spoilage ("diseases") of the wine. There should be little or no growth of organisms during the aging and storage of the wine, but organisms that can grow then may be introduced by contamination from the tanks, barrels, or bottles, and changes such as the malolactic fermentation may take place.

Kinds of Wine

Instead of listing the many names for various types of wines, a few general terms are defined. Most wines are still wines, meaning they do not retain the carbon dioxide produced during fermentation, unlike sparkling wines, which contain a significant amount of carbon dioxide. Some wines may also be artificially carbonated.

Dry wines have little to no unfermented sugar, while sweet wines contain remaining or added sugar. Typically, wines contain between 11 to 16 percent alcohol by volume, though some may have as low as 7 percent. Fortified wines, which have had distilled wine spirits or brandy added, have an alcohol content of about 19 to 21 percent. Table wines are low in alcohol and contain little or no sugar, while dessert wines are both sweet and fortified

French dry sherry is notable because it is made from grapes affected by *Botrytis cinerea,* a gray mold, which causes the grapes to dry and increases their sugar content, resulting in higher alcohol wine. Spanish (Jerez) sherry is known for the growth of a yeast film, likely a species of *Saccharomyces,* which forms while the wine is racked in partially filled barrels after fermentation. This yeast, called "flor," gives the wine its distinct bouquet and flavor

Wine Defects and Microbial Spoilage

Like beer, wine has defects from nonmicrobial causes and spoilage caused by microorganisms. Defects include those due to metals or their salts, enzymes, and agents employed in clearing the wine. Iron, for example, may produce a sediment known variously as gray, black, blue, or ferric casse, and in white wine may be responsible for a white precipitate of iron phosphate termed white casse. Tin and copper and their salts have been blamed for cloudiness. White wines may be turned brown and red wines may have their color precipitated by peroxidase, an oxidizing enzyme of certain molds. Gelatin, used in clarifying wines, may cause cloudiness.

The microorganisms causing wine spoilage are chiefly wild yeasts, molds, and bacteria of the genera *Acetobacter, Lactobacillus, Leuconostoc,* and perhaps *Micrococcus** and *Pediococcus.*

Factors Affecting Growth of Microorganisms in Wine

Several factors influence the susceptibility of wines to microbial spoilage

- **Acidity or pH:** A lower pH reduces the likelihood of spoilage. The minimal pH allowing microorganism growth depends on the organism, the wine type, and its alcohol content. Molds, yeasts, and acetic acid bacteria are not inhibited by normal wine pH levels, but most lactic acid bacteria can only tolerate a pH between 3.3 and 3.5, which is lower than the pH of many wines (California table wines typically have a pH of 3.5 to 4.0).
- **Sugar content:** Dry wines, which contain around 0.1 percent or less sugar, are rarely affected by bacterial spoilage. However, wines with sugar content of 0.5 to 1.0 percent or more are more prone to spoilage.
- **Alcohol concentration:** Alcohol tolerance varies among spoilage organisms. Acetic acid bacteria are inhibited by alcohol content over 14 to 15 percent, while deacidifying cocci are stopped by about 12 percent, Leuconostoc species by over 14 percent, heterofermentative lactobacilli by approximately 18 percent, and homofermentative lactobacilli by around 10 percent. However, *Lactobacillus trichodes* can grow in fortified wines with over 20 percent alcohol.
- **Accessory growth substances:** *Acetobacter* species can synthesize their own vitamins, while lactic acid bacteria require most of these substances to be provided. The primary source of these growth factors in wine is the wine yeast, which releases them upon autolysis. The more growth substances present, the higher the risk of spoilage by lactic acid bacteria.
- **Tannin concentration:** Tannins added with gelatin during clarification help retard bacterial growth, although usually in insufficien amounts to have a significant practical impact as inhibitors
- **Sulfur dioxide concentration:** The greater the amount of sulfur dioxide added, the more it inhibits spoilage microorganisms. The typical 75 to 200 ppm added to the must is usually sufficient The effectiveness of sulfur dioxide increases as the pH and sugar content decrease and is organism-dependent.
- **Storage temperature:** Spoilage is generally most rapid between 20 and 35°C, with the process slowing as the temperature approaches freezing.
- **Air availability:** The absence of air prevents the growth of aerobic organisms, such as molds, film yeasts, and *Acetobacter*. However, lactic acid bacteria thrive in anaerobic conditions.

Spoilage by Aerobic Microorganisms

Film yeasts, which can oxidize alcohol and organic acids, may develop a thick surface layer known as "wine flowers" on must and wines exposed to air. However, they generally do not cause significant issues if the must is regularly mixed and the wine is kept away from air.

In the presence of air, aerobic acetic acid bacteria like *Acetobacter aceti* or *Gluconobacter oxydans* oxidize alcohol in the must or wine to acetic acid, a process called acetification, which is undesirable. These bacteria may also convert glucose in the must to gluconic acid, resulting in a "mousy" or "sweet-sour" taste. Molds, such as *Mucor, Penicillium, Aspergillus,* and others, can grow on surfaces like plant walls, barrels, tanks, hoses, and corks, as well as on grapes or cold must. Mold growth can be minimized through proper cleaning of surfaces and equipment.

Spoilage by Facultative Microorganisms

Wild yeasts, which include all yeasts except wine yeasts added as yeast, can cause abnormal fermentations resulting in low alcohol content, high volatile acidity, off flavors and cloudiness in the wine. These yeasts, which come mainly from the grapes from which the cider is made and are generally of the beekeeping type, are suppressed or eliminated with an active wine yeast, sulfiting or pasteurizing the must before fermentation, and controlling the temperature. of cider during fermentation. Low temperatures, below 70°F, will favor some of the wild yeasts and bacteria that produce scum.

Lactic acid bacteria are the main causes of bacterial spoilage of cider and wine. There is some confusion in the application of names to different types of bacterial wine spoilage, perhaps because several types of bacteria can cause the same defect or because the same organism can cause different defects under different conditions. The most common spoilage is probably shift spoilage, in which acid is formed from the sugars, glucose and fructose present in the wine, mainly by heterofermenting species of *Lactobacillus,* such as *L. brevis, L. hilgardii, L. trichodes** and possibly *L. buchneri*. The growth of lactobacilli produces a silky cloudiness, increases lactic and acetic acids, produces carbon dioxide, sometimes imparts "musty" or other off-flavors and discolors the wine. When fructose fermentation produces a bitter product, mannitol, the fermentation is sometimes called "mannitic," bitterness can also result from the fermentation of glycerol in the wine. Gases resulting from a specific cause, such as the release of carbon dioxide from heterofermentative lactic acids, are called fermentation. Homofermentative. *L. plantarum* mainly forms lactic acid from the sugars of table wines, increasing the fixed acidity and gives a "mouse" taste.

The acidity of wine can be reduced by spoilage bacteria through the oxidation of malic, citric and tartaric acid by *Acetobacter* (aerobic) or through the fermentation of malic and tartaric acid by species of *Lactobacillus, Leuconostoc* or *Pediococcus* or from other cocci.

The viscosity or sharpness of young white wines, accompanied by cloudiness and increased volatile acidity, has been attributed to *Leuconostoc* spp. , *L. mesenteroides* and *L. dextranicum**; *Micrococcus**; and on lactobacilli. The addition of sucrose, when permitted, promotes the production of dextran and therefore viscosity by *Leuconostoc*.

Any bacteria or yeast growing in the wine is likely to cause undesirable haze, and any heterofermentative acetic or lactic bacteria growing in the wine may increase the volatile acidity to a point that makes the product unsaleable. Fermentation of sugars generally results in an increase in acidity, fixed acid if the lactic homo-fermentative organism and fixed and unstable acid if the organism is heterofermentative. Oxidation or fermentation of organic acids in grapes leads to a decrease in the amount of fixed acids. It should be emphasized again that the composition of the wine is important in determining its susceptibility to bacterial spoilage. Thus, white wines with low alcohol content are more susceptible to stickiness and spoilage by bacteria than other wines; ciders and table wines promote the growth of *Lactobacillus hilgardii, L. brevis,* and *Leuconostoc mesenteroides*; while *Lactobacillus trichodes** is the only species known to spoil dessert wines in California and does not grow in cider.

Interestingly, the formation of lactic acid from malic acid in highly acidic wines can improve their quality by reducing acidity. Lactic acid is a weaker acid than malic acid, and only two molecules of lactic acid are formed from three molecules of malic acid. Some bacteria can also form lactic acid, tartaric acid, and glycerin from wine.

Other Wines

Wine from Other Fruits

Wines can be made from most fruits, including apples (hard cider), peaches, apricots, plums, pears (perry), cherries, blackberries, and many others. Berries and most other fruits (except wine grapes) do not have enough sugar to make a good wine and must be "fortified" by adding sugar before fermentation. Otherwise, winemaking is similar to grape wine. The products can be dry, sweet, fortified, carbonated, or sparkling. Wines intended for consumption as such or for distillation to produce alcoholic beverages can also be made from dried fruits such as raisins, dates, figs, and prunes

The production and diseases of apple wine or cider, made from apple juice, have received considerable attention. Much American cider is made locally from apples that are not particularly suited to its production and is fermented by the yeasts present. As a result, it often produces only 4-6% alcohol, some residual sugar remains, and the aroma and bouquet may be muted or nonexistent. British and French ciders and some industrially produced American ciders are made from apples with high sugar and tannin content. Production methods may include sulfiting, the addition of sugars and yeast feed, and the inoculation of a proven yeast culture. Heterofermenting lactobacilli have been reported to be active during must production, malic and citric acid fermentation, sugars and glycerol to produce carbon dioxide; lactic, acetic, propionic and succinic acid; and mannitol.

Most of the diseases in hard cider are similar to those in grape wine; cloudiness, low alcohol content and off-flavor caused by wild yeast; turbidity and bad taste produced by lactobacilli; viscosity or tightness due to bacteria- production of acetic acid, etc. Low acidity and low nitrogen content should encourage the growth of spoilage organisms.

Wines from Other Agricultural Products

Theoretically any edible product that contains sufficien moisture, sugar, and other foods for yeasts can be used to make wine. Honey wine, or mead, is made from diluted honey to which minerals and nitrogenous food for the yeasts have been added. Dandelion wine is a homemade product made by alcoholic fermentation of a water extract of flo ers of the dandelion to which sugar, flavoring substances, and yeast have been added.

DISTILLED LIQUORS

The spirits or distillates we are concerned with here are those produced by the distillation of an alcoholic fermented product. Rum is the distillation of alcoholic fermented sugar cane juice, syrup or molasses. Whiskeys are distilled from the purity of saccharified and fermented grains, for example rye whiskey from rye mash, bourbon or grain whiskey from wheat grain, grain whiskey from corn, etc. Rum and whiskey are made from must fermented by special distillers' yeasts, species of *Saccharomyces cerevisiae* var. *ellipsoideus,* which gives a high alcohol yield. The grain must is usually acidified to favor the yeast. The aging of distilled spirits in charred oak barrels or casks is a chemical, not biological, process. Rakia refers to the distillation of grape wine, unless a qualifying word is added, e.g. for example, apple brandy, peach brandy, and apricot brandy.

VINEGAR

It was pointed out in Chapter 13 that the normal course of changes in fruit juices at ordinary temperatures is an alcoholic fermentation by yeasts, followed by oxidation of the alcohol to acetic acid by acetic acid bacteria. If enough acetic acid is produced, the product is vinegar. Vinegar is defined as a condiment made from sugary or starchy materials by an alcoholic fermentation followed by an acetous one. It must contain at least 4g of acetic acid per 100 ml (or 40 grain) to be legal vinegar.

Kinds of Vinegar

Vinegars can be classified according to the materials from which they are made- (1) those derived from fruit juices, e.g. from apple, grape, orange, pear, berry, etc., (2) those from starchy vegetables, e.g. vegetables rich in starch., potatoes or sweet potatoes, whose starch must first be hydrolyzed into sugars, (3) those of malted grains, such as barley, rye, wheat and corn, (4) those of sugars, such as syrups, molasses, honey , maple syrup, etc., and (5) those of alcohol or alcohol, for example, alcohol (beer) waste from the production of yeast or diluted and denatured ethyl alcohol. In fact, anything that contains enough sugar or alcohol and is not objectionable as food can be used to make vinegar. Vinegar usually gets its descriptive name from the material it comes from- cider vinegar from apple juice, beer vinegar, malt vinegar from malted grains, spirit vinegar from alcohol, etc. In the United States, most table vinegar is apple cider vinegar and therefore, the term vinegar alone usually means apple cider vinegar. Grape (wine) vinegar is most popular in France, and malt (alger) vinegar in the British Isles.

Fermentation

As has been indicated, the manufacture of vinegar from saccharine materials involves two steps:

(1) The fermentation of sugar to ethyl alcohol and (2) the oxidation of alcohol to acetic acid. The first step is an anaerobic process carried out by yeasts, either those naturally present in the raw material or, preferably, added cultures of high-alcohol-producing strains of *Saccharomyces cerevisiae* var. *ellipsoideus*. A simplified equation for the process is:

$$\underset{\text{glucose}}{C_6H_{12}O_6} \rightarrow 2CO_2 + \underset{\text{alcohol}}{2C_2H_5OH}$$

Actually a series of intermediate reactions takes place, and small amounts of other final products are produced, such as glycerol and acetic acid. Also, there are small amounts of other substances, produced from compounds other than sugar, including succinic acid and amyl alcohol.

The second step, oxidation of the alcohol to acetic acid, is an aerobic reaction carried out by the acetic acid bacteria:

$$\underset{\text{alcohol}}{C_2H_5OH} + \underset{\text{oxygen}}{O_2} \rightarrow \underset{\text{acetic acid}}{2C_2H_5OH} + \underset{\text{water}}{H_2O}$$

Acetaldehyde is an intermediate compound in this reaction. Among the final products are small amounts of aldehydes, esters, acetoin, etc.

The eighth edition of Bergey's Manual suggested three groups of *Acetobacter* with a total of nine subspecies. The genus *Gluconobacter* contained species capable of oxidizing ethanol to acetic acid. Volume 2 of Bergey's Manual (1986) suggested a Family called *Acetobacteriaceae* with two genera, *Acetobacter* and *Gluconobacter*. The latter species are differentiated from *Acetobacter* by their inability to oxidize acetic or lactic acid to carbon dioxide. *Acetobacter* is currently described as containing species which can oxidize acetic or lactic acid to carbon dioxide. Many "acetic acid bacteria" are now classified in the genus *Gluconobacter*. Although the majority of the vinegar fermentation "work" may be done by *Gluconobacter* sp., the cultures actually used commercially are not pure but rather are a mixture of strains that have been adapted to the fermentation.

Methods of Manufacture

The ways of making vinegar may be divided into the "slow" methods, such as the home, or "letalone," method and the French, or Orleans, method, and "quick" methods, such as the generator process or the fogging procedure. In slow methods the alcoholic liquid is not moved during acetification, while in quick methods the alcoholic liquid is in motion. For the most part the slow methods utilize fermented fruit juices or malt liquors for acetic acid production, whereas the quick methods are applied mostly to the production of vinegar from spirits (alcohol). Fruit or malt liquors are well supplied with food for the vinegar bacteria, but to maintain active vinegar bacteria in generator methods using alcohol, denatured with ethyl acetate or vinegar, it must be supplemented with a "vinegar food," which is a combination of organic and inorganic compounds that varies with the compounder. Combinations of substances such as dibasic ammonium phosphate, urea, asparagine, peptones, yeast extract, glucose, malt, starch, dextrins, salts, and other substances have been reported in use.

Quick Methods

As previously mentioned, rapid vinegar production methods involve circulating the alcoholic liquid during acetification. Typically, this liquid is passed over surfaces where vinegar bacteria have formed films and where a constant supply of air is provided.

The generator method is widely used today. The standard generator (Figure 22.1) is a cylindrical tank, often made of wood and available in various sizes. It is divided into three sections- the top section, where the alcoholic liquid is added; the larger middle section, where the liquid trickles over materials such as beechwood shavings, corncobs, rattan shavings, charcoal, coke, or pomace, providing a large surface area without compacting; and the bottom section, where the vinegar collects. The alcoholic liquid enters the top through an automatic feed or sprinkling device and trickles over the materials, which have developed a slimy growth of acetic acid bacteria that oxidize the alcohol into acetic acid. Air enters through the bottom of the middle section, rises after warming, and is vented above. Since this oxidation process generates significant heat, it is essential to control the temperature, ensuring it does not exceed 29-30 °C. Cooling coils, adjusting the air and liquid feed rates, or cooling the liquid before entering the generator, or cooling the partially acetified liquid recirculated from the bottom, can manage the temperature.

To start a new generator, the vinegar bacteria slime must first be established. Initially, raw vinegar containing active bacteria is used to inoculate the shavings or is circulated through the generator. Then, an alcoholic liquid, acidified with vinegar, is slowly trickled through the generator to encourage bacterial growth on the shavings before being recirculated. Some makers acidify the entire alcoholic liquid with vinegar before adding it to the generator or leave a portion to acidify the new liquid batch.

Vinegar production may occur with a single pass through the generator, or if insufficien acid is produced or too much alcohol remains, the collected vinegar can be recirculated. Sometimes, generators are operated in series, with liquid from the first tank passing through subsequent generators

The Frings generator is a large, airtight cylindrical tank with a sparger (sprinkler) at the top, cooling coils in the lower part of the middle section containing shavings, and a recirculation system for vinegar from the bottom. Modern generators feature automatic controls for liquid feeding, filtered air introduction, temperature control, and liquid recirculation. These generators provide high acetic acid yields and leave minimal alcohol residue.

In the Mackin process, a fine mist of vinegar bacteria and nutrient alcohol is sprayed through jet nozzles into a chamber. The mist is circulated by filtered air for a while before being allowed to settle for collection. The mist is then cooled, reatomized, and returned to the chamber until the alcohol oxidation is nearly complete.

The dipping generator consists of a tank with a basket filled with beechwood shavings, which can be raised out or lowered into a dilute alcohol solution. When the basket is out, aeration promotes rapid acetification by vinegar bacteria, and when submerged in the liquid, it adds more culture medium and removes some acetic acid.

Submerged Method

In submerged fermentation (Hromatka and Ebner, 1959) a stirred medium containing 8 to 12 percent alcohol (hard cider, wine, fermented malt mash, or spirits) is inoculated with *Acetobacter acetigenum** and is held at 24 to 29 °C with controlled aeration by means of finely divided air. In a subsequent paper, Hromatka described the use of a pure culture of *Gluconobacter oxydans* in a submerged vinegar fermentation (Bergey's Manual, 1984).

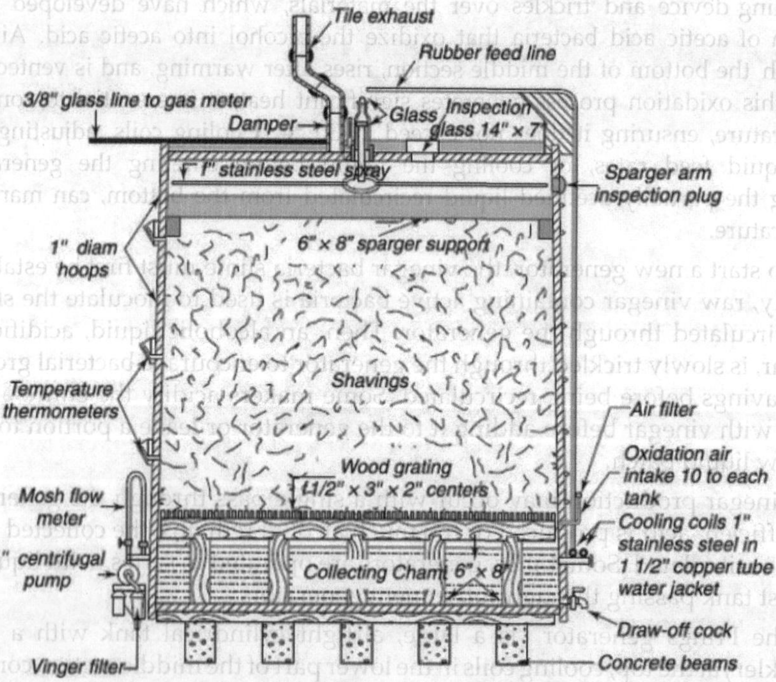

Fig 22.1.Diagram of a quick-method vinegar generator. (Courtesy of Food Engineering.)

Bacteria grow in a suspension of fine air bubbles and fermenting liquid, which is maintained by a specially designed aerator. The aerator consists of a rotor (a) powered by an electric motor (c) located beneath the tank (d). The rotor draws in air, mixes it with water, accelerates the mixture, and evenly distributes the suspension across the tank's cross section. To ensure the uniform distribution of air bubbles, the self-priming rotor is surrounded by a stator (b). An air pipe (e), connected to the rotor, exits the tank near the top and branches into two parts. One branch leads to a rotameter (f), which measures the air entering the tank, while the other connects to a condensate cylinder (g) attached to the exhaust air pipe (h).

Four stabilizer boards (i) are attached to the inner circumference of the tank, to which a stainless steel cooling coil (k) is affixed Cooling water flows into the coil via pipe (l) from a pump (m) equipped with a flowmeter (n). The pump is controlled by a regulating thermometer (o) to maintain a consistent fermentation temperature. The charging pump (p), located near the charging vat, pumps the mash through the charging pipe (q) and directs it into the tank near the center of the top, where it flows directly into the rotor

After each fermentation cycle, the discharging pump (r) near the Acetator empties half the tank. At the top center of the tank is a defoamer (s), which mechanically breaks down the foam (Note- Morton generators do not include a defoamer). The liquid portion of the foam is pumped back into the tank by the defoamer, and the air exits through the exhaust pipe. The controller (t) manages the charging and discharging of the generator.

Slow Methods

In the home or let-alone method, fruit juice, such as apple juice, undergoes spontaneous alcoholic fermentation, typically reaching about 11 to 13 percent alcohol, using yeasts naturally present in the juice. After fermentation, the juice is placed in a barrel, which is partially filled and positioned on its side with the bunghole open and facing upward. This setup allows the juice to undergo acetic acid fermentation, or acetification, driven by the naturally occurring vinegar bacteria until vinegar is produced. A film of vinegar bacteria, known as "mother of vinegar," grows on the surface and oxidizes the alcohol to acetic acid. However, this method often yields low amounts of vinegar due to several factors-insufficient alcohol yield from fermentation, absence of effective vinegar bacteria strains, oxidation of acetic acid when alcohol is in short supply, competitive growth of film yeasts and molds on the surface which consume alcohol and acids, and the presence of undesirable bacteria that impart unpleasant flavors. As a result, the process is slow, and the vinegar produced is often of poor quality.

In contrast, the Orleans, or French, method used extensively in Europe is a continuous process, though it is also carried out in barrels. In this method, raw vinegar from a previous batch is introduced to fill about one-fourth to one-third of the barrel, which serves as an inoculum of active vinegar bacteria and helps acidify the added wine, hard cider, or malt liquor, preventing the growth of competing microorganisms. The remainder of the barrel is filled with alcoholic liquor, leaving an air space above that is open to the outside through the bunghole at the top and a hole in each end of the barrel, all of which are covered with screening. The acetic acid bacteria, which grow as a film on top of the liquid, oxidize the alcohol to acetic acid over several weeks to months, with the temperature maintained between 21 to 29°C. After this fermentation period, part of the vinegar is drawn off for bottling, and the remaining liquid in the barrel is replaced with an equal amount of alcoholic liquor. This cycle is repeated, making the process continuous. The result is high-quality vinegar, although it takes a considerable amount of time.

One challenge with this method is the dropping of the gelatinous vinegar bacteria film, which can slow the acetification process. To address this, a raft or floating framework is sometimes used to support the film. It is believed that an overly thick bacterial film may hinder acetification, so controlling the thickness of the film is crucial

Finishing

The composition of vinegar varies depending on the raw material used, with fruit and malt liquors imparting their distinctive flavors to the vinegar. The production method also plays a significant role in shaping the final product

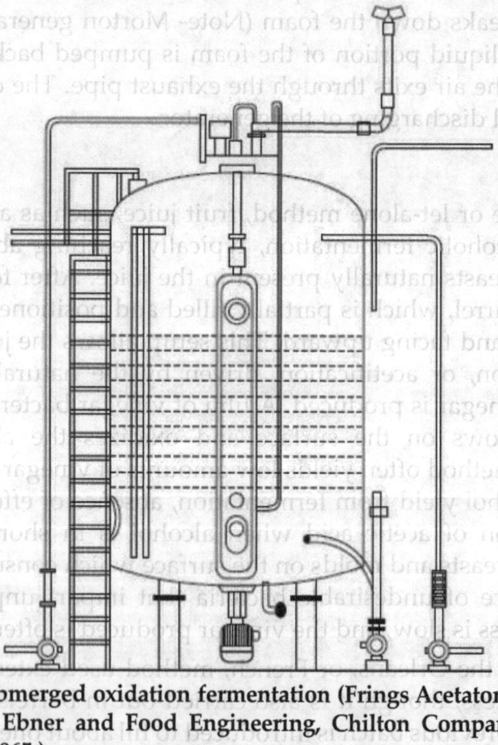

Fig 22.2. Vinegar by submerged oxidation fermentation (Frings Acetator), (By permission from Dr. H. Ebner and Food Engineering, Chilton Company, Philadelphia, Copyright © 1965.)

Vinegars produced through slow methods tend to be less harsh due to the aging process that occurs over a longer preparation time. In contrast, quickly made vinegars can improve in body, taste, and aroma when aged in tanks or barrels. To ensure clarity, vinegar is often subjected to filtration and "fining," which involves removing suspended particles through settling. Most commercially available vinegar is pasteurized, either in bulk or in bottles, with pasteurization times and temperatures varying; for example, heating at 60 to 66°C for a few seconds is a common approach

The strength of the vinegar is expressed in grains, that is, ten times the number of grams of acetic acid per 100 ml of vinegar. Thus 40-grain vinegar contains 4g of acetic acid per 100 ml of vinegar at 20 °C.

Vinegar Defects and Diseases

As in wines, metals and their salts may cause cloudiness and discoloration of vinegar. Ferrous iron may be oxidized to ferric iron and combine with tannins, phosphates, or proteins to produce a haze. Cloudiness also may be caused by salts of tin or copper. Iron acting on tannin or oxidase activity may be responsible for the darkening of vinegar.

Microbial Defects

Microorganisms can cause defects in vinegar by either compromising the quality of the raw materials used or directly affecting the vinegar itself. For instance, wine and hard cider may experience issues similar to those found in wine diseases. *Lactobaci*llus and *Leuconostoc* species in fruit juices can lead to off-flavors, like a "mousy" taste, and may even produce enough acetic acid to hinder yeast-driven alcoholic fermentation. Butyric acid bacteria may also generate undesirable acids under anaerobic conditions. Adding sulfur dioxide to the juices can mitigate some of these issues, but it may inhibit vinegar bacteria. In terms of vinegar defects, excessive sliminess of vinegar bacteria and the reduction of acetic acid are the primary concerns. A thick, slimy bacterial film in slow vinegar production can slow acetification, while in generator processes, it can disrupt aeration. Sliminess tends to occur when the alcoholic liquid is a good culture medium, such as cider or wine,. or when too much rich vinegar food is added. This issue is less problematic when acetification occurs in poor mediums like alcohol-based vinegar. *Acetobacter aceti* subsp. *xylinum* is the main culprit behind this sliminess. Additionally, excessive aeration or insufficien alcohol can lead to the oxidation of acetic acid to carbon dioxide and water, a process facilitated by the acetic acid bacteria themselves. Other organisms like film yeasts, molds, and algae can also oxidize acetic acid under aerobic conditions.

FERMENTED VEGETABLES

The lactic acid fermentation of vegetables undoubtedly originated from the preserving effect on the product. The growth of lactic acid bacteria during vegetable fermentations results in (1) restriction of the growth of undesirable organisms and delay or prevention of the normal spoilage and (2) production of various unique flavors because of the accumulation of organic acids or by-products, giving a characteristic and distinct finished product.

A comparison of some of the various fermented vegetables is presented in Table 22.1. Note that reduced conditions (immersion) and the use of salt are common to all the fermentations listed. The reasons for these conditions will be explained in the discussion of sauerkraut fermentation.

Table. A comparison of Fermented Vegetables

Commodity	Form used	Salt application	Conditions or modifications	Culture used	Resulting dominant lactic acid flora	Acid. %	pH
Carrot	Whole, diced, shredded	Brine, 2%	Immersion	Natural	Homofermentative	1.4	3.3
Celery	Sliced	Brine, $2\frac{1}{2}$%	Immersion	Natural	Homofermentative	1.2	3.5
Olive (green)	Whole						
Old method		Brine,5–8%	Immersion	Natural	Mixed	0.7–1.0	3.8
New method		Brine,10%	Shorter Iye and rinsing times, addiction of lactic acid (3%)	*L.plantarum*	Mixed or homofermentative		3.8
Pickle	Whole					0.6	3.8
Old method		Brine,6–15%	Immersion	Natural	Mixed		
New method		Brine,6.6%	Chlorination,Na acetate (0.5%), N2 purge	*L.plantarum, P.cerevisiae**	Homofermentative		
Sauerkraut	Shredded	Granular, $2\frac{1}{2}$%	Immersion	Natural	Mixed	1.7–2.5	3.5

*Expressed as lactic: After equilibration: Natural, as found in plants: Although olives are fruits, their fermentation resembles that of fermented vegetables. Source- Summarized in Stamer (1973) from numerous references.

Sauerkraut

The federal definition is as follows:

Sauerkraut is a high-quality product with a distinctive flavor, resulting from the complete fermentation of properly prepared and shredded cabbage, primarily through lactic acid fermentation. This process occurs in the presence of 2 to 3 percent salt. Upon completion of fermentation, sauerkraut contains at least 1.5 percent acid, measured as lactic acid. If the sauerkraut is rebrined during canning or repacking, it must still contain a minimum of 1 percent acid, expressed as lactic acid.

General Making Procedure

Whole, fully mature heads of a preferred cabbage variety for making sauerkraut are dried for 1 to 2 days to bring the cabbage to an even temperature and make it easier to cut. Damaged spots and damaged outer leaves are cut off, the heads are washed with clean water, and the core is pierced and chopped to add to the rest of the cabbage. The head is cut into pieces of the desired size, usually quite thin. Then, 2.25 to 2.5 percent salt by weight is mixed with shredded cabbage before transfer to the tank or added during packing of the ground products in the tank.

The first method is preferable because it allows for more uniform salting, gives the salt time to penetrate the cabbage, and makes packing easier. After the pieces are packed in containers, they are packed and finally weighed, so that a layer of squeezed and salted liquid settles on the surface. Some type of coating should protect the surface from contamination from soil insects. The temperature during lactic acid fermentation should be about 21-24 °C. If the temperature is below 15.6°C, fermentation will be slow and incomplete; if it is above 26 to 29°C, abnormal fermentations may occur. During fermentation, yeast or mold will grow on the surface of the pressed juice if the surface of the juice is left uncovered. In the past, they were removed or prevented from growing by covering the surface with mineral oil (or paraffin in small fermenters) after the gas has been stopped or by filling the vessels completely. Today, plastic bags filled with water are placed on the fermentation cabbage to seal the surface and act as a weight. When the desired acidity is reached, fermentation is interrupted by heat treatment during preservation or by low temperatures.

Addition of Salt

Pederson and Ward (1949) have demonstrated that 2.25 to 2.5 percent of salt by weight should be added to the shredded cabbage to obtain kraut of the best quality and that this salt should be distributed evenly. The salt draws out the plant juices containing the sugars and other nutrients, helps control the flora of the fermentation (favoring the lactic acid bacteria), and has a dispersing effect on clumps of bacteria. Undesirable competitors of the lactics, e.g., proteolytic bacteria and aerobic and anaerobic sporeformers, are inhibited more by the salt than are the desired acid formers.

Washing the Heads

Keipper et al. (1932) demonstrated that washing the cabbage heads not only reduces total numbers of microorganisms in the shredded cabbage, it also increases the percentage of desirable lactics in the flora remaining. In their experiments the lactics increased from 24 percent to 35 percent and the percentages of undesirable organisms such as chromogens, coliform bacteria, yeasts, and molds decreased.

Composition of Cabbage

The composition of cabbage varies with the variety and the conditions during its growth. Especially significant in sauerkraut making is the sugar content because of its influence on the maximal acidity that can be produced by fermentation.

Analyses have shown the sugar content to range from 2.9 to 6.4 percent in different lots of cabbage; the higher contents of sugar would permit the production of too much acidity if steps were not taken to stop the fermentation. The sugars are about 85 percent glucose and fructose and 15 percent sucrose.

Fermentation

Anaerobic conditions develop rapidly in the salted, crushed cabbage and the surrounding liquid, mainly due to the removal of oxygen by the respiration of the plant cells, but with the help of bacteria. The juice contains the natural flora of the cabbage, as well as contaminants from the soil and water. Initially, several types of bacteria begin to grow, but the acid-forming types quickly dominate. Among the bacteria that reach significant numbers at the beginning of fermentation, we find coliform bacteria, for example. , *Enterobacter cloacae,* which produces gas and volatile acids, as well as some lactic acid. *Erwinia herbicola* has also been found before fermentation. These organisms are supposed to give a certain aroma. Soon, however, the bacteria *Leuconostoc mesenteroides* begin to outnumber all other organisms and continue to produce acid up to 0.7 to 1. 0 percent acid (such as lactic acid). These streptococci, which occur in pairs or short chains, grow well at 18-21°C and are not inhibited. but are probably also stimulated by 2.5 percent salt. They atta k sugars to form lactic acid, acetic acid, ethanol, mannitol, dextran, esters, and carbon dioxide, which contribute to the flavor of a good sauerkraut, as do the fatty acids produced by the lactic acid bacteria and the lipids of the cabbage. The volatiles inhibit yeast, and the dextran and mannitol (with a bitter taste) are available to the desired successor of leuconostocs, *Lactobacillus plantarum,* but not to most competing organisms. *Streptococcus faecalis,* which can grow during the fermentation of sauerkraut, especially if the salt content is high (for example, 3.5%), produces mainly lactic acid.

Then, lactobacilli that do not produce gas, mainly *Lactobacillus plantarum* species, continue the production of acid and can increase the acidity to 1.5 to 2. 0 percent. These bacteria mainly produce lactic acid during the fermentation of sugars. They also use mannitol manufactured by *Leuconostoc* and thus eliminate the bitter taste. *L. plantarum* completes the desired fermentation in the production of sauerkraut. Experience has shown that a final acidity of about 1.7 percent lactic acid is most desirable. Fermentation can be stopped at this point by canning the sauerkraut or putting it in the refrigerator

If there is enough sugar and mannitol after *L. plantarum* has finished its work, the gas-producing lactobacilli, mainly of *L. brevis,* can grow and continue to produce acid up to 2.4 percent, an acidity that, however, is rarely reached due to the lack of sugar and mannitol. Gas-producing lactobacilli, which produce the same products as leuconostocs, give sauerkraut an undesirable and pronounced sour taste.

Good sauerkraut should be light in color and fresh, with an acidity of about 1.7 percent and a strong, acidic flavor. Small amounts of diacetyl are present to add a pleasant aroma and flavor. According to Pederson (1931), the average finished sauerkraut has a pH of 3.4 to 3.6, a lactic acid content of 1.25 percent, or about 0.01 percent. 3 percent acetic acid and 0.58 percent ethyl alcohol. When 3.5 percent salt is used instead of the usual 2.25 percent, or when the temperature is 32 to 37°C instead of lower, *Pediococcus cerevisiae** can play an important role in fermentation, but the sauerkraut is likely to be of lower quality than that produced. under normal conditions of salt content and temperature. A low salt content, for example 1.0 percent, promotes *Leuconostoc mesenteroides* and heterofermentative *Lactobacillus brevis.*

Experiments have shown that it is not necessary or even beneficial to add lactic acid bacteria to the production of sauerkraut. Sauerkraut can be canned by heating the cans to 150°F, emptying, sealing, and refrigerate.

Sauerkraut Defects and Spoilage

The quality of sauerkraut can be reduced due to abnormal fermentations. Too high a temperature can inhibit the growth of *Leuconostoc* and therefore the production of odors by this organism and can allow the growth of *Pediococcus cerevisiae** and the development of undesirable odors. Too low a temperature can prevent the proper activity of the desired lactic acid bacteria succession and encourage the growth of soil contaminants, e.g. *Enterobacter* and *Flavobacterium*. Long-term fermentation can promote the growth of *Lactobacillus brevis,* a gas-forming bacteria that produces a very acidic taste. Too much salt can promote the growth of microorganisms other than those desired, such as *Pediococcus cerevisiae** and yeasts. Abnormal fermentation of cabbage can result in a cheesy odor caused by propionic, butyric, caproic, and valeric acids, as well as isobutyric and isovaleric acids.

Soft kraut may result from a faulty fermentation and from exposure to air or from excessive pressing or tamping.

- **Dark-brown or black kraut** usually is due to oxidation during exposure to air and is caused by the combined action of plant enzymes and microorganisms. Destruction of acid by film yeasts and molds makes conditions favorable for proteolytic and pectolytic organisms to rot the kraut rapidly. Darkening is encouraged by uneven salting ("salt burn") and a high temperature. A brown color may result from iron in hoops and tannin from barrels.
- **Pink kraut** often is caused by red, asporogenous yeasts in the presence of air and high salt and is found especially when the salt has been distributed unevenly. The development of pink color is favored by high temperature, dirty vats, low acidity, and iron salts. A light-pink color has been attribute to the pigments in some varieties of cabbage.
- **Slimy or ropy kraut** is caused by encapsulated varieties of *Lactobacillus plantarum*. The product is edible but unsalable. The sliminess may disappear on longer holding and usually disappears during the cooking of the kraut.

Sauerkraut, then, is especially subject to spoilage at its surface, where it is exposed to air. There film yeasts and molds destroy the acidity, permitting other microorganisms to grow and causing softening, darkening, and bad flavors.

Pickles

Cucumber pickles can be prepared without fermentation or with partial or complete fermentation. Unfermented, partially fermented, or fully fermented cucumbers can be pasteurized to improve their keeping quality. Typically, pickled and acidified cucumbers (natural or artificial are heated so that the interior of the cucumbers is maintained at 150°F for at least 15 minutes. Heating and cooling must be fairly rapid. We will not attemp to describe here the various methods of pickle preparation, as they vary greatly, and will confin ourselves to pickles produced by fermentation. There are two main types of fermented pickles- salted or savoury with meat broth and dill pickles. Savory pickles are prepared for use in the production of specialty products such as sour, sweet and sour, and mixed pickles and savouries.

Salt or Salt-Stock Pickles

In the preparation of fermented salt or salt-stock pickles immature cucumbers are washed, placed in barrels or tanks, and brined. Sometimes about 1 percent of glucose is added if the cucumbers are low in sugar, but some workers claim that the addition of sugar will favor the production of gassy pickles, or "bloaters."

Addition of Salt

The rate of salt addition and the total amount added vary considerably among producers. Two general methods of salting are used, the low-salt method and the high-salt method. In the low-salt method, a relatively small amount of salt is added and the concentration is gradually increased until it is sufficien to stop all bacterial growth. For example, a 30°-salometer brine (about 8 percent NaCl) may be added to cucumbers at 9 pounds of salt per 100 pounds of cucumbers. Some producers start with less than 8 percent salt, but risk abnormal fermentation or spoilage; 6 percent salt has been found to be the minimum concentration to contain undesirable spore-forming bacteria. In the high salt method, the first brine is 40° salt meter (about 10.5 percent salt) and 9 pounds of salt are added per 100 pounds of cucumbers.

The cucumbers are "drowned" under a shallow layer of brine and fermentation begins. In both methods, salt is added at weekly intervals to increase the saltometer reading from about 3° saltometer to 60° (about 15.9 percent salt). In the low salt method, the increase is about 2° per week up to 50° and 1° per week up to 60° salometer. In warm climates, the salt content of the brine can increase more rapidly, and in cold climates, a lower salometer of 30° can be added initially.

The Traditional Fermentation

Only recently has the controlled fermentation of cucumbers with homofermenters inoculated with *L. plantarum* and *P. cerevisiae** been suggested.

However, before discussing this latest advance, a description of the traditional method of pickle fermentation will be given.

The traditional process generally takes 6 to 9 weeks to complete, depending on the salting method and temperature used.

All or some of a number of salt-tolerant bacterial species may initially grow on fresh pickled cucumbers. In fact, there may be marked differences in the types of bacteria that grow in different batches of cucumber brine, depending on the number and types introduced from the cucumbers or the soil left in them and from the brine, the initial concentration of sodium chloride and the rate of growth of this concentration and the temperature of pickled cucumbers. In general, the lower the salt concentration, the more bacterial species that initially grow, the lower the rapid acid production will be and the higher the total acidity produced. In most cases, the first to grow is a mixture of species from the genera *Pseudomonas* and *Flavobacterium* , species considered undesirable because they are classified as spoilage bacteria rather than acid bacteria. Similarly, Bacillus spp, coliform bacteria (*Enterobacter*), *Leuconostoc mesenteroides, Streptococcus faecalis* and *Pediococcus cerevisiae* * may grow and form acid during the first few days of fermentation, and in 15 percent brine, unidentified gas-producing bacteria may produce acid. Later, *Lactobacillus brevis* may contribute to acidity if the salt concentration is not too high. In most cured meats, *L. plantarum* is the most important bacterium, developing acidity at both low and high salinity. It begins to reach significant values a few days after the start of fermentation. As the salt concentration increases to about 10 to 15 percent, plantarum becomes less and less active. The total titratable acidity, as lactic acid, is about 0.6 to 0.8 percent at the end of fermentation. Fermentations in which heterofermentative lactic acid bacteria have been relatively effective generally produce strong pickles with better density than those in homofermentative fermentations.

To further complicate the fermentation, yeasts may begin to grow after a slight acid has been formed by the bacteria. These yeasts are of two general types, skin or oxidizing yeasts, which grow on the surface of the brine and destroy the lactic acid by oxidation, and fermentative yeasts, which grow in the brine and ferment the sugars to alcohol and carbon dioxide. Film-forming yeasts of the genera *Debaryomyces, Endomycopsis,* and *Candida* have been found. Various methods of reducing or eliminating yeast scum in the brine during fermentation include daily agitation of the surface or the addition of mineral oil, sorbic acid, mustard oil, or other substances. Brine tanks are often located in direct sunlight, which prevents the growth of the brine surface. In order of frequency of occurrence, the following genera of fermenting yeasts have been found in pickles- *Torulopsis, Brettanomyces, Zygosaccharomyces* (a subgenus of *Saccharomyces*), *Hansenula, Torulaspora,* and *Kloeckera*. The gas produced by these yeasts bubbles in the brine and may be responsible for the swelling of pickles.

A fermentation as variable, complex, and unpredictable as that of pickles is difficult to summarize. Most of the acid is normally produced by *Lactobacillus plantarum,* but it can also be formed by *Leuconostoc mesenteroides, Lactobacillus* *brevis, Streptococcus faecalis, Pediococcus cerevisiae**, and possibly coliform bacteria. The acid is destroyed by the tops in the film. The gas can be produced by *Leuconostoc mesenteroids*, fermenting yeast, and coliform bacteria.

When cucumbers are first salted, they are chalky white and dark in cross section, but during fermentation and drying, the color changes from the original bright green to olive green or yellow, and the flesh becomes increasingly translucent. Pickles pickled in a 15 percent salt brine can be stored for long periods if the growth of the film yeasts is inhibited. They are too salty to eat and must be "refreshed" by soaking before they are made into pickles, sweet and sour pickles, or mixed with spices or other products.

The Controlled Fermentation

Numerous mishaps and problems can develop during the traditional fermentation by the indigenous cucumber flora, as will become evident in the section on pickle defects and spoilage. Years of research and experience by investigators at the U. S. Food Fermentation Laboratory, Southern Region, USDA, have resulted in a suggested procedure for the controlled fermentation of brined cucumbers (Etchells et al., 1973). Briefly, the process is designed to eliminate or at least minimize the usual defects of the traditional or natural fermentation. First the cucumbers are washed and sanitized (chlorine 80 ppm) in the vat. The chlorinated brine is then acidified with glacial acetic acid (6 ml per gallon). These two processes (chlorination and acidification) effectively suppress the growth of undesired bacteria during the initial salt addition and equilibration of the brine and cucumbers. Following a purge with nitrogen, sodium acetate is added (0.5 percent) to buffer the brine. This ensures effective utilization of all the fermentable carbohydrate present. About 10 to 24 hr following equilibration of the brine and cucumbers, they are inoculated with special cultures of *P. cerevisiae** and *L. plantarum*. During the active fermentation (10 to 14 days), nitrogen purges are repeated and additional salt is added to maintain 25° salometer (6.6 percent NaCl).

Dill Pickles

Dill pickles are so named because they are flavored by the addition of dill weed in one form or another; spices are also usually added, and for kosher varieties, garlic or onion. Dill pickles may be unfermented or fermented or made from brine, but only the fermented types, "overnight" and "true" dill pickles, will be considered here.

Fermentation for dill pickle production differs from that for pickling in that a lower salt concentration is used than in pickling and The pickling is usually acidified with vinegar (acetic acid) first. Low salt promotes an increased rate and amount of acid production, but increases the risk of undesirable microbial changes. Flavoring materials, fennel, spices, garlic, etc., do not significantly stimulate or inhibit acid-forming bacteria, but can be the source of significant numbers of undesirable microorganisms and therefore the cause of abnormal fermentation or spoilage of pickles. Processed species containing small numbers of microorganisms are now available.

Overnight Dill Pickles

Overnight dill pickles are prepared by slow, low-temperature acid fermentation in a relatively weakly acidified brine. For example, one formula calls for a 20-degree brine (5.3 percent salt), 10 pounds of dried fennel, 1 pound of mixed spices, and 1 quart of 100-grain barrel vinegar. The pickles are then stored at about 3.3°C, where they undergo slow lactic fermentation down to 0.3 to 0.6 percent acidity is developed. Currants must be kept fresh and have a relatively short shelf life due to their low salt and acid content. Higher acidity can be achieved by allowing fermentation to occur before storage, but the risk of fermentation or spoilage is higher and the green color is not preserved as in the usual process.

Genuine Dill Pickles

To make genuine dill pickles, cucumbers are placed in a brine containing approximately 7.5 to 8.5 percent salt (28 to 32° salometer), typically in a 45-gallon barrel, ensuring that the final salt concentration in the pickles will be around 3.5 to 4.5 percent. Dill and pickle spices are also added, and most producers include vinegar, such as 1 quart of 100-grain vinegar per barrel, to prevent abnormal fermentations. The ideal temperature range is between 15 and 30°C, with cooler conditions preferred. Due to the relatively low salt concentration, various soil bacteria first begin to grow. However, acid production likely starts with bacteria like *Leuconostoc mesenteroides*, *Streptococcus faecalis*, and *Pediococcus cerevisiae**, continuing with *Lactobacillus plantarum*, and possibly aided by *L. brevis*. The final acidity of the pickles ranges from 1.0 to 1.5 percent as lactic acid.

Pickle Defects and Spoilage

Fermented pickles can develop several defects or "diseases," most of which are caused by microorganisms. Shriveling occurs when too strong salt, sugar, or vinegar solutions are used. Hollow pickles are believed to form when cucumbers are left to stand too long after harvest before fermentation, though some experts suggest improper fermentation conditions, such as loose packing in the vat, inadequate weighting, too rapid fermentation, or imbalanced brine, may also cause hollow pickles. Floaters, or bloaters, can occur due to hollow cucumbers or gas production by yeasts, heterofermentative lactic acid bacteria, *L. plantarum*, or coliforms, which produce carbon dioxide. Carbon dioxide from the pickles themselves may also cause bloaters, which can be controlled by purging the brine with nitrogen to remove dissolved gas. Factors that favor floaters include thick skins that trap gas, rapid gas production, high initial salt, added acid, and sugar. Bloating is worsened when brine absorption is hindered. Slippery pickles result from cucumbers being exposed to air, allowing the growth of encapsulated bacteria. Slipperiness can also stem from broken scums of film yeasts, which grow on the brine's surface and fall onto the cucumbers. Softening in its early stages gives pickles a slippery surface. Soft pickles are softened by pectolytic enzymes, primarily from molds and cucumber flowers, which enter the fermentation vat. Common molds include *Penicillium, Fusarium, Ascochyta, Cladosporium,* and *Alternaria.* The breakdown of cucumber pectin starts with the removal of methoxyl groups to form pectic acid, aided by pectinesterase from brine yeasts and cucumber parts. Molds produce polymethylgalacturonase, converting pectin into intermediate uronides, which are further broken down into galacturonic acid by polygalacturonases from molds and cucumber flowers. The flowers, often with a dense fungal population, are believed to be a primary source of pectolytic enzymes. Pectolytic bacteria from the *Bacillus* and *Aeromonas* genera, along with coliforms, play a minor role in pickle softening. Final hydrolytic enzymes may assist in the degradation of pectic substances. Softening may also be caused by molds on the cucumbers and enzymes from the cucumber itself, or weak or strong acids. Yeasts that deesterify pectic substances can speed up softening. Softening is encouraged by (1) insufficient salt, leading to abnormal fermentation, (2) high temperatures, which also affect acid production, (3) low acidity due to insufficient acid formation or destruction by yeasts or molds, (4) exposure to air that promotes the growth of yeasts, molds, or pectin-fermenting bacteria, and (5) the presence of cucumber blossoms, which support mold growth and polygalacturonase production, leading to softening.

- Black pickles may owe their color to the formation of hydrogen sulfide by bacteria (or less commonly by chemical reaction) and combination with iron in the water to yield black ferrous sulfide. Therefore, water for pickles should have a low iron and gypsum ($CaSO_4$) content. The defect is favored by low acidity of the brines. Another cause of black pickles is the growth of black-pigmented *Bacillus nigrificans**, a variety of *Bacillus subtillis,* which is favored by (1) presence of an available carbohydrate like glucose, (2) a low level of available nitrogen, and (3) a neutral or slightly alkaline brine.

Ropy pickle brine, caused by various unidentified motile, gram-negative encapsulated rods, is favored by (1) low salt, (2) low acid, and (3) high temperature.

Green Olives

Although olives are classifie as fruits, not vegetables, they are included here because their fermentation process is similar to that of fermented vegetables.

Green olives are harvested when fully developed but still green or straw-yellow, ensuring they are not bruised to avoid product defects. The olives are initially treated with a 0.9 to 2.0% lye solution at temperatures between 15 to 21°C, keeping them submerged until the lye penetrates halfway to three-quarters of the way toward the pit. They are then washed multiple times with minimal exposure to air to prevent darkening, removing most of the bitterness caused by the glucoside oleuropein. Afterward, the olives are placed in barrels and covered with salt brine, with the concentration varying depending on the type of olive. Manzanillo olives are recommended to be submerged in a 10 to 15% brine (40 to 50° salometer), leading to a salt concentration of 6 to 9 percent after stabilization, which is maintained at 7 to 8 percent throughout fermentation. For Sevillan olives, a brine with 5 to 6.25 percent salt (20 to 25° salometer) or less is used, resulting in a 2.5 to 4% brine, which is later adjusted to 6 to 8 percent salt. Any lost brine due to leakage, evaporation, or gas production is replaced promptly, keeping the olives always submerged in brine.

The lactic acid fermentation process of the olives may last between 6 to 10 months, depending on atmospheric temperatures. Vaughn, Douglas, and Gilillang (1943) divided the fermentation process into three stages- (1) the first stage, lasting 7 to 14 days, when the brine stabilizes, microorganisms leach nutrients from the olives, and potential spoilage organisms, such as *Enterobacter* and *Pseudomonas*, may grow until *Leuconostoc mesenteroides* begins to grow; (2) the intermediate stage, lasting 2 to 3 weeks, when *Leuconostoc* becomes dominant in growth and acid production, and *Lactobacillus plantarum* and *L. brevis* begin to grow and produce acid; and (3) the final stage, when *Lactobacillus*, especially *L. plantarum*, predominates. Gas production from yeasts, coliforms, *Leuconostoc*, and heterofermentative *L. brevis* occurs, particularly in the early stages of fermentation. An average temperature of about 24°C promotes rapid fermentation. The final acidity is typically 0.7 to 1.0 percent lactic acid, and the final pH is around 4.0 to 3.8 or lower. Sometimes, due to damage from the lye treatment, the normal lactic fermentation is delayed or halted. Olives may have insufficient sugar or have leached out too much during the lye treatment and washing, necessitating the addition of glucose for proper lactic fermentation.

Recent developments in olive fermentation suggest using a 10% brine acidified with 3% lactic acid to lower the pH and neutralize residual lye. Heating the olives before inoculation enhances the fermentation. A heat-sensitive bacterial inhibitor has recently been identified in green olives. Two hydrolysis products of oleuropein, aglycone and elnolic acid, inhibit a few lactic acid bacteria and other species (Fleming et al., 1973).

Olives that are pitted and stuffed with brined pimento are then barreled, brined, and left to ferment for about a month until the pimento flesh has fermented.

After fermentation, the green olives are sorted and graded. They may be rebarreled and rebrined or washed, then packed into glass jars or other containers under vacuum, and rebrined with brine of about 28° salometer (7% salt). Edible lactic acid may be added to the final brine. The olives may also be pasteurized at around 60°C in the container or brined at 79 to 82°C to enhance their shelf life.

Defects and Spoilage

Gassy spoilage in green olives is typically caused by coliform bacteria, particularly *Enterobacter* spp., but can also result from *Bacillus* spp. and *Clostridium* spp. Gas formation leads to blister-like spots or fissures under the skin, or gas pockets within the olives, which creates a defect known as "fishe" or "fish-eye" and causes the olives to float. Gas-forming yeasts and heterofermentative lactics are less frequently the cause of gassy defects.

If conditions are not ideal for normal lactic fermentation, an abnormal butyric fermentation by *Clostridium* spp., such as *C. butyricum*, can occur, producing foul odors and tastes. A pH above 4.2 may lead to a "sagy" off-odor and taste, referred to as "zapatera" spoilage, caused by *Clostridium* species in combination with propionic bacteria. The odor may range from mildly cheesy (butyric) to foul and putrid (fecal).

Softening of the olives, resulting from the breakdown of pectic substances, can be caused by physical or chemical factors or by pectolytic coliform bacteria, as well as species of *Bacillus, Aeromonas,* or *Achromobacter,* yeasts like *Rhodotorula,* or molds such as *Penicillium* and *Aspergillus.*

Raised white spots or pimples on the olive surface, sometimes called "yeast spots," are actually colonies of *Lactobacillus plantarum* or *L. brevis.* These spots can also appear on fermented cucumber pickles.

Cloudiness in the brine of glass-packed olives can be caused by microorganisms- (1) lactics, if fermentation of residual sugar resumes; (2) salt-tolerant bacteria; or (3) film yeasts or molds, if air is present. During processing, surface growths of film yeasts may destroy lactic acid and create off-flavor and odors that affect the finished product

Storage olives, which are held in brine for weeks or months before processing, undergo lactic acid fermentation and, when exposed to air, can soften due to pectinolytic action from aerobic film yeasts and molds that develop on the surface. Most of these molds belong to the *Fusarium* and *Penicillium* genera.

Ripe Olives

Olives for the production of ripe olives are picked when green to straw-colored, shipped in boxed or bins to the factory, and held before processing in the factory in a 5 to 10 percent brine. A lactic acid fermentation usually takes place while the olives are being held in the brine. After grading and sorting of the olives they are given the following "pickling" process- a first lye treatment with 0.5 to 2.0 percent lye to barely penetrate the skin; an aeration treatment with stirring or administration of compressed air to darken the skin; and more lye treatments, followed by further aeration. Finally the lye is allowed to penetrate to the pit, dehydrolyzing all the bitter glucoside oleuropein, and then the olives are leached with water to remove all the lye. Then comes stabilization of the ripe olives in a 2 to 3 percent brine for 2 or more days, during which fermentation may take place although it is not desired because it may lead to color defects. Ripe olives usually are canned in weak brine and are processed in the glass or tin container at about 115.6°C for 60 min.

- **Defects and Spoilage:** Spoilage of ripe olives may take place while they are in the holding brine, with bleaching of the color and perhaps some softening. Coliform bacteria have been blamed for such defects, as well as for blistering or "fisheye" spoilage. Unless the temperature of the wash water is below 21°C or is in the range 49 to 60°C during the removal of lye from the olives, bacterial growth may take place with softening of the fruit. It has been demonstrated that pectolytic enzymes of *Bacillus subtilis* and *B. pumilus* can cause the defect.

Other Fermented Vegetables

Leafy vegetables such as spinach and chard and "greens" such as beet, mustard, and turnip may be prepared in a manner similar to that for making sauerkraut from cabbage. The addition of 2.5 percent by weight of dry salt causes moisture to be drawn from the vegetable and permits a lactic acid fermentation similar to that for sauerkraut. Lettuce kraut prepared in this way has been compared favorably with sauerkraut. Sauerruben are made from unpeeled, shredded young turnips to which about 2.2 percent salt by weight is added. The salted turnips, packed in half-gallon fruit jars, are held at 21 to 24 °C to undergo a lactic acid fermentation like that for sauerkraut.

Fermented green tomatoes may be prepared for incorporation in relishes and mixed pickles. The fermentation is similar to that for sauerkraut but slower, the same succession of bacteria being involved. The skins of the tomatoes may be punctured to hasten the process.

A number of Oriental fermented foods are made from vegetable products, and some of them will be discussed later.

FERMENTED DAIRY PRODUCTS

The numerous varieties of cheeses and fermented milks cannot be adequately covered in this book. We mention only briefly some of the fermented dairy products. The student should consult the references at the end of the chapter for a broader understanding and appreciation of the scope of the fermented-dairy-products industry. Fermented milks include cultured buttermilk, yogurt, Bulgarian buttermilk, acidophilus milk, kefir, kumiss, skyr, and taette as well as numerous others very similar to or identical with the ones listed. Cultured sour cream is a similar product. In all these fermented milks lactic acid bacteria carry on the main fermentation to produce lactic acid. Table 22.2 lists some of the cultures used in fermented dairy products.

Cultured buttermilk and sour cream employ the action of mixed cultures; one strain is usually responsible for the production of lactic acid, while another strain provides the aroma-forming bacteria. In both these products *Streptococcus lactis* subsp. *cremoris** or *S. lactis* subsp. *lactus** could be used to produce the acidity (0.7 to 0.9 percent as lactic acid), and *Leuconostoc mesenteroides* subsp. *cremoris* or *Streptococcus lactis* subsp. *diacetylactis* as the flavor- or aroma-forming strain to produce diacetyl, the characteristic flavor compound of buttermilk.

Bulgarian buttermilk is made with a pure culture of *Lactobacillus delbrueckii* subsp. *bulgaricus,* while yogurt employs a mixed culture of *Streptococcus thermophilus* and *L.delbrueckii* subsp. *bulgaricus*. The starter for kefir is kefir grains, which are aggregates of a mixture of microorganisms, chiefly *Lactobacillus brevis* and several yeasts. In addition to acid, a small amount of alcohol, 0.5 to 1.0 percent is produced, and enough carbon dioxide to carbonate the drink if it is kept tightly sealed during fermentation. Kumiss, ordinarily made from mare's milk, results from fermentation by a mixture of lactics and yeasts carried over from a previous lot. Acidophilus milk, prepared for its therapeutic properties for intestinal disorders, utilizes a pure culture of *Lactobacillus acidophilus* grown in milk that has been sterilized or nearly sterilized. Recently, the addition of large numbers (a frozen concentrate) of *L. acidophilus* has been used to make a nonfermented "sweet acidophilus" milk. Taette is a ropy buttermilk made with a ropy variety of *Streptococcus lactis* subsp. *lactis**, and skyr is a semisolid fermented milk in which chiefly *S. thermophilus* and *L. delbrueckii* subsp. *bulgaricus* have been active.

Table. Cultures Used in Major Fermented Dairy Products

Culture	Culture function	Product use
Propionibacterium freudenreichii	Flavor and Eye Formation	Emmental (Swiss) cheese
Lactobacillus delbrueckii subsp. *bulgarius*	Acid and Flavor	Bulgaraian buttermilk, yogurt, kumiss, and Emmental (Swiss) and Italian cheese
L. lactis		
L. helvectius		
L. brevis	Acid and Flavor	Kefi
L. acidophilus	Acid	Acidophilus buttermil
Streptococcus thermophilus	Acid	Emmental, Cheddar, and Italian chesse and yogurt
S.lactis subsp. *diacetylactis**	Acid and Flavor	Sour cream, ripened cream butter, cheese, buttermilk, and starter cultures
S. lactis subsp. *lactis**	Acid	Cultured buttermilk, sour cream, cottage cheese, all types of cheese, domestic and foreign, and starter cultures
Leuconostoc cremoris	Acid	Cultured buttermilk, sour cream, cottage cheese, ripened cream butter, and starter cultures
S. faecium, S. faecalis	Acid and Flavor	Soft Italian, Cheddar, and some Swiss cheeses

The acidity of the fermented milks is sufficien to prevent spoilage by proteolytic or other bacteria that are not acid-tolerant. Chilling is necessary to stop acid formation by the starter bacteria at the desired stage and packaging and sealing to avoid mold growth.

A lactic acid fermentation is involved in making most kinds of cheese. Unripened cheeses, such as cottage cheese and cream cheese, are made by starters similar to those used for cultured buttermilk. They must be chilled and kept cold until consumed and have a comparatively short keeping time. Ripened cheeses have an initial acid fermentation by lactic acid bacteria followed by action of their enzymes and those of other microorganisms; in some cheeses there is the additional action of rennet, a and in certain Italian cheeses the action of added animal lipases. The chief compounds contributing to the flavor of ripened cheeses are salt, lactic acid, fatty acids, amino acids, and carbonyl compounds (e.g., aldehydes and ketones). The soft, ripened cheeses, such as Lim-burger, are more perishable than the harder cheeses, e.g., Cheddar and Swiss, but all completely cured cheeses require storage at chilling temperatures to aid in their preservation. Cheeses with hard rinds, such as natural Cheddar and Swiss, are protected by these rinds to some extent from drying and spoilage. Chilling also is necessary for most kinds of cheese, as well as packaging for perishable cheeses and cut pieces of larger, more stable cheeses. Packaging is done to minimize losses of moisture and penetration of oxygen, which otherwise would permit growth of molds.

In general, the curing or ripening processes do not greatly improve the keeping quality, although losses in moisture occur during the aging of long-cured hard cheeses and a protective rind forms on most of them. The chemical products formed during ripening have little preservative effect for the most part, although fatty acids repress the anaerobes; in fact, most cheeses become more alkaline as they age and hence more susceptible to spoilage by bacteria. the propionate formed in the ripening of good Swiss cheese delays the growth of most molds on the cheese, and the surface "smear" of organisms on surface-ripened cheeses such as brick or Limburger may produce products that are inhibitory to other organisms.

SPOILAGE AND DEFECTS OF FERMENTED DAIRY PRODUCTS

Fermented milks and cheese depend on a desired fermentation or succession of fermentations for their manufacture. Therefore, any abnormality in these fermentations will affect the quality of the product and may even spoil it. The finished product, too, may be subject to spoilage by microorganisms.

Fermented Milks

In the manufacture of most fermented milks a starter is added to pasteurized milk, which is incubated until the desired acidity is attained. The chief product of the fermentation is lactic acid, Food Fermentations 340 but lesser amounts of flavoring substances may be produced or added. If the starter bacteria are inactive, other bacteria may grow and damage the curd and the flavor. Proteolytic bacteria, which ordinarily cannot compete with the lactics, may cause a poor curd and off-flavors. Coliform bacteria and lactose-fermenting yeasts should not be present but may enter from equipment and other sources to produce bad flavors and gas. The finished product is susceptible to spoilage by molds from air or equipment if air is available at the surface.

Cheese

Defects of cheese may have mechanical or biological causes, but only the latter will be discussed. The types of spoilage can be divided into those developing during the manufacture and ripening of cured cheese and those occurring in the finished product

Spoilage During Manufacture

During the manufacture of most types of cheese or while the cheese is draining, a lactic acid fermentation is encouraged. If the lactics are ineffective or contamination with other microorganisms is unduly heavy, abnormal changes may take place that affect the quality of the cheese adversely. In cheese made from raw milk the gas-forming organisms may be producing off-flavors as well as gas holes in the curd. Lactose-fermenting yeasts, although not commonly present in appreciable numbers, also can cause gassiness. Sporeforming gas producers, especially species of *Clostridium,* can cause trouble in either raw-milk or pasteurized-milk cheese if the lactic starter bacteria are not functioning properly; less commonly, the aerobacilli*, spore-forming species of *Bacillus* such as *B. polymyxa,* may produce gas and other defects. These sporeformers also can cause defects in ripening cheese.

Other bacteria may compete with the starter organisms with results that do not become evident until during the curing process, where body and flavor may be affected. Thus, acid proteolytic bacteria may produce a bitter flavor, or *Leuconostoc* spp. may cause holes or openness in Cheddar cheese from pasteurized milk.

Cottage cheese especially is subject to spoilage during storage before consumption. If the starter bacteria produce insufficien acid or yield it too slowly, a usable curd will not result or the cheese will be inferior because of the growth of undesirable organisms. Proteolysis, gas production, sliminess, and off-flavor may ruin the product. Cheese with too low an acidity because of the addition of cream or the failure of the starter often is made gelatinous or slimy by soil or water bacteria such as *Pseudomonas*, *P. fragi*, and *Alcaligenes metalcaligenes**.

Spoilage During Ripening

During ripening or curing, cheeses normally undergo physical and chemical changes resulting from the action of enzymes released from the autolyzed cells of bacteria that grew during manufacture and from the action of microorganisms that increase during the ripening period. The growth of organisms other than the desired ones results in inferior or, in extreme cases, even worthless cheese because of alterations in texture, body, general appearance, or flavor. The most important kinds of spoilage differ enough, however, with the kind of cheese concerned to discourage generalization. Most kinds may be subject to "late gas," usually caused by heterofermentative lactic acid bacteria, or by lactate-fermenting *Clostridium* spp. but possibly by bacilli, propionic bacteria, or heterofermentative lactics. Gas holes, or eyes, are desirable in Swiss and related cheeses but not to any extent in other varieties. Especially bad in Swiss and similar cheeses is the cracking or splitting of the cheese by gas or the production of too many, too small, or misshapen eyes. Gas formation by the sporeformers is accompanied by the production of undesirable flavors, e.g., butyric acid from the anaerobes.

Bitterness may be caused by certain lactic streptococci; the proteolytic bacteria, e.g., the acidproteolytic types; coliforms; micrococci*; various other bacteria; and (rarely) yeasts, which usually give a sweet, fruity, or yeasty flavor

Putrefaction may occur locally or generally in cheese where insufficien acidity has been produced by the lactics or the acid has been destroyed by a lactate fermenter, e.g., *Clostridium tyrobutyricum*. Putrefactive anerobes, such as *C. sporogenes* or *C. lentoputrescens**, may be involved.

Discolorations of the ripening cheese may result from the action of microorganisms on compounds produced during curing or on added coloring material, such as the annatto used in Cheddar cheese, or may result from the development of pigmented colonies or organisms on or in the cheese. Blue, green, or black discoloration may be produced by the reaction of hydrogen sulfide produced by organisms with metals or metallic salts. Bacterially formed sulfhydryl groups give a pink to muddy appearance to annatto. Reddish-brown to grayish-brown colors sometimes result from the oxidation of tyrosine by bacteria growing in soft cheese. Rusty spots of Cheddar and similar cheese are caused by colonies of *Lactobacillus plantarum* var. *rudensis** or *L. brevis* var. *rudensis**, while yellow, pink, or brown spots in Swiss cheese, mostly on the surface of the eyes, are colonies of pigmented species of *Propionibacterium*.

Spoilage of the Finished Cheese

In general, the perishability of cured cheeses increases with their moisture content. Therefore, soft cheeses such as Limburger and Brie are most perishable, and hard cheeses such as Cheddar and Swiss are the most stable. Most feared among the spoilage organisms are the molds that tend to grow on the cheese surfaces and into cracks of trier holes. Even cheeses that depend partly on a specific mold for ripening may be demaged by other molds. Most natural cheeses have rinds that serve as some protection to the anaerobic interior but usually are not dry enough to prevent mold growth. The acidity of the cheese is no deterrent to growth, and the storage temperature is not too low for such growth. Most molds grow in colored colonies on the surface or in crevices, without much penetration into the cheese, but some kinds produce actual rots. Products produced by molds, such as mycotoxins and antibiotics, can migrate into the cheese. Not only are discolorations evident, but off-flavors are produced locally. Among the molds that grow on cheese surfaces are the following:

- ***Oospora* (*Geotrichum*) spp:** *Oospora* (*Geotrichum*) *lactis*, called the dairy mold, grows on soft cheeses and during ripening sometimes suppresses other molds as well as surfaceripening bacteria. The curd gradually becomes liquefied under the felt. *O. rubrum* and *O. crustacea* produce a red coloration, and *O. aurianticum* forms orange to red spots. *O. caseovorans* causes "cheese cancer" of Swiss and similar cheeses. Bumps of growth become filled with a white, chalky mass.
- ***Cladosporium* spp:** The mycelium and spores of these molds are dark or smoky and give dark colors to the cheese. Most common is *C. herbarum*, characterized by dark-green to black colors. Other species cause green, brown, or black discolorations.
- ***Penicillium* spp:** *P. puberulum* and other green-spored species grow in cracks, crevices, and trier holes of Cheddar and related cheeses to give a green coloration because of their spores. They may act on annatto to cause

mottling and discoloration. *P. casei* causes yellowish brown spots on the rind, and *P. aurantiovirens* discolors Camembert cheese.

- ***Monilia* spp:** *M. nigra* produces penetrating black spots on the rind of hard cheeses. Species of many other genera may discolor cheeses and give off-flavors, e.g., the genera *Scopulariopsis, Aspergillus, Mucor,* and *Alternaria.*

If the surface is sufficiently moist, yeasts may form colored colonies or areas, and film yeasts may pave the way for the yellow to red growth of *Brevibacterium linens.* The latter is desired in some surface-ripened cheeses but not in others.

TEA, COFFEE, CACAO, VANILLA, CITRON

Tea

Tea can be classified as (1) fermented, or black, (2) unfermented, of green, and (3) semifermented, or oolong. The experts agree that the "fermentation" of tea leaves is the result of the activity of enzymes of the leaves rather than of microorganisms present, although action of microorganisms may harm the flavor and reduce the quality of black tea. Molds of the genera *Aspergillus, Penicillium,* and *Rhizopus* have been reported to cause spoilage.

Cacao

Cacao, or cocoa beans (seeds), when taken from the pod are covered with a slimy or fruity pulp, which is removed by means of a fermentation process. The pulp-covered seeds are placed in piles, in pits, or in a "sweating box," where the beans are covered with banana or plantain leaves. During the 3 to 13 days of fermentation the beans are stirred and turned to aerate them and keep down the temperature. The fermentation has the following purposes- (1) to remove the adhering pulp from the bean, (2) to kill the embryo in the seed, and (3) to give aroma, flavor, and color to the bean. Here again it is difficult to say how much is accomplished by the plant enzymes and how much by the growing microorganisms. According to some reports the fermentation is in several stages- (1) the fermentation of sugars in the pulp to ethanol and carbon dioxide by a variety of yeasts, especially *Candida krusei* and apiculate yeasts, and to acid by lactic acid bacteria, (2) the oxidation of the ethanol to acetic acid by acetic bacteria, (3) chemical changes brought about by the heat of the fermentation, where the temperatures may rise to 44 to 50°C, and by plant enzymes, and (4) further chemical changes during curing or drying of the beans. Molds and actinomycetes can cause spoilage of the beans during curing.

Citron

Halved citron fruits are held for 6 to 7 weeks in seawater or a 5 to 10 percent brine. It has been reported that yeasts improve the aroma by esterification of the essence of citron and that alcoholic fermentation by yeasts followed by an acetic acid fermentation combine to improve the flavor, color, and texture of citron. A yeast, *Saccharomyces citrimedicae,* and a bacterium, *Bacillus citri**, have been found to predominate during the fermentation.

Coffee

The two chief methods of curing coffee are (1) the dry method, in which the berries or "cherries" are spread out and air-dried in the sun or artificially, and (2) the wet, or washed-coffee, method, in which the berries, after removal of outer skin, are soaked in water. The removal of pulpy material in either method is accomplished primarily by pectinolytic bacteria, mostly coliforms, although pectinolytic bacilli and fungi may be present. This is followed by an acid fermentation by lactic acid bacteria such as *Leuconostoc mesenteroides, Lactobacillus brevis* and *L. plantarum,* and *Streptococcus faecalis*. The acids produced may be degraded by oxidizing organisms. After the pulp and its residues have been washed away, the beans are dried and hulled.

There are patents on the fermentation of coffee beans by certain kinds of bacteria before the roasting process to improve the taste and aroma of the roasted product. Also, a pectinolytic enzyme derived from molds has ben utilized in a method for removal of the pulpy layer from the beans, thus avoiding the production of off-flavore coffee that sometimes results from the uncontrolled natural fermentation.

Deterioration of the released coffee beans can occur during drying if this procedure is too prolonged.

ORIENTAL FERMENTED FOODS

Most of the Oriental fermented foods mentioned below have molds involved in their preparation. In the starter, termed koji by the Japanese and chou by the Chinese, molds serve as sources of hydrolytic enzymes, such as amylases to hydrolyze the starch in the grains, proteinases, lipases, and many others. For the most part the starters are mixtures of molds, yeasts, and bacteria, but for a few products pure cultures have been employed.

Soy Sauce

The chief Oriental fermented food imported into the United States and also made here is soy sauce, a brown, salty, tangy sauce used on dishes such as chop suey or as a constituent of other sauces. The methods of preparation of the starter and of manufacture of soy sauce have many variations and may result in different types of products.

The Starter: The starters (koji or chou) may be mixed cultures carried over from previous lots or pure cultures grown separately. The substrate on which the starter is grown varies, although most often it is an autoclaved mixture of soybeans, cracked wheat, and wheat bran; a mixture of wheat bran and soybean flour; or rice. This moistened material is inoculated with spores of *Aspergillus oryzae* (*A. soyae*), spread in small boxes or trays, and held at 25 to 30 °C until the mold growth on the surfaces of the mash is judged to have attained a maximal content of enzymes (usually after about 3 days). A flora of lactic acid bacteria, streptococci and lactobacilli, also develops in the koji and produces lactic acid, and some growth of Bacillus spp. takes place. The starter may be used at once as it is, may be dried and used later, or may be dried and extracted and the extract used.

Manufacture of soy sauce: The mash may consist of autoclaved soybeans or defatted, chemically hydrolyzed soybeans, roasted and crushed wheat, and steamed wheat bran. The mash is inoculated with the koji and incubated in trays for 3 days at about 30°C. Then it is soaked with sterile, 24 percent sodium chloride brine (sometimes the koji is mixed directly with an equal amount of saline water). The brined mash is held for from 2.5 months to a year or longer, depending on the temperature.

Fermentation: The proteinases, amylases, and other enzymes of the koji continue to act throughout the holding period. There are three stages in the curing- (1) lactic acid fermentation by lactic acid bacteria from the koji, followed by more acid production by *Pediococcus halophilus*, (2) alcoholic fermentation by yeasts, such as *Saccharomyces rouxii* and *Zygosaccharomyces soyae*, and (3) completion of the fermentation and aging. The various microorganisms important in the making of soy sauce may be added in pure culture or may come from previous lots of koji and from the ingredients. The chief organisms are *Aspergillus soyae (oryzae)*, the most important organism, which grows in the koji to yield proteinases, amylases, and other enzymes for soy-sauce brewing and contributes aromas and flavors; lactic acid bacteria, e.g., *Lactobacillus delbrueckii*, which makes the koji acid enough to prevent spoilage and acidifies the mash; *Bacillus subtilis* and other bacilli, which grow in the koji to improve flavor and make the soy sauce less turbid; *Pediococcus halophilus*, which increases the acid in the mash, thereby stimulating the yeasts, contributing to essential aromas and flavors, decreasing color intensity, and reducing the activity of the mold proteinases; and *Hansenula* spp., *Saccharomyces rouxii*, and other yeasts, which produce alcohol and help the flavor.

Tamari Sauce

This is a Japanese sauce, similar to soy sauce, made by a short fermentation process from a soybean mash to which rice may have been added. A different mold, *Aspergillus tamarii*, is the principal mold involved in the manufacture of tamari sauce.

Tempeh

In the manufacture of tempeh, an Indonesian food, soybeans are soaked overnight at 25 °C, the seed coats are removed, and the beans, split into halves, are boiled in water for 20 min. dried on mats, cooled, and inoculated with a previous lot of tempeh or with mold spores of species of *Rhizopus* (*R. stolonifer, R. oryzae, R. oligosporus*, or *R. arrhizus*). The mash is packed into a plastic container or a hollow tube or is rolled in banana leaves. It then is incubated at about 32 °C for 20 hr until there is good growth of mycelium but little sporulation. The product is sliced thin , dipped into salt water, and fried in vegetable fat to a golden brown.

Ang-khak

Ang-khak, or Chinese red rice, is produced by growth of *Monascus purpureus* on autoclaved rice and is used for coloring and flavoring fish and other food products.

Natt

In the manufacture of natto, boiled soybeans are wrapped in rice straw and fermented for 1 or 2 days. The package becomes slimy on the outside. *Bacillus natto**, probably identical with *Bacillus subtilis,* grows in natto, releasing trypsinlike enzymes that are supposed to be important in the ripening process.

Soybean Cheese

Soybean cheese, tou-fu-ju, or tofu, is a Chinese fermented food made by soaking soybeans, grinding them to a paste, and then filtering them through linen. The protein in the filtrate is curdled by means of a magnesium or calcium salt, after which the curd is pressed into blocks. The blocks, arranged on trays, are held in a fermentation chamber for a month at about 14°C, during which period white molds, probably *Mucor* spp., develop. Final ripening takes place in brine or in a special wine.

Miso

The koji for miso is a culture of *Aspergillus oryzae* grown at about 35°C on a steamed polishedrice mash in shallow trays until the grains are completely covered but the mold has not sporulated. The koji is mixed with a mash of crushed, steamed soybeans, salt is added, and the fermentation is allowed to proceed for a week at 28°C and then for two months at 35°C, after which the mixture is ripened for several weeks at room temperature. Involved in the main fermentation are the enzymes of the koji, yeasts (*Saccharomyces rouxii and Zygosaccharomyces* spp.), lactic acid bacteria, and bacilli. The final product is ground into a paste to be used in combination with other foods.

Minchin

Fermented minchin is made from wheat gluten from which the starch has been removed. The moist, raw gluten is placed in a closed jar and allowed to ferment for 2 to 3 weeks, after which it is salted. A typical specimen was found to contain seven species of molds, nine of bacteria, and three of yeasts. The final product is cut into strips to be boiled, baked, or fried.

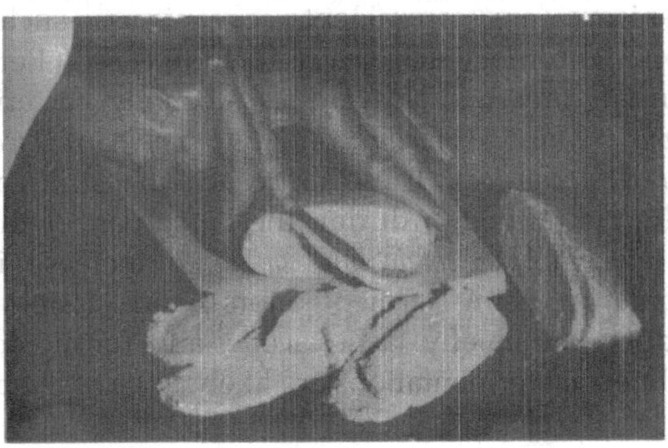

Fig 22.3. A tempeh cake. (Photography Division, USDA.)

Idli

Idli, a fermented food of India, is made from rice and black gram mungo in equal parts. The ingredients are washed and soaked separately, ground mixed, and finally allowed to ferment overnight. When the batter has risen enough, it is cooked by steaming and served hot. *Leuconostoc mesenteroides* grows first in the batter, leavening it,. and is followed by *Streptococcus faecalis* and finally *Pediococcus cerevisiae**, all of which contribute to the acidity.

Fermented Fish

The Japanese prepare a fermented fish by cutting it into strips, cooking it, and then encouraging fermentation by molds, chiefly species of *Aspergillus*. The strips then are dried. The Chinese have a fermented fish product preserved in lao-chao, a fermented rice product. Molds and yeasts are involved in the fermentation of the steamed rice, and some alcohol is produced.

Preserved Eggs

Pidan, or the Chinese preserved egg, is made from duck eggs coated with a slurry of soda, burned straw, salt, and slaked lime and covered with rice husks. The eggs then are kept in sealed clay jars for a month or longer. An assortment of bacteria grow in the egg, but coliform bacteria and species of *Bacillus* apparently are predominant.

Poi

Poi, although Hawaiian rather than Oriental, will be mentioned here. In the preparation of poi, the corms (bulblike, fleshy stems) of the taro plant are steamed at 70 to 100°C for 2 to 3 hr, cooled, washed, peeled, trimmed and scraped, and then finely ground. This ground mass, after being mixed with water to attain a desired consistency, is fresh poi that is ready for consumption. The sour or fermented poi is prepared by the incubation of barrels or other containers of fresh poi at room temperatures for at least 1 day and at most not more than 6 days. During the first 6 hr of the fermentation, the poi swells or puffs slightly and the color changes. During this period a mixture of soil and water microorganisms are prominent, organisms such as coliforms, Pseudomonas spp., chromogenic bacteria, and yeasts. Between 6 hr and 4 days the flora consists predominantly of acid-forming bacteria, among which are *Lactobacillus pastorianus**, *L. delbrueckii, L. brevis, Streptococcus lactis* subsp. *lactis*, and *S. kefir* (*Leuconostoc*). These lactic acid bacteria carry on the main fermentation in the poi, although during the latter part of the process, yeasts, film yeasts, and the mold *Geotrichum candidum* increase in numbers and probably contribute pleasing fruity odors and tastes (bouquet). The fermentation products are chiefly lactic, acetic, and formic acids, alcohol, and carbon dioxide. Abnormal fermentations are likely to be of the butyric acid type.

23 Microbial Enzymes and Their Applications in Food

Microbial enzymes play a crucial role in food production and processing, offering efficienc and specificity. Enzymes like amylases, produced by bacteria and fungi, are used in baking and brewing to break down starches into sugars. Proteases, from microbes like *Bacillus* species, aid in tenderizing meat and producing cheese. Lipases are used to enhance flavors in dairy products. Microbial enzymes improve food texture, flavor, and shelf life, while being cost-effective and sustainable. Their applications span industries, making them vital for innovative food processing and quality enhancement.

Microorganisms can be utilized as food for humans or animal feed, as a source of enzymes for food processing, or as producers of additives for food products.

MICROORGANISMS AS NUTRITION-SINGLE-CELL PROTEIN

Although various microorganisms, such as yeasts, molds, and algae, have been suggested for human consumption, only yeasts have been widely utilized, primarily under specific circumstances. For instance, during World War II, yeast and the mold *Geotrichum candidum* were produced in Germany to address protein and vitamin shortages. Post-war, the British established a yeast production facility in Jamaica. Currently, food and feed yeast plants operate in countries like Germany, Switzerland, Finland, South Africa, Jamaica, Taiwan, and the United States, especially in regions with abundant carbohydrates but limited protein and vitamin resources. Historically, yeast for feed and pharmaceuticals in the U.S. was primarily recovered as a by-product from brewers and distillers, but direct yeast cultivation for such purposes has grown significantly. Yeast strains are classified as primary when cultivated specifically for consumption and secondary when recovered as by-products from fermentation.

Secondary yeasts from alcoholic fermentation include brewers' yeasts (*Saccharomyces cerevisiae* or *S. carlsbergensis*) and distillers' yeasts (*S. cerevisiae* var. *ellipsoideus*). Brewers' yeast is debittered, pH-adjusted, salted, and dried, often fortified with vitamins such as thiamine, riboflavin, and niacin before drying. Alternatively, primary yeast may be produced by further cultivating yeast cells from breweries or distilleries in a molasses medium. However, consuming viable yeast cells, such as in "yeast cakes," can result in the yeast scavenging vitamins, making "dead" yeast products, like single-cell protein (SCP), a better nutritional supplement.

SCP refers to microbial cells cultivated specifically for animal or human food. The term "single-cell protein" is preferred over alternatives like bacterial, algal, or microbial protein, which are less appealing. SCP research has gained traction as a potential solution to future global food shortages, driven by concerns about increasing population pressures. Microbial fermentation and the SCP industry are viewed as viable means to address protein deficits when agricultural and fishing outputs are insufficien

The advantages of SCP production include (1) the ability to use non-human food substrates, (2) high protein content in microorganisms (up to 60–70% of cell weight), (3) rapid biomass production due to short microbial generation times, and (4) independence from climatic conditions. Many SCP processes, are designed for use in animal feeds (feed grade) or human food (food grade). Further insights into SCP can be explored through the references provided at the end of this chapter.

Microorganisms Used

A variety of yeasts, bacteria, fungi, and algae can produce SCP, as indicated in Table 23.1. Two algae have been utilized in culture ponds or basins: *Spirulina maxima* and *Scenedesmus* acutus (267-3A). Due to their need for warm temperatures and lots of sunlight in addition to carbon dioxide, as well as the fact that their cell wall is indigestible, their use may be somewhat restricted in two ways: (1) geographically. *S. maxima* is cultivated commercially in Mexico's Lake Texcoco. *Alcaligenes* spp. (use H_2 and CO_2), *Cellulomonas* spp. (break down cellulosic material), and *Pseudomonas* spp. (used in the UK and by the Chinese Petroleum Corp., Taiwan) are examples of potentially helpful bacteria.

Bacteria are capable of growth on a wide variety of substrates, have a short generation time, and are high in protein content. Their use is somewhat limited by (1) poor public acceptance of bacteria as food, (2) small size and difficult of harvesting, and (3) high content of nucleic acid on a dried-weight basis . Yeasts are probably the most widely accepted and used microorganisms for SCP production. These include strains of *Candida utilis* (*Torula* yeast), which grows rapidly, utilizes pentose as well as hexose sugars, and synthesizes its accessory foods for growth from simple compounds, making possible its production from raw materials that are comparatively poor culture media. This is in contrast to *S. cerevisiae*, which utilizes only hexose sugar and otherwise is more fastidious in its growth requirements. Two special varieties of *Candida utilis* have been used, *C. utilis* var. major, which has larger cells than the original strain, and *C. utilis* var. *thermophila*, a high-temperature strain which can be grown at 36 to 39°C rather than at 32 to 34°C. *C. arborea* (*Monilia candida*), *C. pulcherrima*, and other yeasts also have been employed. A lactose fermenting yeast is required if yeast is to be grown in whey. *Candida lipolytica* strains are used for processes using alkanes and gas oil as substrates. Yeasts in general have several advantages over bacteria and algae including (1) better public acceptance, (2) lower content of nucleic acid, (3) easier harvesting because of size and concentration, and (4) growth in substrates of low pH.

Other studies on SCP production have used the yeasts *Rhodotorula* and *Saccharomyces* and the fungi *Aspergillus, Penicillium,* and *Fusarium.*

Table. SCP Production Processes from Different Substrate Using Various Type of Microorganism

Type	Company	Plant location	Substrate	Type of organism	Plant Size (thousands of tons per year)
Feed grade	British Petroleum	U.K.	n-Paraffin	Yeast	4
	Chinese Petroleum	Taiwan	n-Paraffin	Yeast	1
	Dai Nippon	Japan	n-Paraffin	Yeast	?
	ICI	U.K.	Methanol	Bacteria	1
	Kanegafuchi	Japan	n-Paraffin	Yeast	5
	Kohjin	Japan	?	Yeast	2.4
	Kyowa Hakko	Japan	n-Paraffin	Yeast	1.5
	Milbrew	U.S.	Whey, beer wort	Yeast	10
	Shell	Holland	Methane	Bacteria	1
	Svensa Socker	Sweden	Potato starch	Yeast	2
	British Petroleum	France	Gas oil	Yeast	20
	United Paper Mills	Finland	Sulfite aste	Yeast	10
	USSR	USSR		Yeast	20
	British Petroleum	Italy	n-Parffin	Yeast	100
	Liquichimica	Italy	n-Parffin	Yeast	100
	LSU-Bechtel		Cellulose waste	Bacteria	
	Tate & Lyle		Citric acid Waste	Fungi	
	ICAITI	Guatemala	Coffee aste	Fungi	
	IFP		CO_2+ sunlight	Algae	

Type	Company	Plant location	Substrate	Type of organism	Plant size, thousands of tons per year
	General Electric		Feed-lot waste	Bacteria	
	Mitsubishi		Methanol	Yeast	
	Finish Pulp and paper		Paper-pulp waste	Fungi	
Food grade	AMOCO	U.S.	Ethanol	Yeast	7.5
	Boise Cascade	U.S.	Sulfite aste	Yeast	6
	St. Regis Paper	U.S.	Sulfite aste	Yeast	5
	Slovnaft-Kojetin	Czecho slovakia	Ethanol	Yeast	1
	Exxon-Nestle`		Ethanol	Bacteria	
	Dai Nippon		Molasses	Yeast	
	Kraft Co.		Starch	Fungi	
	Kraft Co.		Whey	Yeast	
	Anheuser-Busch	U.S.	Beer wort	Yeast	5
	Yeast Prodcuts, Inc.	U.S.	Beer wort	Yeast	

Raw Materials Used as Substrates

Materials that have been employed include (1) molasses from sugar manufacture or hydrolysis of starch, (2) spent sulfite liquor, which is a waste product of the sulfite-pulping process in the paper industry, (3) the acid hydrolyzate of wood, (4) agricultural wastes, e.g., whey from the dairy industry, hydrolyzed starchy foods, e.g., grains and cull potatoes, and fruit wastes, e.g., fruit juice or citrus-peel hydrolyzate, (5) methane, (6) methanol and ethanol, as a carbon source for yeast, (7) paraffi or alkanes, (8) gas oil, the petroleum fraction between lubricating oil and diesel fuel, and (9) combustion gas, a source of carbon dioxide for algal cultures.

Conditions for Growth and Production

Since numerous processes are being used or experimented with, this discussion will be limited to the use of yeasts in commonly utilized raw materials.

For the most part, yeasts are produced by a continuous process which requires (1) establishment of active yeast growth in the fermentor, (2) feeding of carbohydrates and sources of nitrogen, phosphorus, and potassium at increasing rates until a maximal level of yeast growth is maintained continuously, (3) application of optimal aeration and agitation, and (4) withdrawal of liquor (beer) containing the yeast cells at rates and volumes equaling the additions of fresh medium.

Optimal conditions for yeast production vary with the yeast employed and the raw material used. Aeration should be considerable but at an optimal level; too little encourages alcohol production rather than growth, and too much favors increased respiration and heat production and hence lowered yields of the yeast cells. The optimal temperature depends on the yeast strain. The pH should be kept on the acid side, usually between 4.5 and 6.0. The concentration of fermentable sugar is maintained at a level no higher than that necessary for a good yield of cells. The amounts and kinds of inorganic nutrients to be added depend on the substrate. Cane- or beet-sugar molasses, for example, usually is high in potassium and fairly well supplied with available phosphorus and nitrogen, but spent sulfite liquor is deficient in all three of these elements, which are needed in relatively large amounts. Nitrogen usually is added in the form of ammonia or ammonium salts.

Yields are 45 percent or more of dry yeast on the basis of the sugar fed. The yeast cells are centrifuged from the medium, washed, concentrated, and dried. All food yeasts are killed before use.

Special pretreatments are required before some of the raw materials can be used to grow yeast. Most of the sulfur dioxide must be removed from the spent sulfite liquor by steam stripping or by aeration and treatment with lime. The treated liquor remains selective enough to favor the yeasts over competing organisms so that troubles with contamination are negligible throughout a long period of continuous yeast production. Wood hydrolyzate similarly requires pretreatment.

Nutritive Value and Use of SCP

Nutritive value varies with the microorganism used. Protein digestibility values, expressed as a percentage, range from 65 to 96 for the various cultures tested. Protein efficienc ratio (PER) values range from 0.6 to 2.6. The method of harvesting, drying, and processing has an effect on the nutritive value of the finished product. Food yeast is high in protein and in most of the B complex vitamins but may be deficient in methionine and perhaps cysteine. Also, the thiamine content may be lower than in secondary yeast, and there is a deficiency of vitamin B12.

Furnished by food yeast in varying amounts are thiamine, riboflavin, biotin, niacin, pantothenic acid, pyridoxine, choline, streptogenin, glutathione, and perhaps folic acid and p-aminobenzoic acid.

The United Nations Protein Advisory Group has summarized the major concerns over the use of SCP for human beings as follows- (1) high concentration of nucleic acids (6 to 11 percent) elevating serum uric acid levels and resulting in kidney stone formation or gout, (2) possible skin reactions from consuming foreign proteins, (3) possible carryover of carcinogenic factors from the diverse substrates, and (4) possible gastrointestinal reactions resulting in nausea and vomiting.

CONCEPT OF PROBIOTICS

The concept of probiotics is the colonization of beneficial bacteria in the intestinal tract, promoting efficien functioning of digestion, helping prevent digestive upsets, and stimulating and maintaining the natural immunity of the body. Probiotic bacteria are normal inhabitants of the intestines and are normally found in the healthy gut of all humans.

Probiotics have been in use for as long as people have consumed fermented milks, but their association with health benefits dates only from the turn of the century when Metchnikoff drew attention to the adverse effects of the gut microflora on the host and suggested that ingestion of fermented milks ameliorated this so-called auto-intoxication. Later work, based on the assumption that colonization of the gut was essential for the maximum effect, used intestinal strains of *Lactobacillus acidophilus* for treatment of constipation.

The use of the term 'probiotic' to describe food supplements specifically designed to improve health, however, dates from 1974 when Parker used it to describe growth-promoting animal-feed supplements. He defined the term as 'organisms and substances which contribute to intestinal microbial balance'.

Composition of Probiotics

Lactic acid bacteria (lactobacilli, streptococci, and bifidobacteria), constitute the probiotic currently used preparations. These three genera have been shown to be important components of the gastrointestinal microflora, which are all relatively harmless. It has also been shown in recent experiments that administration of *Escherichia coli* to infants can prevent the colonization of the gut by the antibiotic resistant strains of *E. coli.* A probiotic preparation may contain one or several of the different strains of bacteria.

- **Lactobacilli:** Fermented foods and dairy products like yogurt contain the species of Lactobacilli. There are three types of lactobacilli, including *Lactobacillus plantarum, Lactobacillus casei,* and *Lactobacillus sporogenes.* It has been established that according to the Environmental Illness Resource, the benefits that lactobacilli can provide include preventing and treating diarrhea caused by antibiotics; prevention of vaginal- and urinary-tract infections; prevention of overgrowth of bacteria like *H. pylori, Salmonella* and *E. coli;* and help with the digestion of lactose products. In addition to these benefits, *L. sporogenes* has also been shown to reduce LDL cholesterol levels, which is the "bad" cholesterol, and raise HDL cholesterol levels, making it a supplement for treating high cholesterol levels and heart disease.
- **Bifidobacteria:** The most common kind of intestinal bacteria found in infants include bifidobacteria. As individuals get older, the level of the

bacteria decreases, and they can be naturally found occurring in the vagina as well as the intestines. The most commonly seen species of these bacteria in humans include *Bifidobacterium longum, B. infantis, B. breve, B. adolescentis,* and *B. pseudocatenulatum*. The group of bifidobacteria contains several kinds of probiotics, all of which are beneficial. These probiotics are known to help protect the intestinal lining; they produce acids to keep the pH in the intestine balanced; they help decreases side effects of antibiotics; ensures regular bowel movements, and helps build B-complex vitamins.

- ***Streptococcus thermophilus*:** The most important lactic acid bacteria for commercial purposes, typically used as a starter culture for dairy foods other than yogurt, like mozzarella cheese is *Streptococcus thermophilus*. The only probiotic in the *Streptococcus* group is *S. thermophilus*. This bacterium is known to help an individual with malnutrition, resulting due to fasting. It reduces intestinal atrophy from short-term fasting and also possesses antioxidant properties. This probiotic prevents nitrates from changing into nitrates that are known to cause cancer and has shown to protect the intestines from mucositis during chemotherapy treatment.

The different strains of lactic acid bacteria used in probiotics are mostly intestinal isolates of importance such as *L. acidophilus, L. casei, Enterococcus faecium,* and *Bifidobacterium bifidum*. Starter bacteria for yogurt (*L. bulgaricus* and *Streptococcus thermophilus*) are also included because yogurt has always been associated with health benefits in the past. The ability of the starter bacteria in yogurt to colonize the gut is extremely doubtful, although they can persist and remain viable throughout the gastrointestinal tract of rats. The necessity for continuous ingestion in these cases is obvious. Even with intestinal isolates such as *L acidophilus*, it is necessary to regularly give doses rather than to assume that a few doses will allow the organisms to help colonize the gut permanently. Work in the USA illustrates this point- when *L. acidophilus* was fed to human patients, there was a significant reduction in the activity of the bacterial enzymes glucuronidase, nitroreductase, and azoreductase. This reduced activity, however, persisted only as long as the lactobacillus supplement was being fed; when it was stopped, the enzyme activity slowly returned to the pre-supplementation values.

Similarly, experiments have revealed that if lactobacilli are administered to newborn rats, there is a significant decrease in intestinal coliform count, but on stopping the treatment, this returns to normalcy after a few days. It seems unlikely, therefore, that the probiotic bacteria will permanently colonize the intestine; thereby indicating that continuous feeding is necessary if a persistent effect is required.

The following mechanisms have shown that probiotics do work:

- **Competition for Nutrients:** Utilization of the same types of nutrients by the beneficial as well as pathogenic microorganisms is seen within the gut. Thus, there exists a general competition for these nutrients by the groups of microbes to grow and reproduce. Hence, if the gut is flooded with beneficial microorganisms, more competition is created between beneficial and pathogenic microorganisms.

- **Competition for Adhesion Sites:** Most intestinal pathogens rely on adhesion to the gut wall. Adhering to adhesion sites along the gut wall is an important factor in colonization to prevent the pathogenic forms from being swept away by peristaltic movement of the food along the gastro intestinal tract. One of the most important functions of these probiotic bacteria is to help prevent or limit the growth and colonization of potentially pathogenic bacteria such as *E. coli, Salmonella, Listeria, Campylobacter,* and *Clostridia* within the gut. Major disturbances within the gut are caused by pathogenic bacteria, thus preventing efficient digestion and ineffective nutrient absorption within the gut and may result in diarrhea or vomiting. When the gut microflora are well balanced with the beneficial microorganisms, colonizing the gut helps reduce the risk of pathogenic.
- **Stimulation of Immunity:** An optimum balance of the microflora is maintained by the use of probiotics in order to stimulate and maintain the natural immune system of the host. It has been observed that when probiotics are used regularly, the enhanced immune effects help prevent illness.
- **Direct Antimicrobial Effect:** Bacteriocins are known to be produced by many species of lactic acid bacteria. Also, the production of organic acids by these organisms can either have a direct effect or operate by reducing the pH of the gut, thus displaying an antimicrobial effect
- **Improvement in Digestion:** Enzymes help in the breakdown of polysaccharides such as carbohydrates, thereby ensuring enough of nutrient flow is governed by t he presence of the probiotics, which act effecti ely in the production of the requisite enzymes. The microflora also helps ferment the carbohydrates which have not been digested in the upper gut and produce vitamins which are a secondary source to the host.

Why Take Probiotics?

If you eat a well-balanced diet without a lot of processed foods and live a stress-free life, probiotics may not be necessary as an additional aid in maintaining your overall health and immunity. However, in today's world, we face daily stress from our environment and the foods we eat. In addition, we also tend to consume many different forms of chemicals, such as antacids, antibiotics, food additives, alcohol, and other foods and medications that can ultimately lead to disruption and reduction in the concentrations of beneficial bacteria in our digesti e tract.

By the age of two or three, most children have developed some intestinal balance and a fairly effecti e immune system. However, with age, environmental and nutritional factors often disrupt this balance and create the need for probiotic supplementation. This results in dysbiosis, disruption of the microflora and potentially increased susceptibility to pathogenic bacteria. Dysbiosis can be caused when we are subjected to stressful factors such as:

Changes in Food and Water Normally Associated With Travel

When we travel, our bodies must endure the time taken during flights or other means of travel, which make us tired, and any time changes which might occur. Ultimately, this puts stress on our bodies. Taking drugs such as antimalarial tablets affects the gut microflora. In addition, the food and water sources will be different and varied in many cases, which may lead to digestive upsets associated with travel to foreign countries or even within the country.

Antibiotic Therapy, Anti-inflammatory Steroids or Chemotherapy

The use of antibiotics, steroids, or chemotherapy can adversely affect gut flora. For instance, when antibiotics are used, a proportion of the beneficial microorganisms becomes disrupted and can lead to diarrhea and an increased susceptibility of the gut to the colonization of pathogenic bacteria such as *E. coli, Salmonella,* etc. The proportion of beneficial microorganisms generally killed in the gut (by an antibiotic) will depend on the action of the antibiotic (narrow or broad spectrum). The duration and the frequency of the course also is important.

Hormonal Fluctuations Around puberty, During Menstruation, Pregnancy, Post Natally or During the Menopause

Hormonal effects during the different stages of our lives are such that the balance of the intestinal microflora can be disturbed at any time. The levels of beneficial bacteria such as *Bifidobacterium* and Lactobacilli decrease with age, the production of stomach acid decreases, which reduces the acidity of the gastrointestinal tract and thus increases the levels of coliforms and other pathogenic bacteria in the intestine.

- **Immunological compromise:** stress can reduce the immune response of animals and humans and the use of certain antibiotics has been shown to significantly reduce the immune response, leading to a decrease in the weight of the spleen and thymus. Withdrawal of these antibiotics in these cases can help restore the intestinal flora and return to normal immune functions. Antibiotics are often known to reduce the population of lactobacilli.
- **Unhealthy diet:** Changes in diet and lack of a healthy diet can affect the balance of microflora. intestines, thus predisposing us to digestive disorders. A balanced diet, sufficien in energy and nutrients, as well as in dietary fiber, is also of great importance to maintain a healthy intestine. In addition, eating behavior that leads to indigestion will disrupt the balance of microflor
- **Stress / modern lifestyle:** There is strong evidence that stress can affect the composition of the intestinal microflora. Stress can be described as a factor that stimulates homeostatic, physiological and behavioral responses beyond the norm. Stress increases blood levels of adrenal corticosteroids, which affects peristaltic movement and mucus production in the intestine. All the

stressful situations to which we are exposed contribute to the increase in the pH of the intestines (more alkaline), and therefore, the gastrointestinal tract is likely to favor the development of pathogenic species such as *E. coli* to the detriment of beneficial species

- **lactase deficiency:** A large part of The world's population is unable to use lactose. The enzyme responsible for digesting lactose, although present in breastfed infants, disappears after weaning. In parts of the world where milk is not a staple food, this does not pose a problem, but if people from these areas migrate to Europe or the United States, problems arise because the intake of lactose in one form or another is difficult to avoid. It has been known for some time that subjects suffering from lactase deficiency can tolerate lactose containing yogurt better than the same.
- **The amount of lactose contained in milk:** this has been confirmed by experiments analyzing exhaled hydrogen air. Although the mechanism is not known, it has been suggested that yogurt provides either preformed lactase or lactase-producing bacteria as it enters the small intestine. It has been possible to demonstrate an increase in lactase activity in the small intestine of mice fed yogurt; the microbial origin of this increase is demonstrated by the large increase in activity in the intestinal contents compared with the intestinal wall. The first The experiments with *L. acidophilus* improved lactose intolerance, but the results of subsequent trials have been variable. This variation may be due to the differences between the strains of *L. acidophilus* used. An intestinal infection can lead to lactase deficiency. Yogurt has been used to restore lactase activity in the intestines of children with *Giardia lamblia* infection.
- ***Pseudomembranous colitis*:** This disease, caused by *Clostridium difficile*, can be cured by giving fecal enemas. for healthy adults. It is therefore concluded that resistance to this disease depends on the presence of a good intestinal flora. There is now evidence that a particular strain of *Lactobacillus* is effective in preventing the recurrence of *p. colitis* in patients treated with antibiotics. Another approach that has shown some success is the administration of non-pathogenic strains of *Clostridium difficile*, which apparently take the place that the pathogen would expect to find available. The use of probiotics in the treatment of *p. colitis* has potential because patients "at risk" can be easily identified and treatment can be started before the onset of the disease.

Infections or diseases caused by pathogenic microbes that cause symptoms such as diarrhea, excessive gas production, and constipation. Additionally, an imbalanced microflora can lead to an overgrowth of harmful and pathogenic bacteria and yeasts, such as *Candida albicans, Clostridium difficile* etc.

In some cases, pathogenic bacteria may be able to colonize the intestines, causing symptoms such as diarrhea. In this case, the number of pathogens in the intestine will be high enough to cause such symptoms.

Malabsorption or chronic inflammatory bowel disease, such as Crohn's disease, ulcerative colitis, diverticulitis- Intestinal problems such as irritable bowel syndrome, ulcerative colitis, and sometimes Crohn's disease are usually associated with dysbiosis. An imbalanced microflora can also lead to arthritis, headaches and migraines, eczema, chronic fatigue, sinus problems or psoriasis.

Probiotics can benefit people in many ways:

- Assist in stimulating peristaltic intestinal movement (reduces constipation and significantly improves digestion)
- Helps in the distribution of digestive enzymes (breakdown of most food products)
- Help reduce the effects of stress
- Reduce cases of diarrhea and other digestive disorders
- Help improve immunity and provide resistance to disease
- Reduce symptoms such as digestive diseases. lactose intolerance and irritable bowel syndrome
- Reduces cholesterol absorption
- Promotion of B vitamins, niacin B2, pyridoxine B6

What Makes a Good Probiotic?

- Safety
  - o Probiotic components must consist of non-pathogenic and non-toxic microorganisms to ensure safety.
- Multistrain
  - o A high-quality probiotic should include multiple species of beneficia microorganisms, enhancing its activity spectrum within the gut and providing maximum benefits to a broader range of host species
- Viability
  - o The microorganisms in a probiotic must remain viable during storage and throughout the digestive process to ensure proper colonization and effecti eness.
- Minimum Dose
  - o A good probiotic should have a concentration sufficien to deliver 10^7 to 10^8 CFU per dose (10 million to 100 million beneficial bacteria per dose).
- Quality Assurance
  - o Probiotics must be free from contamination by other microorganisms during all stages, including fermentation, manufacturing, transport, and storage, to maintain quality and effecti eness.

Probiotic Products

Yogurt

Yogurt is perhaps the most recognized probiotic food. It contains *Streptococcus thermophilus* and various strains of *Lactobacillus* bacteria. Some brands include additional bacterial strains for enhanced benefits. To gain full probiotic advantages, yogurt must have live and active cultures, as pasteurization can destroy beneficial bacteria.

Miso

Miso, a staple in Japanese cuisine, is made by fermenting soybeans with a fungus called koji. It is the main component of miso soup, which can be prepared quickly with miso paste and hot water. Miso also serves as a condiment and is rich in sodium, zinc, copper, and protein. It is readily found in supermarkets.

Kefir

Kefir is a milk-based fermented beverage similar to yogurt, created using kefir grains, which are primarily *Lactobacillus kefiri* bacteria. These bacteria ferment the milk, making it thicker and slightly fizzy due to carbon dioxide production. Kefir comes in various flavors like yogurt and is widely available in both health-food and conventional supermarkets.

Kombucha

Kombucha is a fermented tea drink made using a symbiotic culture of bacteria and yeast. It has been consumed for centuries worldwide and recently gained popularity in the United States. While many attribute health benefits to kombucha, the FDA has not evaluated these claims. Kombucha is sweet, tangy, and fizzy, with various flavors a ailable in health-food stores.

CASE STUDY

Probiotics

Sintesi Research Services conducted a study to evaluate the effecti eness and tolerability of a probiotic for treating acute diarrhea. The primary objective was to measure the time taken for symptom resolution (in days) during the treatment phase, comparing the probiotic group to a group receiving a standard treatment. The study also aimed to monitor the onset of related symptoms or relapses during the follow-up period. Tolerability was assessed by recording any adverse effects occurring during both the treatment and follow-up phases.

The study involved 200 adult patients (aged 18 and above) of both genders in Italy who were experiencing acute diarrhea. The probiotic treatment lasted for 10 days, followed by a one-week follow-up. A therapeutic success was defined as a reduction of at least 20% in the average duration of diarrhea in the probiotic group compared to the standard treatment group.

FATS FROM MICROORGANISMS

Fats (more properly lipids) are synthesized in appreciable amounts by certain yeasts, yeastlike organisms, and molds, but production in this manner has been employed only during periods of emergency, e.g., a state of war, when cheaper and more easily available animal and plant lipids were not available in sufficien quantity.

Organisms Used

Among the yeasts, *Candida pulcherrima, Torulopsis lipofera, Saccharomyces cerevisiae,* and *Rhodotorula glutinis* have been studied for their fat production, and the first was used for this purpose in Germany and Sweden during World War II. The yeastlike *Trichosporon pullulans* was used by the Germans during World War I, as were special strains of the mold *Geotrichum candidum.*

Raw Materials

Media for fat production should in general have a high carbon-to-nitrogen ratio, a god supply of phosphates, and for most organisms a pH on the acid side. In fat production by *Trichosporon pullulans,* good growth first is obtained in a mash with a high ratio of nitrogen to carbon, and fat production is carried out in a medium with a high ratio of carbon to nitrogen. Molasses, cellulose waste, hydrolyzed wood, and spent sulfite liquor are among the sources of carbohydrate employed. Nitrogen can be in the form of ammonium salts, urea, urine, yeast water, molasses slop, or extracts of grains. Salts to be added include potassium chloride, monopotassium phosphate, and magnesium sulfate. Addition of small amounts of alcohol or sodium acetate increases yields of lipids. The choice of a yeast will depend on its ability to utilize both pentoses and hexoses or only the latter. *Geotrichum candidum* is able to utilize the lactose in whey, to which some additional nitrogenous food and salts may be added.

Production of Fat

Since all the previously mentioned organisms grow best under aerobic conditions, their growth for fat production has been in thin layers on trays or other flat areas when *Trichosporon pullulans* or a mold was employed and in well-aerated tanks when yeasts were grown submerged. The optimal temperature varies with the organism employed, ranging from 15 to 20 °C for *T. pullulans* to 25 to 30 °C or slightly higher for molds and yeasts. A fairly long period is required for maximal fat production by most of the organisms mentioned. *T. pullulans,* for example, requires 2 to 3 days to attain growth and 6 to 8 days more for maximal yields of lipids. Fields of lipids vary widely with the organisms and with methods of production. Recovery of lipids is by extraction with solvents, with or without autolysis.

PRODUCTION OF AMINO ACIDS

Commercial fermentation for producing glutamate has advanced significantly since monosodium glutamate (MSG) was recognized as a key flavor enhancing food ingredient, with annual production nearing 200,000 tons. Strains of *Corynebacterium glutamicus* (including species such as *Corynebacterium, Arthrobacter, Brevibacterium,* and *Micrococcus*) are used in these processes. These strains lack α-ketoglutarate dehydrogenase, an enzyme in the Krebs cycle that converts α-ketoglutarate to succinyl-CoA. As a result, α-ketoglutarate, in the presence of ammonia, is redirected to form glutamate via transamination, leading to its accumulation. Similarly, lysine production through fermentation is a significant industry, primarily addressing its deficiency in cereal-based foods. Lysine is widely used to fortify foods low in this essential amino acid. Fermentation processes have also been developed to produce other amino acids, including aspartic acid, threonine, isoleucine, phenylalanine, proline, tryptophan, valine, homoserine, ornithine, leucine, arginine, histidine, and tyrosine.

PRODUCTION OF OTHER SUBSTANCES ADDED TO FOODS

Microorganisms may be employed to produce dextran, xanthan, lactic and citric acids, and perhaps other substances added to foods.

Dextran and Xanthan

Dextran, a gummy polysaccharide and neutral glucan, is produced by *Leuconostoc mesenteroides* using a molasses or refined-sucrose medium. It is utilized as a stabilizer in sugar syrups, ice cream, and confections, and also serves as a plasma extender. Commercial production is feasible with sucrose or sucrose-rich media since the enzyme responsible for its polymerization is extracellular, allowing for the use of cell-free filtrates. Xanthan, on the other hand, is a polyionic hydropolysaccharide produced by *Xanthomonas campestris* when grown in a glucose-based medium. Widely used in the food industry, particularly as a stabilizer, xanthan differs from dextran in that it is not hydrolyzed or metabolized by humans or animals and is excreted unchanged.

Lactic Acid

For the most part, lactic acid is produced industrially by homofermentative lactic acid bacteria or bacteria resembling them. A simplified equation for the production of lactic acid $C_3H_6O_3$ from glucose by such organisms is

$$C_6H_{12}O_6 \xrightarrow[\text{bacteria}]{\text{lactic acid}} 2CH_3CHOH\,COOH$$

Actually a series of steps are involved, and small amounts of other products are produced. It has been estimated that edible lactic acid makes up about half of the commercial acid produced by fermentation.

- **Microorganisms Used:** The microorganism used depenpds on the raw material to be fermented. *Lactobacillus delbrueckii* was most often employed in the past for lactic acid production from glucose, maltose, or sucrose, although increasing use is being made of a flat sour bacterium such as *Bacililus coagulans*. *Lactobacillus delbrueckii* subsp. *bulgaricus* has been selected for making lactic acid from whey. The pentose-fermenting *L. pentosus (L. plantarum)* is recommended for use in spent sulfite liquors, and *L. brevis (L. pentoaceticus)* for hydrolyzed corncobe, cottonseed hulls, etc. Molds, e.g., *Rhizopus oryzae*, have been used experimentally to produce lactic acid from a glucose-salts medium.

- **Raw Materials:** It is advantageous in the manufacture of lactic acid by fermentation to start with a relatively simple medium or mash in order to facilitate the recovery of the product. When glucose, sucrose, or maltose is the carbohydrate fermented, as with a molasses or a starch hydrolyzate mash, *Lactobacillus delbrueckii* or a flat sour bacillus usually is employed. Nitrogenous food, minerals, and various growth factors required by the bacteria may be added in the form of malt sprouts, corn-steep liquor, milk, etc, Similar addition must be made to spent sulfite liquor for the growth of *L. plantarum*. The production of lactic acid from whey by *L. delbrueckii* subsp. *bulgaricus* also has been carried out on an industrial scale. Other raw materials that have been suggested are cull fruits, Jerusalem artichokes, molasses, beet juice, hydrolyzed starchy materials, e.g., potatoes or grains, and hydrolyzed corncobs, corn stalks, cottonseed hull, and straw.

Production of Lactic Acid

The heat-treated mash is maintained at an optimal temperature based on the inoculated organism- approximately 45°C for *L. delbrueckii*, 45–50°C for *L. delbrueckii* subsp. *bulgaricus* or *Bacillus coagulans*, and 30°C for *L. plantarum*. The ideal sugar concentration ranges from 5 to 20 percent, depending on the raw material and the fermenting microorganism. Anaerobic conditions are ensured throughout fermentation.

The pH is kept slightly acidic, with lactic acid neutralized periodically using calcium hydroxide or calcium carbonate during the multi-day fermentation process. The calcium lactate formed can either be crystallized or converted to lactic acid by adding sulfuric acid. Producing edible-grade lactic acid involves more extensive refinement compared to the technical grade

Uses of Edible Lactic Acid

In the food industry, lactic acid is employed to acidify jams, jellies, confectionery, sherbets, soft drinks, extracts, and other products. It is also used in brines for pickles and olives, as well as in horseradish and fish for preservation purposes. Additionally, it improves milk digestibility for infants and is a component of some baking powders in the form of calcium lactate.

Citric Acid

In the United States most citric acid is produced by fermentation.

Organisms Used

Aspergillus niger is the principal mold used in citric acid production, although various other molds are known to be able to make the acid and many have been tried experimentally- molds such as *A. clavatus, A. wentii, Penicillium luteum, P. citrinum, Mucor pyriformis,* and others. Apparently different strains of *A. niger* are preferred for surface methods of citric acid production than for methods involving submerged growth. A simplified theoretical equation for the production of citric acid from glucose is

$$C_6H_{12}O_6 + 1\frac{1}{2}O_2 \rightarrow C_6H_8O_7 + 2H_2O$$

A series of intermediate steps are involved, and other products are produced.

Raw Materials

Citric acid is primarily produced using molasses, with beet molasses being preferred over cane molasses. Other raw materials include cane blackstrap, cane invert molasses, or solutions of glucose or sucrose combined with nitrogen and mineral sources. Nitrogen is typically supplied through simple compounds like ammonium salts or urea. The concentration of minerals, particularly iron, zinc, and manganese, plays a crucial role in achieving high yields. A slight deficiency in nitrogen and phosphate enhances production. Factors that limit the formation of mycelium often lead to higher citric acid yields. Additionally, conditions promoting citric acid production tend to inhibit oxalic acid formation.

Production of Citric Acid

Earlier methods of producing citric acid involved surface growth, where mold mycelium was grown on shallow layers of medium in trays. Modern approaches rely on submerged growth of the mycelium. The choice of mold strain and production medium varies depending on the cultivation method. Typically, sugar concentrations of 14 to 20 percent are used, with a low pH (more acidic in the surface method), temperatures between 25 and 30°C, and fermentation periods of 7 to 10 days for surface methods or shorter durations for submerged methods.

Uses of Citric Acid

In the food industry, citric acid is widely used in flavoring extracts, soft drinks, and candies. It is also added to fish to adjust the pH to around 5.0 for better preservation, to artichokes to enable milder heat treatments during canning, and to crabmeat to prevent discoloration. Additionally, it serves as a synergist with antioxidants for oils and as a dip for sliced peaches to delay browning. A significant portion of citric acid is also utilized for medicinal applications.

PRODUCTION OF ENZYMES

The protein biocatalysts, called enzymes, used by living cells are responsible for numerous metabolic processes of the cell. The use of microbial enzymes, although only recently understood, has been going on for centuries. Since microorganisms are responsible for the fermentations of beer, wine, bread, cheese, and various vegetables, all these processes are examples of cell-mediated conversions or applications of enzymes. Current technology makes it possible to isolate, purify, and even immobilize (bind to a fixed support) the specific enzyme needed for a desired function. Several enzymes used in the food and fermentation industries and their respective sources are presented in Table 23.2, accompanied by a discussion of several of the more important groups of enzymes.

Table. Microbial Enzymes, Source, and Use

Enzyme	Source	Industry	Application
Amylase	*Aspergillus oryzae, Bacillus subtilis*	Food, Brewing	Starch hydrolysis, alcohol production
Invertase	*Saccharomyces cerevisiae*	Food, Confectionery	Sucrose hydrolysis in sweets and syrups
Protease	*Bacillus subtilis, Aspergillus niger*	Detergent, Food	Protein breakdown in cleaning, tenderizing meat
Lipase	*Candida rugosa, Rhizopus oryzae*	Dairy, Detergent	Fat hydrolysis, cheese flavor enhancement
Cellulase	*Trichoderma reesei, Aspergillus niger*	Textile, Paper	Fiber softening, cellulose breakdown
Pectinase	*Aspergillus niger, Penicillium* spp.	Fruit Processing	Juice clarification, pectin removal
Lactase	*Aspergillus oryzae, Kluyveromyces lactis*	Dairy	Lactose hydrolysis for lactose-free products
Xylanase	*Trichoderma reesei, Aspergillus niger*	Paper, Textile	Bleaching, improving paper quality
Glucose Isomerase	*Streptomyces* spp., *Bacillus coagulans*	Food, Beverage	Conversion of glucose to fructose (HFCS)
Phytase	*Aspergillus niger, Pseudomonas* spp.	Animal Feed	Phosphorus availability enhancement

Amylases

Amylases, enzymes that hydrolyze starches, are categorized based on their specific actions on starch molecules. Starch consists of two glucans- linear amylose, made of D-glucose units connected by α-1,4 linkages, and branched amylopectin, which also has α-1,6 linkages at branching points. The main types of amylases are:

- **α-Amylase:** Randomly breaks α-1,4-glucosidic linkages in amylose or amylopectin but does not affect the α-1,6 linkages in am lopectin.
- **β-Amylase:** Specifically cleaves the second α-1,4-glucoside linkage from the non-reducing ends of starch chains, releasing maltose molecules one at a time and leaving behind limit dextrins.
- **Amyloglucosidase:** Hydrolyzes both α-1,6 and α-1,4 linkages, breaking starch down into glucose without producing intermediate dextrins or maltose.

Additionally, maltase (α-glucosidase), which is not classified as an amylase, converts maltose into glucose. While much of the industrial amylase supply traditionally comes from grain malt, which contains varying proportions of amylases, there is a growing trend toward producing amylases from molds and bacteria. These microbial sources can produce either specific types of amylases or mixtures tailored to industrial needs.

From Molds

Molds are utilized as sources of amylases and other hydrolytic enzymes, with specific species and strains selected for their intended purpose. *Rhizopus delemar*, *Mucor rouxii*, and related species are commonly used in the Amylo process, where starchy grain mash is saccharified by mold-produced amylases. This method is primarily employed to prepare mashes for yeast-based alcoholic fermentation. For producing amylase-rich preparations, *Aspergillus oryzae* is the most widely used mold, although *A. niger* is preferred for submerged production methods. The preparation of koji, the *A. oryzae* starter rich in amylases and other enzymes for soy sauce production, was discussed in Chapter 22.

In the tray method for amylase production, *A. oryzae* is grown on moistened, steamed wheat or rice bran spread in thin layers within trays. Alternatively, the drum method involves tossing bran in a rotating drum. Optimal yields are achieved using the tray method after 40 to 48 hours of incubation at approximately 30°C, under conditions of high humidity and proper ventilation. Amylases are extracted from the mold's mycelium and can be purified through precipitation and washing or concentrated as needed. These preparations also contain other hydrolytic enzymes.

From Bacteria

Bacillus subtilis is the primary bacterium used for amylase production, though other bacterial species also produce these enzymes. Most bacteria generate more α-amylase than β-amylase. Amylase production can be carried out using the surface-growth method, involving shallow layers of mash in trays, or the submerged method.

The culture media for *B. subtilis* vary from complex substrates like thin stillage—a by-product of alcohol production from grains—to simpler mixtures containing soluble or hydrolyzed starch, ammonium salts, and buffers. Other media may include hydrolyzed soybean cake, peanut cake, or casein for nitrogen, hydrolyzed starch for energy, and various mineral salts. Additionally, wheat bran is used in bran-salts media. For the tray method, incubation typically occurs at temperatures between 25°C and 37°C over 2 to 6 days, whereas the submerged method operates at 30°C to 40°C for 24 to 48 hours.

Purification and concentration of bacterial amylase involve processes such as dialysis, condensation, and fractional precipitation.

Uses

In the food industries, fungal amylases have been employed to remove starch from fruit extracts, e.g., in the production of pectin from apple pomace; to clarify starch turbidities in wines, beer, and fruit juices; to convert acid-modified starches to sweet sirups; to substitute for malt in breadmaking in aiding leavening and improving dough consistency and hence gas retention (proteinases also are involved); and to saccharify starch in mashes for alcoholic fermentation. Bacterial amylase, chiefly the alpha type, has been used in brewing to produce dextrins of low fermentability and also to clarify the beer and in the manufacture of corn sirup and chocolate sirup to prevent thickening by dextrinizing the starch present.

Invertase

Invertase facilitates the breakdown of sucrose into glucose and fructose. In yeasts, invertase functions as a fructosidase, targeting the fructose portion of the sucrose molecule, whereas in molds, it acts as a glucosidase, attacking the glucose portion. Industrial production of invertase primarily involves cultivating specific strains of *Saccharomyces cerevisiae* (bottom-fermenting type) in a medium containing sucrose, an ammonium salt, phosphate buffer, and other essential minerals, maintained at approximately pH 4.5. The incubation process is carried out for about 8 hours at temperatures ranging from 28 to 30°C.

To extract invertase, yeast cells are filtered, compressed, plasmolyzed, and subjected to autolysis. The enzyme is then recovered and either dried with sugar, stored in sucrose syrup, or further purified through methods such as dialysis, ultra iltration, adsorption, and elution. However, most commercial invertase products are not extensively purified.

Uses

Invertase is used in the confectionery industry to make invert sugar for the preparation of liqueurs and ice creams in which the crystallization of sugars from high concentrations is to be avoided. In soft-center, chocolate-coated candies, e.g., Maraschino cherries, invertase incorporated in the centers softens the fondant after it has been coated with chocolate. Invertase is added to sucrose sirups to hydrolyze that sugar and in this way to prevent crystallization on standing. It also has been used in the manufacture of artificial honey.

Pectolytic Enzymes

Pectin, a methylated form of polygalacturonic acid, plays a vital role in the food industry due to its gel-forming properties when combined with sugar and acid. While this feature is desirable for making jellies, it is undesirable in fruit juices. It is widely accepted that two primary enzymes are responsible for breaking down pectin- pectinesterase, which converts pectin into methanol and polygalacturonic acid (pectic acid), and polygalacturonase, which further breaks down polygalacturonic acid into monogalacturonic acid. Continued hydrolysis can produce sugars and other by-products.

The collective term "pectinase" (also referred to as pectase, pectinols, or filtragols) is often used for a mixture of pectolytic enzymes, particularly those derived from microorganisms. Pectinase is produced by various molds and bacteria, including clostridia associated with retting. However, the fungal type of pectinase is the only one widely produced on an industrial scale, primarily from molds such as *Aspergillus, Penicillium,* and related genera. In production, molds are cultivated on a medium containing pectin or a similar compound, along with a nitrogen source such as plant extract, yeast extract, malt extract, ammonia, or peptone, as well as mineral salts. The resulting mycelium is collected, macerated, and extracted to obtain a crude enzyme mixture, which can then be concentrated and precipitated for use.

Uses

Pectinases from extracts of plant materials or from fungi are used in the food industries for the clarification of fruit juices, wines, vinegars, sirups, and jellies that may contain suspended pectic material. Treatment of fruit juices with pectinase helps prevent jelling of the juices upon concentration. The addition of pectinase to crushed fruit, e.g., grapes, aids in the expression of the juice and results in wines that clarify readily. Partial deesterification by means of pectinesterase to yield modified pectins which set slowly is employed in the manufacture of candy jellies of high sugar content.

Proteolytic Enzymes

The proteolytic enzymes, or proteases, include the proteinases, which catalyze the hydrolysis of the protein molecule into large fragments, and the peptidases, which hydrolyze these polypeptide fragments as far down as amino acids. The proteolytic enzyme preparations from microorganisms are proteases, i.e., mixtures of proteinases and peptidases. Proteases also are prepared from plant or animal sources. Papain, for example, from the papaya fruit, is injected into meat animals before slaughter, so that the meat will be tenderized by the enzyme during coking.

From Bacteria

For the most part, bacterial protease is prepared from cultures of Bacillus subtilis, although many other bacteria yield proteases. A high-yielding strain is selected, special culture media are employed, and temperature and degree of aeration are adjusted to favor the production of protease over that of amylase. The medium or mash has a fairly high content of carbohydrate (2 to 6 percent), as well as of protein, and also contains mineral salts. Incubation is for 3 to 5 days at about 37°C with adequate ventilation. The filtrate from the culture is concentrated, and the enzymes are used in this form, purified further, or absorbed onto some inert material, such as sawdust. The enzyme mixture also contains varying amounts of amylases.

From Molds

Mold protease preparations also contain other enzymes. Thus, koji for soy sauce or Takadiastase for pharmaceutical use contain a number of enzymes. However, it is possible to select fungal strains that give high yields of protease and relatively low yields of other enzymes. Molds can also be selected for their ability to produce proteases active under acidic conditions or active under alkaline conditions. The methods for preparing mold proteases are similar to those used for the production of amylase. *Aspergillus oryzae* is a good source of protease, although other molds have been recommended. Many different media have been suggested, including those containing wheat bran, soybean meal, alfalfa meal, feed, yeast, and other materials. The enzyme is recovered by extraction, concentration, and precipitation, as for other hydrolytic enzymes.

Uses

Proteases from microorganisms are primarily used for their protease activity. Bacterial proteases have been applied to the digestion of fish liver to release fish oil, tenderize meat, and clear, mature malt liquors. Fungal proteases are active in the production of soy sauce and other mold-based fermented oriental foods and can be added to bread dough, where, with amylase, they help improve the consistency of the dough. They can also be used to freshen beer and ale by removing protein haze (fungal tannase present may also be useful), to tenderize meat, to thin egg white so that it can be filtered before drying, and to hydrolyze the gelatinous protein material in fish waste and press out the water for ease. concentration. and drying.

Glucose Oxidase

Glucose oxidase is produced by the submerged growth of *Aspergillus niger* or other molds. It is used to remove glucose from egg whites or whole eggs to facilitate drying, prevent spoilage, and improve whipping properties (of reconstituted dry whites). It has also been used to extend the shelf life of canned carbonated beverages by delaying iron absorption and discoloration. The oxidation of glucose by glucose oxidase forms gluconic acid and hydrogen peroxide, the latter then broken down by catalase in the same preparation. A combination of glucose oxidase and catalase is used to remove the little oxygen remaining in packaged foods.

Other Enzymes

Cellulase, which catalyzes the hydrolysis of cellulose into cellulodextrins and glucose, has been recommended for the production of more fermentable sugar in beer mash, the clarification of orange and lemon and concentrates, and the softening of pods. Microbial lipase removes fat from egg residue in dried egg whites, helps mold spores produce a blue cheese flavor in the spread, and adds flavor to milk chocolate. Dextran-sucrose increases viscosity by producing dextran in foods containing sucrose. Enzymes that produce flavor, from raw foods and from microorganisms, receive special attention. Lactase from *Saccharomyces fragilis* can be used in the hydrolysis of lactose in milk to glucose and galactose, which are less laxative sugars. Catalase, the enzyme that converts hydrogen peroxide to water and oxygen, is commercially prepared from *Aspergillus niger, Penicillium vite,* and *Micrococcus lysodeliticus*. Catalase is used in many applications where the removal of hydrogen peroxide is desired, such as in baking, irradiated foods, and hydrogen peroxide sterilization. Glucose isomerase converts glucose to fructose and is used in the grain industry. In the market, we use *Streptomyces* or *Bacillus coagulans*. It is undeniable that other types of enzymes can be added to those mentioned.

CASE STUDY

Enzymes in Foods

Milk is a nutritious food, providing an important source of protein, fat, vitamins and minerals. Enzymes can break down lactose and allow everyone to enjoy dairy products.

Milk and other dairy products are one of the fi e basic food groups that make up the food pyramid, a popular chart that suggests optimal daily nutritional recommendations. The pyramid recommends consuming two to three servings of dairy products each day, especially to ensure adequate calcium intake. Calcium is essential for the growth and maintenance of healthy bones and teeth, and is also important for muscle and nerve control, blood clotting and blood pressure control. Although calcium is found in other food groups, such as vegetables such as broccoli and spinach, calcium from dairy products is more easily absorbed by the digestive tract than calcium from other sources.

Almost all infants are born with the enzyme lactase, which gives them the ability to digest lactose, the predominant carbohydrate in milk. However, mammals, including humans, experience a decline in lactase production late in the weaning period. This means that the ability to digest lactose decreases in early childhood for many people around the world. The persistence of lactase, which allows lactose digestion into adulthood, is genetically determined. This characteristic appears to have evolved to suit dairy-drinking populations with a traditional pastoral lifestyle, as evidenced in Northern Europe, where only a small percentage of the population is lactose intolerant. It is estimated that approximately 70% of the world's population suffers from some degree of lactose intolerance. Increased awareness of the benefits of calcium, largely due to widespread advertising about osteoporosis, has led to an increase in the consumption of milk and other dairy products worldwide. Strong promotional campaigns for dairy products are currently underway in China illustrate this trend. This means that society at large is looking for a solution that removes lactose and allows everyone to enjoy and benefit from these products

One method of removing lactose from milk is filtration technology, but this procedure can be expensive because it involves a significant investment in equipment, which limits the flexibility of the plant to adapt to ever-changing customer demands. Another effecti e and more economical alternative is to treat milk and dairy products with a lactase enzyme. Lactases work by breaking down lactose into a mixture consisting mainly of glucose and galactose, which can be safely digested by almost everyone. In addition to removing lactose, the resulting dairy product has a naturally sweeter taste. In fact, lactase is traditionally used in the production of ice cream. Since glucose and galactose are sweeter than lactose, they improve the taste while helping to provide a smoother texture. In fact, lactose generally crystallizes at low temperatures, which gives the ice a sandy appearance, but its components, glucose and galactose, remain dissolved.

Novozymes Lactozym Pure® is an extremely pure lactase that offers a host of unique benefits. It is available in a variety of different product concentrations, providing immediate process flexibility. It is robust and able to operate in the pH ranges found in most dairy and milk products, such as regular fresh milk, UHT milk, ice cream, lassi and dulce de leche. What really sets this product apart is its purity. Not only does its high purity improve filtration, but above all, it reduces the risk of the dairy product developing unpleasant odours. This is particularly useful in the production of UHT milk, a growing industry. UHT milk is popular throughout Europe, especially in countries where dairy farming is centralised and consists of several large units. In these situations, milk often has to be transported over long distances and UHT milk is preferred over pasteurised milk because it saves on the high costs and eliminates the difficulties of refrigerated transport. Before opening, UHT milk typically has a shelf life of six to nine months. Lactozym Pure ensures that off-flavor do not develop, helping to preserve the pure and authentic flavor of UHT dairy products during extended storage.

With the growing desire to consume milk and dairy products worldwide, it makes sense to implement an effective and natural solution that breaks down lactose and allows everyone to consume and enjoy these products. Lactozym Pure is an effecti e and natural way to do this, and its purity supports the development of premium lactose-free dairy products.

Part-V

Impact of Nutrition on Disease Prevention and Management

It is essential for every food microbiologist to understand how diseases can be transmitted through food and the methods to prevent such occurrences. Particular attention should be given to modern agents of foodborne illnesses, including their habitats, origins in food, commonly affected food items, mechanisms of pathogenicity, and strategies for control.

Bacterial Contamination and Foodborne Diseases

24

Gastrointestinal problems caused by eating foods can be due to a variety of factors, including overeating, allergies, nutritional deficiencies poisoning by chemicals, toxic plants or animals, bacterial toxins, infestations by animal parasites, and infections by microorganisms. These conditions are often classifie together because of their similar symptoms, which can sometimes lead to confusion between them. This chapter focuses on foodborne illnesses caused by bacterial agents.

ILLNESSES LINKED TO FOOD CONSUMPTION

The term "food poisoning" is often used broadly to encompass illnesses caused by consuming toxins produced by microorganisms as well as infections acquired through the intestinal tract. Food-borne diseases can be categorized into two main groups- poisonings and infections. (Figure 24.1) Poisonings may result from chemical contaminants or the ingestion of a toxic substance (intoxication). Such toxic substances can naturally occur in specific plants or animals (refer to Chapter 25) or be produced as metabolic by-products of microorganisms. Bacterial food intoxications refer to illnesses caused by bacterial toxins present in food, while bacterial food infections arise from the ingestion of contaminated food, leading to bacterial entry into the body and subsequent reactions to their presence or metabolites.

This classification identifies two primary bacterial food intoxications- (1) botulism, caused by the toxin produced by *Clostridium botulinum*, and (2) staphylococcal intoxication, resulting from toxins produced by *Staphylococcus aureus*.

Food infections, are divided into two types- (1) those where food acts as a carrier for pathogens, such as those causing tuberculosis, typhoid fever, brucellosis, cholera, or hepatitis, without supporting their growth; and (2) those where food serves as a medium for the growth of pathogens like *Salmonella* spp, *Vibrio parahaemolyticus*, and enteropathogenic *Escherichia coli*, which can proliferate to levels that significantly increase the risk of infection. Outbreaks of the second type are typically more severe and rapid than those caused by other intestinal pathogens. Example of bacterial food-borne diseases are given Figure 24.2

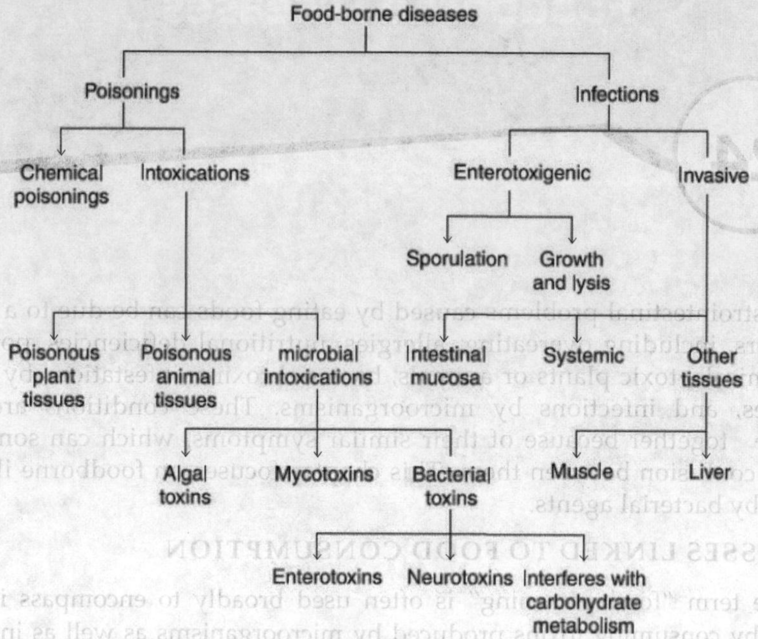

Fig 24.1. A classification of Food-borne Diseases. (Adapted from Br an, F L. 1976. Diseases Transmitted by foods. DHEW Pub. No. (CDC) 76-8237, Center for Disease Control, Atlanta, Ga.)

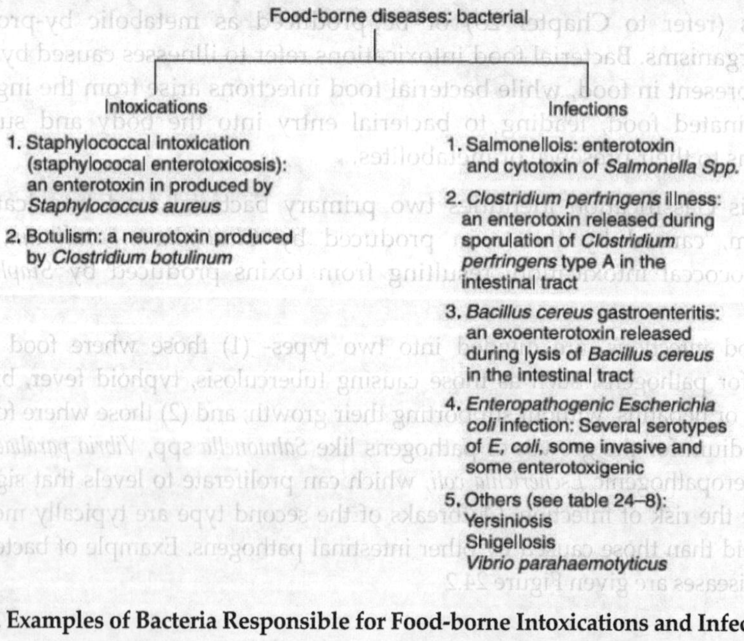

Fig 24.2. Examples of Bacteria Responsible for Food-borne Intoxications and Infections.

Some researchers argue that *Clostridium perfringens* food-borne illness and *Bacillus cereus* gastroenteritis should be classified as food intoxications rather than infections because *B. cereus* may release toxins in food due to cell autolysis, and *C. perfringens* may do so during sporulation in food. If the toxins are indeed released in the food, these illnesses would align more with the definition of food intoxications. However, both illnesses typically require the consumption of a large number of viable cells, suggesting that the toxins are primarily released in vivo rather than in the food. This ambiguity highlights the complex and sometimes controversial classification of these diseases

The broader distinction between food infections and intoxications has also become less clear-cut. For instance, while *Staphylococcus aureus* is traditionally considered a classic food intoxication due to its production of enterotoxin in food, some gram-positive bacteria, including *S. aureus, C. perfringens,* and *B. cereus,* can colonize the intestinal mucosa and contribute to chronic diarrhea. Similarly, the pathogenicity of *Salmonella* is linked to enterotoxins and possibly cytotoxins, further complicating these categorizations. Therefore, these terms should be used with caution.

Table 24.1 presents data on outbreaks and cases caused by bacterial agents over a four-year period in the United States. However, these figures likely underestimate the true number of cases, as many individuals with diarrheal illnesses do not seek medical attention, and such incidents go unreported. The majority of outbreaks and cases were attributed to staphylococcal intoxication, salmonellosis, and *C. perfringens* gastroenteritis. Despite ongoing prevention efforts, food-borne outbreaks remain a concern. Table 24.2 provides data on the locations of food mishandling leading to reported outbreaks between 1968 and 1976. While food processing plants accounted for 5% of outbreaks, food service establishments were responsible for over one-third, with many incidents lacking a clearly identified site of mishandling

Table. Some Food-borne Illnesses Reported in the United States, 1978-1982

Disease	1978	1979	1980	1981	1982
Staphlococcal intoxication	–	3,391(34)	944(27)	2,934(44)	669(28)
Clostridium perfringenes gastroenteritis	617(9)*	1,110(2)	1,463(25)	1,162(28)	1,189(22)
Salmonellosis	1,921(45)	2,794(44)	2,381(39)	2,456(66)	2,056(55)
Botulism	58(12)	9(7)	18(14)	22(11)	30(21)
Bacillus cereus gastroenteritis	248(6)	–	187(9)	74(8)	200(8)
Shigellosis	159(4)	356(7)	1,184(11)	351(9)	116(4)

Vibrio parahaemolyticus gastroenteritis	86(2)	14(2)	12(4)	13(2)	39(3)
Escherichia coli gastroenteritis	35(1)	–	500(1)	–	47(2)

*Number of cases followed by number of outbreaks in parentheses. Source- Center for Disease Control, U.S. Department of Health, Education and Welfare. Foodbome Outbreak Annual Summaries.

Table. Places Where Foods were Mishandled 1968–1976

Place	Number	Percent
Food service establishments	1,283	39
Homes	504	15
Food processing plants	163	5
Unknown or unspecifie	1,354	41
Total	3,304	100

Source- Center for Disease Control, U.S. Department of Health, Education and Welfare, Foodborne Outbreak Annual Summarles.

Botulism

Botulism is a disease caused by the ingestion of food containing the neurotoxin produced by Clostridium botulinum.

- **The Organism:** This rod-shaped soil bacterium is saprophytic, spore forming, gas forming, and anaerobic. Seven types are distinguished on the basis of the serological specificity of their toxins; the predominant (or only) toxin from these types is designated by the same capital letter.
- **Type A:** is the one commonly causing human botulism in the western part of the United States. It is more toxic than type B. Type B is found more often than type A in most soils of the world and is less toxic to human beings.
- **Type C:** causes botulism of fowls, cattle, mink, and other animals but not of human beings so far as is known.
- **Type D:** is associated with forage poisoning of cattle in the Union of South Africa.
- **Type E:** which is toxic for humans, has been obtained chiefly from fish and fish products.
- **Type F:** which except for its toxin is similar to types A and B, has been isolated in Denmark and produces human botulism.
- **Type G:** has been isolated from the soil in Argentina but has not been implicated in human botulism.

Not all types produce a single toxin. For example, some type C strains produce predominately C_1 toxin with smaller amounts of D and C_2, or only C_2. Type D strains produce predominately D toxin with lesser amounts of C_1 and C_2 toxins.

Type A strains and most cultures of type B are proteolytic and are putrefactive enough to give an obnoxious odor to proteinaceous foods, but some strains of type B and those of type E are not. Even the first two types fail to give marked indications of putrefaction in low-protein foods such as string beans and corn, although they produce toxin. The organism ferments carbohydrates with gas production, but sometimes this is not evident either.

Separation of the various strains of *C. botulinum* solely on the basis of toxin types results in very heterogeneous groups. For this reason, *C. botulinum* strains frequently are divided into three general groups, based on cultural and physiological characters, as follows:

- Group I includes all type A strains (proteolytic) and the proteolytic strains of B and F.
- Group II includes all type E strains (nonproteolytic) and the nonproteolytic strains of B and F
- Group Ill includes types C and D; they are nonproteolytic and share a common metabolic pattern.

Growth and Toxin Production

Toxin production by *Clostridium botulinum* depends on the organism's ability to grow in a food matrix and undergo autolysis, as toxins like types A, B, E, and F are synthesized as inactive proteins that require hydrolysis for full toxicity. Factors influencing toxin production include the food's composition, moisture, pH, oxidation-reduction potential, salt content, and storage temperature. For example, glucose or maltose is essential for toxin production, and minimal pH or temperature for growth is often food-dependent. Variations in toxin potency are observed across different media and foods, such as meats, fish, and low- or medium-acid canned foods. Additionally, dissolved tin in canned vegetables can inhibit growth and toxin formation.

Sodium chloride concentration plays a critical role in preventing growth and toxin production, with higher salt levels needed at higher temperatures. Sodium nitrate and disodium phosphate can reduce the required salt concentration. A pH of 4.5 or lower generally prevents toxin production, though growth has been observed in foods with initially lower pH values due to the influence of other microorganisms that raise the pH locally. Notably, outbreaks of botulism have occurred in high-acid foods, such as tomatoes and blackberries, possibly due to factors like pH stratification or interactions with other microbes

Temperature significantly affects toxin production rates. Proteolytic strains optimally produce toxins at around 35°C, while non-proteolytic strains prefer 26–28°C. Spore germination requires a higher temperature than vegetative growth, with 15°C being the general minimum for germination. However, some type E strains can produce toxins at temperatures as low as 3.3°C. These interactions between factors such as pH, redox potential, and temperature are complex and continue to be studied to better understand the conditions under which C. botulinum can grow and produce toxins.

The Toxin

The toxin produced by *Clostridium botulinum* is an exceptionally potent protein that can cause fatal paralysis by targeting the involuntary muscles. It is primarily absorbed in the small intestine. Despite its lethality, the toxin is comparatively thermolabile, with specific heat treatments required for inactivation. For instance, type A toxin is destroyed by heating for 5–6 minutes at 80°C, while type B requires 15 minutes at 90°C. However, relying on cooking to neutralize toxins in suspect foods is not advisable, as some contaminated foods, particularly acidic or low-protein ones, can become toxic without obvious signs of spoilage. Nonproteolytic strains, in particular, produce fewer sensory indicators of spoilage, such as foul odors or gas production, making visual or olfactory assessments unreliable.

Gamma radiation can effectively destroy the toxin in specific contexts, such as 7.3 Mrad for cheese or 4.9 Mrad for broth. The toxin remains stable in foods stored at low temperatures but degrades at pH levels above 6.8. Nonproteolytic strains produce toxins that may require trypsin activation to reach full potency. Immunologically, the seven toxin types (A to G) are antigenic, prompting the production of specific antitoxins when injected. Toxoids have been developed for certain types, providing active immunization for individuals, such as researchers, who may risk accidental exposure to botulinum toxin.

Toxicity and Bacteriophages

It is not unusual to find nontoxigenic colonies from a known toxigenic strain of *C. botulinum*. Recent research on the link between toxigenicity (the ability to produce the toxin) and temperate bacteriophages (phage nucleic acid integrated into the bacterial genome) suggests that the toxin production may be controlled by the genome of an integrated temperate bacteriophage rather than the bacterial genome itself. This could explain why some strains occasionally lose their ability to produce the toxin. Experimental studies have shown that types C and D can be "cured" of their temperate bacteriophages and become nontoxigenic. On the other hand, types A, B, and F, although "cured" of their bacteriophages, remain toxigenic. It appears that certain bacteriophages are responsible for imparting toxigenicity to *C. botulinum*. Additionally, some strains may contain multiple temperate bacteriophages, which could explain why they produce more than one type of toxin.

Heat Resistance of Spores

The spores of some putrefactive anaerobes, such as *C. botulinum*, are relatively resistant to heat when compared to the spores of the majority of other *Clostridium* species. The type of food, the type and strain of *C. botulinum*, the medium in which the spores were formed, the temperature at which they were produced, the age of the spores, and the quantity of spores present all influence the amount of heat treatment required to eradicate all of the spores in a food. For a discussion of the variables affecting spores' resistance to heat, the reader should consult Chapter 6. The following heat treatments have been suggested by Esty and Meyer (1922) to eradicate all *C. botulinum* spores from a food:

Temperature °C	Time, minutes
100	360
105	120
110	36
115	12
120	4

In general, spores of organisms of types C, D, and E are less heat-resistant than those of types A and B, type E spores being inactivated in 15 min at 80 °C.

Types A and B spores have D_{121C} values of 0.21 min while the D_{100C} value for type E has been reported to be 0.003 to 0.017 min. A comparison of type C spores has shown that marine strains are more heat-resistant than are terrestrial strains (D_{104C} of 0.4 to 0.9 min for the former and D_{104C} of 0.02 to 0.08 for the latter).

Distribution of Spores

The habitat of *C. botulinum* is believed to be the soil, for spores have been found in both cultivated and virgin soils all over the world. Tests have shown that type A spores are found more in western soils in this country and type B spores elsewhere. Plant crops may become contaminated from the soil, and intestinal contents and hence manure of animals after consumption of such plants. Type E spores are found in soil, in sea and lake mud, and in fish, primarily in their intestinal tracts.

Incidence of Botulism

Botulism is fortunately a rare occurrence, but it garners significant attention due to its historically high mortality rate. The fatality rate has decreased over time—from over 60% in the United States between 1899 and 1949 to approximately 23% between 1970 and 1973. An analysis of 688 outbreaks reported from 1899 to 1973 showed that 23.1% were linked to type A, 6.3% to type B, and 3.2% to type E, while the type remained unidentified in 67.3% of cases. However, the proportion of outbreaks with undetermined toxin types has declined in recent years; for instance, only 19% of outbreaks between 1970 and 1973 were untyped.

Foods Involved

In the United States, inadequately processed home-canned foods are most often the cause of botulism (Table 24.3); in Europe the main causes are preserved meats and fish. Commercially processed foods have accounted for less than 10 percent of the outbreaks (Table 24.3), while homeprocessed foods were responsible for 72 percent of the outbreaks.

Table Outbreaks of Food-borne Botulism Attributed to Commercially Processed or Home processed Foods, 1889–1973

Year	Source of food			
	Home processed	Commercially processed	Unknown	Total
1889	1	0	0	1
1990-1909	1	1	0	2
1910-1919	48	14	8	70
1920-1929	77	26	13	116
1930-1939	135	6	13	154
1940-1949	120	1	13	134
1950-1959	50	2	51	103
1960-1969	42	10	26	78
1970-1973	21*	2	7	30
Total	495	62	131	688

*Includes one outbreak in which the vehicle was canned by the owner of a restaurant and sold to his customers. Source- Center for Disease Control (1974).

Table. Home-canned Foods Causing Six or More Outbreaks of Botulism, 1899–1947 (United States)

Food	Number of outbreaks	Food	Number of outbreaks
String beans	94	Beet greens	9
Corn	46	Chili papers	9
Beets	22	Beans	7
Asparagus	21	Tomatoes	7
Spinach and chard	12	Mushrooms	6
Peas	10	Sausages	9
Figs	10	Fish	10

Home-canned foods most frequently associated with botulism include string beans, sweet corn, beets, asparagus, spinach, and chard(Table 24.4). However, many other food types have been linked to one or more outbreaks, with 50 different canned fruits and vegetables involved in incidents between 1899 and 1947. Table 24.4 lists home-canned foods that have caused six or more botulism outbreaks in the U.S. from 1899 to 1947. Typically, low- and medium-acid canned foods are the main culprits, but there have been rare cases of botulism from acid foods like tomatoes, apricots, pears, and peaches. These acid foods were poorly processed, allowing other microorganisms to grow and support *C. botulinum* growth and toxin production. Table 24.5 summarizes all foods involved in outbreaks from 1899 to 1973, both commercial and home-processed, along with the toxin types identified. Vegetables were implicated in 56% of these outbreaks. Studies have shown that *C. botulinum* spores can survive extended storage in raw and precooked frozen foods and can grow and produce toxins if these foods are stored improperly at high temperatures after thawing. Therefore, temperature abuse of potentially contaminated foods should be avoided.

The Disease

People are so susceptible to botulism that if appreciable amounts of toxin are present, everyone who eats the food becomes ill and consumption of very small pieces of food, a pod of a string bean or a few peas, can cause illness and death. The typical symptoms of botulism usually appear within 12 to 36 hr, although a longer or shorter time may be required. The earliest symptoms usually are an acute digestive disturbance followed by nausea and vomiting and possibly diarrhea, together with fatigue, dizziness, and a headache. Later there is constipation. Double vision may be evident early, and difficult in swallowing and speaking may be noted. Patients may complain of dryness of the mouth and constriction of the throat, and the tongue may become swollen and coated. The temperature of the victim is normal or subnormal. Involuntary muscles become paralyzed, paralysis spreads to the respiratory system and heart, and death usually results from respiratory failure. Symptoms are similar for types A, B, and E poisoning, although nausea, vomiting, and urinary retention usually are more severe with type E toxin. In fatal cases, death usually comes within 3 to 6 days after the poisonous food has been ingested, but the period may be shorter or longer.

The only known method for the successful treatment of botulism is the administration of antitoxin. Unfortunately, this injection usually is not successful if made after the symptoms of botulism have appeared, but it should always be used at the earliest possible moment since it may prove helpful. Other treatments include artificial respiration, keeping the patient quiet, maintaining the fluid balance in the body, and, perhaps, elimination treatments.

Conditions Necessary for an Outbreak

An outbreak of botulism requires the following conditions- (1) the presence of *C. botulinum* spores of types A, B, or E in the food being canned or processed, (2) a food environment that allows the spores to germinate and the clostridia to grow and produce toxin, (3) the survival of spores due to inadequate heating or processing, (4) environmental conditions after processing that enable the spores to germinate and the organism to grow and produce toxin, (5) insufficien cooking to deactivate the toxin, and (6) the ingestion of food contaminated with the toxin.

Table. Food Products Causing Botulism Outbreaks- 1899-1973

Food	Botulinum toxin type					
	A	B	E	F	A and B	Total
Vegetables	115	31	1		2	149
Fish and fish product	11	4	25	–		40
Fruits	22	7		–	–	29
Condimentst †	17	5	–	1	–	22
Beef ‡	6	1	–	–	–	8
Milk and milk products	3	2	–	–	–	5
Pork	2	1		–		3
Poultry	2	2	–	–	–	4
Other§	8	3	3	–		14
Total	186	56	29	1	2	274

Includes only outbreaks in which the toxin type was determined: Includes outbreaks traced to tomato relish, chili peppers, chili sauce, and salad dressing: Includes one outbreak of type F in venison and one outbreak of type A in mutton: Includes outbreaks traced to vichyssoise, spaghetti sauce, and corn and chicken mash.
Source- Center For Disease Control (1974).

Prevention of Outbreaks

The methods and precautions for the prevention of botulism that have been mentioned in the preceding discussion include (1) use of approved heat processes for canned foods, (2) rejection of all gassy (swollen) or otherwise spoiled canned foods, (3) refusal even to taste a doubtful food, (4) avoidance of foods that have been cooked, held, and not well reheated, and (5) boiling of a suspected food for at least 15 min. To this list might be added avoidance of raw or precooked foods that have been frozen, thawed, and held at room temperatures. To prevent botulism from smoked fish it has been recommended that (1) good sanitation be maintained throughout production and handling, (2) during smoking or thereafter the fish be heated to at least 82 C for 30 min in the coldest part, (3) the fish be frozen immediately after packaging and kept frozen, and (4) all packages be marked "Perishable-Keep Frozen."

Infant Botulism

In the late 1970s, infant botulism was identified as a separate condition, with several hundred cases confirmed since then. Unlike food-borne botulism, the toxin in infant botulism is thought to be released in the body after the organism grows in the intestines. Many affected infants have had a history of constipation.

Clinical symptoms include weakness, difficult sucking, loss of head control, and a weakened gag reflex. Studies show that when infant mice are infected with *C. botulinum* spores, about 50 percent produce toxin in their intestines, while adult mice cannot be infected in the same way. However, infection can occur in adult germ-free mice, suggesting the role of normal microbial flora in the development of the disease, especially since many human infants with botulism show signs of constipation before the infection. The number of reported cases has steadily increased since the 1970s and is now typically higher than the cases of food-borne botulism.

Staphylococcus Food Intoxication

One of the most commonly occurring food poisonings is caused by the ingestion of the enterotoxin formed in food during growth of certain strains of *Staphylococcus aureus*. The toxin is termed an enterotoxin because it causes gastroenteritis or inflammation of the lining of the intestinal tract.

The Organism

The organism is a typical *Staphylococcus*, appearing in clusters resembling grapes or in pairs and short chains. When grown on solid media, it typically displays a golden or yellow color, although some strains may be unpigmented. Most enterotoxin-producing *S. aureus* strains are coagulase-positive (they coagulate blood plasma), produce a heat-stable nuclease, and are facultative in oxygen requirements, thriving better aerobically than anaerobically in a complex glucose medium. However, not all coagulase-positive staphylococci are enterotoxigenic. Some toxigenic strains are highly salt-tolerant (10-20% NaCl), able to survive in curing solutions and on cured meats if other conditions are suitable. They are also tolerant of dissolved sugars (50-60% sucrose), fermentative, and proteolytic, but generally do not produce unpleasant odors or make foods unappealing. *S. aureus* produces six distinct enterotoxins (A, B, C1, C2, D, and E), with type A being the most common cause of food poisoning. Enterotoxin-producing strains of *S. aureus* also produce additional toxins. The range of conditions that allow growth and toxin production varies by food type.

Generally, the more suitable the food is for the bacteria, the broader the temperature, pH, or aw (water activity) range for growth. The optimal temperature range for growth and toxin production is between 4°C and 46°C, depending on the food. S. aureus grows most rapidly between 20°C and 45°C, with growth being four times faster at 45°C than at 20°C. The minimal temperature for growth in foods like custard, condensed milk, and chicken à la king is about 6.7-7.8°C, whereas it's around 10°C for beef-heart infusion and higher in ham salad. Growth at these lower temperatures is slow, meaning it typically takes longer to reach toxin-producing levels than the storage time for most refrigerated foods. The minimal pH for growth is lower under aerobic conditions (pH 4.8) than under anaerobic conditions (pH 5.5), with the maximum pH for growth being about 8.0. The minimal aw is about 0.86 under aerobic and 0.90 under anaerobic conditions. A sublethal heat treatment can decrease salt tolerance.

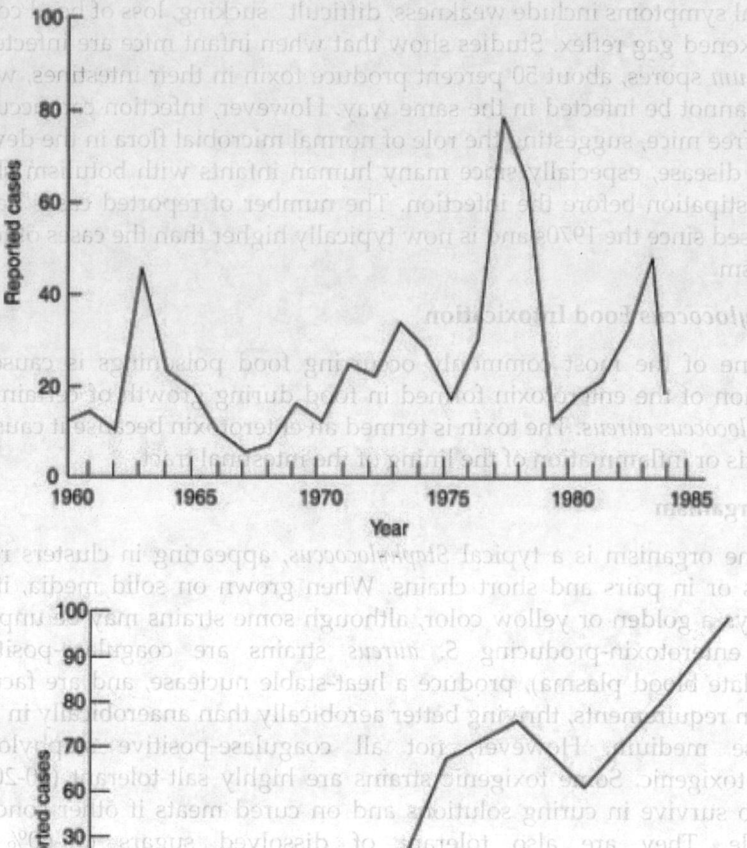

Fig 24.3. Reported cases of botulism per year in the United States. (A) Food-borne. Sixteen outbreaks (19 cases) of food-borne botulism were reported for 1984. Two of these outbreaks involved four individuals and were associated with eating fermented foods. Type E toxin was implicated. Type A toxin was associated with thirteen of the remaining cases. Type B toxin was associated with one case, and for the other case a toxin type was not determined. (B) Infant botulism. Of the ninety-nine infant botulism cases reported in 1984, slightly more than half (fifty-six) ere in females. The age range for all petients was 3 to 37 weeks. Type A toxin was found in forty-two (42 percent) of the cases, type B toxin in fifty-six (5 percent), and both type A and type B toxins in one. (Center for Disease Control, Annual Summaries for 1984, 1986.)

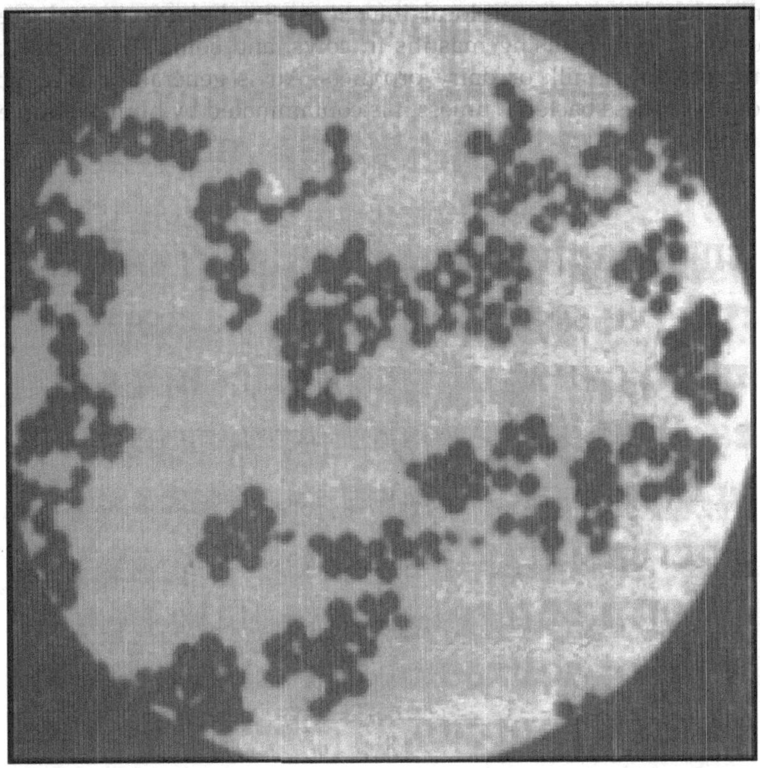

Fig 24.4. Photomicrograph of *Staphylococcus aureus*, (From J. Nowack.)

- Other food bacteria may inhibit the growth of *Staphylococcus* enough to delay or prevent toxin production, or spoilage bacteria may render the food inedible before it becomes hazardous. The extent of this inhibition depends on factors like the types and quantities of competing organisms, the food type, temperature, and time. Typically, staphylococci enter foods in small numbers and are usually outnumbered by other bacteria in raw foods. However, this competition may not occur in heated foods, allowing *Staphylococcus* to grow unchecked. A concentration of one million staphylococci per milliliter or gram in perishable foods can be inactivated by maintaining a temperature of 66°C for at least 12 minutes or 60°C for 78 to 83 minutes. Heat resistance varies slightly with the food and strain of *Staphylococcus*. For example, D values at 60°C in custard are about 7.7 to 7.8 minutes, while in chicken à la king, they are about 5.2 to 5.4 minutes. Gamma radiation (0.37 to 0.48 Mrad) on moist foods can kill most staphylococci. The primary sources of food-poisoning staphylococci are human or animal carriers. The nasal passages of many individuals are colonized by these bacteria, which are also common causes of sinus infections. Boils and infected wounds can serve as additional sources. The human skin is a source of these bacteria primarily when they originate from nasal passages or local infections. Staphylococcus is increasingly responsible for causing mastitis in cows, and some strains can produce enterotoxin in milk or dairy products. Air is generally not a significant source of these bacteria, unless it is contaminated by human sources.

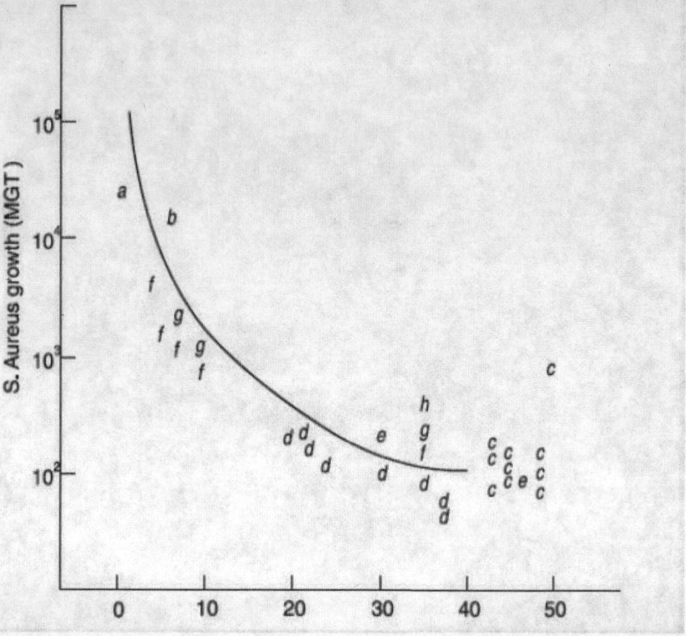

Fig. 24.5. Mean Generation Times (MGT)of *Staphylococcus aureus* in (A) rawgroundbeef, (B) freshraw eggs, (C) roast beef, (D) skim, whole, and raw milk, (E) barbequed chicken, (F) egg custard, (G) chicken á la king, and (H) ham salad. Regression coefficient, r=0.89. (Fr RMtuso and Synder, 1980.)

Incidence of the Disease

Reported cases in the United States are presented in Table 24.1. There probably are no reliable figures on the numbers of cases of staphylococcus poisoning in the United States or in any of the states for any given period. The poisoning usually is not reported or publicized unless the outbreak is fairly large, as at a picnic, large dinner, or convention. It is known, however, that a large percentage of all cases reported as food poisoning or food infection actually are staphylococcus poisoning and that many of us encounter this illness during our lifetime.

The Enterotoxin

Staphylococcal enterotoxins are simple proteins with molecular weights between 26,000 and 30,000. These proteins consist of single polypeptide chains cross-linked by a disulfide bridge, forming a characteristic cystine loop. Many of the amino acids in this loop are similar across different enterotoxin types, which is thought to be the toxic part of the molecule. Types A and D are most commonly associated with food poisoning outbreaks. Significant levels of enterotoxin are produced only after substantial growth of *Staphylococcus*, typically requiring a population of millions of bacteria per milliliter or gram. Conditions that favor toxin production also support bacterial growth. Toxin production occurs efficientl at temperatures between 15.6°C and 46.1°C, with optimal production at 40°C. Under ideal conditions, enterotoxin can be detected within 4 to 6 hours. At lower temperatures, it takes longer to produce enough toxin for poisoning. For example, enterotoxin production was observed in 3 days at 18°C, in 12 hours at 37°C, but not in 3 days at 15°C, 7 days at 9°C, or 4 weeks at 4-6.7°C. Toxin production is more likely when competing microorganisms are absent, few, or inhibited. Foods contaminated with *Staphylococcus* after a heat process are particularly conducive to toxin production. Antibiotic treatment that disrupts competitive bacteria in the intestines may also lead to toxin production by *Staphylococcus*.

The type of food affects the amount of enterotoxin produced; for instance, little toxin is produced in salmon, while meat products and custard-fille baked goods produce much more. Starch and protein in foods are thought to enhance toxin production. A key feature of the enterotoxins is their heat stability. The interpretation of data on heat inactivation should consider factors such as the initial concentration of the toxin, the medium in which it is heated, and the temperature used. Some studies suggest that enterotoxins are more readily inactivated at lower temperatures, a phenomenon possibly due to low-temperature aggregation. Moreover, heat-inactivated enterotoxins may undergo reactivation in certain foods. Pasteurization (72°C for 15 seconds) and ultrahigh-temperature heating (143.3°C for 9 seconds) generally do not inactivate the enterotoxins. Type B enterotoxin is the most heat-resistant, as indicated by its higher z-value. Normal cooking of foods will not destroy the toxin formed prior to the heat process, meaning such foods could still cause poisoning even if no live Staphylococcus is present.

Foods Involved

Staphylococcus food poisoning has been most commonly associated with custard- and cream-filled bakery goods, ham, and poultry. About 75% of these outbreaks occur due to improper cooling of foods. Other implicated foods include various meats and meat products, fish and fish products, milk and milk products, cream sauces, salads, puddings, custards, pies, and salad dressings. Bakery fillings, in particular, provide an excellent medium for bacterial growth when these items are stored at room temperature. Toxin production has even been noted in imitation cream fillings. Hams, especially those that are tongue, mildly cured, rapidly cured, tenderized, or precooked, are often stored without sufficien refrigeration, unlike traditional country-cured hams. Contaminated leftover turkey, poultry, gravy, and dressing can lead to poisoning if left unrefrigerated. Additionally, foods that are typically too acidic for *Staphylococcus* growth may become suitable for bacterial proliferation if their acidity is lowered by ingredients like eggs or cream. In places like cafeterias, restaurants, and food vending machines, where foods are kept heated for long periods, staphylococcal growth and toxin production can occur if proper temperature and time controls are not maintained.

Table . Thermal Inactivation Characteristics of Staphylococcal Enterotoxins

Type of caterotoxin	Assay sytem used	Sensitivity or amount Injected or fed	Initial toxin concentration, mg/ml	Heating medium*	Heating temp., F	F250 mln	z value, F
A	Monkey feeding	47.25 mg	7	Distilled water	212-250	8	46
A	Cat-intravenous injection	2.3 mg	7	Distilled water	212-250	11	48
B	Serological-double diffusion tube	0.7 mg/ml	30	0.04 *M* veronal buffer, pH 7.2	204-259	19-16.4	55-58
	Cat-intravenous injection	2.0 mg	30	0.04 *M* veronal buffer, pH 7.2	240	32.5	
A	Serological-single diffusion tube	1 mg/ml	21	0.04 *M* veronal buffer, pH 7.2	212-250	22	50
B	Serological single diffusion tube	1 mg/ml	10-100	0.04 *M* veronal buffer, pH 7.2	250-320	62	52
					320	2.8	

Dialyzed growth material dissolved in listed solvent: Source- Summarized from various workers by Tatini (1976).

The Disease

Individuals have varying levels of susceptibility to staphylococcal food poisoning. In a group consuming food contaminated with the toxin, some may experience severe symptoms, while others may be minimally affected or not at all. The incubation period for this type of poisoning is typically short, ranging from 1 to 7 hours, with most cases showing symptoms within 2 to 4 hours. This is much faster compared to other foodborne illnesses, which usually have longer incubation periods.

Common symptoms include salivation, nausea, vomiting, retching, abdominal cramps, and diarrhea. In severe cases, blood and mucus may be found in the stools and vomitus. Additional symptoms such as headache, muscle cramps, sweating, chills, weakness, shock, and shallow breathing may also occur, with subnormal body temperature often seen instead of fever. The illness generally lasts only a day or two, with recovery being swift and complete, and mortality is very low. Treatment is rarely required, though severe cases may be managed with saline solutions to restore electrolyte balance and address dehydration.

Food poisoning outbreaks are often linked to staphylococci based on the type of food, the short incubation period, and the presence of the bacteria in the food. To confirm a diagnosis, staphylococci must be isolated, and it must be demonstrated that they are capable of producing enterotoxins, or the enterotoxins themselves must be detected.

Prevention of Outbreaks

Preventing outbreaks of staphylococcal food poisoning involves several key strategies:

- **Prevention of contamination:** This can be achieved through proper sanitation practices, such as ensuring clean environments and using ingredients that are free from staphylococci, such as pasteurized milk instead of raw milk. It is also crucial to keep food handlers away from food when they have staphylococcal infections like colds, boils, or carbuncles, which can be sources of contamination.
- **Prevention of staphylococcal growth:** Staphylococcal growth can be inhibited by maintaining adequate refrigeration, which slows down the bacteria's ability to proliferate. Additionally, adjusting the pH of the food to be more acidic can help prevent growth. In some cases, bacteriostatic substances, such as serine or antibiotics, may be added to food to control bacterial growth.
- **Killing the bacteria:** Foods can be pasteurized before exposure to regular temperatures, effecti ely killing staphylococci. For example, custard-filled puffs and eclairs can be pasteurized by heating them in an oven at temperatures between 190.6 to 218.3°C for 30 minutes. This treatment helps eliminate the bacteria before the food is exposed to potentially favorable conditions for bacterial growth.

By implementing these preventive measures, the risk of staphylococcal food poisoning can be significantly reduced

Conditions Necessary for an Outbreak

The following conditions are necessary for an outbreak of staphylococcus food poisoning- (1) The food must contain enterotoxin-producing staphylococci, (2) the food must be a good culture medium for growth and toxin production by the staphylococci, (3) the temperature must be favorable to growth of the cocci, and enough time must be allowed for production of enterotoxin, and (4) the enterotoxin-bearing food must be ingested.

Salmonellosis

Salmonellosis can occur after consuming viable cells of a *Salmonella* species. It is the most common bacterial foodborne infection and, in certain years, the leading bacterial foodborne illness (as shown in Table 24.1). Besides the typical food-poisoning symptoms, two additional disease syndromes may result from *Salmonella* consumption, which are compared in Table 24.7. The classification of the genus *Salmonella* is complicated, and its naming conventions do not adhere to standard rules. Initially, the names given to *Salmonella* isolates were based on their pathogenicity in humans or animals—for example, *S. typhimurium*, which causes typhoid in mice, and *S. typhi*, which causes human typhoid. Over time, the naming system shifted to reflect the location of the initial human infections, leading to names like *S. london, S. panama,* and *S. stanleyville*. Currently, *Salmonella* isolates are identified using the Kauffman-White scheme, a serological method that classifies organisms based on their antigenic sites-O (somatic), Vi (capsular), and H (flagella). This method identifie only diagnostic antigens, not the complete antigenic profile of the organism. The term "serovar" is used to differentiate strains with different antigenic compositions. Further classification can be made into biovars, which are distinguished by differin sugar fermentation patterns within the same serovar. This classification helps in epidemiological investigations, as serovars and biovars can act as markers to trace the source of outbreaks. There are currently over a thousand known serovars. Food poisoning caused by *Salmonella* can result from numerous serovars (as shown in Table 24.7). Typically, the bacterium grows in food to high numbers, increasing the chances of infection and often leading to outbreaks within families or larger groups. In contrast, other intestinal pathogens, such as those causing dysentery or typhoid and paratyphoid fevers, tend to have longer incubation periods and occur in isolated cases unless there is an epidemic.

The Organism

Salmonellae are gram-negative, non-spore-forming rods that ferment glucose, typically with gas production, but generally do not ferment lactose or sucrose. They grow better in a nutrient-rich culture medium compared to a poor one, thriving across a broad range of temperature, pH, and water activity (aw). For example, the minimum temperature for growth in foods ranges from 6.7°C to 7.8°C in chicken a la king and over 10°C in custard and ham salad. Their maximum growth temperature is about 45.6°C, and they grow best at around 37°C. *Salmonella* can grow in a pH range of 4.1 to 9.0, preferring low-acid foods, but growth is unfavorable in salads with a pH between 5.5 and 5.7. The lowest aw for growth, which varies with the food, is generally between 0.93 and 0.95. Different species and strains of *Salmonella* exhibit varying levels of heat resistance and responses to environmental factors. For example, D60°C values (the time required to reduce the population by 90% at 60°C) range from 0.06 to 11.3 minutes, depending on the food and serotype. To destroy salmonellae in perishable foods, recommendations are similar to those for staphylococci, such as heating to 66°C and maintaining that temperature for at least 12 minutes, or 78 to 83 minutes at 60°C. F140 values (the time required at 140°F to reduce the inoculum to an undetectable level) for two species in custard were 78 and 19 minutes, and for chicken a la king, they were 81.5 and 3.1 minutes. These results show how the required heat treatment varies depending on the *Salmonella* species and the food being processed.

Table. The Salmonellosis Syndromes in Humans

Disease	Etiological agent	Nature of organism	Incubation period, signs, and symptoms	Source, reservoir, and epidemiology
Salmonellosis	*Salmonella choleraesuis, enteritids, typhimurium, hidelberg, derby, java, infantis, enteritids, montevideo*	Has O (somatic) and two phases of H(flagella) antigens, over 2,000 known serovars, but only about 50 occur commonly	5-72 hr, commonly 12-36hr, diarrhea, abdominal pain, chills, fever, vomiting, dehydration, prostration, anorexia, headache, malaise; duration of several days; enteritis or local infection may also occur	Feces of infected domestic or wild animals and humans beings; infants, aged, and malnourished persons and those with concomitant disease are more susceptible; carrier state usually lasts a few days to few weeks, but sometimes for months
Typhoid fever (enteric fever)	*Salmonella typhi*	Similar to other salmonellae more or less adaptedto human host; Has VI (capsular) an-tigens as well as O and H antigens	7-28 days, mean 14 days; in food out-breaks may be in shortest incubation range; septicemia lymphoid tissue involvement; malaise, headache, high continued fever, cough, anorexia, nausea, vomiting, constipation, slow pulse rate, tender and distended abdomen, enlarged spleen, nosebleed, rose spots on chest and trunk, perspiration, chills, delirium, dulled, sensorium, diarrhea, bleeding from bowel; relapses occur; slow convalescence	Feces and urine of infected persons; carriers are important in transmission; some are long-term carrier; water also involved in transmission
Paratyphoid fever (enteric fever)	*Salmonella enteritidis, paratyphi A, paratyphi B, paratyphi C, sendai*	Similar to other salmonellae but more or less adapted to human host	1-15 days; bloodstream infection; headache, continued fever, profuse perspiration, nausea, vomiting abdominal pain, enlarged spleen, diarrhea, sometimes rose spots; milder and shorter duration (1-3 weeks) than typhoid	Feces and urine infected persons; carriers important in transmission

Source- Adapted from- Bryan, F.L. 1982. Diseases tranamitted by foods. DHEW No. (COC) 76 8237. Center for Disease Control, Atlanta, Ga.

The likelihood of salmonellal infection from consuming contaminated food depends on factors such as the consumer's resistance, the infectivity of the specific *Salmonella* strain, and the number of organisms ingested. Less infective species, like *S. pullorum,* may require the ingestion of hundreds of millions or even billions of organisms to cause infection. However, more infective strains, such as *S. enteritidis,* typically require fewer organisms— around a million— to cause illness. Salmonellae can proliferate in food without causing noticeable changes in appearance, odor, or taste. The higher the number of pathogens present, the greater the risk of infection for the consumer, and the shorter the incubation period.

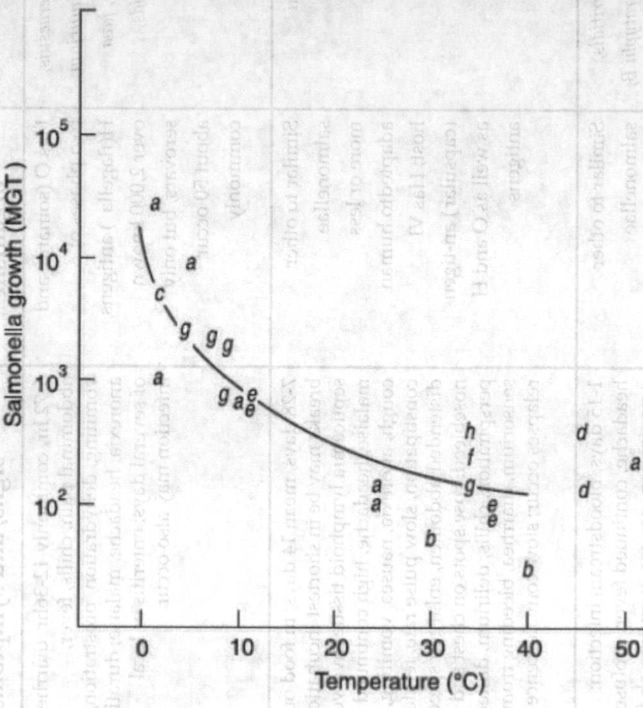

Fig 24.6. Mean Generation Times (MGT) of *Salmonella* in (A) raw ground beef, (B) barbequed chicken, (C) bacon, (D) roast baef, (E) milk, (F) egg custard, (G) chicken á la king, and (H) ham salad. Regression coefficient, r = 0.66. (From Rivituso and ynder, 1981.)

Sources of *Salmonella*

Humans and animals, either directly or indirectly, are the primary sources of Salmonella contamination in food. The bacteria may originate from actual cases of the disease or from carriers. Common serovars like *S. typhimurium* are often responsible for human gastroenteritis, though many other types may also be involved. Animals such as cats, dogs, pigs, and cattle can carry the bacteria, but the main sources of contamination are poultry and their eggs, along with rodents.

Chickens, turkeys, ducks, and geese can harbor various types of *Salmonella,* which are present in their feces, eggs, and meat. Approximately one-third of all *Salmonella*-related food outbreaks involve meat and poultry. Significant attention has been given to shell eggs and processed egg products as potential sources of infection. Infected rodents, such as rats and mice, can contaminate exposed food with their feces, spreading the bacteria. Flies and cockroaches may also contribute to the transmission of *Salmonella,* especially by transferring it from contaminated feces to food. Recent changes in food processing, packaging, and formulation have led to an increase in salmonellosis outbreaks, particularly due to the use of cracked and dried eggs in products like baked goods, candy, ice cream, and convenience foods. The introduction of new ingredients in food production may enable the growth of *Salmonella,* even if it couldn't grow in the original ingredient. Large-scale food handling and vending machines also increase the risk, as do precooked foods. Furthermore, animal feed, especially those derived from meat or fish by-products, can spread *Salmonella* to poultry and other meat animals. Even pet feeds have been linked to transmitting *Salmonella* to domestic animals, which can then infect humans, particularly children.

Incidence of the Disease

Numbers of reported human cases of salmonellosis (other than typhoid and paratyphoid fever) in the United States during recent years. Like most food-poisoning syndromes, the reported number of cases probably represents only a small percentage of the number of cases actually occurring.

Foods Involved

A wide range of foods can be involved in *Salmonella* outbreaks. Meats, poultry, and their products are the most commonly implicated, particularly when they are left unrefrigerated for extended periods. Fresh meats may harbor Salmonella from the infected animals at slaughter or may become contaminated through handling. Processed meat products like pies, hash, sausages, cured meats (such as ham, bacon, and tongue), sandwiches, and chili are often left at room temperature, which encourages *Salmonella* growth.

While poultry, its dressing, and gravy typically don't pose a problem if properly handled and cooked, they are often mishandled, as are fish and seafood products. Milk and dairy items, including fresh milk, fermented milks, ice cream, and cheese, have also been linked to *Salmonella* infections. Since eggs can carry the bacteria, foods made with eggs that are not fully cooked or pasteurized may contain live *Salmonella,* such as pastries with cream or custard fillings, cream cakes, baked Alaska, and eggnog.

The Disease

As with other infectious diseases, individuals differ in their susceptibility to *Salmonella* infections, but in general morbidity is high in any outbreak. As has been stated, the susceptibility of humans varies with the species and strain of the organism and the total numbers of bacteria ingested.

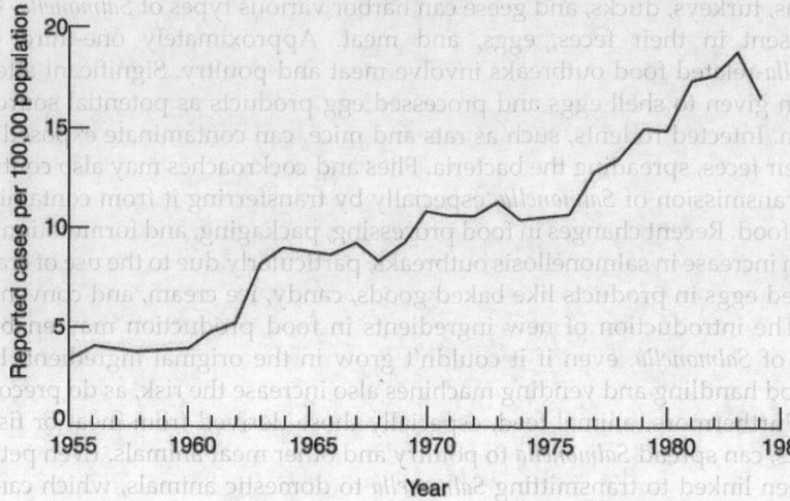

Fig 24.7. Reported cases of salmonellosis by year in the United States, 1955-1984. A slight decrease in reported cases of human salmonellosis was noted in 1984. This decrease most likely represents annual variation rather than a reversal of the secular trend toward increasing rates of salmonellosis in the United States. This steady increase in reported rates is thought to reflect increasing incidence of the disease rathe than more efficient reportin (Centers for Disease Control, Annual Summaries for 1984, 1986.)

Salmonellosis is typically distinguished from staphylococcus poisoning by its longer incubation period, usually between 12 to 36 hours for *Salmonella* infections, compared to 2 to 4 hours for staphylococcus poisoning. In some cases, the incubation period for *Salmonella* can be shorter (as little as 5 hours) or longer (up to 72 hours). The main symptoms of a *Salmonella* gastrointestinal infection include sudden onset of nausea, vomiting, abdominal pain, and diarrhea, often preceded by a headache and chills. Other signs may include watery, greenish, foul-smelling stools, weakness, faintness, a moderate fever, restlessness, twitching, and drowsiness. The mortality rate is low, typically less than 1 percent. The severity and duration of the illness can vary depending on the amount of contaminated food consumed and the individual's response. Symptoms can range from mild discomfort and diarrhea to severe illness or death within 2 to 6 days. Generally, the symptoms last for 2 to 3 days, followed by full recovery, but in some cases, they may persist for weeks or months. Around 0.2 to 5 percent of patients may become carriers of the *Salmonella* bacteria. Diagnosing the disease in the lab can be challenging unless *Salmonella* is isolated from the suspected food and from the stool samples of infected individuals. However, by the time the diagnosis is made, the contaminated food may no longer be available, and the bacteria may have disappeared from the intestines.

Conditions Necessary for an Outbreak

The following conditions are necessary for an outbreak of a food-borne Salmonella gastrointestinal infection- (1) The food must contain or become contaminated with the *Salmonella* bacteria, (2) these bacteria must be there in considerable numbers, either because of contamination or more often because of growth; these high numbers mean that the food must be a good culture medium, the temperature must be favorable, and enough time must be allowed for appreciable growth, and (3) the viable organisms must be ingested.

Prevention of Outbreaks

To prevent outbreaks of food-borne *Salmonella* infections, three key principles are essential:

- **Avoidance of Contamination:** The primary goal is to prevent food from becoming contaminated with *Salmonella*. This can happen through sources like diseased humans, animals, carriers, or contaminated ingredients such as eggs. Proper hygiene during food handling, ensuring that food handlers are healthy and clean, and preventing contact with vermin and insects are all critical steps. Using *Salmonella*-free ingredients, when possible, also helps in reducing the risk.
- **Destruction of *Salmonella*:** Heat treatment, such as cooking or pasteurization, is effecti e at destroying *Salmonella* in foods. Special attention should be paid to foods held over or stored improperly, as they can support bacterial growth. For instance, if food is left at room temperature for too long, cooking it thoroughly can eliminate the *Salmonella* organisms, though it will not neutralize toxins from other bacteria like *Staphylococcus*.
- **Prevention of *Salmonella* Growth:** Keeping food at appropriate temperatures, particularly refrigeration, is essential in preventing Salmonella from growing. Foods should be kept cool to avoid bacterial proliferation, especially in leftovers or canned foods that have been opened but not refrigerated.

Regular inspection of animals and meats in packing houses can reduce some risks, but it is not sufficien on its own to prevent *Salmonella* infections. Therefore, strict adherence to hygiene practices, temperature control, and proper food handling are necessary to minimize outbreaks.

***Clostridium perfringens* Gastroenteritis**

First reported in the United States in 1945, *Clostridium perfringens* gastroenteritis is being detected and reported more frequently than formerly. although it probably is no more prevalent (Table 24.1).

The Organism

The bacterium causing this illness is *C. perfringens* (*welchii*), type A, a gram-positive, nonmotile, anaerobic, spore-forming rod. Maximal temperature for growth is about 55°C, and optimal temperature is about 43 to 47°C. Growth is restricted at 15 to 20°C. The organism will not grow below pH 5.0 or above pH 9.0. It is inhibited by 5 percent NaCI (a_w = 0. 97), and some strains are held back by 2.5 percent sodium nitrate.

The spores of food-poisoning strains differ considerably in their heat resistance; D_{90C} = 0.015 to 8.71 min.

Foods Involved

Spores of *Clostridium perfringens* have been found in a variety of raw foods, as well as in soil, sewage, and animal feces. The most common sources of outbreaks involve meats that have been cooked, allowed to cool slowly, and then held for extended periods before being consumed. Meats and poultry products are responsible for approximately 75% of *C. perfringens*-related outbreaks, with fish paste and cold chicken also implicated.

Because these spores are widespread in raw foods and are heat-resistant, their presence in many foods is often unavoidable. While cooking can destroy the vegetative cells and spores of some strains, surviving spores may still germinate and grow if cooked foods are not properly refrigerated. A typical outbreak could occur with a large cut of roasted meat, where oven cooking may not eliminate all the spores, creating conditions favorable for their growth. If the cooked meat is not cooled correctly, the spores of *C. perfringens* can germinate, multiply, and lead to contamination. The presence of high levels of *C. perfringens* in cooked food typically signals improper handling.

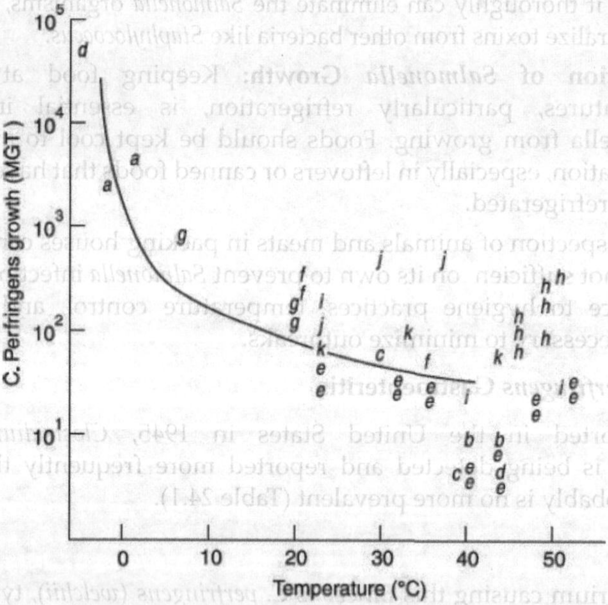

Fig 24.8. Mean Generation Times (MGT) of *Clostridium perfringens* in (A) fresh chicken, (B) rolled beef strips, (C) barbequed chicken, (D) raw ground beef, (E) cooked ground beef, (F) turkey rolls, (G) ground beef casseroles, (B) roast beef, (I) cooked meat, (J)turkey rice soup, and (K) mashed potatoes. Regression coefficient, r = 0.71. (From Rivi so and Synder, 1981)

The Disease

Symptoms of *Clostridium perfringens* infection typically appear 8 to 24 hours (with a median of 12 hours) after ingestion and include acute abdominal pain, diarrhea, and bloating. Fever, nausea, and vomiting are rare. Most outbreaks suggest that millions of viable *C. perfringens* cells per gram of food are needed to trigger symptoms. The illness is caused by a toxin, known as enterotoxin, which is released in the gut during the sporulation of the bacteria. This enterotoxin leads to excessive fluid accumulation in the intestinal lumen. The enterotoxin is relatively heat-sensitive and can be inactivated at 60°C for 10 minutes.

Conditions Necessary for an Outbreak

The following conditions are necessary for an outbreak of *C. perfringens* gastrointestinal infection- (1) The food contains or becomes contaminated with *C. perfringens*, (2) usually the food is cooked and reduced conditions develop, (3) the food is inadequately cooled, and favorable temperatures and enough time are allowed for appreciable growth, (4) the food is consumed without reheating so that large numbers of viable cells are ingested, and (5) the cells sporulate *in vivo* and elaborate the enterotoxin.

Prevention of Outbreaks

Means of prevention of outbreaks of *C. perfringens* food infection include (1) adequate and rapid cooling of cooked meats and other foods, (2) holding hot foods above 60°C, (3) reheating of leftover foods, and (4) good personal hygiene.

Vibrio parahaemolyticus Infection and Other Vibrios

Outbreaks of *Vibrio parahaemolyticus* gastroenteritis have been of significant concern in Japan, where it is one of the most common foodborne illnesses. In recent years, this pathogen has also caused several foodborne outbreaks in the United States (Table 24.1). *V. parahaemolyticus* is a gram-negative, motile rod-shaped bacterium, either straight or curved. It is halophilic, requiring 1 to 3 percent NaCl for growth, and can grow in up to 7.0 percent NaCl. The ideal growth temperature is between 35 to 37°C, though it can grow within a range of 10 to 44°C. Growth is inhibited at pH levels below 5.0 and above 11.0. *V. parahaemolyticus* has been isolated from various seafoods, including oysters, shrimp, and blue crabs. Proper cooking of seafood can kill the organism. Most outbreaks in the United States are linked to the contamination of cooked seafood by raw or undercooked seafood. Holding the contaminated cooked seafood at improper temperatures allows the bacteria to multiply, leading to a high bacterial load, and if the food is not reheated, symptoms will occur.

Vibrio cholerae serovar O1 is responsible for epidemic or Asiatic cholera, a serious worldwide, typically waterborne disease. While a few outbreaks in the U.S. have been linked to seafood transmission, non-O1 serovars of *Vibrio cholerae* do not pose the same health risks but can still cause intestinal infections or gastroenteritis.

These strains, closely resembling O1, are referred to as nonagglutinable (NAG) vibrios because they do not react with anti-O1 serum. Surveys in the Chesapeake Bay and Gulf Coast regions have found that both O1 and non-O1 *Vibrio cholerae* are common in estuary waters, and outbreaks have been associated with oyster consumption.

Vibrio vulnificus is another pathogen that can be isolated from seafood and seawater. This organism is highly invasive, producing both a hemolysin and a cytotoxin, and can lead to primary septicemia in humans.

Enteropathogenic *Escherichia coli*

Escherichia coli (*E. coli*) is generally considered a normal component of the human intestinal flora, as well as that of many animals. However, several outbreaks in the 1940s linked *E. coli* to diarrheal disease in infants. Certain *E. coli* serotypes have been identified as causing human diarrheal illnesses or foodborne outbreaks and are classified as enteropathogenic *E. coli* (EEC). The diseases caused by the ingestion of EEC can be categorized into two main groups. The first group includes strains that produce an enterotoxin, leading to a cholera-like or enterotoxigenic illness. These enterotoxigenic strains typically produce two enterotoxins- a heat-stable (ST) toxin and a heat-labile (LT) toxin. These toxins are thought to contribute to conditions like infantile diarrhea and traveler's diarrhea. To develop enterotoxigenic illnesses, individuals must ingest EEC serotypes capable of producing these toxins, which then colonize the upper small intestine and produce the enterotoxins. These enterotoxins cause a movement of water into the intestinal lumen, leading to fluid accumulation without significant macroscopic changes in the intestinal epithelium or bacterial invasion.

Table .Characteristics of some Food-borne Illnesses

Disease	Etiologic agent	Incubation period, signs, and symptoms	Foods involved	Control measures
Vibrio parahaemolyticus infection	*V.parahaemolyticus*	2-48 hr, usually 12hr; abdominal pain, diarrhea(water stools containing blood and mucus), usually nausea and vomiting, mild fever, chills, headache, prostration; recovery within 2-5 days	Raw foods of marine origin; saltwater fish, shellfish, crustacean, and fish products	Cook foods throughly; chill foods rapidly in small quantities; prevent cross contamination from saltwater fish; sanitize equipment; avoid using seawater for rising foods to be eaten raw or for cleaning

Enteropathogenic *Escherichia coli* infection	*E.coli;* both enterotoxigenic and invasive strains cause illness	8-24 hr, mean 11 hr (invasive type); 8-44 hr, mean 26 hr (enterotoxigenic type-) invasive illness fever, chills, headache, myalgia, abdominal cramps, profuse water diarrhea; similar to shigellosis; enterotoxigenic illness; diarrhea (rice water stools), vomiting dehydration, shock; similar to cholera	Coffe substitute, salmon(?). cheese	Chills foods rapidly in small quantities; cook food throughly; practice personal hygiene; prepare food in sanitary manner; protects and treat water, dispose of sewage in sanitary manner
Bacillus cereus gastroenteritis	Diarrheal, syndrome, diarreagenic toxin	8-16 hr or 1.5-5 hr; nausea, abdominal cramps, watery diarrhea, some vomiting	Custards, cereal products, puddings-sauces, meat loaf	Chill foods in rapidly small quantities; hold hot foods at 62 °C or above; practice personal hygiene; process and prepare food in sanitary manner; reheat leftover foods to 71.1 °C
	Emetic syndrome, emetic toxin	Incubation period 1-6 hr, 2-5 most common, with nausea and vomiting predominant, similar to staphylococcal intoxication); short duration, 1 day or less	Fried rich, mashed potatoes, vegetable sprouts	

Shigellois	*Shigella sennei, S.flexneri, S.dysenteriae, S.boydii*	1-7 days, usually less than 4 days; extremly variable, mild to severe symptoms; abdominal cramps, fever, chills, diarrhea, watery stools (frequently containing blood, mucus or pus) tenesmus, headache, lassitude,prostration, nausea, de-hydration	Moist, mixed foods; milk beans; potato, tuna, shrimp, turkey,and macaroni salads; apple cider; and poi	Practice personal hygiene; Chills foods rapidly in small quantities; prepare food in sanitary manner; cook food throughly; protects and treat water, dispose of sewage in sanitary manner, control flie
Yersiniosis	*Yersinia pseudotuberculosis*	24-36 hr, and longer abdominal pain suggesting acute appendicitis, fever, headache, malaise, anorexia, diarrhea, vomiting, nausea, chills, pharyngitis, leukocytosis, erythema nodousm	Pork and other meats, raw milk, or any contaminated raw or leftover food	Cook food throughly; protect foods from contamination; control rodents
Arizona infection	*Arizona hinshawii*	2-46 hr, usually 24 hr, abdominal pain,diarrhea, nausea, chills, headache, weakness, fever, lasts a few days	Turkey, chicken, cream filled pastry, ice cream, custard containing eggs	Chill foods rapidly in small quantities; practice personal hygiene; cook food throughly; pasteurize milk, exclude workers with respiratory illness or skin lesions
Beta-hemolytic streptococcal infections (scarlet fever, septic sore throat)	*Streptococcus pyogenes*	1-3 days; sore and small throat, pain in swallowing, tonsillitis, high fever, headache, nausea, vomiting, malaise, rhinorrhea; occasionally a rash occurs	Milk, ice cream, eggs, steamed lobster, potato salad, egg salad, custard,and pudding; foods usually contain eggs or milk	Chill foods rapidly in small quantities; practice personal hygiene; cook food throughly; pasteurize milk, exclude workers with respiratory illness or skin lesions

The second major group of *E. coli* consists of invasive strains that produce a cytotoxin, leading to invasive illnesses such as colitis or dysentery-like syndromes. These serotypes are nonenterotoxigenic, grow in the colon, and invade or penetrate the epithelial cells of the colonic mucosa, causing the symptoms outlined in Table 24.8. A large infective dose of enteropathogenic *E. coli* (EEC) is necessary for either enterotoxigenic or invasive illness to develop. Therefore, foods must be heavily contaminated or inadequately preserved or refrigerated to allow for significant bacterial growth.

The optimal temperature for growth is 37°C, with a growth temperature range of 10 to 40°C. The ideal pH for growth is between 7.0 and 7.5, with the minimum being pH 4.0 and the maximum pH 8.5. The organism is relatively heat-sensitive and can be effecti ely destroyed through pasteurization or proper cooking of foods. Table 24.8 provides examples of foods implicated in EEC outbreaks and methods for prevention. In addition to the strains mentioned, there is a group known as hemorrhagic *E. coli,* which can cause severe illness in humans, including bloody diarrhea and intense abdominal pain.

Bacillus cereus

Reports of outbreaks of *B. cereus* food gastroenteritis are quite uncommon in the United States; however, many European countries report frequent implication of this organism in food-borne illness. *B. cereus* is a gram-positive, aerobic, spore-forming rod. Its optimal temperature for growth is 30 °C, with a minimal temperature for growth at 10 °C and a maximum of 49 °C. The pH range for growth is 4.9 to 9.3. B. cereus spores have reported D values (heat resistance) of D_{100}C of 2.7 to 3.1 min in skim milk and D_{100}C of 8 min in phosphate buffer (pH 7.0). Numerous surveys on foods and ingredients have indicated a high percentage of samples containing *B. cereus*. It is undoubtedly widely distributed in nature and our food supply.

Extremely large numbers (10^8 per gram) of viable cells of *B. cereus* must be ingested to develop signs and symptoms (Table 24.8) of the syndrome. Two syndromes are recognized- the diarrheal syndrome and the emetic syndrome. Some of the characteristics of *B. cereus* gastroenteritis are presented in Table 24.8.

Shigellosis

Food-borne outbreaks of shigellosis have been reported in the United States, but most incidents of shigellosis involve contaminated water.

Optimal temperature for growth is 37 °C, with a temperature range of 10 to 40 °C. The organisms tolerate salt concentrations of 5 to 6 percent and are relatively heat sensitive. Pathogenicity involves the release of a lipopolysaccharide endotoxin which affects the intestinal mucosa.

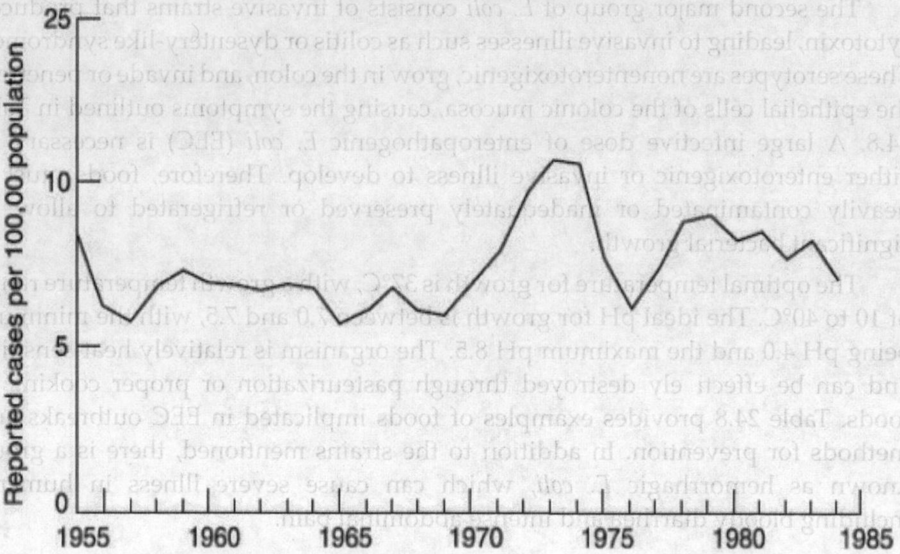

Fig 24.9. Reported cases of shigellosis by year in the United States, 1955-1984. For 1984,17, 371 cases of shigellosis were reported in the United States. Approximately 70 percent of the *Shigella* isolates reported to the CDC each year are *Shigella sonnei*, with *Shigella fexneri* accounting for a large percentage of the rest. (Centers for Disease Control, Annual Summaries for 1984, 1986.)

Yersinia enterocolitica

Yersinia enterocolitica is a small, rod-shaped bacterium that can cause gastrointestinal illness in humans. It has been isolated from the intestines and feces of various animals, including cats, pigs, dogs, deer, raccoons, and horses, with pigs being the primary reservoir for the strains that infect humans. This bacterium has been found in numerous foods, such as beef, pork, liquid eggs, soft cheese, raw milk, pasteurized milk, fish, raw oysters, shrimp, crabs, chocolate milk, turkey, chow mein, powdered milk, and tofu.

Some strains are considered environmental or noninvasive and do not cause illness, while the invasive or virulent strains are responsible for gastroenteritis. The typical symptoms, including severe abdominal pain, fever, and diarrhea, usually appear 24 to 36 hours after consumption of contaminated food, although the incubation period can sometimes be longer. The abdominal pain is often sharp and localized in the lower right quadrant, which has led to the condition being referred to as pseudoappendicitis. In one outbreak, 16 children underwent appendectomies.

Although *Y. enterocolitica* has been found in many foods, there have been relatively few foodborne outbreaks linked to it. The presence of *Y. enterocolitica* in pasteurized milk is likely due to contamination after pasteurization, as even the most heat-resistant strains are typically killed during the pasteurization process. A distinctive feature of this organism is its ability to grow at refrigeration temperatures, below 5°C. A closely related species, *Yersinia pseudotuberculosis*, has also been associated with human illness. Both *Y. enterocolitica* and *Y. pseudotuberculosis* are classified in the *Enterobacteriaceae* family

Campylobacter

Heat-tolerant strains of *Campylobacter*, specifically *C. jejuni* and *C. coli*, are the most commonly linked to acute gastroenteritis in humans. The term "heat-tolerant" is misleading, as it refers to growth at 42°C, not to heat resistance; these strains are inactivated at temperatures above 45-50°C. Key characteristics include a lack of growth below 25°C, sensitivity to oxygen (21% O_2), resistance to cephalothin, a doubling time of around one hour at their optimum temperature (42°C), sensitivity to drying and acidic conditions, and an inability to utilize carbohydrates, making them poor competitors in mixed populations. As a result, it is unlikely that they will proliferate in foods stored at or below room temperature.

C. jejuni is commonly found in warm-blooded animals, and many animal products, including chicken, pork, and beef, are often contaminated. Studies suggest that *C. jejuni* and *C. coli* are significant contributors to bacterial enteritis worldwide, though specific outbreaks are less commonly reported. Contaminated foods include raw milk, raw clams, undercooked chicken, pasteurized milk, cake icing, raw hamburger, and barbecued chicken. The isolation of *Campylobacter* from the feces of patients with gastroenteritis is more common than *Salmonella*, indicating that actual case numbers may be much higher than reported.

While the pathogenic mechanism remains somewhat unclear, some strains of *Campylobacter* produce a heat-labile enterotoxin and are invasive, suggesting a high level of virulence despite their low numbers in contaminated foods. Symptoms of infection include abdominal pain, cramps, diarrhea, headache, fever, and sometimes bloody stools, with an incubation period of 2 to 3 days, though it can extend to 7 to 10 days.

Pasteurizing milk and properly cooking food can prevent many outbreaks. As Campylobacter is commonly found in animal-based foods, it is important to avoid cross-contamination between raw and cooked items.

Plesiomonas shigelloides

Plesiomonas shigelloides is a facultatively anaerobic, gram-negative rod that is typically motile due to its polar flagella. It can grow on minimal media using ammonium salts as a nitrogen source and glucose as a carbon source. This bacterium can cause intestinal disturbances in humans, with diarrhea of varying severity being the primary symptom. *P. shigelloides* has been isolated from aquatic environments, fish, oysters, crabs, and mammals such as cats, dogs, zoo animals, goats, sheep, and monkeys.

The bacterium has been associated with several foodborne outbreaks, particularly involving oysters, crabs, and fish. Although *P. shigelloides* can be found in the feces of individuals without symptoms, it is considered an opportunistic pathogen rather than a normal part of the human intestinal flora.

Studies have shown that *P. shigelloides* strains can grow at pH levels between 4.0 and 8.5, with 58% of isolates growing at pH 4.0, and 22% growing at 8°C and 25% at 45°C. The organism is inactivated when heated to 60°C for 30 minutes. Additionally, all strains grew in 3% sodium chloride, with some even surviving in 5% sodium chloride.

Listeria monocytogenes

Listeria monocytogenes is a gram-positive, motile, short rod that can grow at temperatures as low as 4°C, which makes it particularly concerning for food safety. In cattle, the bacterium can cause abortion and mastitis, with infected animals shedding the organism in their milk. Other animals, including sheep and chickens, can also serve as reservoirs, contaminating the food supply. *L. monocytogenes* has been isolated from various environments, including water, milk, silage, sewage, and the feces of both animals and humans.

Human listeriosis was first reported in 1929, with the disease typically manifesting in pregnant women, fetuses, or newborn infants. In adults, infections are more common in immunocompromised individuals and can present as septicemia, meningitis, or meningoencephalitis. Major foodborne outbreaks of *L. monocytogenes* have been reported globally. For instance, in the United States, a significant outbreak involved contaminated coleslaw made from cabbage fertilized with sheep manure from animals that had ovine listeriosis. After harvesting, the cabbage was stored at low temperatures, which likely promoted the growth of *L. monocytogenes* in the cold environment.

Table Three Outbreaks of *Listeria monocytogenes* in the United States

Date	Location	Food vehicle	Cases	Fatality rate, %
1981	Nova Scotia	Coleslaw	34 P* 7A	44
1983	Massachusett	Milk†	7P 42 A ‡	29
1985	Los Angeles County	Soft cheeses §	93 P 49 A	33

*A = adult; P = perinatal: † Pasteurized: ‡ Most were immunocompromised: Mexican-style.

Listeria monocytogenes, like many gram-positive organisms, can persist in the soil, which raises concerns when manure containing the bacterium is used as fertilizer, especially on crops like fruits or vegetables that may not undergo heat treatments. This is a particular concern since *L. monocytogenes* can grow even at low temperatures.

In pasteurized milk, the presence of *L. monocytogenes* initially raised concerns about the adequacy of milk pasteurization. However, studies (Bradshaw et al., 1985; Donnelly and Briggs, 1986) suggest that proper pasteurization, such as the HTST (High Temperature Short Time) method at 161°F for 15 seconds, can eliminate the organism. Contamination of milk is more likely to occur post-pasteurization, which was highlighted in FDA surveillance of dairy plants in 1986. Environmental sources and finished products were found to harbor *L. monocytogenes* and its inoculum.

The psychrotrophic (cold-tolerant) nature of *L. monocytogenes* makes it particularly concerning in refrigerated foods, as the bacterium can continue to grow at low temperatures. This characteristic implies that contamination of refrigerated foods can pose a significant health risk, e en after pasteurization.

Aeromonas hydrophilia

Aeromonas hydrophilia is a gram-negative motile rod with an optimum temperature of 28°C. It may be pathogenic for frogs, fish, and mammals including humans (Krieg, 1984). The organism has rarely been incriminated in food-borne outbreaks in the United States; however, it is a newly recognized pathogen that may cause food-borne diarrhea. It is ubiquitous in water and has been reported to be the cause of outbreaks in other countries.

OTHER BACTERIAL FOOD-BORNE INFECTIONS

Streptococcus faecalis and similar species have been implicated in foodborne illnesses, though no enterotoxin has been identified, and their role as causative agents remains uncertain. Foods such as barbecued beef, Vienna sausage, ham bologna, and turkey a la king have been associated with outbreaks, with symptoms including nausea, vomiting, and diarrhea, typically appearing 2 to 18 hours after consumption. However, most authorities now consider these organisms innocuous, as volunteer studies with high doses of the bacteria have failed to induce enteritis.

Other bacteria, like *Arizona hinshawii* and *Streptococcus pyogenes,* have more substantial evidence linking them to foodborne outbreaks. Pathogenic bacteria that cannot grow in food may still be carried by it, posing a risk without multiplying. These diseases often involve intestinal or respiratory pathogens, such as those causing typhoid, dysenteries, tuberculosis, scarlet fever, and Q fever.

Contamination sources include food handlers, utensils, air, soil, water, animals, and vermin. Disease transmission can occur through improperly handled or raw foods, especially fruits or vegetables. Foods treated by heat may not always destroy pathogens fully, especially inside the food, leading to potential outbreaks. Preventing foodborne infections involves controlling contamination, such as eradicating vermin, avoiding night soil as fertilizer, washing raw foods, rejecting contaminated shellfish, and ensuring milk is from healthy cows. Detecting pathogens on animals or food handlers is challenging, and ill or carrier workers can unknowingly spread diseases. While regulations exist, enforcement remains difficult, with the empl er generally responsible for worker health checks.

CASE STUDY

Salmonellosis

There have been numerous reports linking raw egg consumption to infections like salmonellosis, with outbreaks often associated with foods like mayonnaise and desserts. These outbreaks have been more common during the summer months due to improper egg handling and refrigeration.

On January 18, 2010, NSW Health informed the NSW Food Authority of a gastroenteritis outbreak affecting 20 people who ate at a local burger bar on January 14 and 15. By January 28, 179 cases of *Salmonella typhimurium* phage type 9 had been connected to the establishment. Interviews with affected individuals revealed that aioli, commonly served during this period, was a likely source of the infection. The business prided itself on homemade ingredients, and the aioli was prepared on-site using raw eggs, without further cooking. DNA fingerprinting confirmed a match between the *Salmonella* isolates from the burger bar and clinical samples. The establishment was ordered to stop serving aioli, and additional samples from food and the premises were tested. No new cases were reported after January 15, and the business resumed normal operations.

On December 12, 2006, a foodborne illness outbreak was reported following a private party where the main meal was catered by a local business. Interviews suggested that the illness was linked to *Clostridium perfringens* or *Bacillus cereus* contamination, potentially from leftover food. During the following week, two more complaints were made from other functions catered by the same business, with roast pork as the common food. Of the 120 party attendees, 80 became ill, and 17 cases were analyzed, showing symptoms consistent with *Cl. perfringens* infection. Fecal specimens from the affected individuals tested positive for *Cl. perfringens,* and high spore counts were found. Leftover roast pork also showed an infective dose of the bacterium. The outbreak was likely caused by improper cooking, slow cooling, and prolonged storage of the roast pork before reheating, allowing *Cl. perfringens* to multiply. Inadequate reheating also contributed to the illness. The evidence from the clinical samples and food strongly indicated temperature abuse as the cause of the outbreak.

Nonbacterial Foodborne Illnesses: Poisonings and Infections

25

Nonbacterial foodborne illnesses arise from viruses, parasites, and natural toxins present in contaminated food or water. These illnesses can cause severe health issues, including gastrointestinal distress and organ damage. Viruses, such as norovirus and hepatitis A, are common culprits of foodborne infections. They spread through contaminated water, food, or infected handlers. Parasites like *Toxoplasma gondii, Giardia,* and *Trichinella spiralis* infect hosts through undercooked meat, raw produce, or unclean water sources, leading to symptoms ranging from mild diarrhea to severe neurological or muscular complications.

Poisonings occur due to natural toxins, such as mycotoxins from fungic molds, marine toxins like ciguatoxins in fish, or plant toxins like alkaloids. These toxins can cause acute or chronic health issues, depending on the exposure level. Preventing nonbacterial foodborne illnesses involves proper cooking, storage, hygiene, and food handling practices, alongside regular monitoring of food sources to ensure safety and reduce risks.

Certain foodborne disease outbreaks are not attributed to bacteria or their toxins but are caused by mycotoxins, viruses, rickettsias, parasitic worms, protozoa, or toxic substances in food. While the full impact on human health is not completely understood for mycotoxins and many viruses, their occurrence and effects in animals arrant their consideration.

MYCOTOXINS

Mycontoxins are metabolites of fungi. Some are extremely toxic to a wide range of animals and may be toxic to humans. Concerns have recently been raised about their carcinogenic properties and the fact that they are found in many foods.

Fungi and Human Beings

Molds, yeasts, mildews, blights, rusts, and mushrooms are examples of fungi. A lot of fungi are beneficial. Some, like yeast's single-cell protein and mushrooms, are edible. Others are commonly employed in food and industrial fermentations; for example, molds aid in the ripening of some cheeses, and *Aspergillus oryzae* is used to produce sake, miso, and soy sauce.

Penicillin, a metabolite of *Penicillium chrysogenum,* has made a significant contribution to human health. Molds have historically been thought to be innocuous, but some mushrooms are toxic or dangerous to people. Numerous fungi, such as *Alternaria, Rhizopus, Fusarium, Cladosporium, Helminthosporium,* and *claviceps,* can be isolated from plants. The two most common fungal genera found in stored goods are most likely *Aspergillus* and *Penicillium,* both of which produce mycotoxins.

The syndrome resulting from the ingestion of toxin in a mold-contaminated food is referred to as mycotoxicosis. Historically, the first documented case of mycotoxicosis attributed to a fungus-containing food was that of rye ergot. *Claviceps purpurea* parasitizes rye and other grains and elaborates many lysergic acid derivatives which are responsible for the syndrome. Consumption of the grain or flour made from it over a period of time can result in gangrenous ergotism. Outbreaks of ergotism were quite common during the Middle Ages. More recent outbreaks of ergotism have been reported in the Soviet Union (1926-1927), England (1928), and France (1951); however, there has not been a major outbreak in the United States since 1925 (Gray, 1970).

Aflatoxin

In 1960, 100,000 turkey poults died suddenly in England. This was followed by the reported death of 14,000 ducklings and nine outbreaks of disease in calves (Gray, 1970). A common factor in each of these episodes was the use of Brazilian peanut meal as part of the animal feed. *Aspergillus flavus* was isolated from the meal, and subsequently a toxic metabolite, or toxin, was isolated and identified. The resulting *A. flavus* toxin was called aflatoxin. The attention and research associated with these outbreaks have greatly stimulated an interest in, and concern for, the presence of aflatoxins and other mycotoxins in foods for human consumption.

Some strains of *Aspergillus flavus* and *A. parasiticus,* among others, produce aflatoxins (Table 25.1). Aflatoxi production is not guaranteed by a fungus's identification as *A. flavus* or *A. parasiticus*. In fact, there is some misunderstanding about *A. flavus* in the literature. The species *A. flavus* and *A. parasiticus* are members of the *A. flavus* group, one of the morphologically distinct groups that make up the genus *Aspergillus*. Each strain produces different amounts and kinds of aflatoxins. For instance, *A. parasiticus* Speare produces both B1 and G1 and their associated metabolites, whereas *A. flavus* Link strains produce B1 and its associated metabolites. Over a mesophilic temperature range, both species can grow on a broad range of substrates. Optimal conditions for the production of aflatoxin would be an a_w of 0.85 and temperature of 25 to 40°C.

Chemistry The two major metabolites or aflatoxins have been designated B1 and G1 because they fluoresce blue (B1) and green (G1) when exposed to long-wave ultraviolet light. Aflatoxins B_2 and G_2 are the dihydroderivatives of B1 and G_1 (Figure 25.1). Other closely related aflatoxins include B_2a, G_2a, and GM1. Aflatoxins M_1, M_2, and P1 are the hydroxylated derivatives of B1 and B_2 which are excreted in the urine, feces, and milk as metabolic products of B1 and B_2 following their consumption by mammals. They are all highly oxygenated heterocyclic compounds.

Table Mycotoxins that May be Significant in Food

			Animals affected	
Mycotoxins	Some molds producing the toxin	Foods or feeds isolated from	Toxic to	Carcinogenic to
Aflatoxin	*Aspergillus flavus, A. parasiticus*, some *Penicillium*	Barley, corn, cottonseed, millet, oats, peanuts, peanut meal, peanut butter, rice, soybeans, wheat, spaghetti, cassa a, cottonseed meal, cowpeas, sorghum, peas, sesame, soybean meal, sweet potatoes	(B_1) quail, cats, chickens, pheasants, salmon, rabbits, monkeys, dogs, hamsters, turkeys, mink, cattle guinea pigs	(B_1), trout, rats, sheep, mice, ducklings
Patulin	*Penicillium expansum, P.clavifrome, P.patalum, P. mlinii, P. leucopus, P. urticase, P.equinum P.cyclopium, Aspergillus clavatus, A.giganteous, A.terreus*	Apple sap, apple cider, apple juice	Mice, rats, cats, rabbits, quail, guppies, brine, shrimp	Mice
Ochratoxin A	*Aspergillus ostianus, A. petrakii, A.alliaceus, A.sclerotiorum, A.sulphureus, A.mellecus, Penicillium cyclopium, P.purpurescens, P.commune, P.viridicatum*	Corn, wheat, barley, white beans, peanuts, dough, bread, hen's eggs	Rats,chicks, ducklings, trout	Rats, trout, chicks
Luteoskyrin	*Penicillium islandicum*	Mold, rice flour	Mice	Mice
Sterigmatocystin	*Aspergillus regulosus, A.nidulons, A.versicolor, Penicillium latium*	Wheat, oats	Mice, monkey, rats	Rats
Penicillic acid	*Penicillium puberulum, P.cyclopium, P.marteusii, P.thomii, P.suavolens, P.madriti, P.baarneuse, Aspergillus quercinus, A.sulphureus, A.ochraceus, A.mellens*	Dried beans, tobacco	Rats	Rats
Alimentary toxic aleukia (ATA)	Species *of Cladosporium, Penicillium, Fusasrium, Mucor, Alternaria*	Grain	Human beings	
Roquefortine	*Penicillium roqueforti*	Blue cheese, Roquefort cheese, Stilton cheese	Mice	

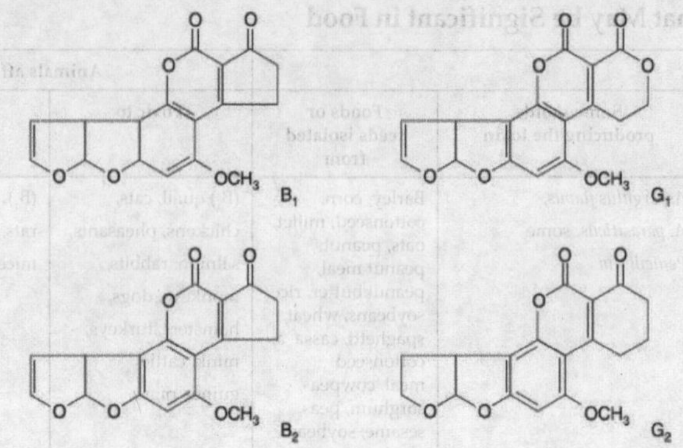

Fig 25.1. Structure of four aflatoxins. (From. D. Gray, The Use of Fungi as Food and in Food Processing. The Chemical Rubber Co., 1970. Used by permission of The Chemical Rubber Co.)

Toxicity

Aflatoxin B_1, the most toxic of the aflatoxins, is toxic to various animals, as summarized in Table 25.1. Many of the other aflatoxins have been shown to be toxic or carcinogenic to different species of fish, mammals, and poultry.

When cows eat feed containing aflatoxin, aflatoxin M1 and M_2 is excreted in the milk. Although M1 and M_2 are less toxic than the parent compounds B_1 and B_2, M1 retains its toxic and carcinogenic ability in many animals. M1 has also been detected in the urine of Philippine women who had consumed peanut butter containing aflatoxin

Significance in Foods

Since the discovery (or at least the identification) ofthe aflatoxins in the early 1960s numerous surveys have been conducted on the detection of the aflatoxins in foods (Table 25.1). Many commodities will support the growth of toxigenic strains if inoculated, including various dairy products, bakery products, fruit juices, cereals, and forage crops.

In most cases, the growth of a toxigenic strain and the elaboration of aflatoxin occurs following harvesting or formulation of the product. Peanuts, cottonseeds, and corn, however, differ significantly in that these products are susceptible to fungal invasion, growth, and mycotoxin production before harvesting. The contamination and potential for aflatoxin production in these crops is related to insect damage, humidity, weather conditions; and agricultural practices. For example, with peanuts it is highly desirable to harvest and dry them as soon as they reach maturity.

The FDA began surveillance activity for aflatoxin contamination in foods and animal feeds in 1963. Originally a guideline of 20 ppb of aflatoxin resulted in action against a food. Improvement in detection methods now makes it possible to measure lower concentrations. In cooperation with FDA, the USDA and the peanut industry began a certification program for aflatoxin-free raw peanuts. The results of an FDA survey in 1973 indicated that 25 percent of peanut butter samples contained detectable levels of aflatoxin. Aflatoxin levels above the 20 ppb guideline were found in 4 percent of the samples of peanut butter and in 2 percent of the raw peanuts sampled. Also during 1973 a survey was made on various dairy products including cottage cheese, nonfat dry milk, and evaporated milk.

Aflatoxin M_1 was found in less than 1 percent of the samples, with a range in concentrations of 0.05 to 0.4 ppb, well below the guideline. However, it is suggested that if a cow consumes feed containing aflatoxin B_1 at a concentration 100 µg per kilogram of feed, the milk will contain aflatoxin M_1 at a concentration of 1 µg per liter. Therefore, only about 1.0 percent of the amount consumed finds its way into the milk. The elimination of aflatoxins in dairy products is really a problem of keeping the aflatoxins out of the animal feed.

International efforts to monitor and control the aflatoxin levels in foods resulted in the establishment of a 30 ppb guideline (FAO/WHO/UNICEF, Protein Advisory Board). This guideline had as its basis a no-effect level in monkeys with a safety factor of 50 (Van Walbeek, 1973). Peanut products and cottonseed products are imported by many countries, and the value of peanut flour as a good protein source for malnourished populations is recognized. However, considering all available data on aflatoxins, it is now suggested that peanut flour not be depended on as a protein source for feeding malnourished infants.

Patulin

First isolated and described as an antibiotic, patulin is structurally synonymous with expansin, penicidin, claviformin, clavatin, clavacin, mycoin C, and gigantic acid. Several molds have been reported to produce patulin, as shown in Table 25.1.

- **Chemistry:** Patulin in the pure state is a white crystal with a melting point of 110.5°C and a molecular weight of 154. It is an unsaturated lactone with the chemical name of 4 hydroxy-4H-furo[3,2c]pyran-2(6H)-one. It is sensitive to $SO_2$and is unstable in alkali but stable in acid.
- **Toxicity:** Originally isolated as an antibiotic, Patulin. (Figure 25.2) it is effecti e against many bacterial species. Concentrations as low as 0.1 percent completely inhibit *E. coli* and *S. aureus*. It also exhibits strong fungistatic activity and is toxic to seeds and seedlings of higher plants including sugar beets, corn, wheat, peas, tomato, cucumber, and flax.

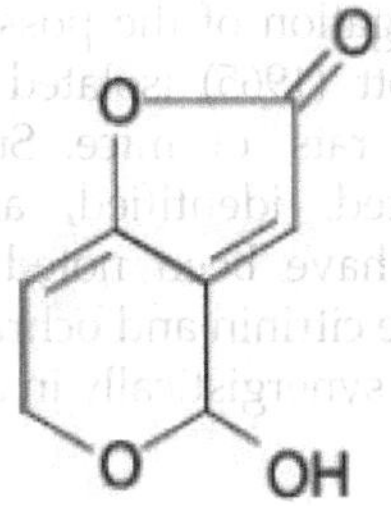

Fig 25.2. Structure of patulin.

Oral and intravenous injections of patulin in concentrations of 0.3 to 2.5 mg per gram of body weight are fatal to mice and rats. Pathological changes included edema of the brain, hemorrhaging of the lungs, and capillary damage of the liver, spleen, and kidney. Carcinogenic and mutagenic properties of patulin have been observed in mice at sublethal doses. Since many other animals are known to be sensitive to patulin, it is considered a potential human carcinogen (Scott and Bullerman, 1975).

Significance in Foods

Many patulin-producing strains have been isolated from food and animal feeds. The presence of patulin has been detected in apple cider and apple juice. Its occurrence in apple products may be related to the fact that over 60 percent of sampled rotted apples have yielded patulin producing strains of *Penicillium expansum*. In most other products patulin producing molds represent only a small percentage of the total isolates.

Another explanation for the inability to detect patulin chemically in foodstuffs which support good growth of patulin producing fungi might be the observed inhibitory effect of several food compounds on patulin. For example, peptone, glycine, methionine, p-aminobenzoic acid, asparagine, sodium sulfate, sodium thiosulfate, and casein hydrolyzate have an inhibitory action on patulin. It is possible, therefore, that some foods which will support patulin-producing fungi do not constitute a problem because of their inherent composition. Of additional interest to the food microbiologist is that several patulin-producing fungi when grown on a synthetic medium will elaborate patulin at refrigeration temperatures. The resistance of patulin to heat also has been noted. This mycotoxin resists boiling; e.g., it is stable at 100 °C for 15 min.

The carcinogenic property of patulin in animals, the isolation of patulin-producing fungi from several foodstuffs, its inactivation in some foods, the potential for toxin production at refrigeration temperatures, and its stability to heat suggest that patulin will be the subject of further study and concern in the food industry.

Ochratoxin

Published work on the aflatoxins and suggestions of a correlation between mold metabolites and a high incidence of liver cancer in the Bantu population of South Africa provided the impetus for investigation of the possible presence of mycotoxins in the cereal grains of that region. Scott (1965) isolated twenty-two fungi (seven species) which were toxic to ducklings, rats, or mice. Subsequently a toxic metabolite of *Aspergillus ochraceus* was isolated, identified, and named ochratoxin A. Other ochratoxin A-producing molds have been noted (Table 25.1). Some strains of *P. viridicatum* and *P. palitans* produce citrinin and ochratoxin A. There is some speculation that these two mycotoxins can act synergistically in animals to result in nephrotoxicity.

- **Chemistry:** Ochratoxin A is structurally a chlorinated isocoumarin derivative with an amide bond to phenylalanine. A dechloro analog of this compound has also been isolated and named ochratoxin B. In addition, there are other minor components including a methyl and ethyl ester of A and B and 4-hydroxyo chratoxin A. Ochratoxin A fluoresces green under ultraviolet light, and ochratoxin B fluoresces blue.

- **Toxicity:** Ochratoxin A is toxic to ducklings, rats, chicks, trout, and other animals. It is about one-third as toxic as aflatoxin B_1 to rats. The other derivatives or analogs are all equally toxic or less toxic than ochratoxin A. They have been shown to produce lesions in the kidneys of rats and lesions in trout and chicks. Citrinin also has a pathological effect on the kidneys of animals. Mold nephrosis, a disease in pigs, has occurred at high rates when the animals were fed grain which had been harvested wet. There is speculation that molds producing ochratoxin A and citrinin are responsible for this syndrome. If these mycotoxin-producing molds are isolated and grown on synthetic media, citrinin is produced. Consumption of the citrinin by rats, rabbits, guinea pigs, and pigs results in kidney damage similar to that observed in pigs with mold nephrosis (Van Walbeek, 1973). A moldy alfalfa-grass mixture was considered to be responsible for a high abortion rate in dairy cows (Still et al., 1971). Although ochratoxin A was not isolated, an ochratoxin-producing *Aspergillus* strain was identified.
- **Significance in Foods:** In addition to their unknown effect on human beings, the ochratoxins are of interest in foods for at least three reasons- (1) They are toxic to some animals, (2) some are very heat resistant, e.g., prolonged autoclaving does not destroy ochratoxin A when heated in oatmeal (Trenk et al., 1971), (3) many ochratoxin- and citrinin-producing fungi are capable of growth and mycotoxin production at temperatures below 10 °C, and (4) ochratoxins have been isolated from numerous foods.

Lúteoskyrin

Penicillium islandicum produces two metabolites, luteoskyrin and cyclochlorotine, which are hepatotoxic to some animals. Although luteoskyrin is not as carcinogenic as aflatoxin B_1, mice seem to be more sensitive to luteoskyrin than to aflatoxin B1. There are no known acute human intoxications attributed to luteoskyrin or cyclochlorotine.

Alimentary Toxic Aleukia (ATA)

In the Soviet Union, outbreaks of this mycotoxicosis have happened; in some areas, between 1942 and 1947, the death toll approached 1,000 per 10,000 people. The toxic metabolites epicladosporic acid, fagicladosporic acid, and fusariogenin are the cause of the syndrome in humans. If grain is harvested and stored correctly, ATA won't be an issue. Consumption of overwintered grain—grain that has been left in the fields throughout the winter and harvested later than expected—has been the cause of all prior outbreaks.

Penicillic Acid

Several molds have been reported to produce penicillic acid, and its carcinogenic ability has been noted. Many commodities, including oats, wheat, rice, corn, and barley, support the growth of penicillic acid-producing strains.

Roquefortine

A toxic substance has recently been detected in commercial blue cheese from several countries. Heavily molded portions of the cheese contain higher concentrations than the white portions, suggesting that *Penicillium roqueforti* may be producing a mycotoxin during curing of Roquefort cheese (blue cheese). The toxic factor, tentatively named roquefortine, acts as a neurotoxin when injected into mice and leads to convulsive seizures.

Sterigmatocystin

Structurally similar to aflatoxin, sterigmatocystin has a carcinogenic potency probably between one-tenth and one-hundredth of that of aflatoxin.

Implications

The above list of mycotoxins is far from complete. Since the isolation and characterization of the aflatoxins, much information has been published on a large number of diverse toxic metabolities of fungal origin.

There is little question that many fungi produce and elaborate toxic metabolites. Of major concern is their carcinogenic property. This topic has been excellently reviewed by Enomoto and Saito (1972). Most of the studies on the toxicological and carcinogenic effects of the mycotoxins have, of course, been made with experimental animals, with limited or nonexisting data on human beings. Therefore, clinical evidence and the effect of mycotoxins on people is essentially not known. Studies with human tissue cells for determination of human susceptibility to mycotoxins is now possible and should prove to be a valuable research tool. The possible wide range of effects and susceptibility to carcinogens may make it impossible ever to establish safe dose levels of the mycotoxins in human foods. The abundance of surveys and field and storage studies has definitel established the presence of many of the mycotoxins in our food supply. The actual impact on human health and its long-term implications are still being established.

VIRUSES

Some common characteristics of viruses are that they are (1) ultramicroscopic in size, varying from 10 to 450 nm, (2) able to pass through most bacterial filter (i.e., 0.22 μm), (3) cultivatable only on a susceptible host cell line, (4) incapable of reproduction without a host, and (5) able to infect people, animals, plants, or bacteria; however, they have a very specific target host. Viruses consist of a core of nucleic acid, either deoxyribonucleic acid (DNA) or ribonucleic acid (RNA), and a protein coat. They actually exist in two different states, the intracellular state and the extracellular state. When the virus particle invades a susceptible host cell (the intracellular state), the nucleic acid core and the protein coat separate.

There are two possible responses of the viral nucleic acid in the host cell. In most instances the viral nucleic acid serves as the template to direct the host cell's machinery to synthesize new virus particles. In this way viruses multiply and destroy host cells. Sometimes, however, a stable relationship between the host nucleic acid and the viral nucleic acid is established, and new virus particles are not produced; instead the viral nucleic acid is replicated when the host cell's nucleic acid is replicated.

Classification

Arbitrary and convenient forms for the classification of viruses include subdivisions based on (1) the host in which the virus multiplies, (2) the types of tissue or organs of primary infection, and (3) the mode of transmission. More recent taxonomical approaches include consideration of (1) the nucleic acid present, i.e., RNA or DNA, (2) symmetry, (3) presence or absence of an envelope, (4) diameter of the helical nucleocapsids, and (5) base sequence of the nucleic acid.

Numerous viral infections may result in the death of animals or the destruction of plants. This consequence could be considered a reduction of potential foods available for humans. In addition, many of the animal viruses can cause disease in humans, e.g., encephalitis, hepatitis, measles, mumps, rabies, smallpox, and yellow fever. Those associated with food-borne outbreaks will be discussed subsequently. Many of the enteroviruses, including the coxsackie viruses and ECHO viruses, may result in human gastroenteritis. Since many cases of food-borne human gastroenteritis are not caused by bacteria ("nonbacterial acute gastroenteritis"), it is widely believed that viruses may be responsible for, or implicated in, these outbreaks of food-borne diseases in humans. Several viruses implicated in food-borne outbreaks, their mode of transmission, and measures to prevent their spread are summarized in Table 25.2. Further clarification of possible relationships is hampered by the lack of practical laboratory methodology for detection and isolation of viruses from foods.

Infectious Hepatitis

The hepatitis virus enters a person through the oral route normally as a result of fecal contamination of water or food. The incubation time (onset of symptoms) is long but eventually may result in serious liver complications. There are many documented food-borne outbreaks in people; perhaps the classic outbreak was described by Mason and McLean (1962), who identified the source as oysters harvested from polluted water. Oysters and clams are able to concentrate the numbers of bacteria or viruses during their normal feeding, which is to filter and remove particles from the water. The infectious hepatitis virus has been shown to be stable during refrigerated storage of oysters. The problem is of further concern since many oysters are eaten raw. Cliver (1967) summarized reports over a 20-year period involving 3,000 cases of food-borne infectious hepatitis and noted that in addition to shellfish, raw milk, potato salad, sandwiches, and cold meat cuts also were implicated.

Table. Viruses Implicated in Food-borne Outbreaks

Illnes	Causative agent	Foods usually Involved	Other modes of transmission	Incubation period	Signs and symptoms	Measures to prevent spread by food
Poliomyelitis*	Poliovirus types I, II III	Milk; possibly other beverages and prepared foods	Case or carrier; contaminated water	5-35 days	Fever, vomiting; headache; pain in muscle groups; paralysis	adopting improved hygiene use of properly pusleary food
Infectious hepatitis	Infectious hepatitis virus (or viruses)	Milk and other beverages; shellfish (raw oysters and clams)- specific foods served as part of a meal, such as potato salad	Case or carrier; contaminated water	10-50 days, (mean 25 days)	Jaundice in approximately one-half of cases; loss of appetite, gastrointestinal	Cooking of shellfish; checking personnel handling food; adequate heating of milk and foods; adequate heating or distinfection of water cleanliness of food handlers
Acute nonbacterial gastroenteritis*	Coxsackie and ECHO viruses, viral agents as yet unidentifie	Possible food-borne, but as yet this mode of transmission is unestablished	Case or carrier	27-60 hr (average)	Fever, constitutional symptoms; headache; abdominal pain, vomiting, and diarrhea	Probability the same as for poliomyelitis

*Usually not food-borne: Source- From International Association of Milk, Food, and Environmental Sanitarians, Inc., Procedure for the Investigation of Foodborne Disease Outbreaks, 2d ed., 1966.

Poliomyelitis

There are a limited number of reported food-borne outbreaks of polio. Cliver (1967) noted ten such outbreaks between 1914 and 1949. Milk (both pasteurized and raw) was implicated in eight of the ten outbreaks, and lemonade and a cream-filled pastry in the remaining two. The implication of pasteurized milk (two outbreaks) is noteworthy since the heat required for pasteurization should inactivate the polio virus. It was assumed either that the milk was improperly pasteurized or that it was contaminated following processing.

Other Viruses

The virus responsible for foot and mouth disease in cattle can be transmitte to people in foods. Two viral diseases of poultry, ornithosis and Newcastle disease, have been implicated in human ailments. Workers in poultry processing plants have been known to contract an eye infection, possibly as a result of the splashing of water containing the Newcastle virus. The ornithosis virus produces a respiratory infection in man. Other viruses which are considered good candidates for food-borne transmission are enteroviruses including coxsackie and ECHO viruses.

At least eighty individuals became ill following the consumption of coleslaw in a 1976 outbreak which was attributed to ECHO virus 4. One of the most frequently involved virus in recent years has been the "Norwalk" virus or Norwalk-like agents. Shellfish is the common vehicle for this viral diarrheal syndrome. In 1982 viral agents (hepatitis A and Norwalk virus) accounted for 21 outbreaks and 5,325 cases. Norwalk gastroenteritis was involved in two large outbreaks, one of over 3,000 cases (frosting on bakery items) and one of over 2,000 cases (coleslaw).

Significance in Foods

In addition to the known food-borne viral outbreaks there are many suspected viral implicated food-borne disease outbreaks. The lack of methodology and susceptible host cell lines complicates viral surveys of foods. It is not unreasonable to assume that the enteroviruses (intestinal viruses) can enter our food supply as readily and as frequently as the enteric bacteria, since they can be isolated from feces as readily as the coliforms and the enteric pathogens.

They follow the same oral-fecal route of contamination and dissemination. Although the resistance to heat and the persistence during storage vary considerably between viruses, some do have a greater resistance than vegetative bacteria. Details of some specific viruses in regard to effects of processing and storage can be found in several of the references cited at the end of this chapter.

RICKETTSIAS

The rickettsias may be considered degenerative bacteria since they represent a form of life closely resembling bacteria except that they cannot be cultivated outside of living cells. Like the viruses, they are obligate parasites. The mode of transmission of rickettsias to people is quite variable, but at some point in their normal life cycle rickettsias are associated with fleas, lice, or ticks. Therefore, many of the major human rickettsial diseases are contracted by bites from these bloodsucking arthropods. *Epidemic typhus, rickettsial pox, Rocky Mountain spotted fever*, and *Q fever* are examples of human rickettsial diseases.

Cows infected with the rickettsia of Q fever, *Coxiella burnetii*, are of public health concern, since the organism can be excreted in milk in large quantities and result in human infections. At one time the pasteurization times and temperatures for milk (61.7°C for 30 min) were based on the complete destruction of *Mycobacterium tuberculosis*. When it was shown that *C. burnetii* was able to survive these conditions, the pasteurization temperature was raised to 62.8 °C (30 min) to ensure its destruction in milk.

FOOD-BORNE PARASITES

Although, no attempt will be made to discuss in any detail the numerous parasitic round- or flatworms, protozoa, and flukes occasionally encountered in foods, it is important for the food microbiologist to be aware of their existence. A summary of common parasites is presented in Table 25.3. A comprehensive listing of possible parasites transmitted in foods can be found in Table 25.4.

Trichinosis

Trichinosis, although caused by a nematode worm, *Trichinella spiralis*, usually is discussed along with bacterial food poisoning and infection because all have similar symptoms and all are food-borne. Most human trichinosis results from the consumption of raw or incompletely cooked pork containing the encysted larvae. The larvae are released into the intestinal tract during digestion and invade the mucous membranes of the first parts of the small intestine, where they develop into adults. The fertilized females give birth to numerous larvae, which travel through the blood vessels and lymphatics to skeletal muscle tissue, where they encyst. The worm goes through a similar cycle in hogs, rats, and other hosts, e.g., mice, rabbits, cats, dogs, and bears. Recent trends in the number of cases of trichinosis reported in the United States.

- **Symptoms:** The incubation period between ingestion of the pork and the first symptoms varies widely, being reported to be as short as a day or two and as long as several weeks. The first symptoms, which may be confused with food poisoning, appear when the larvae, freshly released from their cysts in the ingested and digested pork, invade the mucosa. Symptoms may include nausea, vomiting, diarrhea, profuse sweating, colic, and loss of appetite and may continue for days. Later symptoms, resulting from the migration of the newborn larvae to the muscles and their

Table. Important Parasitic Infections Transmitted by Food

Illnes	Causative agent	Foods usually involved	Incubation peroid	Signs of symptoms	Measures to prevent spread by food
Anisakiaias	*Anisakis* spp. (a nematode)	Raw or insufficientl cooked fis	Several days	Irritation of throat and digestive tract	Cook fish throughly
Amedic dysentery (amebiasis)	*Entamoeba histolytica*	Water contaminated with sewage, moist food contaminated with human feces	Several days to 4 weeks	Diarrhea of varying severity; fatalities not common	Protect water supplies; cleanliness in food preparation; ensure proper disposal of human excreta
Beef tapeworm (taeniasis saginata)	*Taenia saginata*	Raw or insufficientl cooked beef containing live larvae	Several weeks	Abdominal pain, hungry feeling, vague discomfort	Use meat processed under veterinary inspection; cook beef throughly
Fish tapeworm (diphyllobothrisis)	*Diphyllobothrium latum*	Raw or insufficientl cooked fish containing live larvae	3-6 weeks	Usually none; anemia in heavy infectious	Cook fish throughly; avoid eating raw smoked fish
Pork tapeworm (taeniasis solium)	*Taenia solium*	Raw or *insufficiently cooked* pork containing live larvae	Several weeks	Varies from a mild chronic, digestive disorder to severe malaise with encephalitis; may be fatal	Use meat processed under veterinary inspection; cook pork throughly
Trichinosis	*Trichinellaspiralis*	Raw or insufficiently cooked pork and pork products; whale seal bear or walrus meat containing live larvae	Usually 9 days but may vary from 2 to 28 days; in heavy infections 24 hr	Nausea, vomiting, diarrhea, muscular pains, fever, labored breathing, swallowing of eyelids; occasionally fatal	Cook pork and pork products throughly; freeze pork at –15 C for 20 days, or –29 C for 12 days; cook garbage fed to swine eliminate rats from hog lots

Source- Chiefly from InternationalAssociation of Milk, Food, and Environmental Sanitarians, Inc., Procedure for the Investigation of Foodborne Disease Outbreaks, 2d ed., 1966.

Table. Endoparasites (Protozoa, Nematode, Cestoda, Treamatoda) Transmissible through Food

Parasites	Potential pathogenicity	Method of infection
Protozoa		
Entamoeba histolytica	+	Food and drink contaminated with cysts
Entamoeba coli	–	Food and drink contaminated with cysts
Endolimax nana	–	Food and drink contaminated with cysts
lodamoeba butschlii	–	Food and drink contaminated with cysts
Dientamoeba fragilis	+	Food and drink contaminated with trophozoites
Retortamonas intestinalis	–	Food and drink contaminated with cysts
Retortamonas sinensis	+	Food and drink contaminated with cysts
Chilomastix mesnili	–	Food and drink contaminated with cysts
Enteromonas hominis	–	Food and drink contaminated with cysts
Enteromonas hervei	–	Probably via food and drink contaminated with cysts
Trichomonas hominis	–	Food and drink contaminated with trophozoites
Trichomonas tenax	–	Food and drink contaminated with trophozoites
Giardia lamblia	+	Food and drink contaminated with cysts
lsospora belli	+	Food and drink contaminated with cysts
lsospora natalensis	+	Food and drink contaminated with cysts
Balantidium coli	+	Food and drink contaminated with cysts
Sarcocystis ssp.	+	Red meat containing cysts
Toxoplasma gondii	+	Meats and milk contaminated with cysts
Nematoda		
Trichinella spiralis	+	Meats containing larvae
Trichuris trichiura	+	Food and drink contaminated with eggs
Capillaria hepatica	+	Food and drink contaminated with eggs

Capillaria philippinensis	+	Ingestion of fish harboring lar ae
Dioctophymae renale	+	Ingestion of fish harboring lar ae
Rhabditis sp.	–	Contaminated drink; molluscs
Syngamus laryngeus	–	Food and drink contaminated with larvae
Trichostrongylus sp.	+	Vegetables contaminated with larvae
Haemonchus contortus	+	Vegetables contaminated with larvae
Enterobius vermicularis	+	Food and drink contaminated with eggs
Syphacia obvelatea	–	Food and drink contaminated with eggs
Ascaris lumbricoides	+	Food and drink contaminated with eggs
Toxocara cati	+	Food and drink contaminated with eggs
Toxocara canis	+	Food and drink contaminated with eggs
Gnathostoma spinigerum	+	Fish and frog legs containing larvae
Echinocephalus sp.	+	Oysters containing larvae
Phocanema decipiens	+	Fish containing larvae
Anisakis spp.	+	Fish containing larvae
Porrocaecum sp.	+	Fish containing larvae
Contracaecum sp.	+	Fish containing larvae
Angiostrongylus cantonensis	+	Vegetables contaminated with larvae or small molluscs harboring larvae; prawns and other paratenic hosts
Angiostrongylus costaricensis	+	Vegetables contaminated with slugs harboring larvae
Cestoda		
Spirometra sp. *larvae*	+	Water containing procercoid infected *Cyclops* sp.
Diphyllobothrium latuerm	+	Fish harboring plerocercoids
Diplogonoporus grandis	+	Fish harboring plerocercoids
Digramma brauni	–	Fish harboring plerocercoids
Ligula intestinalis	–	Fish harboring plerocercoids
Braunia jasseyensis	–	Probably fish harboring plerocercoid
Taenia solium	+	Pork containing cysticerci

Taeniarhynchus saginatus (=*Taenia saginata*)	+	Beef containing cysticerci
Multiceps multiceps (larva)	+	Food and drink contaminated with eggs
Multiceps serialis (larva)	+	Food and drink contaminated with eggs
Echinococcus granulosus (larva)	+	Food and drink contaminated with eggs
Echinococcus multilocularis (larva)	+	Food and drink contaminated with eggs
Echinococcus vogeli (larva)	+	Food and drink contaminated with eggs
Hymenolepis nana	+	Food contaminated with eggs
Hymenolepis diminuta	+	Food contaminated with cysticercoid infected beetles
Trematoda		
Watsonius watsoni	+	Vegetables contaminated with metacercariae
Gastrodiscoides hominis	+	Vegetables contaminated with metacercariae
Fasciola hepatica	+	Vegetables contaminated with metacercariae
Fasciola gigantica	+	Vegetables contaminated with metacercariae
Fasciolopsis buski	+	Vegetables contaminated with metacercariae
Echinostoma spp.	+	Molluscs harboring metacercariae
Himasthla muehlensis	+	Clams harboring metacercariae
Echinochasmus perfoliatus	+	Fish harboring metacercariae
Opisthorchis felineus	+	Fish harboring metacercariae
Clonorchis sinensis	+	Fish harboring metacercariae
Heterophyes heterophyes	+	Fish harboring metacercariae
Metagonimus yokagawai	+	Fish harboring metacercariae

Metagonimus minutus	+	Fish harboring metacercariae
Centrocestus armatus	+	Fish harboring metacercariae
Centrocestus formosanus	+	Fish and frog legs harboring metacercariae
Haplorchis pumilio	+	Fish and frog legs harboring metacercariae
Haplorchis microrchia	+	Fish harboring metacercariae
Haplorchis yokogawai	+	Fish and shrimp harboring metacercariae
Haplorchis taichui	+	Fish harboring metacercariae
Diorchitrema formosanum	+	Fish harboring metacercariae
Diorchitrema amplicaecale	+	Fish harboring metacercariae
Diorchitrema pseudocirratum	+	Fish harboring metacercariae
Nanophyetus salmincola	+	Fish harboring metacercariae
Paragonimus westermani	+	Crabs and other crustacea harboring metacercariae
Isoparorchis hypselobagri	–	Fish harboring metacercariae
Alaria americana	+	Frog legs harboring mesocercariae

Source- Speck (1984).

encystment there, are mostly related to muscular soreness and swelling and would not be confused with food poisoning. Death may follow in severe cases.

- **Diagnosis:** Diagnosis often is based primarily on symptoms since other methods of diagnosis are difficult The suspected food may be examined for encysted larvae, but they usually are hard to find, as are adult worms in stools of patients. Muscle strips from the patient may be examined for cysts, or intradermal and precipitin tests may be positive several weeks after the first symptoms have appeared.
- **Prevention:** The chief method for the prevention of trichinosis is the treatment of pork (or other meat) to ensure the destruction of any trichinae that may be present. This can be accomplished by (1) the thorough cooking of all pork so that every part reaches at least 58.3 °C, (2) quick freezing or storage at –15 °C or lower for not less than 20 days, (3) treatment with 20,000 rep of

ionizing rays, or (4) processing sausage or similar pork products according to recommended schedules of salting, drying, smoking, and refrigeration as formulated originally by the former Bureau of Animal Industry of the USDA. Directions for drying specify 1 part of salt per 30 parts of meat and holding in the drying room for over 20 days at 7.2 °C or above. Smoking should be for 40 hr or more in the drying room at 7.2 °C or above.

Inspection of animals and meats for trichinae at the packing plant is laborious and not always successful, although formerly practiced. Some attempt has been made to reduce the incidence of trichinosis in swine by control of rats and by cooking garbage fed to hogs.

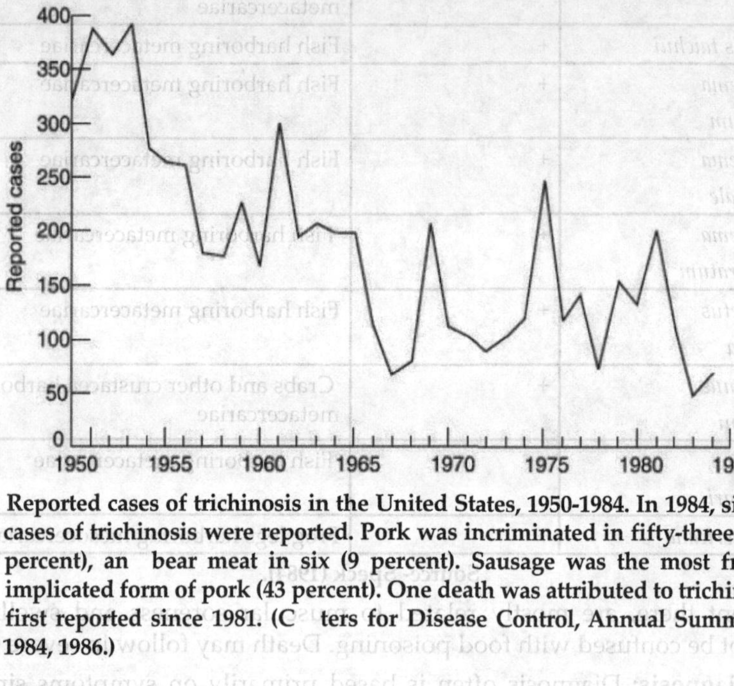

Fig 25.2. Reported cases of trichinosis in the United States, 1950-1984. In 1984, sixty-eight cases of trichinosis were reported. Pork was incriminated in fifty-three cases (82 percent), an bear meat in six (9 percent). Sausage was the most frequently implicated form of pork (43 percent). One death was attributed to trichinosis, the first reported since 1981. (C ters for Disease Control, Annual Summaries for 1984, 1986.)

SEAFOOD TOXICANTS

Shellfish Poisoning

Many shellfish become toxic to humans as a result of feeding on toxic algae, particularly the dinoflagellates, including *Gonyaulax catenella* and *G. tamareusis*. Symptoms include numbness of lips, fingertips, and tongue shortly after consumption of the shellfish. Death can result within 2 to 12 hr as a result of eventual respiratory paralysis.

Ciguatera Poisoning

Numerous species of fish have been implicated in ciguatera poisoning; however, the fish do not produce the poison but acquire it as a consequence of feeding on smaller fish which may have been fed on toxic plankton, plants, or algae. Isolated incidences of fish poisonous to humans have been shown to be a result of the fish feeding on the toxic alga *Lyngbya majuscula*.

Scombroid Fish Poisoning

This poisoning is thought to be caused by the ingestion of histamine, formed in the fish product as a result of bacterial degradation. The name comes from a certain group of fish, i.e., the scombroid fishes (tuna, mackerel, skipjack, and bonito). Symptoms include nausea, facial flushing, vomiting, labial edema, oral burning sensation, and itching of the skin. Bacteria such as *Proteus morganii* and Klebsiella pneumoniae are thought to be involved.

POISONING BY CHEMICALS

Poisoning by consumption of chemicals is rather uncommon and usually is characterized by appearance of the symptoms within a short time after the poisonous food is eaten. Antimony, arsenic, cadmium, chlorinated hydrocarbons, copper, cyanide, fluoride, nicotinic acid, lead, and zinc in foods have been blamed for food poisoning. Poisonous chemicals may enter foods from utensils, e.g., from cadmium-plated ware or cheap enameled ware containing antimony. The insecticide sodium fluoride has been accidentally added to food in place of baking powder, flour, dry milk, or starch. Lead and arsenic residues from fruit sprays may be on the surfaces of fruits but usually in harmless amounts, especially after washing. Often the source of poison is wrongly attributed to food; methyl chloride poisoning from a leaking mechanical refrigerator, for example, or poisoning from materials that are hazards in some industries has been mistaken for food poisoning.

26 Investigation of Food-Borne Disease Outbreaks

The International Association of Milk, Food, and Environmental Sanitarians' Committee on Communicable Diseases Affecting Man wrote a manual titled Procedures to Investigate Foodborne Illness, which the association published and recommended in 1976. A large portion of the discussion that follows is based on the information in this manual, to which the reader is directed for a more thorough examination of the topic, for the use of standard report formats, and for information that must be left out of a textbook discussion.

Several publications available from the U.S. Department of Health, Education, and Welfare, Public Health Service, and the Center for Disease Control (CDC) are also excellent sources of additional information. Morbidity and Mortality Weekly Report is a weekly summary of diseases (including food-borne disease outbreaks) occurring in the United States.

Specific data on numbers of cases and outbreaks in a given year can be found in the CDC Foodborne Outbreaks Annual Summary. A very completed listing of diseases transmitte by foods, including the etiologic agents, the nature of the organisms, incubation periods, signs and symptoms, source or reservoir, epidemiology, foods involved, and control measures can be found in Center for Disease Control (1976a).

FOOD-BORNE DISEASES

Food-borne diseases include those resulting from consumption of any solid food or of milk, water, or other beverage. The more important diseases and their causes have been mentioned in Chapter 25- staphylococcal intoxication, caused by *Staphylococcus aureus*; botulism, by *Clostridium botulinum*; *C. perfringens* gastroenteritis, salmonellosis, including typhoid and paratyphoid fevers, by *Salmonella* serovars; bacillary dysenteries, by *Shigella* species; and diseases from *Bacillus cereus, Yersinia enterocolitica, Campylobacter jejuni, E. coli,* Vibrio *parahaemolyticus, Listeria monocytogenes,* and others.

These microorganisms or evidences of their presence and growth are sought by the investigators of outbreaks of food-borne diseases. Other food-borne infections are brucellosis, diphtheria, scarlet fever, septic sore throat, tuberculosis, infectious hepatitis, and tularemia. Various nonbacterial parasitic infections, and poisoning by chemicals, plants, and animals and by ionizing radiations may be encountered.

OBJECTIVES OF INVESTIGATION

From the public health viewpoint, the main purposes of the investigation of an outbreak of food-borne disease are to determine how the foodstuff became contaminated and if growth of a toxigenic or infectious organism was involved, to find how such growth could take place so that measures can be taken to prevent a repetition of the same set of conditions.

This requires the location and identification of the causative agent, establishment of the means of transmission, demonstration of the opportunity for growth of the pathogen, and, in instances of infections, proof that the pathogen has infected the victims. Prompt investigation also may help limit the spread of the outbreak and sometimes be of assistance to physicians treating the victims. Publicity given an outbreak and the explanation of its cause may be helpful in educating and warning the public and therefore in avoiding future outbreaks.

PERSONNEL INVOLVED IN INVESTIGATION

The organization of the team to investigate an outbreak of food-borne disease varies with the public health department concerned, but this team will consist ordinarily of a person in charge, a field group, and a laboratory group. The field group interviews persons, both ill and healthy, who consumed the suspected foods, physicians and nurses who are treating the victims, and personnel at the place of exposure to the disease; collects samples of suspected foods and transmits them to the laboratory; collects specimens from patients or food handlers when such sampling is indicated; inspects the premises where the foods were stored, prepared, and served; ascertains where suspected foods were purchased and the conditions there; and fills out appropriate reports on these activities, to be made available to the person in charge and to the laboratory staff

The laboratory group makes such microbiological and chemical tests as are indicated by the reports of the field group and the nature of the suspected food and records its findings on appropriate report blanks. The person in charge or a qualified epidemiologist then can interpret the data from all sources to determine the cause and the source of the disease outbreak. The manual cited at the beginning of this chapter states that, at times, cooperation may be needed between the epidemiologist, the health officer physicians, nurses, veterinarians, sanitarians, sanitary engineers, laboratory technicians, and statisticians in an investigation.

MATERIALS AND EQUIPMENT REQUIRED

The equipment and supplies needed to equip a field kit to take food samples and transmit them to the laboratory include sterile containers and sampling devices for sampling, a thermometer, an alcohol lamp, sterile swabs in diluent, sterile wrapping paper, tape for sealing samples, sterile paper towels, ice, an insulated chest for conveying samples, and forms for recording data.

The laboratory should be prepared, of course, to conduct the necessary microbiological and chemical tests and record results. Prepared materials would include sterile glassware, water blanks, appropriate culture media, test solutions, serological materials and equipment, and hypodermic syringes and needles, as well as experimental animals. If possible, the laboratory staff should be warned far enough ahead to be ready for the samples and specimens on their arrival. Specific examples of food sampling techniques can be found in Speck (1984).

THE FIELD INVESTIGATION

Prompt reporting of an outbreak to the health department is most important if the investigation is to be successful, yet the information often is delayed. Reports usually come from physicians, hospitals, news agencies, or even rumors. Promptness in initiating the investigation also is important because samples or specimens may be available for only a short time, information obtained promptly is usually more reliable than delayed reports, and additional cases in the outbreak may be prevented.

Gathering Information

A complete inspection is made immediately of the place or places where the suspected meal, meals, or beverages were prepared and consumed, and the results are recorded on appropriate forms. Information sought includes the menu for the meal or meals, the source and method of preparation of each item of food on the menu, methods of storage of perishable foods, sources of purchase of foods served, and health of employees serving or preparing foods and their health history. Observations are made on infections on exposed surfaces of the bodies of employees and on the sanitary condition of the establishment.

Theoretically, all persons present at the time the questionable meal was eaten, including those who prepared, served, or ate the meal, and physicians treating victims should be interviewed. Actually, it usually is not practicable to interview all victims of a large outbreak. Geidt (1957) has suggested that in outbreaks where no more than 20 persons are involved, an attempt should be made to question all of them; if about 50 persons were involved, about half of them should be questioned, including proportionate numbers of those who became ill and those who did not; and about 25 percent of a total of 100 or more persons should be interviewed.

The information obtained may be recorded on a form such as that entitled "Case History Questionnaire" in the previously mentioned manual, where there is a place to record age and sex, whether the individual partook of the suspected meal and if so the exact time, whether he or she became ill and if so the incubation time and symptoms, and which of the list of the foods and beverages served were consumed. The case histories are then summarized on a second form, and by means of these data the suspected food is located.

Collection of Food Samples

Samples of all leftover foods and beverages served at the suspected meal or meals should be taken aseptically, and samples of perishable foods should be refrigerated immediately and kept cold in transit to the laboratory. Samples of food should be taken aseptically by means of sterilized sampling devices into sterile containers. Entire packages of foods in small, unopened containers may be taken when available. It is essential to label each sample to give information as to the type of food, the place and time of sampling, the reason for its collection, the organism or chemical suspected, and any other pertinent information. Each sample must be sealed, both inner and outer container, with the date and time of sealing and the name of the person who collected and sealed the sample written on the tape. All the information available at the time of sampling should accompany the samples, and the reasons for suspecting one or more of the foods should be given.

Unfortunately, the food samples sought often are no longer available, such as food scraps from plates on which the food was served or samples from serving containers. Then the collector of samples must settle for what he or she can get—rinsings, garbage, or food handled in the same manner as the suspected food. If a canned food is involved, part of the used can of food is first choice, but only a sample from the same lot may be available. Brand and lot number should be obtained from the can of the commercially canned food, and the method of canning and heating of the home-canned food should be ascertained. Food samples should be taken, labeled, and sealed in the presence of witnesses if legal action is likely.

Collection of Specimens from Human Sources

Whether to identify the causative organism of the outbreak or to determine the ultimate source of the pathogen that entered the food, specimens can be taken from food handlers or patients who have food illnesses. Naturally, the illness in question will determine the kind of specimen that needs to be collected.

Cultures from the nose or throat or from skin lesions of food handlers are made to test for staphylococci able to produce enterotoxin. Fecal samples are used to test for organisms, e.g., *Salmonella* and *Shigella* spp., capable of causing enteric infections; the tests might be to find carriers among food handlers or to identify the cause of illness in patients. Blood specimens from patients may be used for serological tests for the identification and typing of certain pathogens, e.g., *Salmonella* spp. Vomitus may be tested when chemical poisoning is suspected. A complete listing of suggested specimens to be analyzed as indicated by predominant symptoms and incubations periods.

LABORATORY TESTING

The procedure to be followed in testing the samples of food or specimens from human sources upon receipt in the laboratory will depend on the type of food and the information available about the outbreak of food illness (Table 26.1). A suggested guide for testing foods incriminated as a vehicle in food-borne illness is outlined in Table 26.2. The more complete that information is, the better the laboratory can select the type of examination to be used. Especially helpful will be reliable information on the symptoms of those made ill and the incubation period.

The first act in most laboratories is to make a microscopic examination of a preparation of the food stained by the Gram method. The smear is made from liquid or from the sediment from homogenized, centrifuged food. The microscopic examination may give a clue to the causative organism and may indicate the numbers in the original food if the sample has been properly refrigerated. The method of testing for the various causes of important food-borne illnesses is beyond the scope of this text. Recommended procedures can be found in Speck (1984) and in the FDA's Bacterological Analytical Manual.

Table. Guide for Laboratory Tests Indicated by Certain Symptoms and Incubation Periods

Incubation periods	Predominant symptoms	Specimen to analyze	Organism, toxin, or toxic substances
Upper gastrointestinal tract symptoms (nausea, vomiting) occur first or predominate			
Less than 1 hr	Nausea, vomiting, unusual taste, burning of mouth	Vomits, urine, blood, stool	Metallic chemicals
1-2 hr	Nausea, vomiting, cyanosis, headache, dizziness, dyspnea, trembling, weakness, loss of consciousness	Blood	Nitrites
1-6 hr mean 2-4 hr	Nausea, vomiting, retching, diarrhea, abdominal pain, prostration	Vomits, stool	*Staphylococcus cereus* and its enterotoxins
8-16 hr (2-4 hr rarley)	Vomiting, abdominal cramps, diarrhea, nausea	Vomits, stool	*Bacillus cereus*
6-24 hr	Nausea, vomiting, diarrhea, thirst, dilation of pupils, collapse, coma	Urine, blood	*Amanita* mushroom
Sore throat and respiratory symptoms			
12-72 hr	Sore throat, nausea, fever, vomiting, rhinorrhea, sometimes a rash	Throat swab	Streptococcus pyogenes
2-5 days	Inflamed throat band nose, spreading grayish exudate, fever, chills, sore throat, malaise, difficulty i swallowing, edema of cervical lymph node	Throat swab, blood	*Corynebacterium diphtheriae*

Lower gastrointestinal tract symptoms (abdominal cramps, Diarrhea) occur first or predominate			
8-22 hr, mean 10-12 hr	Abdominal cramps, diarrhea, putrefactive diarrhea associated with C perfringenes	Stool	*Clostridium perfringenes, Bacillus cereus, Streptococcus facclias, S.faccium*

Consider chemical tests for such substances as zinc, copper, lead, cadmium, arsenic, antimony: Test for discoloration of blood: Identify mushroom species eaten; test urine and blood for evidence of renal damage (SCOT, SGPT enzyme tests).

Incubation periods	Predominant symptoms	Specimens to analyze	Organism, toxin, or toxic substances
12-74 hr, mean 18-36 hr	Abdominal cramps, diarrhea, vomiting, fever, chills, malaise	Stool	*Salmonella* (including *S.arizone*), *Shigella,* enteropathogenic, *Escherichia coli,* other enterobacteriaceae, *Yerisinia enterocolitica, Pseudomonas aeruginosa*(?), *Aeromonas hydrophila, Plsiomonas, shigelloides, Camphylobacter jejuni, Vibrio cholerae,* (01 and non-01), *V.parahaemolyticus*
35 days	Diarrhea fever, vomiting, abdominal pain, respiratory symptoms	Stool	Enteric viruses
1-6 weeks	Mucoid diarrhea (fatty stools) abdominal pain, weight loss	Stool	*Giardia lamblia*
1-several weeks, mean 3 to 4 weeks	Abdominal pain, diarrhea, constipation, headache, drowsiness, ulcers, variable-often asymptomatic	Stool	*Entamoeba histolytica*

3-6 months	Nervousness, insomnia, hunger, pains, anorexia, weight loss, abdominal pain, sometimes gastroenteritis	Stool	*Taenia saginata, T.solium*
Neurological symptoms (visual disturbances, vertigo, tingling, paralysis)			
Less than 1 hour	Tingling and numbness, giddiness, staggering, drowsiness, tightness of throat, incoherent speech, respiratory paralysis		Shellfish toxin
	Gastroenteritis, nervousness, blurred vision, chest pain, cyanosis, twitching, convulsions	Blood, urine, fat biopsy	Organic phosphate insecticides
	Excessive salivation, perspiration, gastroenteritis, irregular pulse, pulps consticted, asthmatic breathing	Urine	Muscaria-type mushroom

	Tingling and numbness, dizziness, pallor, gastroenteritis, hemorrhage, desquamation of skin, eyes fixed, loss of reflexes twitching, paralysis		Tetraodon toxin (puffer fish poisoning)
1-6 hr	Tingling of numbness, gastroenteritis, dizziness, dry mouths, muscular aches, dilated eyes, blurred vision, paralysis	Blood, urine, stool, gastric washings	Ciguatera toxin
	Nausea, vomiting, tingling, dizziness, weakness, anorexia, weight loss, confusion		Chlorinated hydrocarbons (insecticides)

12-72 hr	Vertigo; double and blurred vision; loss of reflex to light; difficul of swallowing, speaking, and breathing; dry mouth, weakness; respiratory paralysis	Blood, stool	*Clostridium botulinum* and its neurotoxins
More than 72 hr	Numbness, weakness of legs, spastic paralysis, impairment of visions, blindness, coma	Urine, blood, stool, hair	Organic mercury
	Gastroenteritis, leg pain, ungainly high-stepping gait, foot and wrist drop		Triorthocresyl phosphate
Allergic symptoms (facial flushing, itching			
Less than 1 hour	Headache, dizziness, nausea, vomiting, peppery taste, burning of throat, facial swelling and flushing, stomach pain, itching of skin	Vomitus	Histamine
	Numbness around moth, tingling sensation, flushing, dizziness, headache, nausea		Monosodium glutamate (Chinese restaurant)
	Flushing, sensation of warmth, itching, abdominal pain, blood, puffing of face and kne		Nicotinic acis

Incubation periods	Predominant symptoms	Specimen to analyze	Organism, toxin, or toxic substances
Generalized infection sympptoms (fever, chills, malaise, prostration, aches, swollen lymph nodes)			
4-28 days, (mean 9 days)	Gastroenteritis, fever, edema about eyes, perspiration muscular pain, chills, prostration, labored breathing	Muscle biopsy	*Trichinella spiralis*
7-28 days, (mean 14 days)	Malaise, headache, fever, cough, nausea, vomiting, constipation, abdominal pain, chills, rose spots, bloody stools	Stool, blood	*Salmonella typhi*

10-13 days	Fever, headache, myalgia, rash	Lymph node biopsy, blood	*Toxoplasma gondii*
10-50 days, 25-30 days	Fever, malaise, lassitude, anorexia, nausea, abdominal pain, jaundice	Urine, blood	Etiological agent not yet isolated, probably viral
Varying periods (depends on specific illness	Fever,chills, head or joint ache, prostration, malaise, swollen lymph nodes and other specific symptoms of disease in question	Blood,stool, urine, sputum, lymph node, gastric washings (one or more depending or organism)	*Bacillus anthracis, Brucella melitensis, B.abortus, B.suis, Coxiella burnetii, Francisella tularensis, Listeria monocytogenes, Mycobacterium tuberculosis, Mycobacterium* spp., *Pasteurella multcoida, strptibacillus moniliformis, Campylobacter jejuni*

Table. Guide for Test of Foods Alleged, Suspected, or Epidemiologically Incriminated as Vehicles of Food-borne Illness

Food	Oragnism, toxin, or toxic substance
Soft drinks, fruit juices, andconcentrates (in metallic containersor vending machines)	Tests for chemicals such as copper, zinc, cadmium, lead, antimony, tin
Canned foods	*Clostridium botulinum* and its neurotoxins
Cereals, rice, foods containing cornstarch	*Bacillus cereus*, mycotoxins
Cream-filled baked goods	*Staphylococcus aureus* and its enterotoxins, *Salmonella* spp.
Confectionery products	*Salmonella* spp.
Egg and egg products	*Salmonella* spp.
Molluscan shellfis	*Vibrio parahaemolyticus*, shellfish toxin (Saxotoxin), *V. cholerae*, hepatitis A virus (epidemiological implication only)
Raw fruits and vegetables	Parasites, *Shigella* spp.

Mixed vegetable, meat, poultry, fish salad	*Staphylococcus aureus* and its enterotoxins, *Salmonella* spp., beta-hemolytic streptococci.*Shigella* spp., enteropathogenic *Escherichia coli*
Meat and poultry, and mixed foods	*Salmonella* spp., *Clostridium perfringens, Staphylococcus aureus* and its enterotoxins,
Containing meat and poultry	*Taenia* spp.
Ham	*Staphylococcus aureus* and its enterotoxins, *Trichinella spiralis*
Fermented meats	*Staphylococcus aureus* and its enterotoxins
Fish	*Vibrio parahaemolyticus,* histamine (*Proteus* spp.), fish poisons, *V. cholerae* (01 and non-01), V. *vulnificus,* anisakine nematodes, *Aeromonas hydrophilla, Plesiomonas shigelloides, Diphyllobothrium* spp. tapeworms
Crustaceans	*Vibrio parahaemolyticus,* fish poisons, *V. cholerae* (01 and non-01) *V. vulnificus, Aeromonas hydrophilia, Plesiomonas shigelloides*
Cheese	*Staphylococcus aureus* and its enterotoxins, *Brucella* spp., enteropathogenic *Escherichia coli*
Dry milk	*Salmonella* spp, *Staphylococcus aureus* and its enterotoxins
Raw milk	*Campylobacter jejuni, Brucella* spp., *Salmonella* spp., *Coxiella brunetii*

Source- Speck (1984)

INTERPRETATION AND APPLICATION OF RESULTS

The results of the field and laboratory investigations, if complete, can lead to incrimi-nation of the guilty food and location and elimination of the ultimate source of the cause of the food-borne disease outbreak. For reasons previously indicated, data often are incomplete, and circumstantial evidence may have to be substituted for actual proof.

When an outbreak is small, as within a family, the location of the food responsible for the illness may be fairly simple. Table 26.3 summarizes a simplified report on such an outbreak. Chocolate éclairs obviously are the food to be suspected, and because of the nature of the food and the short incubation (2½ to 4 hr), staphylococcal intoxication is probable. The source of the staphylococci would be sought among the food handlers at the bakery from which the éclairs came.

When the number of persons involved in an outbreak is fairly large, it is difficul to obtain complete and accurate data. Not all the persons may be available for interviewing, not all persons are equally susceptible to food illnesses, and people are forgetful about just what they ate. An aid to finding the offending food is a comparison of the percentage of persons who ate each food without becoming ill with the percentage of those who became ill.

A comprehensive tabulation comprises information on the percentage of people who consumed each food and who did not, as well as the percentage of people who consumed each food and fell ill. The group that consumed the offending food should have the highest percentage of sick people; this group should have a significantly higher percentage of sick people than any other group. The group that did not consume the offending food should have the lowest proportion of sick people. Finding the food that caused a significant outbreak can be done with the help of statistical analyses. Only after taking into account the laboratory results are final conclusions made about the food in question

Table . Summary of Data on a Food-borne Disease Outbreak within a Family

Name	Age year	Time of first symptoms, hr*	Food consumed								
			Hamburger	Gravy	Potato	Fruit salad	Chocolate eclairs	Fresh peas	Milk	Coffe	Canned cherries
Jones, John	35	3	✓	✓	✓	✓	✓	✓		✓	✓
Jones, Marry	33	2***	✓	✓	✓	✓	✓	✓		✓	✓
Jones, Wm	4			✓	✓			✓	✓		
Jones, Ruth	8	4	✓	✓	✓	✓	✓	✓	✓		✓
Jones, mabel	6.3		✓		✓	✓		✓		✓	✓

***Nausea, vomiting, abdominal cramping, diarrhea.**

As has been mentioned, the likelihood that an outbreak will come to the attention of local, state, or federal agencies varies considerably and depends to a great extent on the cooperation of the attending physician (if one is consulted) and the general awareness of the public. Usually local health department official are responsible for most of the epidemiological investigations and the completion of initial reports. This information is forwarded to state health departments and reported on standardized CDC reporting forms and sent to the CDC. In some instances, e.g., a botulism outbreak, the CDC will work closely with the initial investigation or be asked to conduct it. Consideration of data for confirmation of outbreaks is based on clinical, laboratory and epidemio-logical criteria, as presented in Table 26.4. Only outbreaks in which sufficien data are available to satisfy these criteria are reported as a confirmed outbreak.

As previously mentioned, one of the primary goals of the inquiry is to identify the source of the foodborne illness in order to eradicate it and stop similar outbreaks in the future. It is typically necessary to analyze both field and laboratory data in order to determine the source's location.

The completely successful investigation of an outbreak of food-borne disease finds the food responsible for the transmission of the disease, identifies the causative agent, finds the source of contamination of the food with the agent, and eliminates that source.

Table. Criteria to be Satisfied before Listing an Outbreak as Confirmed

Etiological agent	Clinical syndrome	Laboratory and/or epidemiological criteria
Bacillus cereus	Incubation period 2-16 hr Gastrointestinal syndrome	Isolation of 10^5 organisms in epidemiologically incriminated food or Isolation of organism from stools of ill person
Clostridium botulinum	Incubation 2 hr-8 days (usually 12-8 hr) Clinical syndrome compatible with botulism (see) CDC Botulism Manual	Detection of botulinal toxin in human sera, feces, or food or Isolation of C.*botulinum* organism from epidemiologically incriminated food or stools or Food epidemiologically incriminated
Clostridium perfringens	Incubation period 9-15 hr Lower-intestinal syndrome-majority of cases with diarrhea but little vomiting or fever	Organisms of same serotype in epidemiologically incriminated food and stool of ill individuals or Isolation of organisms with same serotype in stool of most ill individuals and not in stool or controls or 10^5 organisms per gram in epidemiologically incriminated food provided specimen properly handled
Escherichia coli	Incubation period 6-36 hr Gastrointestinal syndrome-majority of cases with diarrhea	Demonstration of organism of same serotype in epidemiologically incriminated food and stool of ill individuals and not in stool of controls or Isolation of 10^5 per gram organisms or same serotype in implicated food or Isolation of organism of same serotype from stool of most ill individuals, and if possible, organisms should be tested for enterotoxigenicity and invasiveness by special laboratory techniques
Salmonella	Incubation period 6-48 hr Gastrointestinal syndrome-majority of cases with diarrhea	Isolation of salmonellae form epidemiologically implicated food or Isolation of salmonellae from stools of ill individuals

Shigella	Incubation period 12-50 hr Gastrointestinal syndrome-majority of cases with diarrhea	Isolation of *Shigella* from epidemiologically implicated food or Isolation of *Shigella* from stools of ill individuals
Staphylococcus aureus	Incubation period 30 min-8 hr (usually 2-4 hr) Gastrointestinal syndrome-majority of cases with vomiting	Detection of enterotoxin in epidemiologically implicated food or Organisms with same phage type in stools or vomits of ill individuals and, when possible, implicated food and/or skin or nose of food handler or Isolation of 10^5 organisms per gram in epidemiologically implicated food
Vibrio parahaemolyticus	Incubation period 15-24 hr Gastrointestinal syndrome-majority of cases with diarrhea	Isolation of 10^3 organisms from epidemiologically implicated food (usually seafood) or Isolation of Kanagawa-positive organisms of same serotype from stool of ill individuals

Source: Condensed from center for Disease Control (1976b).

PREVENTIVE MEASURES

Means of prevention of food-borne outbreaks of some of the more important intoxications and infections have been discussed in Chapters 24 and 25. The general principles are:

- To keep foods as free as possible from contamination with pathogenic agents by selection of uncontaminated foods, by adequate pasteurization or other heat processing, by keeping away pathogen-bearing vermin, by avoiding contamination from infected food handlers or carriers, and by generally good sanitary practice throughout the handling, preparation, and serving of foods.
- To eliminate opportunities for the growth of pathogens, toxigenic or infectious, in foods by adjustment of the composition, by prompt consumption after preparation, and by adequate refrigeration of perishable foods if they must be held for any considerable time. Keeping foods warm for long periods is especially to be avoided.
- To reject suspected foods.
- To educate the public better concerning the causes and prevention of food-borne illnesses and the dangers involved.

Part-VI
Ensuring Food Safety and Hygiene

Food sanitation, control, and inspection have been considered primarily from the microbiological standpoint.

27 Microbiology in Food Sanitation

The general cleanliness and sanitation of the plant and its surroundings, the health of its workers, and aseptic procedures in the production, processing, and packaging of its food products are the concerns of the food-industry sanitarian. Specific responsibilities related to food products may include raw product quality control and storage, ensuring a clean water supply, preventing contamination of foods at any point during processing by personnel, equipment, and rodents, and supervising the packaging and storage of final goods.

The supervision of cleanliness and sanitation of plant and premises includes not only the maintenance of clean and well-sanitized surfaces of all equipment touching the foods but also generally good housekeeping in and about the plant and adequate treatment and disposal of wastes.

Duties affecting the health of the employees include provision of a potable water supply, supervision of matters of personal hygiene, regulation of sanitary facilities in the plant and in plant-operated housing units, and contact with sanitary aspects of plant lighting, heating, and ventilation. The sanitarian may also participate in training employees in sanitary practices. Only bacteriological aspects of plant sanitation will be discussed here. For other facets of the problem the reader is referred to the references at the end of this chapter.

For the most part, sanitarians concern themselves chiefly with general aspects of sanitation, making inspections, consulting with personnel responsible for details of sanitation and executives directing such work, and training personnel in sanitation. They may or may not be connected with a plant laboratory.

BACTERIOLOGY OF WATER SUPPLIES

The water for drinking purposes and for plant use may be from the same source or from different sources.

Drinking Water

The water that the employees drink must meet public health standards when tested by methods recommended in the latest edition of Standard Methods for the Examination of Water and Wastewater (American Public Health Association, 1985). Coliform bacteria must not be present at levels indicating contamination of the water by sewage. Total plate counts of the water sometimes are made to indicate when trouble may be incipient so that such trouble can be forestalled.

Plant Water

All water that comes into contact with foods should meet the bacteriological standards for drinking water, and preferably all fresh water at the plant should be that good. But this water also should be satisfactory from a bacteriological standpoint for use with the particular food being processed. A water supply may be adjudged potable yet be unsatisfactory for use with a food. Thus, for example, water containing appreciable numbers of psychrotrophs of the genera *Pseudomonas* or *Alcaligenes* might be unsatisfactory without treatment in a dairy plant making butter or cotta e cheese. The slimy growth of iron bacteria in water supplies often leads to trouble in the food plant.

More likely to be important is the chemical composition of the water, which must be suited to the use to be made of it. Thus hard water is undesirable in pea canning and in brewing; iron and manganese are bad in beet canning and in brewing; excessive organic matter may lead to off-flavors, et

Of special interest in canning factories is the bacteriology of the water in which the cans of processed foods are cooled after their heat treatment. If this water contains microorganisms able to spoil the food, it can enter defective cans through minute leaks and increase the percentage of cans of food spoiling during storage. Many canneries routinely chlorinate the cooling water to reduce or eliminate this problem.

The shortage of water in many food plants has necessitated reuse of part of the water, and microorganisms may build up in such reused water. Water employed for the final rinse of a food must be fresh and potable, but after use it may be returned for soaking, first wash, or fluming, preferably after treatment with chlorine, chlorine dioxide, or a similar germicide.

In-plant or continuous chlorination beyond the break point (the point where the chlorine demand has been satisfied) to a residual of 5 to 7 ppm of chlorine is employed for continuous application to areas and equipment where slime bacteria may be a problem, e.g., conveyors or belts, can coolers, product washers, and flumes. The chlorinated water may be applied as a spray, or parts of equipment may be immersed. When operations cease, chlorinated water may be applied to fillers, peelers, dicers, and similar equipment. Contaminated or polluted water lines are held filled with chlorinated water containing 50 to 100 ppm of chlorine for 12 to 48 hr, the strength of chlorine and length of time depending on the extent of pollution (Table 27.1).

Ice used in contact with foods should meet the bacteriological requirements for potable water. Much work has been done on the incorporation of bacteriostatic or bactericidal chemicals in water and in ice to aid in food preservation. It has been noted previously that a chlortetracycline or oxytetracycline dip for dressed poultry had been approved, but approval was later revoked; however, these antibiotics may be incorporated in ice to be applied to fish and other seafood.

SEWAGE, WASTE TREATMENT AND DISPOSAL

The food sanitarian is concerned directly or indirectly with the adequate treatment and disposal of wastes from the industry. Solid and concentrated wastes ordinarily are kept separate from the watery wastes and may be used directly for food, feed, fertilizer, or other purpose; may first be concentrated, dried, or fermented (e.g., pea-vine silage); or may be carted away to available land as unusable waste.

Care is taken to keep out of the waste waters as much wasted liquid or solid food material as possible by taking precautions to avoid introduction into the watery wastes of drip, leakage, overflow, spillage, large residues in containers, foam, frozen-on food, and food dust during the handling and processing of the food. It is recommended that sewage of human origin be kept separate from other plant waters because of the possible presence of human intestinal pathogens and the necessity for a guarantee of their removal or destruction. Such sewage may be turned into a municipal system, if one is available, for adequate treatment and disposal or may be treated separately at the food plant. Other food-plant wastes should not contain human pathogens.

Table. Suggested Concentrations of Chlorine for Various Purposes in Food Processing Plants

Water types	Chlorine *ppm**
Drinking water	0.2
Processed water	0 –0.5
Cleaning	10 –20
Sanitizing	100 –250
Rinse water	1.0 –5.0
Cooling (can)	0.5 –10.0
Conveying water	0.5 –5.0
Belt sprays	1.5 –3.0
Hydrocooling meat	5.0 –200
Fish thawing	5.0 –10.0

*As total residual chlorine. Source: Troller (1983).

Wastes from food plants ordinarily contain a variety of organic compounds, which range from simple and readily oxidizable kinds to those which are complex and difficul to decompose. The strength of the sewage or food waste containing organic matter is expressed in terms of biochemical oxygen demand (BOD), which is the quantity of oxygen used by aerobic microorganisms and reducing compounds in the stabilization of decomposable matter during a selected time at a certain temperature. A period of 5 days at 20°C is generally used, and results are expressed as 5-day BOD. The BOD is determined by dilution of a measured quantity of waste with water that has been saturated with oxygen and incubation of the mixture at 20°C, along with a control of dilution water alone. After 5 days, the residual oxygen in both control and test sample is measured by titration. The difference represents the oxygen-consuming capacity of the waste and is calculated to be expressed as parts per million (ppm) of oxygen taken up by the waste. The strength of the waste in terms of pounds of BOD is calculated as follows:

$$\frac{\text{ppm 5-day BOD} \times \text{gallons of waste} \times 8.34}{1{,}000{,}000} = \text{pounds BOD}$$

This value can be converted to population equivalent (PE) by assuming that the domestic sewage of one person is equivalent to one-sixth of a pound of BOD per day.

Whenever appreciable amounts of wastes high in oxidizable organic matter (high BOD) are emptied into natural waters, such as streams, ponds, or lakes, the 7 to 8 ppm of free oxygen normally present in the waters is used up soon by oxidation processes carried out by aerobic or facultative microorganisms. When the oxygen drops below 3 ppm, the fish either leave or die, and when anaerobic conditions have been attained, hydrolysis, putrefaction, and fermentation by microorganisms will follow, with the result that the body of water will become malodorous and cloudy and hence unsuited for recreational use and unfit for drinking and for use in the food plant. Wastes from a food plant to be emptied into a body of water must either be so greatly diluted by that water as to be innocuous or must be treated first to reduce the oxidizable compounds to a harmless level. Even the effluen from an efficientl operated sewage treatment system will encourage the growth of algae and higher aquatic plants in the water and make it less attractive for recreational purposes.

Preliminary treatments of food-plant wastes by chemical means may be employed, but most systems of treatment and disposal depend on (1) screening out of large particles, (2) floating off of fatty and other floating materials, (3) sedimentation of as much of the remaining solids as practicable, (4) hydrolysis, fermentation, and putrefaction of complex organic compounds, and finally (5) oxidation of the remaining solids in the water to a point where they can enter a municipal sewage treatment and disposal system, a plant disposal system, a lake or stream, or soil. The completeness of oxidation required will depend on the disposal to be made. Thus less oxidation might be required for feeding to a municipal system or for irrigating soil than for entering a stream or lake.

Chemical Treatment

Chemical pretreatments involve adding a chemical or combination of chemicals to the sewage or waste to create a flocculent precipitate, which carries a large amount of the suspended and colloidal material, including bacteria, with it when it settles After that, the wastewater is discharged into a biological treatment system, soil, or a body of water. Commonly used chemicals include lime and soluble iron or aluminum salts, like ferrous sulfate or alum, which result in a flocculent precipitate of ferric hydroxide or aluminum. It could be challenging to dispose of the sludge (settlings) in this way.

Biological Treatment and Disposal

The general biological methods for waste disposal and/or treatment include: (1) dilution, by running waste waters into a large body of water, (2) irrigation, in which waste waters are sprayed onto fields of open-textured soil, (3) Iagooning, by running the waste waters into shallow artificial ponds (with or without other treatments), (4) use of trickling filters, made of crushed rock, coke, filter tile, etc., (5) use of the activated-sludge method, in which waste water is inoculated heavily with sludge from a previous run and is actively aerated in tanks, and (6) use of anaerobic tanks of various kinds, where settling, hydrolysis, putrefaction, and fermentation take place, usually to be followed by some aerobic treatment.

The dilution method seldom is practicable because a sufficiently large or rapidly moving volume of water rarely is available or because the location is such that sewage decomposition cannot proceed without objections from nearby populations. Irrigation is increasing in popularity and is especially adaptable to use by plants located in rural areas and near open-textured soil. Lagooning has been used especially for seasonal wastes, as from canning factories. The wastes are decomposed slowly in these shallow ponds or lagoons until the liquid part can be run into a stream or other body of water during the rainy season or time of melting snow, when there is a good volume of water.

Usually, sodium nitrate is added to reduce obnoxious odors. Sometimes the liquid is pumped from and returned to a lagoon, or it may be pumped from one lagoon to another in a series of lagoons. Trickling filters and activated sludge systems are probably the most effecti e of the systems listed, but they are expensive to run and require supervision by an expert. Anaerobic tanks yield an effluen that needs further treatment and should be either turned into a municipal system or given an aerobic treatment.

Types of Food Wastes

An extended discussion of the nature and composition of wastes from the different food industries cannot be given here. It should be noted, however, that each type of waste has a characteristic BOD that may be high, low, or intermediate and that each presents its own problems of treatment and disposal. Dairy wastes, for example, are usually high in protein and lactose and contain many microorganisms. Such wastes, if not already acid, will turn acid if kept under anaerobic conditions and then will be more difficul to treat. Some wastes may be acid originally, e.g., wastes from fruit canneries.

Malthouse, brewery, distillery, sweet-corn cannery, and corn-products plant wastes are high in carbohydrates and likely to become acid under anaerobic conditions. Wastes high in proteins, e.g., pea- or fish-cannery and packing-plant wastes, are likely to putrefy under anaerobic conditions. Other wastes may contain antiseptic chemicals, such as the sulfite in waste sulfite liquors from paper mills, and therefore may be difficul to decompose by means of microorganisms. Ranges of 5-day BOD values reported for wastes from various types of food-processing plants are shown in Table 27.2. Most industry-related wastes have been the subject of extensive research on waste utilization.

Table. Range of 5-day BOD Values for Wastes from Various Food Processing Plants

Source of waste	5-day BOD, ppm	Source of waste	5-day BOD, ppm
Dairy plants	500-2,000	String bean cannery	160-600
Meat-packing plants	Up to 2,500	Lima bean cannery	190-450
Poultry plants	300-7,500	Sweet-corn cannery	625-6,000
Sugar processing plants	500-1,500	Pea cannery	380-4,700
Fruit cannery	200-2,100	Pumpkin cannery	2,800-6,900
Tomato cannery	180-4,000	Spinach cannery	280-730
Brewery	420-1,200	Sauerkraut cannery	Up to 6,300

MICROBIOLOGY OF THE FOOD PRODUCT

To reduce contamination with microorganisms to a minimum and obtain good keeping quality of the product, the raw materials are examined; the equipment contacting the food is adequately cleaned, sanitized, and tested; the preserving process is checked; and packaging and storage are supervised.

The Ingredients

The raw product is inspected and tested for quality, but this does not necessarily involve bacteriological laboratory testing in all instances. Some of the ingredients of some products may contain numbers and kinds of microorganisms that can affec the keeping quality of the product or even its acceptability. Some ingredients, such as sweetening agents, starch, and spices, can be purchased on specification as to maximal allowable content of microorganisms or of numbers of certain kinds. The numbers of bacteria in ingredients are important in foods for which there are bacterial standards. Large numbers of spores of aerobes are undesirable in dry milk to be used in breadmaking because of the increased risk of ropiness developing; heat-resistant spores in sugar and starch may add to the difficult in adequately heat-processing canned vegetables to which sugar or starch is added; and large numbers of bacteria in spices may favor the spoilage of summer sausage.

The microbiology of the main raw product often is important. Excessive mold mycelium in the raw fruit, which is indicative of the presence of rotten parts, may lead to condemnation of the canned or frozen product. Large numbers of thermoduric bacteria in raw milk may yield a pasteurized milk that will not meet the bacterial standards for numbers as estimated by the standard platecount method. Large numbers of bacteria on vegetables or in fruits may indicate inferiority that will carry over into the frozen product. Laboratory examination may be employed to detect these undesirable organisms and estimate their numbers.

Often there is opportunity for microorganisms to grow in a food product during handling and processing in the plant. Examples are the buildup of thermophiles where foods are kept hot, as in forewarmers and blanchers, and increases in total numbers of bacteria in vegetables between blanching and freezing. Line samples may be tested in the laboratory to ascertain where appreciable growth of microorganisms is taking place.

Packaging Materials

Packaging materials are a possible source of contamination of foods with microorganisms, but ordinarily the penetrability of nonmetallic materials to moisture and to gases is of more significance in the preservation of foods than the microbiology of these materials, for they harbor mostly low numbers of innocuous microorganisms or no organisms. Also, as indicated previously, wrappers may be treated or impregnated with bacteriostatic or fungistatic compounds, e.g., cheese wraps with sorbic or caprylic acid.

Paper and paperboard used for milk cartons contain mostly bacilli and micrococci, and occasionally other rods, actinomycetes, and mold spores, but no organisms of public health significance. Wax paper is practically sterile as produced, as are most plastic packaging materials. All packaging materials should be protected from contamination with dust or other sources of microorganisms in handling.

According to federal regulations a food is deemed to be adulterated "if its container is composed, in whole or in part, of any poisonous or deleterious substance which render its contents injurious to health."

The Equipment

Unless the equipment that comes in contact with foods is adequately cleaned and sanitized, it may be an important source of contamination of foods with microorganisms. Not only may organisms persist on equipment, they may increase in numbers when treatment has been inadequate.

Cleaning From a bacteriological viewpoint: Cleaning equipment is primarily to remove as much food for microorganisms as is practicable. Equipment may be disassembled for cleaning and sanitizing, although this is difficul with some pieces. To aid in the cleaning action of water, cleaning agents called detergents are employed. These agents may serve to soften or condition the water, improve the wetting ability of the cleaning solution, emulsify or saponify fats, solubilize minerals, deflocculate or disperse suspended materials, and dissolve as much soluble material as possible. At the same time the detergents should be noncorrosive and readily rinsed from the surfaces. Among the detergents used alone or in mixtures are the alkaline varieties, such as lye, soda ash, sodium metasilicate, trisodium phosphate, and the polyphosphates; acid detergents, usually organic acids, such as hydroxyacetic, gluconic, citric, tartaric, and levulinic acids; and wetting agents

These wetting agents may be anionic (NaR), such as the hydrocarbon sulfonates; nonionic, e.g., polyether alcohol; or cationic (RC1), for example, the quaternary ammonium compounds. Cleaning is often made easier by using brushes and water under pressure. High-pressure cleaning eliminates many problems associated with hand scrubbing. Commercially available systems for cleaning or sanitizing generate water sprays at 300 to 1,000 psi.

Sanitizing: The sanitizing process is an attempt to reduce the number of microorganisms on equipment surfaces. The kind of sanitizer, the concentration employed, the temperature of the sanitizer, and the method of application vary with the kind of sanitizing agent, the conditions during use, the type of equipment to be treated, and the microorganisms to be destroyed. Among the sanitizing agents in common use are hot water, flowing steam or steam under pressure, halogens (chlorine or iodine) and halogen derivatives, and the quaternary ammonium compounds.

Steam under pressure: It is the most effecti e way of applying heat as a sanitizing agent, but its use is limited to closed systems that can withstand pressure. Steam jets, flowing steam, or hot water may be used, but jets are ineffecti e except at very short distances, flowing steam may condense and drop in temperature as it passes through equipment, and hot water may undergo a similar drop in temperature. All microorganisms and their spores can be killed by adequate treatment with high-pressure steam. Effecti ely applied flowing steam and boiling water will kill all but some of the more resistant bacterial spores. The lower the temperature of hot water, the less effecti e it will be in killing organisms.

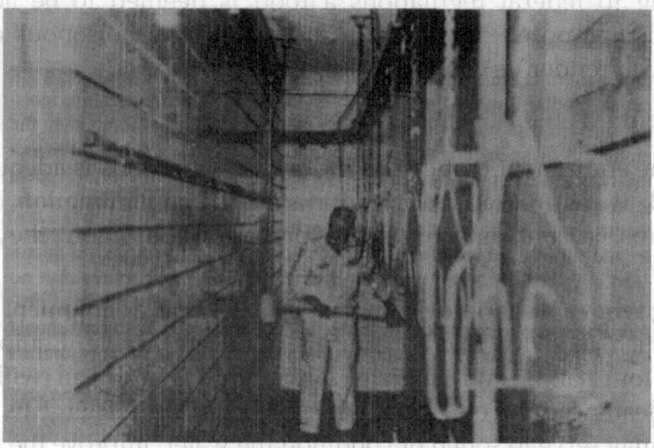

Fig 27.1. General cleanup in a food processing plant. (KJenzade Products. Beloit, Wise.)

Chlorine, iodine, and their compounds (hypochlorites, chloramines, iodophors, etc.): These are effecti e germicides if in proper concentrations and if given enough time to act. Usually, more sanitizer is necessary in the presence of organic matter. Bacterial spores are especially resistant to these sanitizers. Chlorine is used to destroy undesirable bacteria in water for drinking, for use in foods, for washing foods or equipment, and for cooling. Hypochlorites are more labile but more effective at acid pH values than at alkaline ones. As stated earlier, in-plant or continuous chlorination beyond the break point (where chlorine demand has been satisfied) to a residual of 5 to 7 ppm is employed for continuous application to areas where slime bacteria may be a problem, e.g., on conveyors, belts, or product washers. Chlorine (50 to 100 ppm) also is used to treat contaminated or polluted water lines.

Quaternary ammonium compounds: These are in general more effecti e against gram-positive than gram-negative bacteria. These compounds have a residual effect— i.e., they adhere to equipment surfaces and deter bacterial growth—but they rinse off onto foods coming into contact with these surfaces and, if they are present in detectable concentrations, might be considered undesirable. Many of these compounds are active under alkaline conditions. Most are affected by hardness of water.

Detergent sanitizers: These usually are a combination of an alkaline detergent and a quaternary ammonium compound, sometimes are used to clean and sanitize utensils or equipment in one operation.

Cieaned-in-Place Systems: Some industries, especially the dairy industry, leave pipelines permanently connected and clean and sanitize them in place. Apparatus is available for accomplishing this automatically. Different sequences of treatments are recommended for different cleaned-in-place (CIP) systems. Milk pipelines, for example, are rinsed first with tepid water, which is pushed or pulled through the system. Then hot (71 C) detergent solution may be passed through, followed by rinsing water and finally a sanitizing agent, such as hot water (77 °C or over), chlorine solution (200 ppm), or a quaternary ammonium compound (200 ppm). Often a sanitizing treatment is given immediately before use.

References listed at the end of this chapter should be consulted for more detail on detergents and sanitizers and their selection and use.

The Preservation Process

Typically, the sanitarian's only involvement in food processing is to verify the processing's efficac in a laboratory, if one is available. For instance, the lab may perform bacterial counts on frozen foods, pasteurized milk, dry milks, and canned foods as well as keeping-quality tests.

Vending Machines for Foods and Beverages

With the rapid expansion of the use of vending machines to dispense perishable foods has come increased interest in the sanitation of these machines and dispensed foods. The United States Public Health Service Ordinance and Code (The Vending of Foods and Beverages) covers sanitation of foods and machines, operation of machines, and inspection. "Readily perishable foods" are defined as those consisting in whole or in part of milk, milk products, eggs, meat, fish, poultry, etc. These are foods which can support rapid growth of microorganisms and can cause food infections or intoxications. Adequately dried or canned foods are excepted. Perishable foods include sandwiches, pastries, hot coffee, tea or chocolate, malted milk, fluid milk, ice cream, frozen desserts, and hot-food plates (meat, stews, soup, baked beans, poultry, fish, etc.).

During transportation from the commissaries and in the machine, perishable foods should be kept either cold (3.3 to 4.4 °C) or hot (66 °C or above). Slow growth of psychrotrophs can take place at the lower temperatures and of thermophiles in the hot foods if these recommendations are barely met, and excessive heat will deteriorate many foods. All parts of vending machines in contact with readily perishable foods should be cleaned and sanitized periodically, daily if the above temperature limitations are not met. Water used in connection with the foods should be potable, and waste disposal should be adequate. Most machines dispensing perishable foods are equipped with safety devices to stop dispensing food when refrigeration or heating fails.

Food Handling on a Large Scale

Large-scale food handling by caterers, restaurants, institutions, airlines, camps, and similar establishments requires adherence to common guidelines. The Food Service Sanitation Manual, published in 1962 by the U.S. Public Health Service under the Department of Health, Education, and Welfare, provides general recommendations and the Food Service Sanitation Ordinance and Code. The ordinance specifies "safe" food storage temperatures as 7.2°C or below, or 60°C or above, except during preparation and service.

It mandates washing raw fruits and vegetables and thoroughly cooking certain foods- stuffing poultry, and stuffed meats to at least 74°C, and pork products to at least 66°C before serving.The ordinance also includes regulations on the health and hygiene of personnel, the cleanliness and sanitization of food utensils, and the potability of water. It requires food to be clean, wholesome, unspoiled, free from adulteration and misbranding, safe for consumption, and compliant with quality and inspection standards. Additionally, it provides guidelines for handling pastry fillings and puddings

Sandwiches

Sandwiches and other foods may be retailed without vending machines. Such foods may be a potential food-poisoning hazard, for they often are held at ambient temperatures for 18 to 24 hr before being sold. One survey (Adame et al., 1960) indicated that the wrapped sandwiches examined showed signs of contamination during preparation and of growth of bacteria before vending. All sandwiches showed high total numbers of bacteria per gram, no salmonellae or *Clostridium perfringens,* and considerable numbers of staphylococci (most of which, however, were coagulase-negative), with higher numbers in the moist sandwiches than in the dry, and appreciable numbers in those heated to 55.5 C and served hot. Similar results were obtained by McCroan et al. (1964), who concluded that spiced-ham sandwiches and cheese sandwiches were more hazardous than sandwiches containing mayonnaise, e.g., egg-salad and chicken-salad sandwiches, for contact with the acid dressing helped repress the staphylococci. A more recent survey by Christiansen and King (1971) stated that 60 percent of the sandwiches examined contained coagulase-positive staphylococci.

GOOD MANUFACTURING PRACTICES

Several recent regulations promulgated by the Department of Health, Education, and Welfare, Public Health Service, Food and Drug Administration (FDA), specify current good manufacturing practices (GMPs) in the manufacturing, processing, packing, or holding of human foods. These can be found in the Code of Federal Regulations, Title 21. Of particular interest are the "umbrella GMPs" since they cover many aspects of the food industry in a general way. The code does cover regulations that would be of interest to the food sanitarian including plant and grounds, equipment and utensils, sanitary facilities and control, sanitary operations, processes and controls, and personnel. In addition, there are specific GMPs written for fish and seafood products; cacao products and confectionery; bottled water; bakery foods; tree nuts and peanuts; pickled, fermented, acidified, and low-acid foods (proposed); and thermally processed low-acid foods packaged in hermetically sealed containers.

HAZARD ANALYSIS AND CRITICAL CONTROL POINTS (HACCP)

Product processing lines in industry usually are distinct entities producing one item under constant control. In this type of operation, a careful analysis of microbiological hazards can be made and an in-house, effecti e monitoring system for quality assurance applied. HACCP is basically a statement of a preventive system of controls based on the hazard analysis and critical control points. Hazard analysis involves the identification of ingredients and products which might have a pronounced effect on food safety- might be consumed by special populations such as infants or the elderly; or might have no history of implication as the source of pathogens. Once the sensitivity of the ingredients is known, various critical control points can be identified. This involves the identification and control over those processing parameters whose loss of control would result in an unacceptable risk to consumers. Microbiological critical control points have been summarized for frozen foods and canned foods. Ito (1974), Peterson and Gunnerson (1974), and Bauman (1974) should be consulted for more detail.

The HACCP concept is really a sophisticated food-control option that incorporates many of the traditional approaches that have been attempted over the years. As outlined in Table 27.3, many government agencies and other organizations have relied on various food control measures, including (1) education and training, (2) inspection of processing facilities or food handling operations, and (3) microbiological surveys and testing. The HACCP concept is a new approach, but it also utilizes some of the above principles.

How is a hazard analysis done?

Knowledge that a food represent a hazard suggests that adequate epidemiological information is available (indicating that the food is potentially a health hazard) or that there is sufficien technical information on hand to indicate that the product poses a health hazard. If neither the epidemiological information nor the technical information is available or if one is concerned about a new product, information and knowledge about that product must be obtained. The report of the World Health Organization/International Commission on Microbiological Specification of Foods (Subcommittee on Microbiological Criteria, Committee on Food Protection, Food and Nutrition Board, National Council, 1985) suggests that the following questions be asked in an attempt to gather the necessary information

Table. Principal Food Control Options Available

Approach	Components
Education and training	Develop an understanding of food hazards Develop an appreciation of personal hygiene, sanitation, and food hygiene Develop an understanding of microbial contaminants and control measures Introduce factors affecting microbial growth and survi al
Inspection of processing facilities, food handling operations, warehouse etc.	Monitor adherence to a recommended or required food handling practice Follow a recommended or required guideline such as a good manufacturing practice (GMP) Cite violations or make recommendations for improving performance
Microbiological surveys and testing of product	Sample and analyze ingredients, components, and finished product Monitor for pathogens, indicators, total numbers, etc. Compare to a standard, a guideline, a defect action level, etc., and advise or regulate accordingly
"New approaches"	Combinations of the above to improve upon the prevention of foodborne diseases HACCP concept

Hazard Analysis and Critical Control Points (HACCP) is a process-control system designed to identify and prevent microbial and other hazards in food production. It includes steps designed to prevent problems before they occur and to correct deviations as soon as they are detected. Such preventive control systems with documentation and verification are widely recognized by scientific authorities and international organizations as the most effecti e approach available for producing safe food.

HACCP is endorsed by the scientific and food-safety authorities such as the National Academy of Sciences and the National Advisory Committee on Microbiological Criteria for Foods (NACMCF), and by international organizations like the Codex Alimentarius Commission and the International Commission on Microbiological Specifications for Foods.

Hazard Analysis Critical Control Points (HACCP) is a tool that can be useful in the prevention of food-safety hazards. While extremely important, HACCP is only one part of a multi-component food-safety system. Implementation of HACCP along with other practices such as good manufacturing practices, sanitation standard operating procedures, and a personal hygiene program are required to ensure the success of the program.

HACCP was introduced as a system to control safety as the product is manufactured, rather than trying to detect problems by testing the finished product. This new system is based on assessing the inherent hazards or risks in a particular product or process and designing a system to control them. Specific points where the hazards can be controlled in the process are identified.

The HACCP system has been successfully applied in the food industry. The system fits in well with modern quality and management techniques. It is especially compatible with the ISO 9000 quality assurance system and just in time delivery of ingredients. In this environment, manufacturers are assured of receiving quality products matching their specifications. There is little need for special receiving tests and usually time does not allow for extensive quality tests.

SEVEN PRINCIPLES

There are seven discrete activities that are necessary to establish, implement, and maintain a HACCP plan, and these are referred to as the 'seven principles' in the Codex Guideline (1997).

The seven principles are the following:

Principle 1: Conduct a Hazard Analysis

Identify hazards and assess the risks associated with them at each step in the commodity system. Describe possible control measures. Hazards (biological, chemical, and physical) are conditions which may pose an unacceptable health risk to the consumer. A flow diagram of the complete process is important in conducting the hazard analysis. The significant hazards associated with each specific step of the manufacturing process must be listed. Preventive measures (temperature, pH, moisture level, etc.) to control the hazards are also listed.

Principle 2: Determine the Critical Control Points (CCPs)

A critical control point is a step at which control can be applied and is essential to prevent or eliminate a food-safety hazard, or reduce it to an acceptable level. A Critical Control Point (CCP) is a point, step, or procedure in a food process at which control can be applied and, as a result, a food-safety hazard can be prevented, eliminated, or reduced to an acceptable level. A food-safety hazard is any biological, chemical, or physical property that may cause a food to be unsafe for human consumption.

Principle 3: Establish Critical Limits

Each control measure associated with a CCP must have an associated critical limit which separates the acceptable from the unacceptable control parameter. A critical limit is the maximum or minimum value to which a physical, biological, or chemical hazard must be controlled at a critical control point to prevent, eliminate, or reduce the hazard to an acceptable level.

Principle 4: Establish a Monitoring System

Monitoring is the scheduled measurement or observation at a CCP to assess whether the step is under control, i.e. within the critical limit(s) specified in Principle 3. Monitoring is a planned sequence of measurements or observations to ensure the product or process is in control. It allows processors to assess trends before a loss of control occurs. Adjustments can be made while continuing the process. The monitoring interval must be adequate to ensure reliable control of the process.

Principle 5: Establish a Procedure for Corrective Action, when Monitoring at a CCP indicates a Deviation from an Established Critical Limit

These are actions to be taken when monitoring indicates a deviation from an established critical limit. The final rule requires a plant's HACCP plan to identify the corrective actions to be taken if a critical limit is not met. Corrective actions are intended to ensure that no product injurious to health or otherwise adulterated as a result of the deviation enters commerce. HACCP is intended to prevent product or process deviations. However, should loss of control occur, there must be definite steps in place for disposition of the product and for correction of the process. These must be preplanned and written If, for instance, a cooking step must result in a product center temperature between 165°F and 175°F, and the temperature is 163°F, the corrective action could require a second pass through the cooking step with an increase in the temperature of the cooker.

Principle 6: Establish Procedures for Verification to Confirm the Effectiveness of the HACCP Plan

Such procedures include auditing of the HACCP plan to review deviations and product dispositions, and random sampling and checking to validate the whole plan. The HACCP regulation requires that all plants maintain certain documents, including its hazard analysis and written HACCP plan, and records documenting the monitoring of critical control points, critical limits, verification activities, and the handling of processing deviations. The HACCP system requires the preparation and maintenance of a written HACCP plan together with other documentation. This must include all records generated during the monitoring of each CCP and notations of corrective actions taken. Usually, the simplest record keeping system possible to ensure effecti eness is the most desirable.

Principle 7: Establish Documentation Concerning all Procedures and Records Appropriate to these Principles and their Application

Validation ensures that the industry or the plant complies with the required design or plan; that is, they are successful in ensuring the production of safe products. Plants will be required to validate their own HACCP plans. FSIS (Food

Safety and Inspection Service) will not approve HACCP plans in advance, but will review them for conformance with the final rule.

Verification ensures the HACCP plan is adequate, that is, working as intended. Verification procedures may include such activities as review of HACCP plans, CCP records, critical limits, and microbial sampling and analysis. Requirement of FSIS is that the HACCP plan includes verification tasks to be performed by plant personnel. Further, verification tasks would also be performed by FSIS inspectors. Both FSIS and industry will undertake microbial testing as one of several verification activities.

Verification has several steps. The scientific or technical validity of the hazard analysis and the adequacy of the CCPs should be documented. Verification of the effecti eness of the HACCP plan is also necessary. The system should be subject to periodic revalidation using independent audits or other verification procedures

HACCP offers continuous and systematic approaches to assure food safety. In light of recent food-safety-related incidents, there is a renewed interest in HACCP from a regulatory point of view. Both FDA and USDA are proposing umbrella regulations, which will require HACCP plans of industry. The industry will do well to adopt HACCP approaches to food safety whether or not it is required.

HACCP system verification activities include the following:

- Review of the HACCP system and its records
- Observation of operations at CCPs
- Asking employees questions, especially those that monitor CCPs
- Routine checks of monitoring procedures and equipment
- Review of critical limit deviations and non-conforming product handling and dispositions
- Internal auditing of the HACCP system
- External third-party auditing of the HACCP system
- Microbiological sampling of product contact surfaces
- Microbiological sampling of the product
- Official aluation of the product

CASE STUDY

Conducted for HACCP

A case study was conducted by Paa-Nii, T. Johnson et al., to develop appropriate quality assurance systems for cassava-based foods in Ghana.

Based on the HACCP principle, the pre-requisite programmes of the two companies were first assessed, HACCP teams were constituted, flow diagrams constructed and verified, and critical control points with accompanying critical limits, monitoring procedures, corrective actions, verification procedures, record keeping and documentation procedures were established. The study clearly highlights some difficultie that potential cassava-based factories might face in ensuring safe and quality products.

Description of Products and Intended Use

Fufu flour is a convenience form of pounded fufu, made from cassava and plantain, cocoyam, or yam flour (Johnson, et al., 2006a). Its moisture content is 6% (w/w) and has a stable shelf life of 1.5 to 2 years. It is made into a thick paste by adding boiling water and eaten immediately with soup.

Freshly harvested cassava roots

↓

Wash→Peel→Wash in plentiful water→Slice (< 9 mm) →Solar-dry at 50-60°C (Partial fermentation during drying); mill and sift through a 250-micron sieve kokonte flour

Kokonte Flour is made from partially fermented cassava chips, sun/solar-dried and milled into flour. Its moisture content (6 % w/w), pH 4.6, shelf-stable (1.5-2 years) and used as in fufu flour.

Baseline audits of the pre-requisite programmes for the implementation of HACCP were carried over a period of one month. The ten pre-requisite programmes assessed were the structure and fabrication, storage facilities, raw materials, process equipment, personnel standards, food-handling practices, quality assurance, pest prevention, cleaning systems, and management control.

Each programme had ten sub-programmes expected to be satisfactorily performed by the company. A 5-point scoring system, starting from "not performed" to "very well performed "was used. As part of the assessment, samples of raw materials, in-process materials as well as finished products were taken and analyzed at the microbiology and chemistry laboratories of the Food Research Institute of Ghana. A report on non-compliances identified and the recommended corrective actions was prepared for implementation by each company.

Preliminary steps for HACCP Implementation

The HACCP implementation was carried out a year after the baseline audits, after the two companies had the chance to correct most of the non-compliances identified during the baseline audit. The HACCP system was based on the methods by the Codex Alimentarius. To start it all, a HACCP team was first constituted for each factory. Each team was made of production and quality-control managers, three production supervisors, a purchasing officer and the cleaner. Several sessions were held with these teams to explain the principles and methods used in HACCP systems. The expected role of each member of the team in the HACCP implementation programme was carefully explained. For each product, a full description and its intended use were documented together with team. Next, the terms of reference of the management of the two companies in respect of the HACCP systems were fully defined.

HACCP Steps and Analysis

Hazard identification implies listing of the hazards of potential significance. For inclusion in this list, establishing Critical Control Points (CCPs). The HACCP implementation began with construction of the Process Flow Diagrams (PFDs) of the two products with the teams, followed by on-site verification of the PFDs. During this exercise, and for each process step, all potential hazards, their sources, and possible control measures were discussed and documented in the form of worksheets. The hazard analysis included any previous reports the two factories had earlier regarding safety of their products, recall of products as well as results of the analysis carried out on samples taken during the baseline audit. The critical control points (CCPs) were then established using the Codex decision tree (Codex Alimentarius 1997). Critical limits and monitoring procedures for each of these limits were then established. Corrective actions that need to be undertaken in the event of something going wrong and verification procedures were established. Finally, the type and procedures for record keeping and documentation were established.

Establishing Standard Operating Procedures and Quality Manual

The two companies' HACCP teams received assistance in creating standard operating procedures and working instructions for production personnel in the primary processing sections to aid in appropriate monitoring. These were printed in bold letters and displayed as posters in different sections. Additionally, the HACCP team received assistance in identifying and cataloging the laboratory analyses that must be performed on a regular basis to confirm the safety and quality of two products. A quality manual contained documentation of each of these.

Instituting Internal Audit Scheme

To assist periodic monitoring of the HACCP Plan, the managements of the two companies were also introduced to the principles and procedures for internal auditing. Two of such internal audits were carried out with the companies during the two-year period during the implementation of the HACCP plan.

HEALTH OF EMPLOYEES

The duties of the sanitarian play a crucial role in safeguarding the health of employees within a plant. These responsibilities encompass the provision of potable drinking water, oversight of personal hygiene practices, regulation of sanitary facilities such as sewage treatment and disposal systems, and ensuring sanitation in both eating establishments and plant-operated housing units. Many of these duties require the sanitarian's attention to the sanitary design of plant and housing facilities, hiring qualified personnel for managing these operations, and training employees in proper sanitary practices.

While the bacteriology of drinking water and sewage treatment has been covered, sanitation in plant dining areas deserves particular focus. Designating specific areas for employees to eat carried lunches ensures these spaces remain clean and hygienic. In cases where the plant offers meals in a cafeteria or restaurant, the sanitarian is tasked with overseeing sanitation during food preparation, handling, serving, and storage. This responsibility is essential to prevent the spread of infectious microorganisms and minimize the risk of foodborne illnesses. To further reduce the risk of food poisoning, food service equipment and utensils must be handled, washed, and sanitized following guidelines outlined in the U.S. Public Health Service's Food Service Sanitation Manual.

CASE STUDY - FOOD SAFETY CHALLENGES: INSIGHTS FROM CASE STUDIES

Studies have revealed that ice cream's microbiological quality is poor in several parts of India (Pednekar et al., 1997). *Listeria monocytogenes* and *Yersinia enterocolitica* were found in 3% of 30 ice cream samples from two distinct brands and flavors in Mumbai, according to a thorough analysis of the samples. High concentrations of aerobic bacteria and coliforms were found in a number of samples, which did not satisfy Indian guidelines (Warke et al., 1999). Both irradiated and non-irradiated samples were stored at 4°C for two hours in order to analyze them for aerobic mesophilic bacteria, molds, coliforms, *Staphylococcus aureus, Bacillus* cereus, and pathogens such as *Listeria, Yersinia,* and *Salmonella.* This was done in order to determine the effect of irradiation on the microbiological quality. A week's worth of sensory assessments were carried out.

The findings showed a significant reduction of microbial load by approximately 1–2 log cycles after exposure to 1–2 kGy of radiation. The initial count of *Bacillus cereus* (3×10^2 cfu/ml) dropped to 30 cfu/ml after a 2 kGy dose and was undetectable at doses above 5 kGy. Similarly, *Staphylococcus aureus* levels (1.9×10^3 cfu/ml) were reduced to 6×10^2 and 1.6×10^2 cfu/ml after exposure to 1 and 2 kGy, respectively. *Listeria* species were absent in the ice cream treated with 1 kGy. No significant difference in taste was noted between irradiated and non-irradiated samples (Anu Kamat, 2000). This suggests that a 1 kGy dose of radiation is effective in eliminating most naturally occurring pathogens without compromising the sensory qualities of the ice cream, providing a feasible solution to managing microbial contamination in India.

Listeria monocytogenes is a psychrotrophic pathogen prevalent in the environment, often found in animal products. It has caused numerous listeriosis outbreaks, with raw milk and dairy products being significant sources. Consuming contaminated food can lead to symptoms such as persistent fever and gastrointestinal issues. In severe cases, listeriosis can take days to weeks to manifest. A study conducted in Central India from 2002 to 2004 analyzed 2,060 raw milk samples and found 6.74% positive for *Listeria* spp., with higher isolation rates in autumn and summer compared to winter and spring (D. R. Kalorey et al., 2008). Sources of contamination include fecal matter environmental factors during milking and storage, and infected cows. Maintaining proper hygiene and pasteurizing milk are essential to reduce the risk of listeriosis transmission.

Vibrio species, such as *Vibrio cholerae* and *Vibrio parahaemolyticus,* are responsible for gastroenteritis, with symptoms like abdominal pain, diarrhea, vomiting, and fever. Contaminated seafood or water often serves as the infection source. In India, cholera outbreaks caused by *Vibrio cholerae* O1 and O139 are significant public health issues, especially in coastal regions. For instance, a cholera epidemic in southern India in 1992 involved a new *V. cholerae* serotype, leading to widespread illness and fatalities (M. Shahadat Hossain et al., 2000). In 2007, outbreaks in Punjab and Haryana affected several individuals, particularly adults, and led to a shift in the disease's epidemiology (N. Taneja et al., 2009).

Food safety hazards are also present when sweetmeat is prepared in India, especially in rural areas with poor hygiene standards. Poor practices like sporadic hand washing, a lack of protective gear, and pest contamination were found in a study on sweetmeat producers and handlers. These elements play a part in the microbial contamination of desserts like kalakand and sandesh. Because of these unhygienic conditions, sweetmeat producers in rural areas had higher rates of contamination than those in urban areas (S. Chakraborty, 2005). This emphasizes how crucial it is to teach food handlers good hygiene practices in order to avoid foodborne illnesses.

28 Regulating Food Safety

Regulating food safety is essential to prevent contamination, ensure quality, and protect public health. Food safety regulations establish standards for the production, processing, and distribution of food to minimize risks from microbial, chemical, and physical hazards. Agencies like the FDA, USDA, and international bodies such as the WHO and FAO, play critical roles in developing and enforcing these regulations. Key measures include Good Manufacturing Practices (GMP), Hazard Analysis and Critical Control Points (HACCP), and regular inspections of food facilities. These frameworks ensure hygiene, proper labeling, and adherence to temperature and storage requirements.

Consumer education, along with monitoring and testing for contaminants like pathogens, toxins, and allergens, further enhances safety. Compliance with food safety regulations is vital to reduce foodborne illnesses, maintain consumer confidence, and ensure global trade standards

The main goals of food control, regulation, and inspection are to ensure that the food received by consumers is safe, healthy, and meets the quality standards it claims to offer

REGULATORY AND OVERSIGHT BODIES

Enforcement and control agencies range from international to private, as the following brief outline will illustrate.

International Agencies

Several branches of the United Nations are involved in international food commerce, including the Food and Agriculture Organization (FAO), the World Health Organization (WHO), and the International Children's Emergency Fund (UNICEF). While they are not primary enforcement or regulatory bodies, they share a common goal of ensuring access to adequate, safe, and nutritious food. The FAO focuses on improving food production, processing, preservation, and distribution methods, while the WHO is concerned with consumer health and maintaining food wholesomeness.

Food regulation is a responsibility of every nation, leading to diverse standards and regulations across countries. The FAO/WHO Food Standards Commission serves as a platform for international collaboration to create and agree upon food industry standards. These standards are published in the Codex

Alimentarius, a collection of regional and global food standards. Membership in the Codex Alimentarius Commission is voluntary, and by 1986, it included around 150 international standards. Subsidiary groups have developed codes on general food hygiene principles and hygienic practices for specific commodities

The International Commission on Microbiological Specifications for Foods (ICMSF) is another voluntary organization focused on creating international sampling plans and analysis methods. It has conducted collaborative studies on sampling and laboratory techniques in partnership with other organizations like the International Dairy Federation (IDF) and the Association of Official Analytical Chemists (AOAC). ICMSF's first publication, which includes sampling plans and methodologies, was revised in 1985.

FEDERAL AGENCIES

Only foods produced in or transported into territories, or foods transported interstate, are under the jurisdiction of U.S. federal enforcement agencies. Nearly every day, the Federal Register publishes news announcements from federal agencies about food inspection and standards. Such data is compiled and obtained from the Federal Register by the Code of Federal Regulations. The Agricultural Marketing Service updates rules and guidelines pertaining to the inspection, standards and grades of different foods through periodic publications of separate listings.

The Food and Drug Administration (FDA)

The Food and Drug Administration (FDA), part of the Department of Health, Education, and Welfare (HEW), enforces the Federal Food, Drug, and Cosmetic Act as amended in 1980. The FDA's primary responsibilities involve ensuring the safety and quality of foods and ensuring they are labeled accurately and informatively. Two key programs under the FDA include the FDA Compliance Policy Guides and the FDA Food Defect Action Levels.

The Compliance Policy Guides outline specific microbiological criteria for various foods and animal feeds, including total or aerobic plate counts, coliforms, coagulase-positive staphylococci, foodborne pathogens, mycotoxins, bacterial indicators, and *Escherichia coli*. The Food Defect Action Levels primarily focus on tolerable levels of natural defects in foods or commodities, not directly linked to health risks. These levels specify the threshold at which products may be removed from the market. The concept of defect action levels has been applied to microbiological criteria, as seen in a survey of shrimp-breading plants, which helped establish a microbiological defect action level for raw breaded shrimp.

United States Department of Agriculture (USDA)

Through various acts, such as the Agricultural Marketing Act, the Egg Products Inspection Act, the Wholesome Meat Act (Federal Meat Inspection Act), and the Wholesome Poultry Products Act (Poultry Inspection Act), the USDA has the authority to ensure the marketing of safe and high-quality agricultural products. The USDA's Agricultural Marketing Service (AMS) and the Food Safety and Inspection Service (FSIS) oversee egg, meat, poultry, and dairy products. The AMS has set microbiological standards for processed milk and raw milk products, as well as a single microbiological criterion for egg and egg products, primarily ensuring they are free of salmonella. The FSIS is responsible for overseeing meat and poultry products, with specific microbiological criteria established for these items, which are outlined as USDA meat and poultry advisory criteria.

National Marine Fishery Service (NMFS)

The United States Department of Commerce/National Marine Fishery Service (USDC/NMFS) is a fee-for-service fisheries products inspection program. Most of the criteria applied have to do with organoleptic evaluation of the product and examinations of the processing facility. However, USDC/NMFS is involved through several memorandums of understanding with federal agencies to establish microbiological criteria for food.

United States Army Natick Research and Development Center

Food procurement and food protection for military purposes involve problems that are not always encountered in civilian food service. Therefore, the Department of Defense, through the Defense Standardization and Specification Program, has established numerous microbiological criteria for the procurement of foods.

The Natick Microbiology Branch is concerned with microbiological problems involved in military ration development and the establishment of microbiological criteria for initial procurement.

State Agencies

State Departments of Agriculture, Public Health, or Sanitary Engineering are typically in charge of enforcing state food laws. There are microbiological guidelines or standards for food in some states. Similar to the Federal Register, many states publish their own state-level publications. The Maryland Register, for instance, is a weekly publication published by the state of Maryland that includes a wealth of announcements from the various state agencies.

Commercial Agencies

Food associations and institutes often take the initiative to make recommendations or even regulate within their respective industries. For instance, the National Food Processors Association has set microbiological standards for sugar and starch used in canning. Similarly, the American Dry Milk Institute has established bacteriological standards for dry milk, while the American Bottlers of Carbonated Beverages has set bacteriological standards for the sweetening agents used in soft drinks.

Private Agencies

Several private agencies approve and list tested foods, e.g., the Good Housekeeping Institute.

The Processing Industry

Many specific food processing industries and/or companies have established their own in-house microbiological criteria for both finished products and raw materials and ingredients. Usually the larger the company, the more sophisticated its microbiological testing program.

Professional Societies

The American Public Health Association has published many recommended methods for the bacteriological and microbiological examination of foods; the International Association of Milk, Food and Environmental Sanitarians has also published Recommended Procedures for the Investigation of Foodborne Illnesses. (International Association of Milk, Food, and Environmental Sanitarians, 1976).

Agency Cooperative Programs

The Food and Drug Administration (FDA), state agencies, and the private shellfish industry collaborate through the National Shellfish Sanitation Program (NSSP). This partnership focuses on standardizing regulations for shellfish sanitation and maintaining a list of participating countries.

Additionally, the FDA and USDA jointly run a *Salmonella* surveillance program for dry milk products, while the FDA's Retail Food Protection Program exemplifies another federal-state cooperative initiative. Several resources, such as Vending of Food and Beverages (FDA, 1978), Retail Food Store Sanitation Code (FDA, 1982c), and Food Service Sanitation Manual (FDA, 1976), provide technical assistance to state agencies.

The U.S. Public Health Service and the FDA have established the Grade A Pasteurized Milk Ordinance (PMO). States that cooperate with the FDA use the PMO as their primary standard for certifying interstate milk shippers, and individual milk processors also refer to it for guidance on milk sanitation.

As mentioned earlier, the National Marine Fisheries Service (NMFS) works closely with other federal agencies, including the FDA and the Department of Defense, and has specific agreements with numerous state agencies. Microbiological criteria for shellfish and other seafoods developed by federal and state agencies are outlined in the National Fisheries Institute Handbook (Martin and Pitts, 1982).

MICROBIOLOGICAL CRITERIA FOR FOODS

The primary objectives of microbiological criteria for foods are to ensure (1) the food is safe from a public health perspective, meaning it won't contribute to the spread of infectious diseases or food poisoning, (2) the food maintains satisfactory quality, consisting of good materials that haven't deteriorated or become overly contaminated during processing, packaging, storage, handling, or marketing, (3) the food meets aesthetic standards by preventing contamination with filth like fecal matter, vermin parts, pus cells, or mold, and (4) the food retains the expected shelf life.

Establishing and implementing microbiological standards for foods is challenging. Sampling is complicated due to the lack of uniformity in many foods, making the size, location, and number of samples crucial. Standards often focus on total organism counts, numbers of indicator organisms, or the presence or absence of pathogens, but there's ongoing debate over what counts should be significant, which organisms should serve as indicators, and whether pathogens can be identified. The correlation between the presence of indicators and pathogens is often uncertain, and high organism counts don't always indicate a public health risk.

Additionally, the number and types of organisms generally decrease during storage in dry or frozen conditions. If an "average standard" is used, half of the samples might be excluded, and in legal situations, differing counts from prosecutors, defendants, and neutral agencies may lead to disagreements.

The particular food types to which microbiological standards apply must be taken into consideration. When it comes to raw food versus food that will be cooked or processed, they might be different. For instance, yeast counts are a requirement for ingredients in soft drinks, while heat-resistant bacterial spores are the focus of canned low-acid foods, and aerobic spore-formers, which can make bread ropy, may be a concern for flour standards. Each food type has a different pathogen risk; for example, coliform bacteria can be used as an indicator for oysters but not for frozen orange juice. Trichinae are examined in raw pork, whereas salmonella is tracked in eggs or egg products.

The National Academy of Sciences, Food Protection Committee, offers the following definitions for microbiological criteria- a. A microbiological specification refers to the maximum acceptable number of microorganisms or specific types, as determined by prescribed methods, in food purchased for a firm's or agency's use. b. A microbiological standard is part of a law or regulation specifying the maximum acceptable number of microorganisms or specific types in food produced, packed, stored, or imported into the jurisdiction of an enforcement agency. An additional definition by Elliott (1970) describes a microbiological guideline as a level of bacteria in a final or shipped product that triggers identification and correction of underlying issues in production or handling.

An authoritative text on establishing and implementing microbiological criteria is the report by the National Academy of Science, Food Protection Committee (1985). It recommends (1) adapting testing procedures and standards to specific foods, (2) demonstrating a numerical relationship between the standard and the hazard, (3) allowing tolerances for sampling and analysis inaccuracies, where multiple samples over time are considered in setting and interpreting standards, and (4) testing any proposed criteria on a voluntary basis. Increased consumer awareness and pressure, along with confusion over the implications of high bacteria counts, have driven demand for bacterial criteria in certain foods. However, challenges in correlating bacteria levels or indicators with health risks and the perceived low risks in many foods have caused hesitation in adopting such standards.

Part-VII

Detection of Microorganisms in Food

Microbial populations in foods, varies greatly depending upon the source of contamination and storage, level of sanitation used at all phases, the degree of abuse leading to the microbial growth, and the processing and preservation method used, resulting to foodborne outbreaks due to Infection and/ or poisoning in humans. Determining the microbial type (qualitative),number/ population of microorganisms (quantitative) in a food involved in an outbreak, is an important aspect of food microbiology. Chapter 29 deals with the detection of foodborne pathogens, such as bacteria, fungi, protozoa, helminths and viruses using conventional techniques (e.g., culture-based method, biochemical methods, immunological-based detection methods, nucleic-acid based methods) ;rapid methods based on traditional methods ; and advanced methods (e.g.,hybridization, DNA microarray, spectroscopy and biosensor-based methods).

29 Conventional and Advanced Detection Techniques of Foodborne Pathogens

FOODBORNE OUTBREAK

Foods are complex matrices of carbohydrates, fats, proteins, preservatives and other chemicals; and vary with regard to their physical nature: solid, semisolid, dry or liquid. Microorganisms are omnipresent and inhabit our environment, our body and body of animals. They occur in the air we breathe, in the food we eat, and in the water we drink. Microbial population in foods and food contact environment normally constitute varied microbiota (yeasts, molds, bacteria, viruses and protozoa) coming from different sources. The total microbial load in a food varies greatly depending upon the level of sanitation used at all phases, the degree of abuse that leads to microbial growth and the processing and preservation method used to kill and prevent microbial growth. Similarly, contamination of food by specific types or species of microorganisms is dependent on the presence or source of these microorganisms and their entrance into the food, often due to poor sanitation, during handling and processing. An illness experienced by two or more persons after ingestion of a contaminated/spoiled food and epidemiologic analysis implicates the food as the source of the illness, is called *"foodborne outbreak"*. The steps involved in a foodborne outbreak through consumption of contaminated food are shown in Figure 29.1.

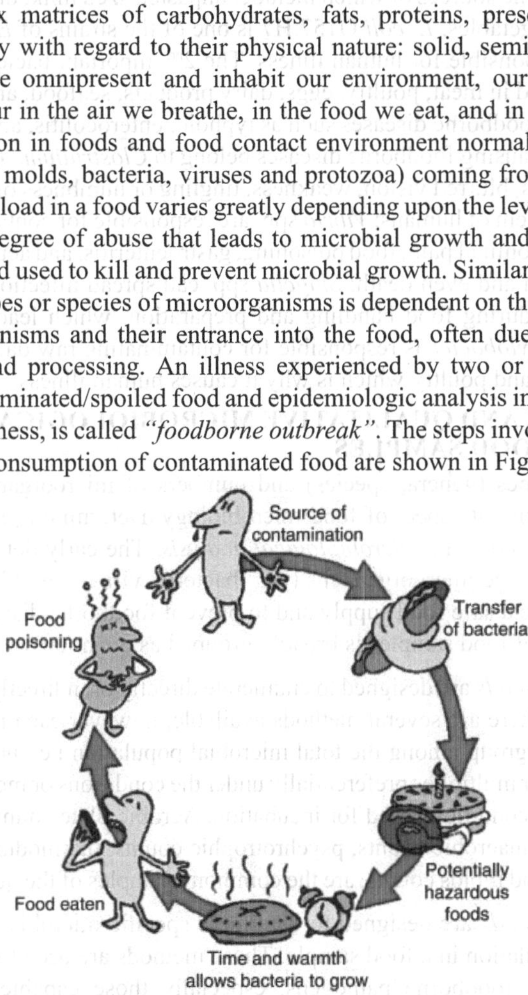

Fig. 29.1. Steps involved in foodborne outbreak

MAJOR BACTERIA INVOLVED IN FOODBORNE POISIONINGS/ DISEASES

Pathogens such as bacteria, viruses, fungi, and parasites are commonly responsible for foodborne diseases. They contaminate the food products (freshly produced and raw foods, including fish, meat, poultry, eggs, and dairy) during growth, harvesting, processing, storage, shipping, and preservation. These pathogens enter the human body through gastrointestinal tract routes and cause many foodborne diseases/outbreaks. *Escherichia coli, Salmonella* spp., *Clostridium* spp.,*Bacillus* spp., *Vibrio* spp., *Shigella* spp., *Pseudomonas* spp., *Listeria* spp., *Cyclospora* spp., *Campylobacter* spp., *Staphylococcus* spp., *Klebsiella* spp., and *Acinetobacter* spp. are key bacterial species which cause foodborne diseases in humans by pathogenic effects. One of the major bacterial pathogens responsible for foodborne diseases, is *Escherichia coli*, the sources of which include: unpasteurized milk, undercooked and raw meat, fruits, and vegetables. *E. coli* O157:H7 is one of the strains of *E. coli* that produces the Shiga toxin responsible for human illness. The 2nd important bacterium is *Salmonella* whose spp. are found in meat, poultry, eggs, dairy products, seafood, and other products of animals that cause foodborne diseases such as typhoid, enterocolitis, and diarrhea. Another important bacteria causing foodborne diseases belong to *Clostridium. C. botulinum* causes headaches, dizziness, blurred vision, weakness, tingling or numbness of the skin, paralysis, and the nervous system of humans; *Vibrio* spp. are responsible for contaminating water and food that causes abdominal pain, food poisoning, gastroenteritis, and acute dysentery, which leads to dehydration and even death; *Shigella* spp. can spread infection by contaminating the food materials during food handling and preparation, which leads to gastroenteritis and diarrhea; *Campylobacter* is responsible for contaminating raw dairy products, raw or undercooked meat, and poultry which is why it causes human illness.

QUANTITATIVE AND QUALITATIVE MICROBIOLOGICAL ANALYSIS OF FOOD SAMPLES

Determining the types (genera, species) and numbers of microorganisms (populations) in a food is an important aspect of food microbiology. Determining levels of bacteria in food samples is termed as its *microbiological analysis.* The early detection of foodborne pathogenic and spoilage microorganisms (e.g., bacteria, viruses, molds, protozoa, prions) is essential to ensure a safe food supply and to prevent foodborne diseases and outbreaks. Microbial analysis of food samples is broadly grouped as quantitative and qualitative.

The *quantitative methods* are designed to enumerate directly or indirectly the microbial load in a food sample. There are several methods available, however each method enumerates/ estimates a specific group among the total microbial population i.e., normally present in a food, which grows or multiplies preferentially under the conditions or methods of testing, the media used and the conditions used for incubation. Aerobic plate count (APC) or standard place count (SPC), anaerobic counts, psychrotrophic counts, thermoduric counts, coliform counts, and yeasts and molds counts, are the common examples of the quantitative methods.

The *qualitative methods* are designed to determine specific microbial species among the total microbial population in a food sample. These methods are used to detect the possible presence of certain foodborne pathogens, especially those capable of inflicting high fatality rates among the consumers. Examples of the category of microorganisms in this group belong to *Escherichia coli* 0157:H7, *Salmonella, Clostridium botulinum*, *Listeria monocytogenes* in ready-to-eat food.

CLASSIFICATION OF DETECTION METHODS

The detection methods of foodborne pathogens have been classified into two major groups: *conventional methods* and *advanced detection methods* (Fig. 29.2) based upon their principal advantages and disadvantages. A third category, in which traditional methods form the basis of rapid methods, has been used for the enumeration of foodborne organisms.

Conventional Methods

The conventional methods provide high selectivity and sensitivity; however, they take a long time and are labour-intensive. The conventional surface test methods are essential to know whether the food contact surfaces are being maintained in a hygienic state. These are classified as under:

- **Culture-based methods:**
- **Biochemical methods:**
- **Nucleic acid-based methods:** (polymerase chain reaction (PCR), multiplex PCR, real-time PCR, quantitative real-time PCR (qPCR), and reverse transcriptase PCR);
- **Immunological-based methods** :(enzyme-linked immunosorbent assay (ELISA), lateral flow immunoassay, immunomagnetic separation assay, and immunofluorescence assay); and
- **Ultrasound technique**:

The conventional culture-based method is considered a gold standard for detection of foodborne pathogens, since it is highly sensitive, cheaper and can provide both qualitative and quantitative estimation of the number and types of microorganisms. However, it is labour intensive and lengthy, requiring 7-10 days.

Advanced Methods

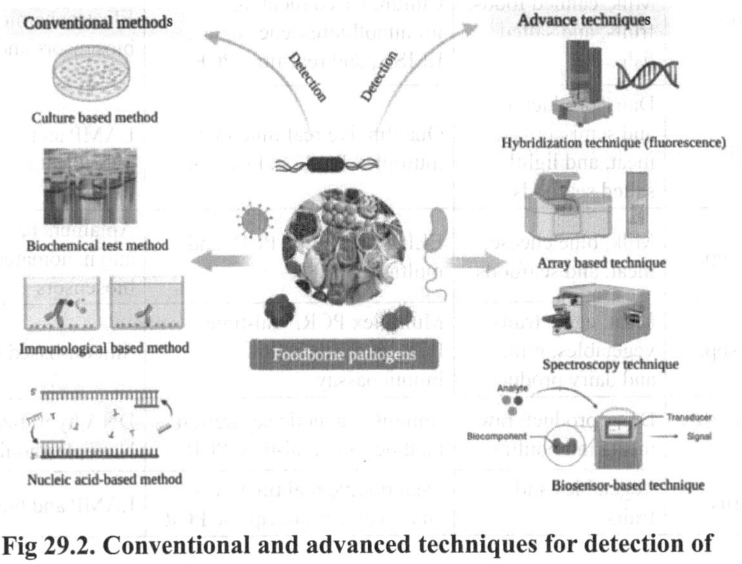

Fig 29.2. Conventional and advanced techniques for detection of pathogens in foods.

The advanced foodborne pathogen detection methods are non-labour intensive and could meet the parameters, such as accuracy level, efficiency, quickness, specificity, sensitivity for industrial food applications. However, they are expensive and require well-trained operators for running the sophisticated instruments. These include:

- **Biosensor-based methods**: and
- **Nucleic acid sequence-based detection techniques:** (DNA microarray, DNA hybridization, spectroscopic technique, instrumental-based methods, aptamers-based method, loop-mediated isothermal amplification (LAMP) based method, and metagenomic assay) have been devolved into the platform for detection and identification of foodborne pathogens.

The list of foodborne pathogens' detection methods, both conventional and advanced, is presented in Table 29.1.

Table. Conventional and Advanced Methods for Detection of Foodborne Pathogens*

Pathogen	Source	Detection method	
		Conventional	Advanced
E. coli O157:H7	Unpasteurized milk, raw meat, fruits, and vegetables	Lateral flow immunoassay, ELISA, multiplex PCR, and real time PCR	Electrochemical biosensor, LAMP, and aptamers-based method
Salmonella spp.	Meat, poultry, egg, dairy products, and seafood	Immunomagnetic separation assay, real-time PCR, and multiplex PCR	Biosensor (optical, electrochemical, piezoelectric), aptamers-based method, and LAMP
Clostridium spp.	Milk, canned foods, fruits, and salted fish	Culture based method, immunofluorescence assay, ELISA, and real-time PCR	Electrochemical biosensors and LAMP
Vibrio spp.	Dairy product, raw and semi-cooked meat, and lightly salted seafoods	Quantitative real time PCR, multiplex PCR, and ELISA	LAMP and DNA hybridization
Shigella spp.	Milk, blue cheese, meat, and seafoods	ELISA, real time PCR, and multiplex PCR,	Aptamers based method and nanomaterial-based biosensors
Bacillus spp.	Meat, eggs, fruits vegetables, milk, and dairy products	Multiplex PCR, real-time PCR, and lateral flow immunoassay	Silicon-based biosensor
Campylobacter spp.	Dairy product, raw meat, and poultry	Immunomagnetic separation methods and real-time PCR	DNA hybridization and Nanoplasmonic sensor
Adenovirus	Vegetables and fruits	Quantitative real time PCR and reverse transcriptase PCR	LAMP and biosensor

Pathogen	Source	Detection method	
		Conventional	Advanced
Norovirus	Fruits, vegetables, meat, poultry, and dairy product	Immunoassay based method, quantitative real time PCR, and reverse transcriptase PCR	Aptamers based method and photoelectrochemical biosensor
Hepatovirus	Poultry, meat, and meat products	Reverse transcriptase PCR and ELISA	Biosensor and LAMP
Aspergillus spp.	bread, jams, fruit cake, dried fruit, and grain	PCR	Electrochemical biosensor
Ascomycetous spp.	–	PCR	Biosensor

PCR: polymerase chain reaction, *ELISA*: enzyme-linked immunosorbent assay, *LAMP*: Loop-mediated isothermal amplification.

---

* Kabiraz, M.P. *et al.* (2023). Conventional and advanced detection techniques of foodborne pathogens: A comprehensive review. *Heliyon*: **9**(4), April 2023, e15482.

CONVENTIONAL METHODS

Culture-based Method

The *culture-based method* is the oldest technique that confirms the presence of foodborne pathogens in contaminated foods. It is a sequential cultural enrichment method consisting of selective and differential plating, confirmation, and strain typing. The details of this method have been discussed earlier in Chapter 18. Several foodborne pathogens from various food sources have been identified using different selective media along with incubation period and temperature (Table 29.2).

Table. Foodborne Pathogens Identi ied Using Culture-Based Method

Pathogen	Food source	Media used	Incubation temperature/ Time
E. coli	Meat, dairy product, fruit, and vegetables	Tryptic soy broth (TSB), brain-heart-infusion (BHI), eosin methylene blue agar (EMB), and xylose lysine dextrose agar (XLD).	35–37 °C/18–48 h
Vibrio spp.	Vegetables, dairy products, raw and dried fish, and seafoods	TSB, marine broth (MB), blood agar, thiosulfate citrate bile salts sucrose (TCBS) agar, and CHROM agar Vibrio (CV).	37 °C/24 h
Salmonella spp.	Meat, poultry, egg, dairy products, and seafood	xylose lysine deoxycholate agar, Hekaton enteric agar and bismuth sulphite agar, *Salmonella Shigella* agar, and McConkey agar.	37 °C/24 h

Pathogen	Food source	Media used	Incubation temperature/ Time
Clostridium spp.	Canned food, dried, and liquid food	Prototype chromogenic medium, CLO medium, cycloserine-cefoxitin-fructose-egg yolk agar (CCFA), Oxoid medium, and *Clostridium difficile* agar.	37 °C/24 h
Bacillus spp.	Meat, vegetables, and dairy products	Mannitol egg yolk polymyxin (MYP) medium and polymyxin pyruvate egg yolk mannitol bromothymol blue agar (PEMBA), and chromogenic agar.	37 °C/4–18 h
Norovirus	Fruit and vegetables	Dulbecco's modified Eagle's medium (DMEM-F12).	37 °C/10 min
Hepatovirus	Raw and slightly cooked food	Sea Kem LE agarose medium.	37 °C/24–48 h
Aspergillus spp.	Bread, dried fruit, grain and tomato paste	Sabouraud's dextrose broth/agar.	25 °C/2-5 days

Biochemical Methods

There are a variety of biochemical tests which confirm the presence of particular pathogens in food samples, such as the oxidase test, catalase test, indole production test, methyl red, Voges-Proskauer, triple sugar iron agar, blood agar plates, motility agar, mannitol salt agar, starch hydrolysis test, galactose hydrolysis test, carbohydrate fermentation, citrate utilization, urase test, hydrogen sulfide production test, nitrate reduction test, optochin sensitivity test, and bacitracin sensitivity test. Several foodborne pathogens have been identified based on the biochemical tests. Examples include: Lactic acid bacteria (LAB) isolated from fish and prawns can be identified by producing different enzymes, acids, ammonia, indole, and gas. Analysis of volatile compounds (e.g., alcohols, fatty acids, ketones, hydrocarbons), and aromatic compounds are used to detect pathogens in food samples. Ethanol and acetic acid can identify *Saccharomyces* spp., *Aspergillus* spp. and *E. coli,* in canned tomatoes.

Immunological-based Detection Methods

The immunological-based detection of foodborne pathogens is based on antibody-antigen interactions where a particular antigen binds to a specific antibody (monoclonal or polyclonal antibody). Monoclonal antibodies are more suitable than polyclonal antibodies for the selective detection of pathogens due to their specificity, sensitivity, reproducibility, and reliability. It is a rapid and robust method compared to the culture-based method to detect pathogens and their toxins (i.e., mycotoxin). It detects the pathogen's protein toxin and metabolic substances like protein, glycoprotein, and polysaccharides related to the pathogen growth. Immunological methods used for the detection of the pathogen in food include:

- Enzyme-linked immunosorbent assay (ELISA):
- Lateral flow immunoassay:
- Immunofluorescence assay:
- Immunomagnetic separation:
- Latex agglutination:
- Immunodiffusion assays:
- Immunochromatographic assay:
- Immunoglobulin G (IgG) assay: and
- Gold-labelled immunosorbent assay (GLISA).

Examples of foodborne pathogens using different immunological methods are given in Table 29.4.

Table. Foodborne Pathogens Identi ied Using Immunological-Based Method

Immunological assay	Pathogen	Food sample	Detection time	Detection limit
Enzyme-linked immunosorbent assay	*Escherichia coli* O157: H7	Vegetables	3 h	1×10^4 CFU/mL
	Salmonella typhimurium	Milk	10 min	1.25×10^6 CFU/ mL
	Cronobacter sakazakii	Fruits	4 h	1×10^4 CFU/mL
Lateral flow immunoassay	*Listeria monocytogenes*	Raw food	20 min	1×10^4 CFU/mL
	Shigella boydii	Bread, milk, jelly	5–10 min	1×10^6 CFU/mL
Immunofluorescence Assay	*Escherichia coli* O157: H7	Meat	1 h	1.2×10^3 CFU/ mL
Immunomagnetic separation	*Salmonella* spp.	Poultry	2 h	1×10^2 CFU/mL
Latex agglutination assay	*Campylobacter* spp.	Milk, poultry, and meat	48 h	2.18 to 10.17 log10 CFU/mL
Immunodiffusion assays	*Salmonella* spp.	Dairy product	14 h	1×10^5 CFU/mL
Immunochromatographic assay	*Vibrio parahaemolyticus*	Sea food	4.5 h	1.58×10^2 CFU/ mL
Immunoglobulin G assay	*Staphylococcus aureus*	Meat	70 min	3.1×10^2 CFU/ mL
Gold labelled immunosorbent assay	*Bacillus cereus*	Spices and herbs	NA	1.6–2.0 × 10^3 CFU/mL

Nucleic Acid-based Methods

Nucleic acid amplification is a molecular method based on identifying and quantifying specific pathogen genome (DNA/RNA). It is a better method than any other conventional detection method for food pathogens because of its rapidity, sensitivity, accuracy, specificity, robustness, minimized risk of contamination, and capacity to identify small amounts of target nucleic acid in food samples. This method's principle amplifies various pathogen's genomes where specific primer sets are used for replication by following three desired range of temperature steps: denaturation, annealing, and extension, where buffer systems in different thermocycler machines are used. Agarose gel electrophoresis and ethidium bromide staining detect nucleic acid products.

There are various types of nucleic acid amplification-based methods-

- Polymerase chain reaction (PCR):
- Nested PCR:
- Real-time PCR:
- Quantitative real-time PCR (qPCR):
- Reverse transcriptase PCR (RT-PCR):
- Real-time reverse transcription PCR (Rti-RT-PCR): and
- Multiplex PCR that has been used for the identification of foodborne pathogens.

Foodborne pathogens identified by using various nucleic acid-based methods are as follows:

- **PCR** - *E. coli, Salmonella typhimurium, Vibrio parahaemolyticus* and *Aspergillus flavus.*
- **Nested PCR** - *Yesinia enterocolitica* and *Salmonella enterica.*
- **Real-time PCR** - *E. coli* O157:H7, *Y. enterocolitica,* Campylobacter jejuni.
- **qPCR** - *E. coli, Listeria monocytogenes* and *Salmonella enterica.*
- **RT-PCR** - *Vibrio* spp., *E. coli and* Hepatitis A virus.
- **Rti-RT-PCR** - Yeasts and molds, *Salmonella enterica,* L. monocytogenes.
- **Multiplex PCR** - *Clostridium perfringens, Salmonella* spp., *E. coli* O157:H7, *Staphylococcus aureus* and L. monocytogenes.

RAPID METHODS BASED ON TRADITIONAL METHODS

A variety of rapid methods based on the traditional methods have been developed, such as *Petrifilm system (3M), hydrophobic grid membrane filter (HGMF)* and *SimPlate system.* 3M is one of the most widely used method to detect and enumerate bacteria in foods.

Petrifilm system, an all-in-one plating system, is a more efficient culture method to detect and enumerate microorganisms as compared to conventional plating techniques. Petrifilm plates are widely used because of their cost-effectiveness, simplicity, convenience, and ease of use. For example, conventional plating would require preparing agar for pour plating, or using agar plates and vial inoculum loops for streak plating; but for Petrifilm plates, the agar is completely housed in a single unit (Figure 29.3) so that only the desired sample has to be added, which saves time. An added advantage of this system is that images of plates can be stored for future viewing and analysis. For incubation, Petrifilm plates can be safely stacked and incubated just like Petri dishes.

Petrifilm system consists of rehydratable nutrients and cold-water-soluble gelling agent, and indicators for activity and enumeration embedded in a disposable cardboard. A typical Petrifilm plate has a 10 cm (H) × 7.5 cm (W) bottom film which contains a foam barrier accommodating the plating surface, the plating surface itself (a circular area of about 20 cm^2), and a top film which encloses the sample within the Petrifilm. A yellow grid (1 cm × 1 cm) is printed on the back of the plate to assist enumeration.

For inoculating a Petrifilm, a sample is prepared through standard serial dilution, massage using a stomacher and pH adjustment, if needed. For rehydrating the film to support the microbial growth, the top layer is lifted to expose the plating surface, and 1-ml of the diluted sample is dispensed onto the centre of the film using a sterile pipette (Figure 29.3A). The inoculum is then evenly distributed over the film using a specially designed plastic spreader (Figure 29.3B), allowed to gel taking one minute for gelling to occur, and is incubated under appropriate conditions. The bacterial colonies developed on the surfaces are counted directly on a standard colony counter and colony forming units (CFUs) are calculated based on the standard dilution used. Identification (Qualitative analysis) can also be done by picking out individual colonies because the top film can be lifted quite effortlessly to expose the gel. The results of 3M Petrifilm of coliforms/*E.coli* are shown in Figure 29.3 C&D.

3M has been used for testing of foodstuff for a variety of microorganisms. Types of Petrifilm plates available are:

- Aerobic plate count:
- Aerobic plate count with lactic acid bacteria:
- Lactic acid bacteria:
- Coliform:
- Rapid coliform:
- High - Sensitivity coliform:
- *E. coli*/coliform:
- *Enterobacteriaceae*:
- *Staphylococcus* aureus:
- Yeasts and molds: and
- Environmental *Listeria*.

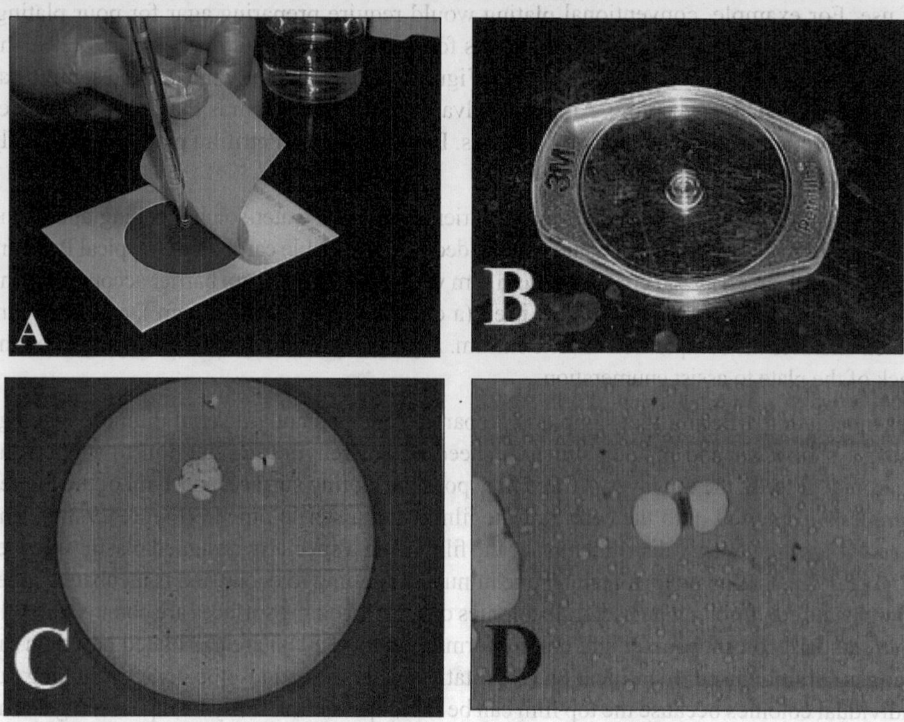

Fig. 29.3. Petrifilm system. (A) Inoculating the Petrifilm; (B) Plastic spreader; (C) Petrifilm tested positive for coliforms and (D) Individual colony of a coliform.

ADVANCED METHODS

Hybridization Technique (Fluorescence)

The hybridization-based method is an advanced molecular method based on complementary DNA and RNA sequences to detect the presence of specific genes of pathogens. Synthetic complementary DNA fragments (single or double-stranded), called probes, are labelled with fluorescent dyes and used to target the nucleic acid of specific pathogens. It is a rapid, stable, and sensitive fluorescence-based detection method to detect the pathogen by the signal of its presence in the amplification. Hybridization can be used in the assay of fluorometric, colorimetric, electrochemical, and chemiluminescent. Examples of foodborne pathogens detected through these assays include:

- *Listeria monocytogenes* in ready-made food:
- *Salmonella* spp. in spiked lettuce: and
- *E. coli* O157:H7 from milk.

Array-based method

An array technique detects the pathogen by DNA sequences, RNA transcripts, and proteins by *in situ* and *ex-situ* synthesis of biomolecules on the solid substrate surface. It identifies the interaction between the target and probe, which addresses spatial screening of the microarray format. Array technology is essential with the advantages of rapidity, sensitivity, high accuracy, and throughput. detection of Pathogens in food samples are detected by:

- **DNA-based array** also called **DNA microarray:**
- Carbohydrate-based array: and
- Lectin-based microarray.

DNA microarray is a well-established tool for detecting and quantifying pathogens that measure the genes expression level. DNA microarray is an advanced technology where immobilized nucleic acids (oligonucleotides, genomic DNA, and cDNA) are exposed to nucleic acid probes on solid surfaces (i.e., nylon membranes, glass slides, and silicon chips). It can be used to confirm and characterize microbes in an easy, fast, cost-effective, and reliable way that is better than the polymerase chain reaction. Nucleic acid probes with fluorescent are amplified with test oligonucleotides and hybridized to surface chips with target immobilized single-stranded nucleotides where each chip can hold hundreds of target nucleotides. It allows the determination of multiple species simultaneously, which provides the virulence gene data. There are four chromosomal loci: 16S rRNA, dnaJ, recA, and gyrB are targeted by 853 probes to detect the bacterial and viral genome sequences in shrimp and fish samples. Amplification and labelling of the nucleic acid of pathogens are done by multiplex PCR and the Klenow fragment-based method. However, the confusion of first-time users and non-reproducible results are the main disadvantages of this method. The pathogens identified through DNA microarray technique are: *E. coli, Salmonella* spp., *Campylobacter jejuni* and *Listeria monocytogenes*.

Carbohydrate-based array is one of the powerful methods to detect pathogens by the carbohydrate-mediated interaction with the proteins of pathogens. The mannose-coated microarray detects *E. coli* and *Salmonella* spp., which shows the allelic variation of pathogens.

Lectin-based microarray detects pathogens using a glycan which interacts with the lipopolysaccharide of bacterial cells. This lectin array provides rapid identification and differentiation of various bacteria by glycosylation. Gram negative bacterial cells such as *Campylobacter jejuni, Escherichia coli, Lactobacillus* spp., and *Pseudomonas* spp. are identified by lectin-based microarray

Spectroscopy Technique

Loop-mediated isothermal amplification (LAMP) is a spectroscopy technique used for detecting food-borne pathogens. LAMP uses four sets of primers to identify six distinct zones on the desired gene. This method requires Bst polymerase, deoxynucleotide triphosphates (dNTPs), betaine, magnesium sulphate, and a buffer. It is a more rapid, sensitive, and reliable technique for the detection of pathogens than conventional PCR due to its ability to produce a considerable number of amplicons, which is around 10^3 times higher than conventional PCR products in a short period (almost 1 hour). Foodborne pathogens such as *E. coli, Vibrio cholerae,* and *Salmonella* spp. can be detected in chicken and meat products within 1 h using the LAMP technique.

LAMP can be quantitative by correlating turbidity signals with the number of DNA copies in the sample. This method has been applied to detect multiple bacterial and viral agents such as *E. coli, Campylobacter* spp., *Salmonella* spp., *Vibrio* spp., and norovirus in food.

The fluorescent DNA-binding dye-based LAMP method helps to detect the amplification and quantify the accurate number of reactions. A visual-mixed-dye (VMD) containing calcein (precombined with $MnCl_2$) and hydroxynaphthol blue (HNB) for LAMP is used for the detection of foodborne pathogens such as *Vibrio* spp. and *Staphylococcus aureus* in food samples.

Real-time electrochemical LAMP is an electrochemical microsystem device that uses microfluidic chips or DNA sensors to differentiate targeted nucleic acid sequences of pathogens. This microdevice is small, stable, portable, and easy to detect pathogens in food. Examples of the foodborne pathogens that can be detected by rapid real-time LAMP are *E. coli* O157:H7 and *Salmonella* DNA in food samples.

Biosensor-based Technique

A *biosensor* is an analytical device that is designed to detect an analyte (target pathogen) by biological sensing elements for a specific, measurable signal, and a physical transducer store, amplifies, manipulates, and analyses the signal. The biosensor beaded detection method is easy, low cost, rapid, and highly selective for identifying foodborne pathogens. The biological sensing elements that recognize the target foodborne pathogen are called *bioreceptors* (e.g., antibodies, enzymes, aptamers, antimicrobial peptides, bacteriophage, biomimetic cell, tissue, and nucleic acid probe). They are immobilized on the surface of the transducer to interact with selective analyte molecules. A biosensor is established on a supporting matrix where bioreceptors are attached to detect analytes. The most commonly used sensor matrices are paper, carbon paste, graphite, glassy carbon electrode (GCE), indium tin oxide (ITO), and screen-printed electrodes (SPE), which are selected based on the analyte and mechanism of the transducer. A *transducer* is a detector element of a biosensor that converts recognition element signals into a measurable form. The signal can be measured either directly or indirectly. Direct detection is the identification of a target by a single ligand (i.e., antibody), and indirect detection is the identification of a target by a double ligand where the primary ligand bounds on the surface of the sensor to capture the analyte and the secondary ligand generates signal.

Examples of foodborne pathogens that can be detected through different types of biosensors are presented in Table 29.5.

Table. Different Types of Biosensors Used to Identify Foodborne Pathogens

Biosensor wtype	Target pathogen	Source	Bioreceptor	Electrode	Detection limit	Assay time
Amperometric biosensor	*Escherichia coli* O157: H7	Milk	Antibody	Nickel oxide thin film	10 cells/ mL	–
	Salmonella Typhimurium	Milk	Antibody	Gold screen-printed	10 CFU/ mL	125 min

Biosensor wtype	Target pathogen	Source	Bioreceptor	Electrode	Detection limit	Assay time
Voltammetric biosensor	*Listeria monocytogenes*	Dairy products, meat	Enzyme	Gold nanoparticles carbon	9 CFU/ mL	1 min
	Salmonella spp.	Milk	Antibody	Urease coated gold nanoparticles	10^1 CFU/ mL	14 min
Potentiometric biosensor	*Salmonella typhimurium*	Apple juice	Antibody	Paper-based strip	5 cells/ mL	1 h
	Staphylococcus aureus	Pig	Cell	Aptamer based graphene	8×10^2 CFU/mL	–
Impedimetric biosensor	*Salmonella* spp.	Milk	Cell	Nisin molecules with gold	1.5×10^1 CFU/mL	1 min
	Escherichia coli O157:H7	Culture	Cell	Fabricated affinity peptides	20 CFU/ mL	30 min
Colorimetric biosensor	*Staphylococcus aureus*	Culture	DNA	Aptamer based	81 CFU/ mL	5.5 h
	Campylobacter jejuni	Chicken, meat	Antibody	Lactoferrin-based	10 CFU/ mL	20 min
Fluorescent biosensor	*Escherichia coli* O157:H7	Apple juice	Protein	Magnetic DNAzyme-copper	1.57 CFU/mL	1.5 h
	Listeria monocytogenes	Culture	Cell	Aptamer-functionalized up conversion nanoparticles	8 CFU/ mL	2 h
SPR biosensor	*Campylobacter jejuni*	Chicken	Antibody	surface plasmon resonance	131 ± 4 CFU/mL	–
	Listeria monocytogenes	Milk	Carbohydrate	Wheat germ agglutinin	3.25 log CFU/100	–
SERS biosensor	*Salmonella typhimurium*	Culture	DNA	Gold modified magnetic nanoparticles	4 CFU/ mL	40 min
	Staphylococcus aureus	Orange juice	Cell	Aptamer-Fe_3O_4@Au magnetic nanoparticles	21.1 ± 1.5 cell/mL	50 min
Piezoelectric biosensor	*Campylobacter jejuni*	Poultry	Antibody	Magnetic nanobeads	20–30 CFU/mL	30 min
QCM biosensor	*Escherichia coli* O157:H7	Culture	DNA	Aptamer based quartz crystal microbalance	1.46×10^3 CFU/ mL	50 min

Biosensor wtype	Target pathogen	Source	Bioreceptor	Electrode	Detection limit	Assay time
SAW biosensor	*Escherichia coli*	Packaged food	Antibody	Aluminium nitride based	6.54 × 10^5 CFU/mL	10 min
Magnetostrictive biosensor	*Salmonella Typhimurium*	Poultry and meat	Cell	Carbon-coated copper grid	10^8 CFU/mL	25 min

SPR: Surface plasmon resonance, *SERS:* Surface-enhanced Raman scattering, *QCM:* quartz crystal microbalance, *SAW:* surface acoustic wave, *CFU:* colony forming unit.

Nanomaterial-based Biosensor

A *nanomaterial-based biosensor* is a novel biosensor with electricity, optics, mechanics, and thermal properties developed as a sensing platform for detecting pathogens in food samples. It provides rapid, portable, sensitive, and direct on-site detection of the target pathogen. Examples of nanomaterials used in this biosensor are

- **Metallic nanomaterials** - Gold (AuNPs), silver (AgNPs), platinum (PtNPs), and palladium (PdNPs);
- **Metal oxide nanomaterials -** Erium dioxide (CeO_2) and copper oxide (CuO);
- **Magnetic nanomaterials (MNPs)** - NiO, CO_3O_4, and Fe_2O_3;
- **Carbon nanomaterials** - Carbon nanotubes (CNTs) and graphene;
- **Polymer nanomaterials** - Dendrimers, conducting polymers, and molecularly imprinted polymers;
- **Quantum dots (QDs)**;
- **Upconverting nanomaterials (UCNPs)**; and
- **Transition metal dichalcogenides (TMDs)**.

The nanomaterials can interact with target pathogens to produce a measurable signal. Examples of foodborne pathogens detected include *Listeria monocytogenes, Salmonella enterica,* and *Vibrio parahaemolyticus*.

Appendix A

Since the writing of the third edition of this textbook, many changes have been made in the classification and taxonomy of bacteria. The importance of codes of nomenclature is obvious, but we continue to use the names of organisms as they appeared in the literature by the original authors. Several of these original names have been changed or eliminated in later editions of *Bergey's Manual*. For one reason or another, the following are no longer "accepted" names. In all instances, lack of acceptance is based on *Bergey's Manual of systematic Bacteriology*, Vol. 1 (1984) and Vol. 2 (1986), unless otherwise stated. A brief statement on the current status of each organism is presented.

- ***Acetobacter aceti:*** subsp. *suboxydans* was not given any taxonomical status in Vol. 1.
- ***Acetobacter aceti:*** subsp. *xylinum,* a cellulose-synthesizing strain, is considered a synonym of *A. pasteurianus.*
- ***Acetobacter acetigenum:*** was an accepted species in the 6th ed. of Bergey's Manual but did not appear in the 7th or 8th eds. or in Vol. 1.
- ***Acetobacter capsulatum:*** was listed as a synonym of *Gluconobacter oxydans subsp. industrius* in the 8th ed. of Bergey's Manual. However, subsp. industrius was not recognized in Vol. 1.
- ***Acetobacter oxydans:*** was listed as a synonym of *Gluconobacter oxydans* in the 8th ed. of Bergey's Manual.
- ***Acetobacter suboxydans:*** was listed as a synonym of *Gluconobacter oxydans* subsp. *suboxydans*. However, the latter subsp. was not recognized in Vol. 1.
- ***Acetobacter turbidans:*** was listed as a synonym of *Acetobacter pasteurianus* in the 8th ed. of Bergey's Manual.
- ***Acetobacter viscosum:*** was listed as a synonym of *Gluconobacter oxydans* subsp. *industrius* in the 8th ed. of Bergey's Manual. However, the latter subsp. as not recognized in Vol. 1.
- ***Acetobacter xylinum:*** was listed as a synonym of *Acetobacter aceti* subsp. *xylinum* in the 8th ed. of Bergey's Manual; the latter was listed as a synonym of *A. pasteurianus* in Vol. 1.

- ***Achromobacter:*** many of the species previously listed in this genus are now species in the genera *Alcaligenes* and *Zymomonas*.
- ***Achromobacter anaerobium:*** was listed as a synonym of *Zymomonas anaerobia* in the 8th ed. of Bergey's Manual. *Z. anaerobia* was listed as synonym of *Z. mobilis* in Vol. 1.
- ***Achromobacter perolens:*** was listed as a synonym of *Pseudomonas perolens* in the 7th ed. of Bergey's Manual. It was not listed in Vol. 1.
- ***Aerobacillus:*** the species of this previously proposed genus (8th ed.) were listed as species of the genus *Bacillus*.
- ***Aerobacter:*** the species previously listed in this genus were incorporated into species in the genera *Enterobacter* and *Klebsiella* in the 8th ed. of Bergey's Manual.
- ***Aerobacter cloacae:*** was listed as a synonym of *Entobacter cloacae* in the 8th ed. of Bergey's Manual.
- ***Alcaligenes metalcaligenes:*** was an accepted species in the 7th ed. but was not listed in the 8th ed. or in Vol. 1.
- ***Alcaligenes viscolactis:*** was an accepted species in the 7th ed. of Bergey's Manual. It was not listed in the 8th ed., and it is not listed in Vol. 1.
- ***Bacillus betanigrificans:*** was listed as a synonym of *B. macerans* in the 8th ed. of Bergey's Manual.
- ***Bacillus citri:*** was listed as a synonym of *Xanthomonas citri* in the 6th ed. of Bergey's Manual but did not appear as a synonym of *X. citri* in the 7th ed.; *X. citri* is listed in the 8th ed. as a nomenspecies of *X. campestris; Xanthomonas (Bacillus)* citri is therefore distinguishable from *X. campestris* only by plant-host reactions.
- ***Bacillus globigii:*** was not listed in Vol. 2. (1986).
- ***Bacillus mesentericus:*** was listed in the 8th ed. of Bergey's Manual but it lacked a type culture and was thought to be indistinguishable from *B. subtilis*. Vol. 2. did not list *B. mesentericus*.
- ***Bacillus natto:*** was listed as a synonym of *B. subtilis* in the 8th ed. of Bergey's Manual.
- ***Bacillus nigrificans:*** was listed as a synonym of *B. subtilis* var. *atterrimum* in the 6th ed. of Bergey's Manual. The latter var. was not recognized in Vol. 2 but was included in the species *B. subtilis*.
- ***Bacillus subtilis:*** var. niger was considered by Vol. 2. (1986) as *B. subtilis* and not given separate taxonomical status.
- ***Bacillus vulgatus:*** was listed in the 8th ed. as not having a type culture and being indistinguishable from *B. subtilis*. It was not listed in Vol. 2.
- ***Brevibacterium erythrogenes:*** was listed as a species incertae sedis in the 8th ed. of Bergey's Manual; it was not listed in Vol. 1. (1984).

- ***Clostridium calidotolerans:*** was not given any taxonomical status in Vol. 2 (1986).
- ***Clostridium lentoputrescens:*** is homologous with type strain *C. cochlearium.*
- ***Clostridium nigrificans:*** was listed as a synonym of *Desulfotomaculum nigrificans* in the 8th ed. of Bergey's Manual.
- ***Clostridium putida:*** was not listed as a species name in Vol. 2.
- ***Enterobacter oxytocum:*** was not listed in Vol. 1 (1984).
- ***Erwinia carotovora:*** subsp. *betavasculorum*: a new subspecies proposed.
- ***Flavobacterium proteus:*** is now *Obesumbacterium proteus.*
- ***Flavobacterium rhenanum:*** was listed as a synonym of *Erwinia* herbicola in the 8th ed. of Bergey's Manual.
- ***Gluconobacter oxydans:*** subsp. *suboxydans* and subsp. *industrius* were not considered subsp. in Vol. 2. (1986). All are referred to as G. oxydans.
- ***Halobacterium cutirubum:*** is listed as a synonym of *Halobacterium salinarium.*
- ***Lactobacillus arabinosus:*** was listed as a synonym of *Lactobacillus plantarum* in the 8th ed. of Bergey's Manual. It was not listed in Vol. 2.
- ***Lactobacillus brevis:*** var. *rudensis* was not listed in Vol. 2. (1986).
- ***Lactobacillus bulgaricus:*** is now a subspecies of *L. delbrueckii.*
- ***Lactobacillus diastaticus:*** was not listed in Vol. 2.
- ***Lactobacillus lactis:*** is now a subspecies of *L. delbrueckii.*
- ***Lactobacillus leichmanii:*** is listed as *L. delbrueckii* subsp. *lactis.*
- ***Lactobacillus pastorianus:*** was listed as a species incertae sedis in the 8th ed. of Bergey's Manual; it is not given any taxonomical status in Vol 2.
- ***Lactobacillus plantarum:*** var. *rudensis* was listed as a synonym of *L. plantarum* in the 8th ed. of Bergey's Manual.
- ***Lactobacillus salinmandus:*** is not given any taxonomical status in Vol. 2.
- ***Lactobacillus thermophilus:*** was originally described as producing endospores. It was suggested to be similar to, if not identical to, *Bacillus coagulans* in the 8th ed. of Bergey's Manual. It was not given any taxonomical status in Vol. 2.
- ***Lactobacillus trichodes:*** was listed as a junior subjective synonym of *L. fructivorans* in Vol. 2.
- ***Lactobacillus vermiformis:*** was listed as *B. vermiforme* in the 6th ed. of Bergey's Manual, as a slime-forming *lactobacillus,* but did not appear in the 7th or 8th eds. or in Vol. 2.
- ***Leuconostoc citrovorum:*** was listed as a synonym of *Leuconostoc cremoris in the 8th ed.; however, L. cremoris is now listed as L. mesenteroides subsp. cremoris.*

- ***Leuconostoc cremoris:*** is now listed as *L. mesenteroides* subsp. *cremoris*.
- ***Leuconostoc dextranicum:*** is now listed as *L. mesenteroides* subsp. *dextranicum*.
- **Microccoci***:* see the following category.
- ***Micrococcus:*** this genus has been extensively altered in recent publications of Bergey's Manual. The number of species in the 8th edition had been reduced from sixteen to three; the genus *Sarcina* was retained for the anaerobic packet-forming cocci. Bergey's Manual. Vol. 2 (1986), lists nine species but suggests that the micrococci should probably be in the genus *Arthrobacter*.
- ***Micrococcus candidus:*** was not listed in Vol. 2.
- ***Micrococcus caseolyticus:*** was listed as an accepted species in the 7th ed. of Bergey's Manual; it was not listed in the 8th. In Vol. 2 it is mentioned in the section dealing with *Staphylococcus caseolyticus*.
- ***Micrococcus freudenreichii:*** was listed as a species incertae sedis in the 8th ed. of Bergey's Manual. It is not given any taxonomical status in either Vol. 1 or Vol. 2.
- ***Micrococcus lipolyticus:*** was listed in the 6th ed. of Bergey's Manual for historical interest as a fat-splitting micrococcus from salted fis
- ***Paracolobactrum:*** according to the 8th ed. this genus was proposed to include late or non-lactose-fermenting coliform bacteria; this is no longer justified. These organisms should have been place in the genera *Escherichia, Citrobacter*, or *Klebsiella*.
- ***Pediococcus cerevisiae:*** as a species name has been rejected by Vol. 2, and the genus name *Pediococcus* is conserved by the species name damnosus. P. damnosus occurs in beer and the brewing industry, *P. pentosacens* is used in meat fermentations, and *P. halophilus* occurs in pickling brines.
- ***Pediococcus soyae:*** was listed as synonym of *Pediococcus halophilus* in the 8th ed. of Bergey's Manual.
- ***Propionibactacerium shermanii:*** was listed as a synonym of Propionibacterium freudenreichii. Vol. 1 has listed as *P. freudenreichii* subsp. *shermanii*.
- ***Proteus melanovogenes:*** was listed as a synonym of *Aeromonas hydrophila* in the 8th ed. of Bergey's Manual.
- ***Pseudomonas graveolens:*** was listed as synonym of *P. taetrolens* in the 7th ed. The 8th ed. of Bergey's Manual listed *P. taetrolens* as a species *incertae* sedis. Vol. 1 has given *P. taetrolelns* species status.
- ***Pseudomonas nigrifaciens:*** is listed as a *speciesincertae* sedis and is said to be more closely related to the genus *Alteromonas*.

- ***Pseudomonas putrefaciens:*** was listed in the 8th ed. of Bergey's Manual as a *Speciesincertae sedis*. Vol. 1 lists the organism under *Alteromonas putrefaciens,* which is currently a species incertae sedis.
- ***Pseudomonas sapolactica:*** was listed as a *speciesincertae sedis* in the 8th ed. of Bergey's Manual; it was not listed in Vol. 1.
- ***Pseudomonas syncyanea:*** was listed in the 8th ed. of Bergey's Manual as a *speciesincertae* sedis; it was not given any taxonomical significance in Vol. 1.
- ***Pseudomonas visosa:*** was listed in the 6th ed. of Bergey's Manual but has not appeared since.
- ***Sarcina lutea:*** was not listed as a valid species in Vol. 2. *S. lutea* is a packet-forming gram-positive aerobic cocci; only the anaerobic species were retained in the genus *Sarcina.* Aerobic non-spore-forming *Sarcina* were assigned to the genus *Micrococcus.*
- ***Serratia salinaria:*** was listed as a synonym of *Halobacterium salinarium* in the 8th ed. of Bergey's Manual.
- ***Streptococcus cremoris:*** is now considered a synonym of *S. lactis.* A new subsp., *S. lactis* subsp. *cremoris,* has been proposed.
- ***Streptococcus durans:*** was listed as a synonym of *S. faecium* in the 8th ed. of Bergey's Manual; it was not given any taxonomical status in Vol. 2.
- ***Streptococcus faecalis:*** subsp. *liquefaciens* is now considered a synonym of *S. faecalis.*
- ***Streptococcus faecalis:*** subsp. *zymogenes* is now considered a synonym of *S. faecalis.*
- ***Streptococcus faecium***: subsp. *durans* is not given any taxonomical status in Vol. 2.
- ***Streptococcus lactis:*** was a recognized species in Vol. 2. However, a new subsp., *S. lactis* subsp. *lactis,* has been proposed.
- ***Streptococcus lactis:*** subsp. *cremoris* was not recognized in Vol. 2, but it is proposed as a subsp.
- ***Streptococcus lactis:*** subsp. *diacetylactis* was listed as a synonym of *S. lactis.* A subsp., *S. lactis* subsp. diacetilactis has been proposed.
- ***Streptococcus lactis:*** subsp. *lactis* was not recognized in Vol. 2, but it is proposed as a subsp.
- ***Streptococcus lactis:*** var. *maltigenes* was not a recognized name in Vol. 2 (1986).

Appendix B

International Microbiological Specifications

The following tables are reprinted from An Evaluation of the Role of Microbiological Criteria for Foods and Food Ingredients, 1985, National Academy Press, Washington, D.C., with permission. The letters symbols in the tables are defined as follows:

n = number of sample units analyzed which are chosen separately and independently.

c = maximum allowable number of sample units yielding unsatisfactory test results, e.g., the presence of the organism, or a count above m.

m = a microbiological criterion that in a 2-class plan separates good quality from defective quality, or in a 3-class plan separates good quality from marginally acceptable quality.

M = a microbiological criterion that in a 3-class plan separates marginally acceptable quality from defective quality. Values at or above M are unacceptable.

case = a set of circumstances related to the nature and treatment of a food, categorized into 15 such sets which influence the anticipated hazard from the presence of specified bacterial species or groups within a food (ICMSF, 1974).

Table . FAO/WHO Expert Consultation on Microbiological Specifications for Foods- Egg Products

Product	Test	n	c	m	M
Dried frozen whole egg	Mesophilic aerobic bacteria	5	2	5×10^4	10^6
	Coliform	5	2	10	10^3
	Salmonella	10	0	0	–
Other egg product	*Salmonella*	10	0	0	–
Any egg product intended for special purpose	*Salmonella*	30	0	0	–

Source: CAC/RCP 15, 1976

Table. FAO/WHO Expert Consultation on Microbiological Specifications fo Foods- Foods for Infants and Children

Product	Test	Case	n	c	m	M
Dried biscuit, plain, coated	None	–	–	–	–	
	Coliform	5	5	2	<3	20
	Salmonella	11	10	0	0	–
Dried instant products	Mesophilic aerobic bacteria	6	5	2	10^3	10^4
	Coliform	6	5	1	<3	20
	Salmonella	10	60	0	0	–

Product	Test	Case	n	c	m
Dried products requiring heating before consumption	Mesophilic aerobic bacteria	4	5	3	10^4
	Coliform	4	5	2	10
	Salmonella	10	5	0	0

Source: CAC/RCP 21, 1979.

Table. FAO/WHO Expert Consultation on Microbiological Specifications fo Foods- Precooked Frozen Shrimp and Prawns

Test	n	c	m	M
Mesophilic aerobic bacteria	5	2	10^5	10^6
Staphylococcus aureus	5	2	5×10^2	5×10^3
Salmonella	5	0	0	–

Source: CAC/RCP 17, 1978.

Table. FAO/WHO Expert Consultation on Microbiological Specifications fo Foods- Ice Mixes

Test	n	c	m	M
Mesophilic aerobic bacteria	5	2	2.5×10^4	10^5
Coliform	5	2	10	10^2
Salmonella	10	0	0	–

Source: Report of 2nd joint FAO/WHO Expert Consultation, 1977.

Table. FAO/WHO Expert Consultation on Microbiological Specifications fo Foods- Edible Ices

Test	n	c	m	M
Mesophilic aerobic bacteria	5	2	5×10^4	2.5×10^5
Coliform	5	2	10^2	10^3
Salmonella	10	0	0	–

Source: Report of 2nd joint FAO/WHO Expert Consultation, 1977.

Table. International Dairy Federation Proposed Microbiological Specifications for Drie Milk, 1982.

Test	n	c	m	M
Mesophilic count	5	2	5×10^4	2.5×10^5
Coliform	5	1	10	100
Salmonella	15	0	0	

Source: IDF- D-Doc 90, 1982.

Table . European Economic Community Standards for Caseins and Caseinates

Organism(s)	M (maximum allowable concentration)
Total bacterial count	30,000/g
Thermophilic organisms	5,000/g
Coliforms	0(in O. 1g)

Source: Regulation (EEC) No. 2940/73, O.J. No. L301/25.

Table .European Economic Community Standards for Natural Mineral Waters

Organism(s)	M (maximum allowable concentration)
Total count	20/ml at 37 °C 100/ml at 22 °C
Parasites and pathogenic microorganisms	Absent
E. coli, coliforms and fecal streptococci	Absent in 250 ml

Organism(s)	M (maximum allowable concentration)
Sulphite-reducing anaerobes	Absent in 50 ml
Pseudomonas aeruginosa	Absent in 250 ml

Source: Council Directive 15 July 1980 (BO/7/7/EEC), O.J. No. L229/1.

Table. European Economic Community Standards for Water for Human Consumption

Organism(s)	m (guide level)	M (maximum allowable concentration)
Sulphite-reducing clostridia	–	MPN ≤ 1
Total count (tap water)	10/ml at 37 °C 100/ml at 22 °C	– –
Total count (bottled ater)	5/ml at 37 °C 20/ml at 22 °C	20 100
Total coliforms	–	
Fecal coliforms		MPN£1
Fecal streptococci	–	
All pathogenic bacteria, viruses, algae, parasites	absent	

Source: Council Directive 15 July 1980 (80/778/EEC), O.J. No. L229/11.

Table .Microbiological Guidelines of Codex Standard for Natural Mineral Waters

Organism(s)	M (maximum allowable concentration)
Aerobic mesophilic count at source	20/ml at 21 °C (72 hrs)
Aerobic mesophilic count after bottling	100/ml at 20-22 °C (72 hrs) 20/ml at 37 °C (24 hrs)
Coliforms (including *E. coli*)*	None in 250 ml (30 – 32 °C and 44 °C)
Fecal streptococci (Lancefield group D)*	None in 250 ml
Sporulated sulphite-reducing anaerobes	None in 50 ml
Pseudomonas aeruginosa, parasites and pathogenic microorganisms*	None in 250 ml

***Applies both at source and during marketing. Source: Appendix 1 CX/FH 79/4—ADD. 1, 1979.**

Table . Proposed Guidelines for Drinking-water Quality

Parameter / organism	Value number per 100 ml	Remarks
1. Microbiological quality Piped water supplies Treated water entering the distribution system		
Feed coliforms Coliform organism	0 0	Turbidity < 1 NTU; for disinfection with chlorine, pH preferably < 8.0, free chlorine residual0.2–0.5 mg/1 following 30 min (minimum) contact

Untreated water entering the distribution system		
Fecal coliforms	0	In 98% of samples exterminated throughout the year for large supplies with sufficient sample exterminated
Coliform organisms	0	
Coliform organisms	0	In occasional sample but not in consecutive samples
Water in the distribution system		
Fecal coliforms	0	In 95% of samples exterminated throughout the year for large supplies with sufficient sample exterminated
Coliform organisms	0	
Coliform organisms	3	In occasional sample but not in consecutive samples
Unpiped water supplies		
Fecal coliforms	0	
Coliform organisms	10	Not occurring repeatedly; repeated occurrence and failure to improve sanitary protection, alternate source to be found if possible
Bottled drinking- ater		
Fecal coliforms	0	
Coliform organisms	0	
Emergency water supplies		
Fecal coliforms	0	Advise public to boil water in case of failure to meet guideline value
Coliform organism	0	
Enterovirus	–	No guideline value set
II. Biological quality		
Protozoa (pathogenic)	–	No guideline value set
Helminths (pathogenic)	–	No guideline value set
Free-living organisms (algae, others)	–	No guideline value set

Methods employed in the United States suggest not to use zeros (0), rather to report results as less than one times the reciprocal of the lowes- dilution

Source: EEP/82.39 (adapted).

Index

D

E

F

G

K

L

M

O

P

Q